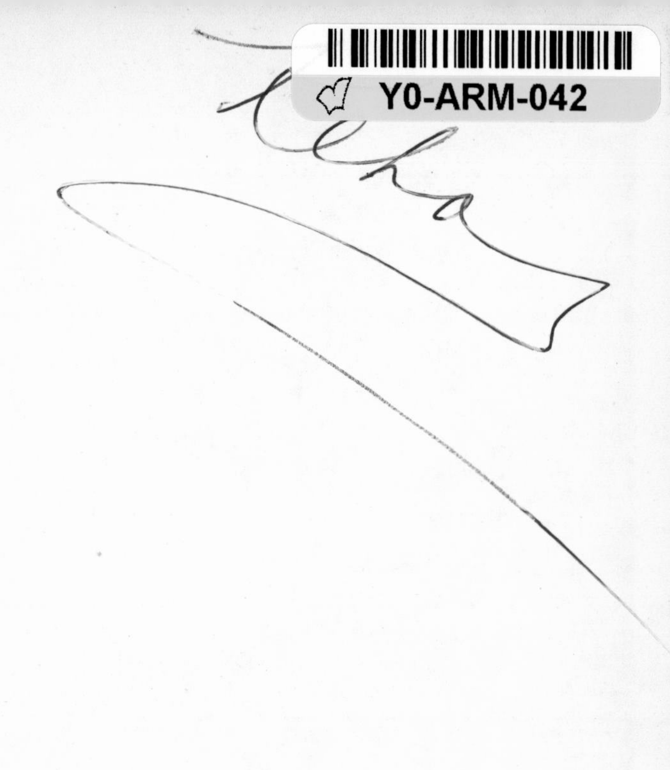

THE YEAR BOOK *of* DRUG THERAPY

(1958-1959 YEAR BOOK *Series)*

EDITED BY

HARRY BECKMAN, M.D.

Director, Departments of Pharmacology, Marquette University Schools of Medicine and Dentistry; Consulting Physician, Milwaukee County General and Columbia Hospitals, Milwaukee, Wisconsin

THE YEAR BOOK PUBLISHERS

INCORPORATED

200 EAST ILLINOIS STREET

CHICAGO 11

THE PRACTICAL MEDICINE YEAR BOOKS

This volume is one of the 15 comprising the Practical Medicine Series of Year Books founded in 1900 by G. P. Head, M.D., and C. J. Head, and published continuously since then. The complete list follows:

Medicine: *Infections*, edited by PAUL B. BEESON, M.D.; *The Chest*, by CARL MUSCHENHEIM, M.D.; *The Blood and Blood-Forming Organs*, by WILLIAM B. CASTLE, M.D.; *The Heart and Blood Vessels and Kidney*, by TINSLEY R. HARRISON, M.D.; *The Digestive System*, by FRANZ J. INGELFINGER, M.D.; *Metabolism*, by PHILIP K. BONDY, M.D.

General Surgery edited by MICHAEL E. DEBAKEY, M.D., with a section on *Anesthesia*, by STUART C. CULLEN, M.D.

Drug Therapy edited by HARRY BECKMAN, M.D.

Obstetrics & Gynecology edited by J. P. GREENHILL, M.D.

Pediatrics edited by SYDNEY S. GELLIS, M.D.

Radiology: *Diagnosis*, edited by JOHN FLOYD HOLT, M.D., and FRED JENNER HODGES, M.D.; *Therapy*, edited by HAROLD W. JACOX, M.D., and MORTON M. KLIGERMAN, M.D.

Ophthalmology edited by DERRICK VAIL, M.D.

Ear, Nose & Throat edited by JOHN R. LINDSAY, M.D., with a section on *Maxillofacial Surgery*, by DEAN M. LIERLE, M.D., and WILLIAM C. HUFFMAN, M.D.

Neurology, Psychiatry & Neurosurgery: *Neurology*, edited by ROLAND P. MACKAY, M.D.; *Psychiatry*, by S. BERNARD WORTIS, M.D.; *Neurosurgery*, by OSCAR SUGAR, M.D.

Dermatology & Syphilology edited by RUDOLF L. BAER, M.D., and VICTOR H. WITTEN, M.D.

Urology edited by WILLIAM W. SCOTT, M.D.

Orthopedics and Traumatic Surgery edited by EDWARD L. COMPERE, M.D., with a section on *Plastic Surgery*, by NEAL OWENS, M.D.

Endocrinology edited by GILBERT S. GORDAN, M.D.

Pathology and Clinical Pathology edited by WILLIAM B. WARTMAN, M.D.

Cancer edited by RANDOLPH LEE CLARK, JR., M.D., and RUSSELL W. CUMLEY, Ph.D.

Dentistry

Printed in U.S.A.

TABLE OF CONTENTS

The designation (Series 1958-1959) used on the cover and title page of this volume is to indicate its publication during the "series year" which begins in September 1958.

INTRODUCTION

Precise count is not kept of the number of journals seen and articles read in making selections for the YEAR BOOK. I do not want to know what these numbers are, as a matter of fact, for they might convict me of some sort of compulsive quirk. Suffice it to say that in the present volume there are 493 articles from 23 countries and 108 journals. Perhaps some users of the book will enjoy seeing the following partial* list of hospitals, clinics, universities and other institutions in which some of the original work, presented in brief essence herein, was done.

Aarhus Amtssygehus, Aarhus, Denmark
Albert Einstein Medical Center, Philadelphia, Pa.
A. N. Brady Hospital, Albany, N. Y.
Ashford Hospital, Middlesex, England
Baptist Memorial Hospital, Memphis, Tenn.
Battey State Hospital, Rome, Ga.
Baylor University, Houston, Texas
Bellevue Medical Center, New York, N. Y.
Beth Israel Hospital, Boston, Mass.
Birmingham Accident Hospital, Birmingham, England
Botleys Park Hospital, London, England
Bowman Gray School of Medicine, Winston-Salem, N. C.
Brooklyn Jewish Hospital, Brooklyn, N. Y.
Carlo Forlanini Institute, Rome, Italy
Cedars of Lebanon Hospital, Los Angeles, Cal.
Charing Cross Hospital, London, England
Charity Hospital of Louisiana, New Orleans, La.
Children's Hospital, Michigan & Wayne State Universities, Detroit, Mich.
City General Hospital, Sheffield, England
Cleveland Clinic, Cleveland, Ohio
College of Medical Evangelists, Loma Linda, Cal.
Columbia University, New York, N. Y.
Cook County Institutions, Chicago, Ill.
Cornell University, New York, N. Y.
County Central Hospital, Örebro, Sweden
Department of Health, New York, N. Y.
District of Columbia General Hospital, Washington, D. C.
Euclid-Glenville Hospital, Euclid, Ohio
Evans Memorial & Massachusetts Memorial Hospital, Boston, Mass.
Facultad de Med., Montevideo, Uruguay
Forest Hills Nursing & Rehabilitation Center, New York, N. Y.
Francis Delafield Hospital, New York, N. Y.
Franklin Square Hospital, Baltimore, Md.

*It is not always possible to identify precisely, from the article published in the journal, the place of origin of some investigations. Therefore, the list, of necessity, is not as complete as it might otherwise be.

Freedman's Hospital, Washington, D. C.
Georgetown University, Washington, D. C.
George Washington University, Washington, D. C.
Gjøvik Fylkessykehis, Gjøvik, Norway
Gloucestershire Royal Hospital, England
Grand View Hospital, Sellersville, Pa.
Grasslands Hospital, Valhalla, N. Y.
Hahnemann Medical College, Philadelphia, Pa.
Harlem Hospital, New York, N. Y.
Harvard University, Boston, Mass.
Hebrew University, Jerusalem, Israel
High Carley Hospital, England
Hosp. Del Rey Para Enfermedades Infecciosas, Madrid, Spain
Howard University, Washington, D. C.
Hudson River State Hospital, Poughkeepsie, N. Y.
Indiana University, Indianapolis, Ind.
Institute of Biology, Montpellier, France
Jackson Clinic, Madison, Wis.
Jersey City Medical Center, Jersey City, N. J.
Jewish Hospital, Cincinnati, Ohio
Johns Hopkins University, Baltimore, Md.
Karolinska Sjukhuset, Stockholm, Sweden
Kings County Hospital, Brooklyn, N. Y.
Lebanon Hospital, New York, N. Y.
Letterman Army Hospital, San Francisco, Cal.
Liber-Institute of American Foundation for Tropical Medicine, Harbel, Liberia
London Chest Hospital, London, England
London Hospital, London, England
Long Island College Hospital, Brooklyn, N. Y.
Louisiana State University, New Orleans, La.
Manchester Royal Infirmary, Manchester, England
Marcy State Hospital, Marcy, N. Y.
Marquette University, Milwaukee, Wis.
Martin Luther University, Halle-Wittenberg, Germany
Massachusetts Eye & Ear Infirmary, Boston, Mass.
Massachusetts General Hospital, Boston, Mass.
Mayo Clinic, Rochester, Minn.
Medical College, Agra, India
Medical College, Amritsar, India
Medical College of Virginia, Richmond, Va.
Medical Corps, U. S. Army
Meharry Medical College, Memphis, Tenn.
Montefiore Hospital, New York, N. Y.
Montreal General Hospital, Montreal, Canada
Montreal Hebrew Old People's Home, Montreal, Canada
Michael Reese Hospital, Chicago, Ill.
Middlesex Hospital, England
Mount Sinai Hospital, New York, N. Y.
National Cancer Institute, Bethesda, Md.
National Institute of Allergy & Infectious Diseases, Bethesda, Md.
National Institutes of Health, Bethesda, Md.
National Jewish Hospital, Denver, Colo.
Newark Beth Israel Hospital, Newark, N. J.
New End Hospital, London, England
New England Deaconess Hospital, Boston, Mass.
New York Hospital, New York, N. Y.

New York Medical College, New York, N. Y.
New York Polyclinic Medical School, New York, N. Y.
New York University-Bellevue Medical Center, New York, N. Y.
New York University Post-Graduate Medical School, New York, N. Y.
Northwestern University, Chicago, Ill.
Ohio State University, Columbus, Ohio
Okayama University, Japan
Oklahoma State Penitentiary, McAlester, Okla.
Oregon State Hospital, Salem, Ore.
Otago University, Otago, New Zealand
Palo Alto Medical Clinic, Palo Alto, Cal.
Point Edward Hospital, Sydney, Nova Scotia, Canada
Postgraduate Medical School of London, England
Queens General Hospital, Jamaica, N. Y.
Rahway General Hospital, Rahway, N. J.
Report & Statistics Service Veterans Administration, Washington, D. C.
Royal Edinburgh Hospital, Edinburgh, Scotland
Royal Free Hospital, London, England
Royal Maternity & Women's Hospital, Glasgow, Scotland
Royal National Orthopaedic Hospital & Institute of Orthopaedics, London, England
Royal Victoria Hospital, Montreal, Canada
Runwell Hospital, Wickford, Essex, England
Sahlgrenska Sjukhuset, Göthenburg, Sweden
San Francisco Department of Health, San Francisco, Cal.
Saskatchewan Hospital, Weyburn, Saskatchewan, Canada
St. Anne's Maternity Hospital, Los Angeles, Cal.
St. Barnabas Medical Center, Newark, N. J.
St. Bartholomew's Hospital, London, England
St. Francis General Hospital, Pittsburgh, Pa.
St. James' Hospital, Leeds, England
St. Louis Hospital, Paris, France
St. Louis University, St. Louis, Mo.
St. Luke's Hospital, New York, N. Y.
St. Mary's Hospital, London, England
St. Peter's Hospital, Albany, N. Y.
St. Thomas's Hospital, London, England
Sefton General Hospital, Liverpool, England
Sheffield Centre, Sheffield, England
South Carolina State Hospital, Columbia, S. C.
State University of New York at Brooklyn
State University of New York at Syracuse
Sylhet Medical School, East Pakistan
Syracuse University, Syracuse, N. Y.
Temple University, Philadelphia, Pa.
Topeka State Hospital, Topeka, Kan.
Tufts University, Boston, Mass.
United Birmingham Hospitals, Birmingham, England
University Department of Clinical Medicine, London, England
U. S. Naval Hospital, Great Lakes, Ill.
U. S. Naval Hospital, Jacksonville, Fla.
U. S. Naval Hospital, Portsmouth, Va.
U. S. Naval Hospital, St. Albans, N. Y.
U. S. Naval Training Center, Bainbridge, Md.
University of Alabama, Birmingham, Ala.
University of Basel, Basel, Switzerland
University of Birmingham, Birmingham, England

University of Buffalo, Buffalo, N. Y.
University of California, San Francisco, Cal.
University of Chicago, Chicago, Ill.
University of Cincinnati, Cincinnati, Ohio
University of Colorado, Denver, Colorado
University of Durham, Durham, England
University of Edinburgh, Edinburgh, Scotland
University of Frankfurt, Frankfurt, Germany
University of Geneva, Geneva, Switzerland
University of Glasgow, Glasgow, Scotland
University of Gothenburg, Gothenburg, Sweden
University of Guadalajara, Jalisco, Mexico
University of Helsinki, Helsinki, Finland
University of Illinois, Chicago, Ill.
University of Iowa, Iowa City, Iowa
University of Kansas, Kansas City, Kan.
University of Malaya
University of Maryland, Baltimore, Md.
University of Melbourne, Melbourne, Australia
University of Miami, Miami, Fla.
University of Michigan, Ann Arbor, Mich.
University of Minnesota, Minneapolis, Minn.
University of North Carolina, Chapel Hill, N. C.,
University of Oxford, Oxford, England
University of Pennsylvania, Philadelphia, Pa.
University of Puerto Rico, San Juan, Puerto Rico
University of Rochester, Rochester, N. Y.
University of Rome, Rome, Italy
University of St. Andrews, St. Andrews, Scotland
University of Sheffield, Sheffield, England
University of South Dakota, Vermillion, S. Dak.
University of Southern California, Los Angeles, Cal.
University of Texas, Galveston, Texas
University of Tennessee, Memphis, Tenn.
University of Wisconsin, Madison, Wis.
Vanderbilt University, Nashville, Tenn.
Veterans Administration Hospital, Brooklyn, N. Y.
Veterans Administration Hospital, Coral Gables, Fla.
Veterans Administration Hospital, Fort Howard, Md.
Veterans Administration Hospital, Phoenix, Ariz.
Veterans Administration Hospital, Oakland, Cal.
Veterans Administration Hospital, Palo Alto, Cal.
Veterans Administration Hospital, Oteen, N. C.
Veterans Administration Hospital, Sunmount, N. Y.
Veterans Administration Hospital, New York, N. Y.
Veterans Administration Hospital, West Haven, Conn.
Victoria Infirmary, Glasgow, Scotland
Wadsworth Hospital, Los Angeles, Cal.
Wake Forest College, Winston-Salem, N. C.
Walter Reed Army Hospital, Washington, D. C.
Washington University, St. Louis, Mo.
Wellcome Laboratory Tropical Medicine, London, England
West London Hospital, London, England
Western Pennsylvania Hospital, Pittsburgh, Pa.
Western Reserve University, Cleveland, Ohio
Yale University, New Haven, Conn.

HARRY BECKMAN

ALLERGIC DISORDERS

Hydroxyzine (Atarax®) in Chronic Urticaria and in Allergic Manifestations: Clinical Observations in Man and Experimental Studies on Asthma in Guinea Pigs Produced by Several Agents. Alan R. Feinberg, Jacob J. Pruzansky, Samuel M. Feinberg and Elmer W. Fisherman[1] (Northwestern Univ.) tried Atarax in 60 patients with various allergic manifestations. Treatment was usually started with 10 mg. 3 times a day. In the absence of appreciable relief, this was often increased to 25 mg. 3 or 4 times daily. If results were obtained with 10 mg., lowering of the dose was attempted to determine the minimum necessary for relief.

Most striking results were seen in patients with chronic idiopathic urticaria. Of 17 patients, 15 obtained complete relief and 2 had fair to good relief. There were no complete failures. In several patients, however, relief lasted only a few weeks, then the drug appeared to lose its effectiveness. A number of the patients who maintained relief were able to take 10 mg. as seldom as every 24-72 hours. In some patients with chronic urticaria, Pyribenzamine® gave good relief from itching but not so much from swellings; however, the effect of each dose lasted only 4-6 hours. In contrast to chronic urticaria patients, only 1 of 4 with acute urticaria had significant relief. One who failed to obtain relief had a serum sickness type of urticaria from penicillin. Of 13 patients with asthma, 7 had fair to good relief and no effect was noted in 6. Better results were obtained in patients with dermographism: 1 had excellent relief and 2 had good relief. One patient with a physical hypersensitivity to cold, who had had only slight relief with antihistamines, obtained excellent results with Atarax. In no case in which good therapeutic results were obtained was it necessary to discontinue this drug because of side effects.

Indirect evidence points to the possibility that there is a mediating mechanism in chronic urticaria besides the possible ones of histamine, acetylcholine or serotonin. Experimental studies in the guinea pig indicate that Atarax is a

(1) J. Allergy 29:358-361, July, 1958.

long-acting, potent, antianaphylactic, antihistamine, antiserotonin and antiacetylcholine agent. Most other tranquilizing or antihistamine drugs have only part or none of these effects.

Treatment of Eosinophilic Lung (Tropical Eosinophilia) with Diethylcarbamazine (Hetrazan®) was studied by T. J. Danaraj[2] (Univ. of Malaya) in 110 patients. The salient features that distinguished eosinophilic lung from other respiratory disorders associated with eosinophilia were massive eosinophilic leukocytosis (over 3,000 eosinophils/cu. mm.), shadows in the chest x-rays and elevated erythrocyte sedimentation rate. Most patients were ill under 6 months.

The dosage of diethylcarbamazine was initially 4 mg./kg. body weight 3 times daily for 4 days. Later, 2 larger dosages were tried: 6 mg. and 10 mg./kg. body weight given thrice daily for 5 days to groups of 57 and 7 patients respectively. Average total adult dose for each of the 3 schedules was 3,200, 6,000, and 10,000 mg. respectively. The drug was given after meals in 50-mg. tablets, the syrup being used for children. Except for 11 who exhibited severe bronchial spasm and were treated with antispasmodics as well, the patients were given only diethylcarbamazine.

The patients were observed 2-4 weeks before treatment began, and up to 14 months thereafter to note any recurrence of symptoms or rise in the eosinophil count. Improvement in symptoms was noted in 107 patients 2-4 days after beginning treatment, while the drug was still being taken, and progressed steadily until, by the end of the 1st week, 59 had complete relief and 48 a residual cough only. Coincident with symptomatic improvement was a general clearing of abnormal lung signs and in most the lungs were clear by the 7th day after start of treatment.

In 98 patients, the leukocyte count showed a marked decrease in eosinophils on the 3d day of treatment; in 12, an increase was noted on the 3d day, followed by a similar rapid decrease, which was apparent on the 5th day.

The erythrocyte sedimentation rate reverted to normal in 19 patients 1 week after completing the diethylcarbamazine course and in 22, 2 weeks later. Although the rates in the other patients were still abnormal, they had decreased from

(2) Quart. J. Med. 27:243-263, April, 1958.

their original high levels and over the period of observation continued to decrease, becoming normal in a further 33; in 25, they were still above normal at the end of the observation period.

Chest x-rays taken 1 week after end of treatment showed distinct improvement in 109 patients in that the striations became less prominent and the pulmonary mottling cleared. Mild toxic effects, which did not require reducing the dosage or discontinuing the treatment, were noted in 12 patients.

The eosinophil response did not vary with the 3 dosage schedules used, a satisfactory decrease in circulating eosinophils occurring with all dosages. Based on this study, the dosage recommended is 6 mg./kg. body weight 3 times a day for 5 days.

► [This is an important contribution since it apparently establishes Hetrazan as less toxic and quite as effective as the organic arsenicals in this disease, which was established as a clinical entity in the tropical Far East about 20 years ago. Most patients improve steadily under arsenotherapy, but some experience exacerbations after the initial treatment, a fairly high proportion suffer relapses (reinfections?), the therapeutic regimen is necessarily a protracted one, and arsenical encephalopathy is a much-feared reaction, in East Indians particularly.—Ed.]

Clinical Evaluation of New Long-Acting Preparation in Allergic Disorders. The antihistamines available until now have been limited by the severity of the side reactions, particularly depression of the central nervous system, drowsiness and short duration of action. Sandostene Spacetabs® is a new long-acting antiallergic drug with chemical structure that differs from most histamine antagonists. It has potent antihistaminic, anticholinergic and antipermeability activity, and local anesthetic properties. This drug is especially effective in allergic dermatitis.

Jerome Miller[3] (Temple Univ.) gave Sandostene Spacetabs to 185 patients (63 males, 122 females) aged 9 months to 73 years. They were observed over 3 months, including the grass hay-fever season, and were seen at least once weekly. Each patient was to take or be given 1 tablet in the morning and 1 in the evening, and the dose was adjusted when necessary according to response and, in children, according to age. Of the 185 patients, 150 (81%) benefited and 63% obtained pronounced relief; results were unsatisfactory in only 35 (19%). The therapeutic response was reported as occurring

(3) Ann. Allergy 16:135-142, Mar.-Apr., 1958.

within at least 30 minutes. Seasonal and perennial hay-fever groups responded especially well, with excellent results in 81 (84.4%). The antipruritic effect was particularly helpful in those with marked itching of the eyes, ears, nose and roof of the mouth. Rhinorrhea and sneezing were modified and nasal blocking was lessened. Of 29 patients with bronchial asthma, 19 (65.5%) were favorably influenced, regardless of cause. Dyspnea and wheezing were abolished. Side effects were reported by 42 patients, but most were so slight and transient that they were no problem; many subsided while medication was continued. In only 5 patients was drowsiness severe enough to require discontinuance of therapy and in only 2 was dryness of the mouth of such severity.

Proper management of allergies calls for removal of the offending allergen from the diet or the environment. If impossible, specific hyposensitization is indicated. When these measures fail, other methods must be used. Sandostene Spacetabs is the most effective agent presently available for symptomatic treatment of allergies.

► [It is entertaining that L. LaMantia *et al.* (Ann. Allergy 5:506, 1957) found Sandostene relatively ineffective but Sandostene with calcium quite effective and well tolerated in treatment of chronic asthma; best results were achieved in elderly patients with complicating cardiac dysfunction.

D. A. Adams and S. Perry have described (J.A.M.A. 167:1207, July 5, 1958) 3 cases of agranulocytosis that occurred in patients who were taking Sandostene.—Ed.]

Prevention of Nonhemolytic Blood Transfusion Reactions with Antihistamine, Chlorpheniramine: Report of 6,131 Cases is presented by Frederick M. Offenkrantz and George Babcock, Jr.[4] (Rahway, N. J., Gen'l Hosp.). In a control series of 3,346 patients, there were 47 allergic reactions, 100 pyrogenic, 21 combined allergic and pyrogenic, and 1 hemolytic reaction. In 2,785 patients in whom 10 mg. chlorpheniramine maleate (Chlor-Trimeton® maleate) was added to the blood before transfusion, there were 2 allergic reactions, 15 pyrogenic, 1 combined reaction and 1 hemolytic. For multiple transfusions, 10 mg. was added every 6 hours. Allergic reactions were thus reduced from 1.40% to 0.07%, pyrogenic from 3.01% to 0.54% and combined allergic and pyrogenic reactions from 0.60% to 0.03%. Incidence of hemolytic reactions was 0.03% in both groups.

There were no undesirable sequelae attributable to the an-

(4) A.M.A. Arch. Surg. 76:379-383, March, 1958.

tihistamine. Drowsiness was observed occasionally, but this was no disadvantage among patients who received blood transfusions. Chlorpheniramine is compatible with whole blood and produces no detectable alteration in fresh or stored blood.

On the basis of the results, the authors recommend routine addition of an antihistamine to flasks of blood immediately before transfusion.

► [M. Hobsley concluded (Lancet 1:497, Mar. 8, 1958) as the result of a controlled trial in 200 transfusions, in 100 of which this drug had been added, that there is no justification for the routine prophylactic use of an antihistamine in each bottle of transfused blood in attempting to prevent pyrogenic reactions unless patients are known to have a history of allergy. In his series the over-all incidence of pyrogenic reactions was 35% in contrast with the 5-6% incidence usually reported; however, the incidence was very little higher, 38 versus 32%, in the control than in the treated cases. He feels that such high incidences might be found in most series if sharply looked for.—Ed.]

Clinical Evaluation of Elixophyllin and Choline Theophyllinate in Management of Chronic Asthma: Control of Asthmatic Attack with Single Oral Dose of Elixophyllin was carried out by Joseph Greenbaum[5] (Englewood, N. J.) as follows:

Method.—Thirty-two patients with chronic asthma were divided into 2 matched groups of 16. All previous medications were discontinued. One group received the alcohol-water solution of theophylline, 2 tablespoonfuls 3 times daily; the other, choline theophyllinate, 200 mg. 4 times daily. Both medications were given 15 minutes before meals. In these dosages, both groups received about the same amounts of theophylline. The alcohol-water solution of theophylline (elixophyllin) contains 80 mg. free theophylline, 3 ml. ethyl alcohol and 12 ml. water per tablespoon. Thus, the total daily dose administered contains 480 mg. theophylline. Each 200 mg. tablet of choline theophyllinate (Choledyl®) (64.4% theophylline) is equal to 129 mg. free theophylline. The total daily dosage of theophylline is thus equal to 516 mg.

Each group was maintained on the original schedule for 1 month. At the end of this period the medications were interchanged and continued for another month. Medications in the 2 groups were again alternated for 2 more months, so that both groups received each medication alternately for 2 periods of 1 months.

Twenty-four patients with an acute attack of asthma were treated with a single oral dose of 2½ oz. alcohol-water solution of theophylline (400 mg. theophylline). Severity of dyspnea, wheezing and cough were estimated before treatment. After medication patients were reevaluated every 3-5 minutes until a half hour had elapsed. The time when symptoms began to be relieved was noted.

Repeated oral use of the alcohol-water solution of theo-

(5) Ann. Allergy 16:312-316, May-June, 1958.

phylline in 32 patients with chronic asthma elicited excellent response in 17, good response in 7 and equivocal response in 8. Of the 8 patients, 5 had not responded previously to any medication administered except steroids.

Oral administration of equivalent doses of theophylline in the form of choline theophyllinate to the same patients with chronic asthma produced 4 excellent results, 13 good and 15 equivocal. All 8 who had previously taken steroids obtained no significant response with choline theophyllinate.

A single oral dose of 5 tablespoonsfuls (2½ oz.) elixophyllin successfully terminated the attacks in 23 of 24 patients with acute asthma. Within 30 minutes dyspnea was controlled, wheezing markedly cleared and prolonged respiration significantly lessened.

Gastrointestinal side effects were few after either medication.

Clinical Evaluation of Isothipendyl Hydrochloride (Theruhistin®). The Committee on New and Unused Therapeutics of the American College of Allergists[6] conducted clinical trials in 602 patients, using Theruhistin, a new type of antihistaminic drug. It is an anticholinergic, antiserotonin agent of the thiophenyl pyridylamine type. Theruhistin gave effective clinical relief in 92% of patients with allergic disease, with an exceedingly low incidence of side effects and no apparent toxicity. Best results were obtained in vasomotor rhinitis and hay fever (up to 96%). It is notable that Theruhistin gave better results in bronchial asthma than did other compounds, probably because it is an effective antiserotonin and anticholinergic as well as antihistaminic agent. The most effective dose was 6-8 mg./day, with a significant clinical effect of about 6 hours' duration.

The compound gave excellent symptomatic relief in patients who had other separate or concomitant allergic manifestations such as gastrointestinal reactions, migraine, iritis or "id" reactions. In urticaria and eczema, the usual dosage range did not produce the desirable results obtained in other categories; however, when the dosage was increased to about 3 times the usual, excellent results were obtained. Theruhistin in doses up to 8 mg. is exceptionally well tolerated

(6) Ann. Allergy 16:237-241, May-June, 1958.

even by infants whereas higher doses produce insomnia rather than sedation.

Chloroquine in Management of Hypersensitivity States. Disseminated lupus erythematosus, periarteritis nodosa, scleroderma and dermatomyositis have widely differing histories and little is known about etiology except for some cases of periarteritis nodosa. They are considered collagen diseases, but it is oversimplification to consider them identical in etiology or pathogenesis. Asthma, serum sickness, rheumatic fever and rheumatoid arthritis are also included as collagen diseases, since in each the collagen is altered, but the etiology and pathogenesis differ markedly.

With introduction of the steroid hormones, these syndromes were grouped on the basis of a common reactive state—hypersensitivity. This too is oversimplification. Neither fibrinoid degeneration nor necrotizing arteritis is exclusively the product of hypersensitivity. Specific fibrinoid degeneration occurs in disseminated lupus erythematosus. The chemistry of fibrinoid degeneration may differ in various collagen diseases.

H. Fuld[7] (Liverpool) treated 9 cases of hypersensitivity diseases: 3 of nonsuppurative subacute panniculitis of the Weber-Christian type, 3 of erythema multiforme (Stevens-Johnson syndrome), 1 of lupus erythromatosus and 2 of nonspecific hypersensitivity states considered to be collagen diseases. The most likely etiology common to all 9 was acquired sensitivity to a bacterial or chemical antigen. The dose of chloroquine was 200-400 mg. 3 times daily in each. The response to therapy was dramatic and after short maintenance therapy, chloroquine was discontinued without relapse.

Woman, 45, had tonsillitis treated with 30 Sulfatriad tablets. Temperature subsided 4 days after onset of sore throat but again rose 2 days later. On the 10th day after onset, she was admitted to hospital with pyrexia, mildly confused. She had microcytic anemia, leukocytosis, elevated sedimentation rate and increased serum globulin with an inverted albumin-globulin ratio. Repeated L.E. cell tests, agglutinin tests, blood cultures and bone marrow examinations were negative.

Pyrexia persisted, blotchy erythema appeared 3 weeks after admission on the trunk and extremities, the general condition deteriorated and weight loss was progressive. Salicylates, penicillin and tetracycline were ineffective during the next month. At the height of the illness, the patient was given chloroquine sulfate, 200 mg. 3 times daily.

(7) Rheumatism 14:12-19, January, 1958.

Within 36 hours temperature decreased for the first time in 5½ weeks and within 10 days of the start of therapy she was afebrile and her general condition rapidly improved. She was maintained on 2 tablets chloroquine daily for the next 3 months. She remained clinically well, and the laboratory findings gradually returned to normal.

Comparative Effects of Aerosol Bronchodilators on Ventilatory Function in Bronchial Asthma and Chronic Pulmonary Emphysema were studied by Lenore Zohman and M. Henry Williams, Jr.[8] (Grasslands Hosp., Valhalla, N. Y.). Three measurements of pulmonary function were made before and after use of the bronchodilators: vital capacity, 1-second vital capacity, and mean midexpiratory flow rate.

The medications used were epinephrine in the form of Vaponefrin, which is a 2.25% solution of racemic epinephrine hydrochloride with 0.5-1% chlorobutanol as a preservative, isoproterenol in the form of Medihaler-Iso®, which is a 0.25% solution of isoproterenol hydrochloride in alcohol with an inert propellant, and isoproterenol-placebo, containing merely the propellant and the vehicle without isoproterenol. The particle size is reported as 2.5 μ for epinephrine and less than 3 μ for isoproterenol, both within the optimum range for nebulization into the smaller bronchi. Epinephrine, 0.5 cc. diluted to 1 cc. with water, was vaporized by means of a Vaponefrin hand nebulizer or an Emerson intermittent positive pressure breathing valve at 10-20 cm. water. Isoproterenol was administered through a plastic adapter and valve which dispensed a uniform dose of 0.06 mg. A similar volume of placebo was administered through the same type of adapter and valve. Patients received no bronchodilator aerosols for at least 3 and usually 6 hours before the test. Only one medication was tested in any one day.

Studies in the 15 patients with emphysema showed a lack of improvement after placebo and, by comparison, a highly significant improvement after isoproterenol in all three tests. Patients with asthma improved slightly after placebo, and the comparative effect of isoproterenol on the mean midexpiratory flow rate was probably significant and on vital capacity and 1-second vital capacity only possibly significant. Cough frequently followed administration of aerosols and was often productive of mucus plugs or small amounts of sputum, but spirograms done after cough induced by the pla-

(8) J. Allergy 29:72-79, January, 1958.

cebo demonstrated no improvement in ventilatory function. Thus isoproterenol has a bronchodilator effect which is independent of the dispersing vehicle, the new mode of administration and the raising of secretions.

Comparison of the effects of isoproterenol with the effects of epinephrine nebulized manually and epinephrine with intermittent positive pressure breathing on the three tests of ventilatory function in patients with emphysema showed two significant results. (1) There was more improvement in 1-second vital capacity after isoproterenol than after epinephrine nebulized manually. (2) There was more improvement in the mean midexpiratory flow rate after isoproterenol than after epinephrine and positive pressure. The mean per cent improvement in the mean midexpiratory flow rate, 1-second vital capacity and vital capacity was greater (though not significantly) after isoproterenol than after epinephrine with or without positive pressure breathing in this group. In asthmatic patients there was no significant difference in any of the three tests with any one type of therapy as compared with the other two.

Comparison of the response of asthmatic patients with that in the emphysema group showed that the mean midexpiratory flow rate improved with all forms of therapy in the former (29.8-33%) and also in the patients with emphysema, but to a lesser extent (3.7-11.1%). The reason for the insignificant difference between improvement of the mean midexpiratory flow rate after isoproterenol in the asthma and emphysema groups may be that this drug was the superior form of bronchodilator therapy in the latter group.

Triamcinolone (Aristocort®), New Corticosteroid Hormone: Its Use in Treatment of Allergic Disease in 70 patients, aged 7-74, was studied by Samuel M. Feinberg, Alan R. Feinberg and Elmer W. Fisherman[9] (Northwestern Univ.). Duration of treatment ranged from one-half week to 40 weeks, with 24 patients treated for 20 weeks or longer. There were 52 patients with asthma. Most had chronic intractable asthma of unknown cause, but a few received treatment during special acute episodes of a seasonal or other unavoidable variety. Thirteen patients had dermatitis: atopic, contact or of unknown cause. Among the treated patients

(9) J.A.M.A. 167:58-59, May 3, 1958.

were 5 with seasonal hay fever and 12 with perennial vasomotor rhinitis. Four patients had urticaria or angioneurotic edema. The initial 24-hour dose varied usually from 8 to 16 mg. Average daily maintenance dose for the entire series was 6 mg.

Triamcinolone (9α-fluoro-16α-hydroxy-Δ^1-hydrocortisone) was found to be a potent antiallergic hormone, producing therapeutic effects with about one half of the dosage required for prednisone. This drug produces most of the usual steroid hormone reactions, such as moon facies, hyperglycemia, muscle cramps and epigastric distress. Unlike some of the other anti-inflammatory hormones it is diuretic and sodium depleting, which may be advantageous in some instances and perhaps disadvantageous in others.

In 12 patients, a peculiar effect was noted: a combination of headache, dizziness, sleepiness and weakness. In some patients, these effects may necessitate withdrawal of the drug. Triamcinolone does not stimulate the appetite and may even depress it, thus commonly causing weight loss.

Treatment of Ragweed Hay Fever with Methylprednisolone (Medrol®): Comparative Effectiveness of Methylprednisolone and Prednisolone. The use of hydrocortisone, prednisone, and prednisolone since 1950 has resulted in lower doses with fewer untoward effects. Methylprednisolone, an analogue of hydrocortisone, is similar to prednisolone except for a methyl group substituted for a hydrogen atom at the sixth alpha position. In animals it is three times as potent as prednisolone.

Earl B. Brown, Thomas Seideman and A. B. Seigelaub[1] (New York) treated 131 patients who had responded poorly to hyposensitization or had received no treatment for ragweed hay fever. Of these, 44 were given 20 mg. prednisolone daily, 42, 15 mg. Medrol daily and 45 were allowed any medication desired except steroids. The study was double blind—neither doctor, nurse nor patient knew what drug was given.

As expected, all patients had the most severe symptoms when the pollen count was highest (Fig. 1) and those on either methylprednisolone or prednisolone had fewer days with severe symptoms than had those in the control group. On days with lower pollen counts, the group on methylpred-

(1) J. Allergy 29:227-232, May, 1958.

nisolone was more comfortable than either the prednisolone group or the control group. Apparently 15 mg. daily of either drug was inadequate to control symptoms caused by pollen counts over 80. Those on methylprednisolone had more symptom-free days than the prednisolone or control group,

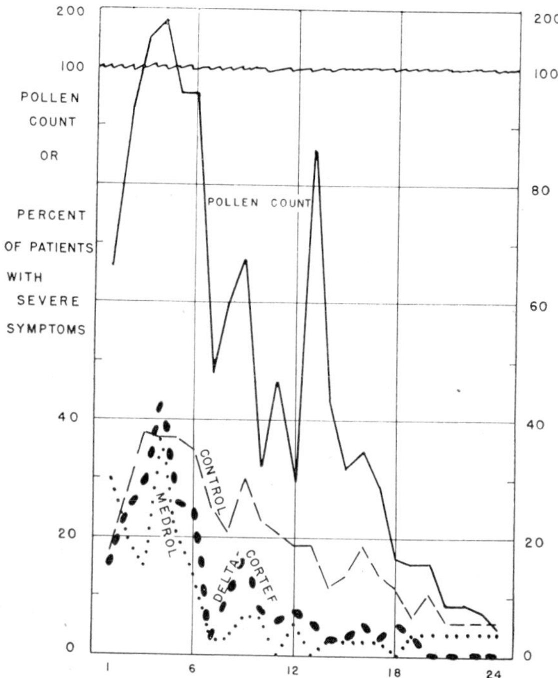

Fig. 1.—Patients with severe symptoms daily during September 1957. (Courtesy of Brown, E. B., *et al.*: J. Allergy 29:227-232, May, 1958.)

but when the pollen count was highest there was no difference between the groups.

Of the 44 patients on prednisolone, 16 had a total of 22 reactions, whereas of 42 on methylprednisolone only 11 had a total of only 13 reactions. No patient had to discontinue either drug because of reactions. These included insomnia, headache, perspiration, palpitation, fatigue, flatulence, dizziness, nausea, abdominal cramps, epigastric distress or heartburn, increased appetite, urinary frequency, nocturia and acneiform eruption.

Medrol® as Effective Agent in Treatment of Allergic Diseases. W. C. Grater[2] administered methylprednisolone (Medrol) in divided doses 4 times daily to 138 patients with various allergic disorders. Three on maintenance therapy with prednisolone were changed to Medrol, and a new minimal effective dose determined. The dosage used varied considerably since the objective was to determine the minimal effective controlling and maintenance dosage for the individual patient.

A satisfactory response was obtained in 92% of the patients (table). Medrol was found about one and a half times

RESULTS OF THERAPY WITH MEDROL

Disorder	Original Series (115 Cases)		New Series (138 Cases)	
	SATISFACTORY	UNSATISFACTORY	SATISFACTORY	UNSATISFACTORY
Allergic rhinitis	21	2	25	3
Asthma	35	4	42	5
Allergic rhinitis and asthma	36	2	43	2
Erythema multiforme	3	0	3	0
Drug reaction	3	0	4	0
Contact dermatitis	7	0	9	0
Eczema	2	0	2	0
Total	107	8	128	10

as potent as prednisolone clinically. To judge its effectiveness in asthma, pulmonary function tests before and after therapy were performed in 29 patients. The results were very satisfactory and correlated closely with the temporary improvement noted on inhalation of epinephrine or isoproterenol.

An antibiotic-steroid combination (Medrol-Panmycin) provided swift and effective therapy for otherwise intractable respiratory tract allergy associated with infection; this may prevent development of chronicity.

Only 6 of 138 patients treated with Medrol demonstrated side effects attributable to it, and these were all minor.

Methylprednisolone (Medrol®), Potent New Anti-inflammatory Steroid: Therapeutic Results in Allergic Diseases. Samuel M. Feinberg, Alan R. Feinberg, Jacob Pruzansky and Elmer W. Fisherman[3] (Northwestern Univ.) administered this drug to 56 patients with intractable asthma or other severe allergic manifestations not responding to usual

(2) Metabolism 7 (pt. 2):481-486, July, 1958.
(3) J.A.M.A. 165:1560-1562, Nov. 23, 1957.

management. Most of the asthmatics had persistent year-round symptoms of the "intrinsic" variety. Duration of treatment with methylprednisolone varied from 1 to 22 weeks.

In 38 patients prednisone and methylprednisolone maintenance dosages could be adequately compared. The average prednisone dose was 10.3 mg., average dose of methylprednisolone 9.5 mg.; range of both drugs was 5-17.5 mg. In 17 other patients, in whom maintenance prednisone dosage was not established, the average methylprednisolone dose was 7.5 mg., range 2-20 mg.

The drugs were about equal in tendency to produce moon face, gastric irritation, hyperglycemia and muscle cramps. Methylprednisolone stimulated excessive appetite least and seemed to promote loss of fluids accumulated from other steroid therapy.

The relative potency of steroid hormones in asthma and other allergic conditions cannot be adequately evaluated by anti-inflammatory studies in rats or inhibition of asthma in guinea pigs.

Role of Adrenocortical Steroids in Treatment of Intractable Bronchial Asthma. John W. Irwin and Walter S. Burrage[4] (Massachusetts Gen'l Hosp.) treated about 60 patients with severe intractable asthma of undetermined etiology continuously with adrenocortical steroids. The early patients received cortisone; later, hydrocortisone, prednisone and prednisolone were used and certain patients were placed serially on each of the 4 compounds.

It is unwise to elect prolonged steroid therapy for a patient unless detailed past history and recent observation indicate that intensive routine treatment is inadequate, in which case treatment with cortisone or similar agents becomes a calculated risk.

Cortisone or hydrocortisone, 300 mg., was given during the first day and then 200 mg. daily thereafter until each patient was subjectively and objectively free from asthma; prednisone or prednisolone, 200 mg. the first day and 100 mg. daily thereafter. Total clearing dose of cortisone was 500-2,700 mg.; of hydrocortisone, 460-3,940 mg.; of prednisone, 200-2,335 mg.

All the drugs were capable of freeing patients from asth-

(4) J. Allergy 29:233-241, May, 1958.

matic symptoms, no one having any advantage over the other three. The total clearing dose varied for each patient and did not depend on severity of symptoms. Daily maintenance dose in milligrams varied greatly; for cortisone, 31-158; hydrocortisone, 31-150; prednisone, 10-100; prednisolone, 7-100.

The most fortunate result of long-term adreno-cortical steroid therapy would be withdrawal of medication without reappearance of severe symptoms. At about yearly intervals each of these patients was separated from maintenance therapy, but only 3 successfully. Three patients died, with the therapy a possible factor in 1 death.

While patients were on steroid therapy, 20 different serious disorders developed. Compressed vertebral fractures appearing in 3 patients at about the same date led to giving most male patients 400 mg. testosterone cyclopentylpropionate intramuscularly at weekly intervals, and postmenopausal women Premarin® in cycles of 10 mg. daily for 28 days with the next 10 days off. No more vertebral fractures appeared after adoption of this regimen. Gastrointestinal bleeding occurred in 3 patients; in none was steroid therapy interrupted. With extensive cellulitis, temporary hyperglycemia and hyperglycuria occurred in 2 patients; prednisone was not stopped.

The commonest disorder was purpura, seen in 23 patients. Its cause was not clear. When steroids were removed, it disappeared. Other disorders included fractured patella, thrombophlebitis, benign hypertrophy of prostate, prostatitis, cystitis, myocardial infarct, pulmonary infarct, muscular back strain, herpes zoster and senile psychosis. The role of concomitant steroid therapy in these disorders was not clear. Clinical edema developed even with prednisone and prednisolone when given for a long time unless dietary salt intake was restricted.

Prednisone in Treatment of Allergic Diseases in Children is discussed by Samuel J. Levin and Philip Adler.[5] Prednisone is an analogue of cortisone, prednisolone an analogue of hydrocortisone. Clinically, these drugs appear to have 3-5 times the efficacy of cortisone and 2-4 times that of hydrocortisone. There seems to be little difference between the clinical effectiveness or dosage of the two.

(5) A.M.A. J. Dis. Child. 95:178-184, February, 1958.

Prednisone exclusively was used in the treatment of various allergic states in 85 children, starting in patients over 5 years old with 10-20 mg. daily in divided doses and subsequently decreasing. Younger children required only slightly lower total dosage. Treatment lasted for 7 days except that 4 children with severe bronchial asthma required longer periods of maintenance; 1 was treated for 4 weeks, 2 for 6 weeks and 1 for 3 months with 2.5-5 mg. twice daily after initially receiving higher doses. No undesirable side effects were noticed in these patients.

This therapy was uniformly excellent in alleviating acute episodes of various allergic states, facilitating earlier allergic investigation, and enabling long-term desensitization therapy to continue uninterrupted. It was almost completely free from undesirable side effects.

Long-term use of this and other steroids in allergic diseases in children should be reserved for the extremely rare patient with intractable asthma or other chronic, debilitating allergic state. Even in such patients, thorough and persistent efforts to uncover and treat specific and nonspecific causes should be continued, so that eventually steroid therapy can be terminated.

Clinical Use of Prednisone and Prednisolone in Allergic States and Collagen Diseases. C. Gregoire and B. Rose[6] (Royal Victoria Hosp., Montreal) treated 146 patients with allergic diseases, mainly asthma, with 4 types of compounds: Meticorten® (prednisone) 5 mg.; Meticortelone® (prednisolone) 5 mg.; Metreton® (prednisone 5 mg., Chlor-Trimeton® 2 mg., ascorbic acid 75 mg.); and Colihist (prednisone 5 mg., carbinoxamine maleate 4 mg.). Results were very good in 34 patients, good in 96 and poor in 16. In ambulant asthmatics, the dosage ranged from 30 to 60 mg. a day in divided doses. After symptoms were controlled, the daily intake was decreased by 5 mg. a day to a maintenance dose that varied from 5 to 15 mg. daily, according to the patient's needs. This regimen varied considerably from one patient to another, depending on the severity of the symptoms and on complications, such as infection, bronchiectasis or emphysema.

Generally, remission was obtained within 24-48 hours and

(6) Canad. M. A. J. 77:833-839, Nov. 1, 1957.

could be maintained as long as steroids were given. In some, 4-5 days elpased before remission was noted. The maintenance dose in some was as low as 2.5-5 mg. a day. However, as much as 30 mg. a day failed to keep some patients free when other medications, such as epinephrine by injection or inhalation, aminophylline or bronchodilators, were not used in conjunction. Patients who failed to respond usually had some complications, such as chronic bronchitis with sputum production, emphysema or chronic vasomotor rhinitis.

On withdrawal of steroids, the duration of remission varied considerably. Most remained clear for periods ranging from 48 hours to 10 days, after which symptoms reappeared. In a few, remission lasted as long as 6 months. This did not apply to those asthmatics with symptoms related to the pollen season because in those the asthma would remit spontaneously once the season was over. Of those treated, some 65% preferred these newer steroids to other forms, such as Hydrocortone® or cortisone.

Reactions were observed in 32.8% of the patients, most of which were minor. Serious reactions, such as diabetes or osteoporosis with spontaneous fracture, occurred in 2%.

In general, prednisone and prednisolone were 3-5 times as potent therapeutically as cortisone and were free from effects on salt and electrolyte metabolism when given in therapeutic doses.

There was little difference in effectiveness among the 4 compounds used. One disadvantage of the combination of the hormone with an antihistamine was that the dose of prednisone might have to be increased. Increase usually was unaccompanied by reactions when prednisone was given alone. Increasing the dose of the antihistamine as well often induced drowsiness.

Comparison of the antihistamines with steroids showed that the steroids provide a more clear-cut degree of freedom from symptoms of seasonal hay fever. One or the other compound should be used, with steroids reserved for the more severe cases that are refractory to antihistamines.

► [In reviewing the principles of management of allergic disorders with prednisone and prednisolone, S. C. Bukantz and L. Aubuchon (J.A.M.A. 165:1256, Nov. 9, 1957) felt it possible that some treated patients are more prone than others to the major complications of such therapy. Severe bacterial infection and the manifestations of hormone excess are likely to develop in any steroid-treated subject, but the arthritic is more prone to angiitis or periarteritis and gastrointestinal ulceration, while the asthmatic tends to develop osteoporosis and infections too, of course, since he is commonly infected before therapy begins. A cardinal principle is that all patients on steroid therapy should be under close clinical and laboratory surveillance, especially those in whom the drugs are to be used for more than a month.

In Bukantz and Aubuchon's experience there seemed to be no difference in clinical effectiveness of prednisone and prednisolone or in development of complications with either of the two drugs.—Ed.]

Comparison of Clinical Effectiveness of Methylprednisolone (Medrol®) to Prednisolone (Delta-Cortef®) was made in a study by Earl B. Brown and Thomas Seideman[7] (Montefiore Hosp., New York). During the 1957 hay fever season 131 patients with proved ragweed pollinosis were divided into 3 groups: 44 were given prednisolone, 42 received methylprednisolone and 45 were not allowed to take corticosteroids. The corticosteroid preparations, 15 mg./day were given by a double-blind method.

Either methylprednisolone or prednisolone, 15 mg./day, was inadequate to control symptoms when the pollen count was over 80. On days with lower counts, patients on methylprednisolone were more comfortable than were those on prednisolone. The former had fewer days with severe symptoms and more symptom-free days. When the pollen count reached its height, neither drug gave better results than did the control.

Side actions in both corticosteroid-treated groups were similar. The commonest reactions were headache, perspiration, fatigue and nocturia. The group on methylprednisolone had about 50% fewer side reactions than did the group on prednisolone.

Comparing Effectiveness of Prednisolone-Hydroxyzine Combination with Prednisolone in Treatment of Allergic Diseases. Because of the importance of psychogenic factors in allergic diseases and because of the observed steroid-induced effects on the nervous system, Earl B. Brown and Thomas Seideman[8] (Montefiore Hosp., New York) studied the effectiveness of a corticosteroid administered in combination with a tranquilizer. Four medications were used in the double-blind study in the following daily dosage: prednisolone, 20 mg.; hydroxyzine, 40 mg.; prednisolone, 20 mg. plus

(7) Metabolism 7 (pt. 2):469-472, July, 1958.
(8) J. Allergy 29:80-84, January, 1958.

hydroxyzine, 40 mg.; and a placebo. The allergic disorders treated in 97 patients, aged 9-76 years, included bronchial asthma, vasomotor rhinitis, allergic rhinitis, urticaria, neurodermatitis, contact dermatitis and conjunctivitis. Most patients had one of the first two disturbances.

The response of patients to each of the medications is shown in the table. Excellent results were obtained with the prednisolone-hydroxyzine combination in a greater proportion of patients (75.6%) than with prednisolone alone (48.3%). This difference is highly significant ($P<0.01$). Both the prednisolone-hydroxyzine combination and prednisolone alone produced a significantly greater proportion of excellent results than either of the other medications ($P<0.05$). The excellent and good categories were grouped to show the proportion of patients in which the medications were of substantial benefit. When this was done, no significant difference was observed between the effectiveness of prednisolone (88.8%) and that of the prednisolone-hydroxyzine combination (95.2%). However, both were significantly more effective than the other medications ($P<0.01$). By this criterion of effectiveness, a highly significant difference ($P<0.01$) in effectiveness between hydroxyzine (58.9%) and the placebo (34.4%) was observed. The results with the placebo were consistent with results published elsewhere in treating a variety of disorders. Elimination of the so-called placebo reactors from the analysis did not materially alter the results of the study.

Response of Allergic Disorders to Therapy

Medication	Number of Patients	Response (Per Cent)				Side Reactions (Per Cent)
		Excellent	Good	Fair	Poor	
Prednisolone-hydroxyzine combination	86	75.6	18.6	3.5	2.3	37.2
Prednisolone	89	48.3	40.5	5.6	5.6	37.2
Hydroxyzine	56	32.1	26.8	19.7	21.4	23.2
Placebo	58	24.1	10.3	19.0	46.6	15.5

Side actions were observed in 37% of patients given prednisolone or the prednisolone-hydroxyzine combination, in 23% given hydroxyzine, and in 15% given the placebo. The incidence of drowsiness caused by hydroxyzine was reduced from 23 to 12% when that drug was combined with prednisolone.

Immediate Therapy for Acute Attack of Asthma: Comparison of Epinephrine and Orally and Intravenously Administered Prednisolone to patients with moderate to severe wheezing due to bronchial asthma is presented by Herman H. Pinkerton, Jr., and Thomas E. Van Metre, Jr.[9] (Johns Hopkins Univ.). Wheezing improved promptly in all 13 patients who received epinephrine intramuscularly, though the amount of relief varied. Their median vital capacity was 0.8 L. before, 1.25 L. 5 minutes after and 1.6 L. 30 minutes after treatment.

Thirteen patients received a single intravenous injection of 33.5 mg. prednisolone. Seven were tested 5 minutes after administration of this drug and were unimproved. Thirty minutes after administration, 7 showed no, 5 slight and 1 marked improvement; the median vital capacity was 0.9 L., compared with a pretreatment median of 0.8 L. Three hours after intravenous administration of prednisolone, there was a slow trend toward improvement, and the median vital capacity was 1.05 L.

Fourteen patients received a single oral dose of 33.5 mg. prednisolone. Four tested 5 minutes after administration of the drug showed no improvement. Thirty minutes after administration, 2 were worse, 9 unchanged, 1 slightly improved and 1 markedly improved, and the median vital capacity had increased from 0.95 to 1 L. Three hours after administration, there was a slow trend toward improvement, and the median vital capacity was 1.3 L.

In 11 cases prednisolone was given 2 or 3 hours before epinephrine. Prednisolone did not seem to potentiate or interfere with the response to epinephrine, which was similar to that observed in the patients receiving epinephrine alone. The median vital capacity was 1 L. before epinephrine, 1.55 L. 5 minutes later and 1.85 L. after 30 minutes.

This study indicates that epinephrine is more rapidly effective against asthma than prednisolone, given orally or intravenously, and that there is no significant difference in the responses to prednisolone given orally or intravenously within 3 hours of administration. Intravenous injection of prednisolone is useful when the oral route is contraindicated.

(9) New England J. Med. 258:363-366, Feb. 20, 1958.

Prednisolone Aerosol in Asthmatic Bronchitis: Preliminary Report. Gustavus A. Peters and Lowell L. Henderson[1] report that 10 of 11 patients treated with an 0.5% solution of prednisolone phosphate, which is completely soluble and well tolerated when used as an aerosol, were benefited. Improvement, however, was less striking than with systemic use. The usual method of administration consisted of 4-6 treatments a day, in each of which 0.25 ml. prednisolone phosphate mixed with 0.25 ml. 1:200 isopropylarterenol hydrochloride (Isuprel®) was nebulized during 15 minutes. Variations included use of water as a diluent instead of Isuprel and use of undiluted prednisolone solution alone. The likelihood of any appreciable absorption of steroid is minimal because the total amount used per day is no more than 7.5 mg., some of which is lost in administration. Courses of treatment ranged from 4 to 25 days. No untoward effect was noted.

Although conventional measures were used concomitantly with prednisolone aerosol, thus making the conclusions less clear cut, it must be remembered that symptoms in the patients had persisted despite conventional treatment until use of prednisolone was started.

Treatment of Ragweed Hay Fever with Powdered Hydrocortisone Applied Intranasally. During August and September 3 children and 15 adults were treated for ragweed hay fever by Clifford F. Lake, George B. Logan and Gustavus A. Peters.[2] Inhalation of powdered hydrocortisone was used. The children and 4 adults had had no desensitization injections. The rest had not responded to such treatment, and all were using an antihistamine without success. Adults were given 15 mg. powder daily, 1 child was given 7.5 mg. and the other 2 were given 5 mg.

Excellent results as judged by congestion, color and moistness of the mucosa, sneezing and condition of the eyes were obtained in 2 of the children and 4 adults. The other child and 7 adults showed a good response, 3 adults fair and 1 poor. The highest pollen counts came during the early part of the study period. Improvement was apparent in 3-5 days and occurred while the pollen count was at a peak.

The daily dose of hydrocortisone was administered in 3 or

(1) Proc. Staff Meet. Mayo Clinic 33:57-58, Feb. 5, 1958.
(2) Ibid. 32:641-644, Oct. 30, 1957.

4 parts over 24 hours. Hypercortisonism under these conditions was not expected or observed. The doses used seemed adequate for the adults, though the 5-mg. dose may have been small for some children aged 7 or 8. In only 1 case was there increased irritation which might be due to the treatment. Intranasal insufflation of hydrocortisone offers effective, convenient therapy for seasonal allergic rhinitis not controlled by other means.

Chronic Asthma Treated with Powder Inhalation of Hydrocortisone and Prednisolone. William Brockbank and C. D. R. Pengelly[3] (Royal Infirm., Manchester, England) report that of 24 patients receiving hydrocortisone acetate powder (3 mg. daily) by inhalation, 17 were improved or much improved, a statistically significant figure compared with results obtained in 13 patients who received a blank, inert powder. There was no evidence in 7 patients that prednisolone (1 mg./day) was of any value used this way. Since the dosage of hydrocortisone was so small, the beneficial effects must have resulted from local action in the bronchial tree and not from a systemic effect after absorption. This action is presumably similar to that of steroids applied topically in skin diseases. When used in this way in dermatology, hydrocortisone is superior to prednisolone. The reason for this is not clear, but it may explain why there was no significant benefit in the patients treated with prednisolone inhalations.

Aerosolized Steroids in Bronchial Asthma are discussed by William Franklin, Francis C. Lowell, Alan J. Michelson, and Irving W. Schiller[4] (Boston Univ.). In an aerosol, (1) the concentration of the steroid should be sufficient for effective dosing in a relatively brief period to avoid excessive demands on the patient; (2) the size of the particles or droplets should be small enough to minimize impingement on tongue and oropharynx and facilitate sufficient entrance into the bronchial tree; (3) the preparation should be tolerable to taste and not irritating on inhalation. Suspensions of finely divided prednisolone and hydrocortisone particles in Freon, delivered through a metered valve and plastic adapter, appear to meet these conditions.

(3) Lancet 1:187-188, Jan. 25, 1958.
(4) J. Allergy 29:214-221, May, 1958.

Strong evidence was obtained, with a double-blind technic, of a topical therapeutic effect of prednisolone in asthma, and clinical experience indicated that this was also true for hydrocortisone. The effect appeared to be about equivalent to that of a daily dose of 40 mg. hydrocortisone by mouth.

The most noticeable subjective effect was relief from cough and irritation, which was sometimes beneficial without change in pulmonary function since inflammation in the larger-caliber tubes of the bronchial tree may have been the principal cause of symptoms.

When bronchial obstruction is severe it may be impossible to deliver much aerosol to the more distal portions of the bronchial tree. Furthermore, particulate matter may be irritating when the asthmatic process is at its height. The chief place of steroid aerosols probably will be in maintenance therapy, not in treatment of acute exacerbations. There is relatively little hazard to short-term steroid therapy such as this and little need to limit systemic absorption.

► [In reporting his experience with a nasal spray containing prednisolone and an antihistamine, chlorprophenpyridamine (Chlor-Trimeton®) in the treatment of allergic rhinitis, W. H. Evans (Ann. Otol., Rhin. & Laryng. 66:716, 1957) said that while most patients preferred the use of the spray bottle to the instilling of drugs it was his impression that in small children the medication could be more effectively applied with a dropper.—Ed.]

BRONCHOPULMONARY DISEASES (GENERAL ASPECTS)

Role of Chlorpromazine in Treatment of Bronchial Asthma and Chronic Pulmonary Emphysema. George L. Baum, Sylvan A. Schotz, Roy C. Gumpel and Catherine Osgood[5] (VA Hosp., Coral Gables, Fla.) studied the effects of chlorpromazine (Thorazine®) given orally, intramuscularly and in combination with other therapy for relief of respiratory distress in 35 patients. Ten had uncomplicated bronchial asthma, 6 bronchial asthma and chronic pulmonary emphysema and 19 primary chronic diffuse obstructive pulmonary emphysema. In addition, laboratory studies were made on 21 patients with the last condition to determine minute volume of respiration, arterial carbon dioxide, oxygen

(5) Dis. Chest 32:574-579, November, 1957.

content and oxygen capacity, and pH immediately before and 1 hour after intramuscular chlorpromazine.

Chlorpromazine was given as a single intramuscular dose of 25-50 mg. to some patients. Others received similar doses orally or intramuscularly in combination with therapy designed to improve ventilation and oxygen transport: intermittent positive pressure breathing (with a nebulized bronchodilator and detergent) with oxygen, antibiotics, expectorants, aminophylline, removal of secretions and, in some instances, ACTH and Diamox®.

A single injection of chlorpromazine caused marked diminution in wheezing and restlessness within ½ hour in 5 patients with uncomplicated bronchial asthma and some relief and relaxation in 2. Drug-induced vomiting (aminophylline) was relieved in 1, and 2 had no response in an hour. In 1 patient with asthma with emphysema, dyspnea and wheezing were reduced after an intramuscular dose. In 2 others these symptoms were relieved when chlorpromazine was combined with bronchodilator therapy. Aminophylline emesis was relieved in 1. Two had no relief from dyspnea, and 1 of these displayed drowsiness. These 2 severely ill patients were given ACTH, and remission followed in each. One patient with primary chronic diffuse obstructive pulmonary emphysema responded to an intramuscular dose of chlorpromazine, and aminophylline-induced vomiting was controlled when the drug was administered orally for 8 days. Eight patients obtained relaxation and control of restlessness on combined therapy. One subject received 4 courses of chlorpromazine combined with intensive therapy during a total of 164 days. Relaxation and control of carbon dioxide intoxication were achieved in 3 of these courses, but the last gave only temporary improvement, and death followed. Despite adequate relaxation, 9 patients were unimproved, and 5 of these died. Deaths were not ascribed to the drug, however.

The head-low position was used when chlorpromazine was given parenterally. A patient who sat up after 15 mg. was injected became pulseless and cyanotic in ½ hour. No jaundice or leukopenia was observed.

No significant changes before and after therapy were found in the laboratory studies. Chlorpromazine, alone or with other treatment, appears to be a safe, effective and use-

before the trypsin or isoprenaline is mixed with trypsin, to produce maximal bronchial dilatation. In later stages of the infection, promethazine is given orally, 10 mg. for children and 25 mg. for adults night and morning.

Even with major atelectasis, bronchoscopy is not done. With the treatment outlined, it may be possible to produce re-expansion in a few days while there is still considerable secretion in the chest; or the patient may recover from the original infection in 1-2 weeks and still have a collapsed area. When the chest becomes dry trypsin is discontinued, but physical therapy, isoprenaline and promethazine are continued. By this routine, collapsed lobes re-expand, although 2 or 3 weeks may be required in some cases.

The following case illustrates the value of the treatment described.

Boy, 15, had been hospitalized with a provisional diagnosis of pneumonia. Figure 2 shows the chest x-ray on admission and Figure 3 the change that occurred in 18 hours with assisted coughing and 2 inhalations of trypsin and isoprenaline. The heart was returning to normal position 15 minutes after starting the first aerosol therapy. Air entry was equal on both sides clinically and to amplification measurement on the electronic stethoscope. Uneventful recovery followed, with the vital capacity increased by 10% over that of 3 months previously.

Comparative Evaluation of Epinephrine and Aminophylline as Bronchodilator Agents was made by Ross C. Kory, Robert A. Pribek and Richard O. Sternlieb[8] (Marquette Univ.). Serial spirometric measurements were used for the objective evaluation of the bronchodilator activity of subcutaneous epinephrine and intravenous aminophylline in 38 men with clinically suspected bronchospasm. After base line studies, the patients were given either 0.3 mg. epinephrine subcutaneously or 0.5 Gm. aminophylline in 20 ml. normal saline intravenously.

Subcutaneous epinephrine showed significant superiority over aminophylline in total vital capacity and maximal breathing capacity tests. Epinephrine was equal to, if not better than, aminophylline in improving timed vital capacities and expiratory flow rates (table). Under the conditions of this study, no appreciable difference could be detected between the two drugs in duration of bronchodilator activity.

(8) Am. Rev. Tuberc. 77:729-736, May, 1958.

Side effects were minimal, but slightly more frequent with intravenous aminophylline.

As the subcutaneous administration of epinephrine is more convenient and is safer than intravenous administration of aminophylline, epinephrine would need only to equal aminophylline in bronchodilator activity to be more useful. Studies of the bronchodilator activity of epinephrine have, with few exceptions, used doses of 0.5-1 mg. subcutaneously. These dosages often result in such side effects as anxiety,

COMPARISON OF BRONCHODILATOR RESPONSE TO EPINEPHRINE AND AMINOPHYLLINE

Determination	Greater Response to Epinephrine	Greater Response to Aminophylline	Equal Response to the Two Drugs
	Number of Patients	Number of Patients	Number of Patients
Total vital capacity	16	7	0
0.5 second vital capacity	11	7	1
1 second vital capacity	15	8	1
3 second vital capacity	13	7	3
Maximal expiratory flow rate (MEFR)	6	4	1
Maximal mid-expiratory flow rate (MMEF)	6	4	1
Maximal breathing capacity	13	6	1

dizziness, pallor, palpitation and headache. Recently smaller doses of epinephrine have been found to be effective clinically, with a much lower incidence of side effects.

Evaluation of the Bronchodilator, Caytine (JB-251). The degree and persistence of bronchodilator activity of Caytine, the 2-(3,4-methylene-dioxyphenyl)-isopropyl derivative of arterenol, its efficacy as compared with that of isoproterenol and patient acceptance were studied by Alan Leslie and Daniel H. Simmons[9] (Los Angeles). Thirty-two men, aged 45-70, who had the chronic emphysema-fibrosis-bronchiectasis triad with varying degrees of bronchospasm and who were experienced subjects for ventilometry were studied immediately before and at intervals up to 2 hours after administration of 1:100 Caytine by nebulizer synchronized with 5 successive deep inhalations.

Statistically significant increases in the inspiratory and expiratory vital capacities—total and timed at 1 and at 3 seconds—were observed in the average values for the group. Single exceptions were noted. Trapped air (difference in ex-

(9) Am. J. M. Sc. 234:321-324, September, 1957.

piratory reserve volume after maximal expiratory effort from the position of normal expiration and from the position of maximal inspiration) was strikingly reduced in 5 patients, though the mean for the group showed no significant reduction.

In half the group, the effects of equimolar doses of Caytine were compared with those of isoproterenol administered by continuous nebulization with a flow of oxygen. The same tests were performed. Statistically, the average values showed that Caytine had a superior effect in each test. Pulmonary airway resistance was also measured and found to be reduced by Caytine but not by isoproterenol. However, there were again pronounced personal variations in response. The patients who were not told which drug was being administered on a particular day did not particularly favor Caytine. Eight expressed a preference for isoproterenol and 4 for Caytine, whereas 4 made no distinction.

With 6 other patients, the foregoing 16 were studied under outpatient conditions. Caytine was administered by a trained nurse, who also made the ventilometric measurements. Other bronchodilators were used and the patients were not told when Caytine was given. Thirteen did not recognize the change. Two had transitory vertigo, in 1 combined with throat dryness. The other 7 commented favorably.

Though the objective aspects of the study favor Caytine over isoproterenol on a statistical basis, the authors note the wide personal variation and recommend that Caytine be included among other bronchodilators which should be given a trial to determine which is most satisfactory for a given patient.

Bronchodilators and Corticosteroids in Treatment of Obstructive Pulmonary Emphysema. The term "obstructive pulmonary emphysema," as used in this study by William Franklin, A. L. Michelson, F. C. Lowell and I. W. Schiller[1] (Boston Univ.), refers to a chronic progressive process manifested clinically by dyspnea, which most commonly appears in middle-aged or elderly men who have had no previous localized or diffuse chronic pulmonary disease and which has generally been regarded as of unknown etiology. In advanced form, the outstanding characteristic is a striking

(1) New England J. Med. 258:774-778, Apr. 17, 1958.

airway obstruction readily recognizable by a reduction in the maximal expiratory flow rate. A second common, but not invariably prominent, feature is chronic cough, often developing several years before onset of obstructive manifestations.

Differentiation of obstructive pulmonary emphysema from asthma is based chiefly on the appearance of symptoms, usually after age 40, and on the relative irreversibility of the obstruction, despite the short duration of symptoms. Heavy smoking, especially cigaret smoking, is a common, and perhaps the specific, cause of the disease in New England. Accordingly, it is assumed that smoking produces a chronic or recurring inflammatory reaction in the airway, and when this occurs in the finer ramifications of the bronchial tree diffuse obstructive pulmonary disease ensues.

The authors treated 58 patients with bronchodilator drugs. Half the group received corticosteroids as well. Though not selected on this basis, all patients were "heavy smokers." Thirteen had peptic ulcer, 6 had congestive heart failure and 1 had both.

Most patients were treated for dyspnea. Steroids were given when the response to bronchodilators was unsatisfactory or, in some cases, when the patient was severely ill. Occasionally, steroids were given to determine the degree of reversibility of pulmonary dysfunction. They were given initially in a daily dose of 8 tablets or more for 2-4 days, followed by 4 tablets or more daily for 1-3 weeks, or until maximum improvement was evident. One tablet contained 25 mg. cortisone, 20 mg. cortisol, 5 mg. prednisone or 5 mg. prednisolone.

In most patients the pulmonary dysfunction could be partially corrected by intensive treatment. Combined treatment with bronchodilator drugs and steroids resulted in a mean increase in vital capacity and 1st second volume of almost 50% of the pretreatment value. Subjective improvement was often greater than was suggested by the change in vital capacity or the maximum expiratory flow rate.

► ↓ Remedial agents in cough, antitussives, are certainly not easy to evaluate. Gregoire *et al.* (Canad. M. A. J. 79:180, Aug. 1, 1958) point out the two principal causes of the difficulty: first, cough is often of sporadic nature and short duration; second, patients who are hospitalized with cough secondary to underlying disease will often have their cough relieved as specific or other symptomatic therapy ameliorates the primary condition. It is fortunate that experimenters in this field have ceased to judge the efficacy of "expectorants" on the basis of the amount of sputum produced, since respiratory tract fluid can be appreciably liquefied, as revealed by postural drainage and bronchoscopic suction, without the action being reflected in the sputum. The newer experimental approach is through production of experimental cough in normal individuals by inhalation of irritant aerosols, and it has already produced some interesting findings.

There is a rash of new antitussives, which are being tried both experimentally and clinically. Unfortunately, most of the articles descriptive of these studies in the following group leave something to be desired, because conclusions appear to be based on too little supporting evidence. More definitive studies are probably already under way.—Ed.

Clinical Evaluation of a New Antitussive Agent. S. J. Shane, T. K. Krzyski and S. E. Copp[2] (Point Edward Hosp., Sydney, N. S.) studied the suppressive action of Tessalon® on induced cough, using a citric acid aerosol as the cough-producing agent. Each of 20 subjects, carefully screened for absence of any spontaneous cough, was given aerosol inhalations of 15% citric acid solution on three separate occasions several days apart. The number of coughs during and for 5 minutes after inhalation of the aerosol was counted. After several days the procedure was repeated on three occasions, the subject having been given ½ gr. codeine 1 hour before testing. Again after several days the procedure was repeated 1 hour after administration of 100 mg. Tessalon on three occasions.

Codeine decreased the frequency of induced cough to 50% of the premedication figure; Tessalon decreased the frequency of induced cough to 20%. This would indicate that in the dosage used, Tessalon is approximately 2½ times as effective in cough suppression as codeine. No undesirable effects resulted from administration of Tessalon. The drug should thus be considered a potent and valuable antitussive agent for routine or specialized use.

Prolonged Cough Suppression. The distressing nature of nocturnal coughing spasms in children is indicated by the 50-60 antitussive preparations stocked by the average pharmacy. However, their popularity depends more on flavor than on antitussive properties. The first successful cough suppressant was opium. Codeine is also effective but habit forming, and constipation is a complication. Dihydrocodeinone is

(2) Canad. M. A. J. 77:600-602, Sept. 15, 1957.

closely related to codeine. It reduces the frequency of coughing without suppressing the cough reflux entirely, reduces the unproductive cough without eliminating cough productive of sputum and is a more potent analgesic and sedative. It may be habit forming and must be prescribed with care.

Antihistamines may potentiate the antitussive effect of dihydrocodeinone. Edward H. Townsend, Jr.[3] (Univ. of Rochester) combined the antihistamine phenyltoloxamine (Histionex) with dihydrocodeinone and an ion-exchange resin to form complexes capable of sustained release of pharmacologically active agents into the gastrointestinal tract. A sulfonic acid resin allows sustained release of the active compounds, independent of pH or enzymatic properties. The level of cation concentration in gastrointestinal secretions determines release of the active compounds, and this remains constant throughout the entire tract. The combination of resin complexes with dihydrocodeinone and phenyltoloxamine in tablet form is available as Tussionex.

The optimal dose was ¼ teaspoonful of the combination (1.25 mg. dihydrocodeinone) every 10-12 hours for infants under age 1, ½ teaspoonful (2.5 mg. dihydrocodeinone) for children age 1-5, and 1 teaspoonful (5 mg. dihydrocodeinone) for those over 5. Personal variations, however, demand adjustment of the dose.

If the combination were given during the early afternoon, the mother might give the aqueous solution of phenyltoloxamine plus dihydrocodeinone at bedtime. The combination, thus potentiated by sleep and the aqueous solution of the effective medicinals, gave complete relief from cough for 10-12 hours. Side effects were rare. Constipation occurred in only 2 of 269 patients treated. Facial pruritus occurred in 5, severe enough to stop the medication in 2. It was due entirely to the dihydrocodeinone. Lethargy seemed related simply to personal dosage variations and diminished when the dose was lowered for the patient so affected.

Use of Noscapine (Narcotine) as Antitussive Agent. Maurice S. Segal, Merrill M. Goldstein and Ernest O. Attinger[4] (Tufts Univ.) administered noscapine to 51 patients

(3) New England J. Med. 258:63-67, Jan. 9, 1958.
(4) Dis. Chest 32:305-309, September, 1957.

with cough due to bronchopulmonary disease. This alkaloid from opium is based on isoquinoline rather than on phenanthrene and also differs pharmacologically from the narcotic alkaloids. Toxicity is low and the effect on the gastrointestinal tract insignificant. The drug has been reported as equal or superior to codeine as an antitussive in experimentally produced cough in normal and asthmatic subjects.

The 27 females and 24 males treated were aged 17-75. Diagnoses included allergic and nonallergic acute bronchitis, tracheobronchitis, chronic bronchial asthma, chronic pulmonary emphysema, bronchiectasis and pulmonary neoplasms. Cough had persisted 1 week to over 30 years.

Dosage, based on patients' needs, ranged from 15 to 30 mg. at bedtime for 17 patients to 60 mg. 6 times daily for 2. Some benefit was obtained by 94%; suppression of cough was graded 3 or 4+ in 48%; 45 reported no side effects. No gastrointestinal symptoms or respiratory depression was observed. Drowsiness was noted in 3, difficulty in raising secretions in 2, and headache in 1 patient. In 3, there was gradual loss of effectiveness. Comparison with other antitussives—dihydrocodeinone bitartrate, X-71, codeine, Dilaudid® and diphenhydramine-aminophylline—showed equal efficacy in 9 trials and greater efficacy in 14.

Comparative Study of Two New Nonnarcotic Antitussive Agents, Tessalon® and Becantex, is presented by S. William Simon[5] (Ohio State Univ.). Tessalon is an esterfied polymericglycol, alkaloid-free, antitussive agent with the chemical formula methoxy-poly(ethyleneoxy)-ethyl-p-butylaminobenzoate. This analogue of local anesthetic drugs acts by anesthetizing the dilation receptors of the lungs, thereby preventing the forcible inspiration with precedes coughing, and causes either marked diminution or complete arrest of the cough. Becantex is sodium 2,6-ditertiarybutylnaphtalene monosulfonate. Its action is also peripheral, probably in the afferent branch of the reflex arc, blocking cough due to irritation of the bronchial tract.

These drugs were given to 59 patients with pulmonary emphysema and chronic asthmatic bronchitis with chronic productive cough. Tessalon in one or two 50-mg. capsules

(5) Ohio M. J. 53:1426-1427, December, 1957.

and Becantex in 30-mg. coated tablets were given 3 or 4 times daily, with additional doses if necessary. Tessalon alone was taken by 18 patients, Becantex alone by 7, and both drugs by 34. Each drug was used a minimum of 2 weeks, and in most cases the drugs were alternated at least 3 times.

Tessalon was considered excellent or good as an antitussive in 83% of patients; 53% obtained this result with Becantex. Sputum was lighter in consistency and less in amount with Tessalon, whereas with Becantex it was more often thicker and unchanged in amount. Results obtained in chronic bronchial infection did not apply when an acute infection was superimposed. Whether this was due to acute inflammation and swelling or to added upper respiratory infection or postnasal drip in unknown. No significant changes in blood count or urinalysis were noted in patients taking these drugs over long periods.

Resin Complex for Prolonged Antitussive Effects is described by Y. T. Chan and Edwin E. Hays.[6] The recently developed principle of using the ion-exchange mechanism to permit sustained, controlled release of active drugs in the gastrointestinal tract was applied to administration of dihydrocodeinone to obtain long-lasting relief from cough with a minimum habit-forming potential. In vitro studies with Tussionex®, a dihydrocodeinone-phenyltoloxamine resin complex, demonstrated that when the complex is percolated with simulated gastric or intestinal juice at the rate of 50 ml./hour, about 76% of the codeine derivatives is released in 8 hours. Studies on dogs demonstrated that the addition of the antihistamine phenyltoloxamine as a resin complex to dihydrocodeinone resin complex gave more complete and sustained antitussive action.

Tablets containing 5 mg. dihydrocodeinone and 10 mg. phenyltoloxamine as their resin complexes were given once every 12 hours to 36 patients who had persistent coughs due to causes ranging from smoke irritation to pulmonary tuberculosis. Fair to excellent relief for 6-12 hours was obtained by each patient. Somewhat longer relief was experienced by 3 when this dosage was doubled. No side reactions were noted, and productive coughing was not prevented.

(6) Am. J. M. Sc. 234:207-212, August, 1957.

CARDIOVASCULAR DISEASES

ARRHYTHMIAS

Stokes-Adams Attacks Treated with Corticotropin. J. W. Litchfield, K. A. Manley and A. Polak[7] (St. Mary's Hosp., London) report immediate improvement in 3 patients treated with corticotropin who failed to respond to atropine and andrenergic drugs. In 1 patient, unstable cardiac rhythm of at least 6 weeks' duration was converted to stable rhythm within 6 days after administration of corticotropin gel, 40 units twice daily, and the Stokes-Adams attacks ceased. In the second patient, attacks occurring 1-40 times a day for many weeks stopped within a few hours. They recurred twice when dosage was reduced. In the third patient, grossly abnormal conduction returned to normal within 6 hours and attacks ceased. Similar results have been reported in the literature.

Corticotropin was used in these cases because it seemed possible that the heart block may have been due to inflammation of the bundle of His. Autopsy on the second patient confirmed the presence of such inflammation. Other hypotheses accounting for the favorable response to corticotropin when atropine and adrenergic drugs fail may be derived from the known effects of the drug on heart muscle metabolism. Infusion of sodium lactate may sometimes produce similar results promptly, but it entails an acute rise in plasma pH. Further study of the relative efficacy and safety of these two methods of therapy is indicated.

► ↓ The following article is a valuable contribution to the drug therapy of Stokes-Adams disease following resuscitation with the external electric pacemaker.—Ed.

Intravenous Drug Therapy of Stokes-Adams Disease: Effects of Sympathomimetic Amines on Ventricular Rhythmicity and Atrioventricular Conduction. Normally the ventricles respond to the sinoatrial pacemaker, and the effects of drugs on ventricular pacemakers are masked by the effect produced on the primary pacemaker. In treating 94 patients with Stokes-Adams disease by external electric stimulation and defibrillation of the heart, Paul M. Zoll, Arthur J. Linen-

(7) Lancet 1:935-937, May 8, 1958.

thal, William Gibson, Milton H. Paul and Leona R. Norman[8] ((Harvard Med. School) studied sympathomimetic drugs and 1M sodium lactate in 21 patients with complete absence of spontaneous ventricular activity. During this time, the only ventricular pacemaker was that supplied by the electronic external stimulator.

Dilute solutions of epinephrine or isoproterenol (Isuprel®)intravenously were equally effective in arousing, accelerating and maintaining intrinsic ventricular activity. The effective dose, 40 µg. epinephrine (8 µg./minute for 5 minutes), was only a small fraction of the usual subcutaneous dose of 200-500 µg. Isoproterenol was effective in doses of 5-43 µg./minute (average 12 µg.). Levarterenol (Levophed®) had a striking vasopressor effect but did not arouse ventricular pacemakers. Once a stable pacemaker was present, it increased the blood pressure, reflexly slowed the sinoatrial rate and independently accelerated the rate of the idioventricular pacemaker. Phenylephrine (Neo-Synephrine®) had only a vasopressor effect. Limited observations of sodium lactate, at the suggested intravenous rates of 7-30 ml./minute, showed it to be less effective than epinephrine and isoproterenol in arousing and accelerating ventricular pacemakers.

In choosing between epinephrine and isoproterenol, the effectiveness of each must be compared with the risk of exciting ectopic ventricular activity. The dose of each drug necessarily varies from patient to patient and at different times in the same patient. There is no striking difference in the cardiac effects of the two drugs. Both require about equal amounts, produce minor toxicity as excessive acceleration and premature ventricular beats which disappear promptly when the drug is stopped. Epinephrine usually had a marked pressor effect, whereas isoproterenol had no effect or lowered the pressure. Isoproterenol usually accelerated the sinoatrial rate markedly, whereas epinephrine had only slight effect. If the first drug was ineffective or toxic, the other was often successful.

With intravenous drip, the effects appear rapidly. When the drip is stopped, they disappear rapidly. This moment-to-moment control allows greater safety but requires constant

(8) Circulation 17:325-339, March, 1958.

supervision and is impractical for long-term administration after the emergency is corrected. For prolonged acceleration and maintenance, the drugs may be given by other routes.

After a patient with Stokes-Adams disease is resuscitated with the external electric pacemaker, stimulation should be stopped promptly to see if intrinsic ventricular activity has returned. If this does not return within an hour and continuous external stimulation is required, epinephrine or isoproterenol should be administered intravenously at 4 μg./minute (4 mg. in 1 L. of 5% dextrose in water at 15 drops/minute). In patients with high blood pressure, isoproterenol is preferable because it has no pressor effect. When blood pressure is normal or low, epinephrine is the drug of choice. The effects should be noted on an ECG during frequent short interruptions of electric stimulation. Every few minutes the rate of infusion should be increased by increments of 4-8 μg./minute until a ventricular pacemaker is aroused or until there are frequent or multifocal ectopic beats, ventricular rate over 50 beats/minute, excessive rise or fall in blood pressure or excessive stimulation of the central nervous system occurs. If the first drug fails or produces toxicity, the other should be tried.

When a ventricular pacemaker is aroused, the rate of drug administration should be adjusted until the idioventricular rate is 35-45/minute, at which time the infusion should be gradually slowed and then stopped if this rate is maintained. Oral ephedrine or sublingual isoproterenol may then be instituted for long-term management.

Strophanthin Therapy in Atrial Flutter. Strophanthin, 0.125-0.5 mg. given intravenously, was used by David Scherf, Edith C. Reid and D. G. Chamsai[9] (New York Med. College) for 22 attacks of atrial flutter in 18 patients. Atrial flutter was converted to atrial fibrillation in 8 attacks and to normal sinus rhythm in 6 others. Six patients did not respond to therapy; 4 of these died of underlying noncardiac disease. One patient showed an increase of atrioventricular block from 2:1 to 4:1. With the doses used, there was only 1 instance of nausea and vomiting and none of ectopic rhythm. The largest permissible dose is 0.5 mg., and this is only to be used if smaller injections have not been followed by extra-

(9) Am. J. M. Sc. 234:180-184, August, 1957.

systoles within 30 minutes. The results showed that strophanthin compares favorably with digitalis in conversion of atrial flutter into normal sinus rhythm or atrial fibrillation.

► [I believe it is generally considered advisable not to attempt conversion of atrial flutter if there is congestive failure and considerable cardiac enlargement.—Ed.]

Place of Methacholine (Mecholyl®) in Management of Paroxysmal Supraventricular Tachycardia is discussed by George S. Husson[1] (State Univ. of New York, Syracuse). Methacholine has a distinct place in management of paroxysmal supraventricular tachycardia, as in the case described.

Infant, aged 10 days, was hospitalized because of labored, grunting respirations and cyanosis for 1 day. The admitting diagnosis was pneumonia. On the 3d and 4th hospital days, the pulse was around 250-300/minute. Digitalization with digitoxin, completed in 24 hours, was effective in terminating the paroxysmal supraventricular tachycardia. On the 6th day tachycardia recurred, followed by congestive heart failure within 3 hours. The maintenance dose of digitoxin was increased by 25%, but this failed to retard the rapid rate, which lasted from the 6th to 11th days. Oral quinidine, 3-4 mg./lb., terminated the tachycardia without evidence of toxicity. A maintenance dose of quinidine (30 mg. every 4 hours) was given; later it was reduced to 15 mg.

The fifth episode of tachycardia failed to respond to higher doses of quinidine and, because of development of toxicity, the drug was discontinued. Digitoxin in high doses was then effective in terminating it. The sixth attack did not respond to higher digitoxin dosage but did respond to quinidine (total dose of 75 mg., 7-8 mg./lb.) given in 5 divided doses every 3 hours. The rate remained normal for 1 week as the quinidine was continued. Extremely high dosage of quinidine and digitoxin failed to terminate the seventh and eighth episodes. Quinidine toxicity developed on these high doses, clinically and by ECG. Pressure on both eyeballs terminated the seventh and eighth bouts of tachycardia while the infant was on maintenance doses of quinidine and digitoxin. The latter drug was discontinued on the 39th hospital day and the infant was discharged on the 45th day, to receive 40 mg. quinidine every 6 hours as prophylaxis.

The infant was readmitted because of tachycardia and congestive heart failure for 1 day. The condition was adequately controlled by continuous intravenous infusion of 5% dextrose in water. A syringe containing atropine in adequate dosage (1/250 gr.) was incorporated into the apparatus for infusion through a 3-way stopcock. Each dose of methacholine was prepared by proper dilution with water just before subcutaneous injection. The injection site was massaged. Methacholine, 0.18 mg./kg., was successful in lowering the pulse to 150/minute after the first 2 doses of 0.045 and 0.090 mg./kg. had failed. The infant was then digitalized (0.035 mg. digitoxin/kg.) and dis-

(1) Pediatrics 21:267-278, February, 1958.

charged 2 days after admission to continue daily maintenance dosage of digitoxin at home.

The infant was next hospitalized with tachycardia (240/minute) and congestive heart failure. Pressure on both eyeballs was unsuccessful in terminating the tachycardia on admission, but was effective the following morning. The maintenance dose of digitoxin was increased from 0.02 to 0.03 mg. daily on discharge.

A few days later, the patient was readmitted with tachycardia and congestive heart failure. Pressure on the eyeballs was unsuccessful. On admission, periods of Wenckebach rhythm occurred after methacholine, 0.33 mg./kg., while the infant was on a large maintenance dosage of digitoxin. Conversion to a normal heart rate was accomplished 1 day later with a dose of 0.32 mg. methacholine/kg. A second episode of tachycardia failed to respond to the same medication. Because of transient, slight bronchoconstriction, further use of this drug was discontinued temporarily.

Oral therapy with quinidine was then started; a total dose of 400 mg. was given within 26 hours. Clinical signs of toxicity and interventricular conduction block, lasting 12 hours, occurred without stopping the tachycardia. On the 3d day, methacholine, 0.36 mg./kg., successfully retarded it.

Because of suspicion of a possible "atropine-like" antagonistic action of digitalis on the cardiac effects of methacholine, digitoxin was discontinued before the successful use of methacholine, 0.39 mg./kg., in terminating a third recurrence of tachycardia. The patient was discharged without any prophylactic therapy.

During the last hospitalization, because of tachycardia and congestive heart failure, methacholine, 0.25 mg./kg., was given. It terminated the tachycardia on the afternoon of the day of admission. The infant was then given quinidine orally as prophylaxis (30 mg. every 6 hours) for the next 4 months. Frequent and regular follow-up has shown no recurrence of the tachycardia to date.

► [Absorption of this drug from the site of its subcutaneous injection may be hastened by massage and delayed by proximal application of a tourniquet. Use of the agent is unquestionably a drastic measure and requires the constant presence of a physician to administer the antidotal atropine if indicated. Electrocardiographic monitoring is desirable, and it is probably advisable to massage the site of the previous injection gently before reinjecting.—Ed.]

Study of Long-Acting Quinidine Preparation: Experience in Normal Subjects and in Patients with Myocardial Abnormality is reported by Samuel Bellet, D. Finkelstein and H. Gilmore[2] (Univ. of Pennsylvania). The expectation that quinidine gluconate, being 10 times as soluble as the sulfate, would produce more satisfactory serum levels was verified experimentally in 10 normal subjects. With administration of delayed-absorption tablets, the blood level rose more slow-

(2) A.M.A. Arch. Int. Med. 100:750-758, November, 1957.

ly, but the peak concentration was maintained for 4½ hours, gradually diminishing thereafter. In 5 normal subjects, 2 doses of 1 Gm. each with 10 hours between produced two peaks, the second higher than the first, with a fairly high level (average, 2.66 mg./L.) remaining 24 hours after the initial dose.

Patients with cardiac arrhythmias—6 with premature contractions, 2 with paroxysmal tachycardia and 4 with atrial fibrillation—were similarly treated. One received smaller doses because of congestive failure and uremia. The long-acting quinidine gluconate successfully abolished extrasystoles in the 6 patients when administered for 3-12 days. The levels at which the extrasystoles disappeared were 1.76-9.44 mg./L. Atrial tachycardia was converted to normal sinus rhythm in 1 of the 2 patients at a plasma level of 5.4 mg. on the 3d day. Therapy was discontinued in the other after 3 days, with a plasma level of 10.54 mg./L. Two patients were relieved of atrial fibrillation, 1 on the 3d day at 2.08 mg./L. and the other the 1st day at 5.82 mg. Smaller doses successfully maintained normal sinus rhythm thereafter. Nausea and vomiting required cessation of treatment in the other 2 patients, 1 of whom, with a plasma quinidine level of 3.76 mg./L., also displayed ventricular extrasystoles.

Long-acting quinidine gluconate, in 1-Gm. doses at 9 a.m. and 7 p.m., gave effective and sustained plasma levels in this limited series, and the effects on cardiac arrhythmias were comparable to those characteristic of quinidine sulfate.

► [When giving 0.4-0.6 Gm. quinidine sulfate every 2 hours for 5 doses, Sokolow and Edgar (Circulation 1:576, 1950) found that in 28 of 30 patients converted from atrial fibrillation or flutter to sinus rhythm the average peak level of the drug at conversion was 5.9 mg./L., three fourths of the patients converting at 4-9 mg./L.—Ed.]

Combined Quinidine and Procaine Amide Treatment of Chronic Atrial Fibrillation was used by Mervin J. Goldman[3] (VA Hosp., Oakland, Calif.) in 18 patients with degenerative heart disease and 20 with rheumatic mitral stenosis or mitral stenosis and insufficiency. When these patients could not be converted to normal sinus rhythm with quinidine alone, as shown by a course of 4-6 Gm. quinidine daily, combination therapy was begun after a lapse of at least 4 days. Minimal doses used were 0.2 Gm. quinidine plus 0.25 Gm. procaine

(3) Am. Heart J. 54:742-745, November, 1957.

amide every 6 hours. Every 3 days the dosage of quinidine or of both was increased. The maximum dose used to date has been 1 Gm. quinidine plus 0.75 Gm. procaine amide every 6 hours.

Successful conversion was obtained in half the cases of degenerative heart disease and in half the rheumatic cases. Normal sinus rhythm was maintained thereafter with smaller doses of quinidine alone or combined with procaine amide. The combination had to be discontinued in 3 patients, because of nausea and vomiting, but 5 who had this difficulty on quinidine alone in larger doses were converted successfully without distress by the combined treatment. Therapy was discontinued in 1 patient because of a 50% increase in the QRS interval. No serious blood pressure drop, ventricular arrythmia or atrioventricular nodal rhythms were encountered. Six patients had had pulmonary or systemic emboli before conversion, but no embolic phenomena took place thereafter. Proper precautions are needed, however, since improper use of these drugs can produce serious toxicity.

Reversion of Atrial Fibrillation to Sinus Rhythm with Digitalis Therapy. Paul B. Jennings, Norman Makous and Joseph B. Vander Veer[4] (Pennsylvania Hosp., Philadelphia) succeeded in 25 patients, aged 33-88, in reverting 33 instances of atrial fibrillation to normal sinus rhythm. Six patients reverted twice and 1, 3 times. Arteriosclerosis or hypertension, or both, were etiologic factors in 23 patients, 3 of whom had concomitant rheumatic heart disease, 2 had acute myocardial infarcts and 1 had had surgery.

All patients had a degree of cardiac failure. There was no evidence of thyroid disease. Patients were generally hospitalized because of heart failure and treated with usual measures, such as digitalization, rest, salt restriction and mercurial diuretics. Digitalis was administered in different forms. Fifteen patients had only oral digitalis. Of these, 10 were already on digitalis previously, and an increase in the daily dosage resulted in reversion to sinus rhythm In the other 5, digitalization was carried out by the oral route. Four received digitalis leaf.

The usual method consisted in giving 1-1.2 Gm. whole leaf in divided doses for the first 48 hours. Then 0.1-0.3 Gm. was

(4) Am. J. M. Sc. 235:702-705, June, 1958.

given daily until full therapeutic results were achieved. One patient was digitalized with digitoxin. Ten were digitalized initially by the intravenous route, 8 with lanatoside C (Cedilanid) and 2 with Digoxin. Cedilanid was given in doses of 0.4-0.8 mg. every 4-6 hours, according to urgency, to a total of 1.2-1.6 mg. The usual dose of Digoxin was 1.5 mg. in divided doses for 6-8 hours. Quinidine or Pronestyl® therapy was not given to any patient.

Many returned to normal sinus rhythm within the 1st week of digitalis therapy. In all patients digitalis was thought to be at least a contributing factor in the conversion to normal. Eleven remained in sinus rhythm for over a year and at least 4 showed a normal rhythm 2 years later. Ten patients eventually started to fibrillate again. Six reverted from atrial fibrillation to sinus rhythm on 2 occasions. Most of them were taking digitalis but were not under adequate control at the time of hospitalization. A slight increase in digitalis as well as other measures to control heart failure again resulted in conversion to sinus rhythm. The only patient who reverted 3 times had a 3-year period with regular sinus rhythm before fibrillating a second time. After the second conversion he was in sinus rhythm 7 months and after the third conversion only 1 month.

Congestive Heart Failure

Use of Prednisone in Congestive Heart Failure. The adrenal cortical steroids lead to retention of sodium and water and excretion of potassium, all of which may be detrimental in patients whose myocardium is already failing. Corticoids have been considered contraindicated in established cardiac failure. However, several cases were reported recently in which excessive edema in patients with congestive heart failure and nephrosis responded to corticotropin and corticoids.

In an attempt to clarify this problem, Leonard B. Gutner, John B. Moses, Sidney Dann and Herbert S. Kupperman[5] (New York Univ.) studied the effect of prednisone on sodium, potassium and water excretion in patients with congestive heart failure treated with digitalis. In each of 11 who were given 5 mg. prednisone 4 times daily, the effect was

(5) Am. J. M. Sc. 234:281-286, September, 1957.

almost entirely favorable. Five reported decreased dyspnea, 3 of whom lost weight; 5 who were well compensated had no untoward alteration in cardiac status; and in only 1 was there questionable increase in exterional dyspnea, associated with weight gain. The 24-hour excretion of sodium was increased in 7, decreased in 2 and unchanged in 2. Potassium excretion was similarly affected.

Prednisone can be used without hesitation for any desired therapeutic end in patients whose myocardial efficiency is reduced and may alleviate massive cardiac edema, especially when response to mercurial and other diuretics is lost. The mechanism of the beneficial effect in congestive heart failure is unknown but the most attractive hypothesis is that it counteracts production of aldosterone.

Acetyl Strophanthidin Used as Measure to Evaluate Status of Digitalization. Dietegen von Capeller and Thomas N. Stern[6] (Univ. of Tennessee) report this cardiac glycoside of ultrashort action to be an extremely accurate measure in digitalis-tolerance tests. No serious toxic effects were encountered. The test was used on 20 patients to determine the status of digitalization. The following case reports illustrate some problems involved.

Case 2.—Man, 53, with hypertension and syphilitic heart disease with aortic insufficiency for 3 years had severe left and right ventricular failure. Before hospital admission he had been maintained for months on digitalis leaf, 1.28 gr. daily. For the first 2 hospital days the dose was doubled, resulting in nausea and vomiting. Potassium chloride was given intravenously without any detectable effect. Since his condition was critical and the status of digitalization doubtful, an acetyl strophanthidin test was performed. Four minutes after a total of 0.3 mg. acetyl strophanthidin had been injected, ventricular premature beats occurred every 6th beat. One minute later the premature beats became multifocal. Thirty minutes after injection the rhythm returned to a normal sinus rhythm. The test was interpreted as indicating that he was overdigitalized. Digitalis was withheld for 3 days and given again on the initial maintenance dose. He improved somewhat on bed rest and diuretics and was discharged, although still considered to be in functional class 4.

Case 7.—Man, 47, had chief complaints of severe shortness of breath, paroxysmal dyspnea at night and orthopnea, gradually increasing over 3 years. He had been digitalized 3 years before and maintained since on 1.28 gr. digitalis leaf daily. Examination revealed blood pressure 170/110 mm. Hg, pulse rate 130 and respiratory rate 28/minute. On admission he received 1.2 mg. digitoxin intramuscular-

(6) Am. Heart J. 55:8-17, January, 1958.

ly and was maintained on digitalis leaf, 2.56 gr. daily, for the next 2 weeks. His condition changed little and his heart rate continued to be elevated. An acetyl strophanthidin test was then performed. After a total dose of 0.7 mg. he felt nauseated and developed rare ventricular premature contractions. This was interpreted as indicating that he was approximately half digitalized. After the test he was put on oral digitoxin 0.4 mg. daily. After 4 days the heart rate decreased to 76 and orthopnea and peripheral edema disappeared. He was discharged on a regimen of 0.2 mg. digitoxin daily and 6 weeks later was still doing well.

The clinical impression before the test was digitalis intoxication, based on the fact that the patient had received large doses of digitalis before the test without apparent improvement. The response to digitoxin afterward confirmed the interpretation of the acetyl strophanthidin tolerance test. The unusually high digitalizing dose in this patient can be explained, perhaps, on the basis of a poor and unpredictable absorption of orally administered digitalis leaf in the presence of severe congestive failure.

Case 16.—Man, 53, with a history of rheumatic heart disease since 1942 and progressive shortness of breath improved markedly after a mitral commissurotomy was performed in 1952. In 1955, however, he again had shortness of breath and had to be maintained on digitalis leaf, 1.28 gr. daily. In 1956 he was again hospitalized with acute pulmonary edema, orthopnea and paroxysmal nocturnal dyspnea. Examination showed blood pressure of 90/60 mm. Hg, extremely irregular pulse and respiratory rate 36. Neck veins were distended. Lungs were full of moist rales bilaterally. The heart showed an absolute irregularity, with a rate of 145 per minute.

Since his condition did not improve after being given morphine, aminophylline and nasal oxygen, and since the digitalization status was not clear, he was given an acetyl strophanthidin test. Initially he received 40 mEq. potassium chloride as an intravenous drip. Under the influence of potassium, ventricular premature contractions disappeared but the general condition deteriorated further. Four and one-half minutes after a total of 1.25 mg. acetyl strophanthidin had been injected, he felt nauseated and vomited. The heart rate fell from 145 to 110. The test indicated that the patient had to be fully redigitalized. Lanatoside C, 0.8 mg., was given intravenously immediately and 9 gr. digitalis leaf during the next 24 hours. He improved markedly on this regimen. After recovery it was revealed that he had omitted to take digitalis for 4 days. X-ray studies and cardiac catheterization, done later, demonstrated that mitral stenosis was the predominant lesion, as confirmed by a second commissurotomy. The patient is relatively asymptomatic at present.

Case 20.—Man, 45, was seen for the first time 6 months before the acetyl strophanthidin test, with chief complaints of fluttering heart and exertional dyspnea for 2 days. Examination was nonrevealing except for tachycardia. An ECG was interpreted as nodal tachycardia, with a rate of 130 and left ventricular strain pattern. Numerous measures including quinidine, procaineamide, Mecholyl®, potassium chloride and lanatoside C, did not stop tachycardia. Since there were symptoms of congestive heart failure, he was digitalized and maintained on 1.28 gr. digitalis leaf daily. Tachycardia persisted unchanged for 6 months, at the end of which acetyl strophanthidin was tried as a measure to convert the ectopic rhythm. After a total dose of 0.9 mg., frequent nodal arrests developed, followed in each instance by a nodal escape of lower origin. This was interpreted as indicating that digitalis-like compounds are not helpful in converting arrhythmia.

Evaluation of Digitalis Tolerance with Acetyl Strophanthidin. Lee Ehrlich, Bernard M. Lipschultz and Joe C. Ehrlich[7] (VA Hosp., Phoenix, Ariz.) report experience with 10 digitalized patients, using the following test. Two cc. acetyl strophanthidin (1.1 mg.) was diluted to 20 cc. with 5% aqueous glucose; 5 cc. was injected intravenously every 5 minutes until the therapeutic or toxic effect appeared on a continuous direct-writing ECG.

The 10 patients were well digitalized with whole-leaf digitalis or digoxin, as shown by slowing of the ventricular rate, subsidence of symptoms of congestive heart failure and maintenance of a dry weight for at least 2 weeks. The digitalis effect on the S-T segment and T wave was evident in the ECG of each. Four had chronic cor pulmonale, 4 arteriosclerotic heart disease and 2 hypertensive cardiovascular disease.

During testing, ECG evidence of toxicity was achieved in only 2 patients. In 1 with arteriosclerotic heart disease, frequent multifocal premature ventricular systoles after 0.82 mg. acetyl strophanthidin indicated incomplete digitalization. In the other with cor pulmonale, a transient nodal rhythm was similarly interpreted. In 6, no change in the ECG pattern was found with 1.1 mg., and 2 tolerated 1.65 mg. without ECG evidence of toxicity.

It was concluded that the test will show whether more digitalis may safely be administered, but it will not show whether the patient has received digitalis or is partially or completely digitalized.

Rapid Digitalization of Ambulatory Patients with Atrial Fibrillation: Use of Intramuscularly Given Deslanoside Followed by Orally Given Acetyldigitoxin. Digitalization by means of a single intramuscular injection of deslanoside (desacetyl-lanatoside C. lanatoside D) was carried out by

(7) Dis. Chest 32:289-294, September, 1957.

Emanuel Hellman and Murray Port[8] (New York) in 19 trials in 16 ambulatory patients. The dose was 1.6 mg. in 16 instances and 1.2 mg. in 3. When a 10% reduction of the control ventricular rate occurred, maintenance therapy was begun with acetyldigitoxin in doses of 0.1-0.2 mg. Maintenance therapy was begun the same day in 12 of the 16 patients. Adequate digitalization was obtained in 15 of the 16 patients. No toxic effects were noted. Moderate to severe pain at the site of injection was noted in 7 of 19 trials, an incidence of 37%.

Digitalis Intoxication: Review and Report of 40 Cases, with Emphasis on Etiology is presented by Morton W. Shrager[9] (Albert Einstein Med. Center, Philadelphia). Digitoxin seemed to produce severer toxicity with fewer warning symptoms than did digoxin. Nausea and vomiting were by far the most prominent symptoms, but anorexia might often be missed as an early symptom of intoxication. Neurologic symptoms occurred in about half the cases but were usually accompanied by gastrointestinal symptoms. Pulse irregularities were present in 93% of patients; bradycardia was found in 25%. The average P-R interval was 0.23 seconds in the intoxicated group, compared to 0.19 seconds in nontoxic controls. The presence of digitalis effects on an ECG was not a significant criterion of the presence or severity of intoxication. Arrhythmias as shown by the ECG were present, however, in 95% of cases. Auricular fibrillation was attributable to digitalis intoxication in only 3 of 14 patients with this arrhythmia and was accompanied by other arrhythmias in 11 of the 14. Bigeminy was present in 25% of cases of intoxication.

Of 6 cases of refractory heart failure, 5 improved with withdrawal of digitalis. Failure to attribute advancing congestive heart failure to digitalis intoxication may be a serious and not uncommon error. When clinical signs and symptoms are compatible with both congestive heart failure and digitalis intoxication and if the congestive failure has not previously responded to adequate digitalis dosage, benefit will often be obtained by stopping or reducing the dosage of digitalis.

Of the 40 cases of digitalis intoxication, 80% were felt to have been preventable by attending physicians, and 88% of

(8) J.A.M.A. 167:215-216, May 10, 1958.
(9) A.M.A. Arch. Int. Med. 100:881-893, December, 1957.

these could be attributed to errors in dosage. A common error, responsible for 9 cases, was an attempt to control intractable failure by exhibiting high-maintenance dosage or by adding frequent small supplementary doses to an already adequate maintenance dose. Small increases of dosage are especially hazardous in patients with any of the well-known limitations to digitalis therapy: poor myocardial status, electrolyte imbalance due to diuresis and congestive failure, acute myocardial infarction, pulmonary embolism, severe kidney disease and advanced liver disease.

A commoner and insidious error was the failure of physicians frequently to follow patients who were receiving relatively normal maintenance dosage of digitalis. The follow-up was inadequate to individualize these so-called normal doses and re-evaluate patients' dosage on the basis of advancing congestive failure and other criteria which may predispose to intoxication. The most frequent offending dosage was 0.2 mg. digitoxin daily and 0.5 mg. digoxin daily, but toxicity developed in patients receiving 0.15 and even 0.1 mg. digitoxin.

Electrolyte imbalance was prominent in 8 cases but seemed to be of etiologic importance primarily in only 4 instances of toxicity. Two cases of toxicity (with 1 death) associated with intravenous calcium therapy were reported. Infusion of hypertonic saline probably precipitated intoxication in 1. Diuresis was felt to be primarily responsible in 4 cases. Acute myocardial infarction seemed to predispose to development of toxicity in 3.

The author emphasizes the gravity of the syndrome of digitalis intoxication. With oral potassium therapy and discontinuation of digitalis, the average time for disappearance of symptoms or signs due to digoxin was 2-3 days in 5 cases. In 9 patients receiving digitoxin, symptoms and signs disappeared in 9-11 days.

► [Considering the long time that digitalis has been in use, it seems to me a severe castigation of cardiovascular practice when the author of a careful study such as this can charge that 80% of the cases of intoxication could have been prevented and that 88% were attributable to errors in dosage. —Ed.]

Effects of Sublingual Administration of Nitroglycerin on Pulmonary Artery Pressure in Patients with Failure of Left Ventricle. John B. Johnson, Jean F. Gross (Howard Univ.)

and Edward Hale[1] (Univ. of Pittsburgh) report that nitroglycerin sublingually, 0.6-1.3 mg., was clinically effective in relieving respiratory and retrosternal distress of paroxysmal nocturnal dyspnea. A physiologic study using catheterization of the right side of the heart was made in 10 patients with hypertensive heart disease and left-sided heart failure to determine the effect of nitroglycerin on pulmonary artery pressure.

Nitroglycerin produced prompt reduction in pulmonary artery hypertension associated with failure of the left ventricle. Fall in systemic arterial pressure also was observed in 9 of the 10 patients during the first 15 minutes and in 7 of 9 patients in 16-30 minutes after nitroglycerin administration. In each of these 2 periods, fall in brachial artery pressure was significant in 5 patients. No relation was found between the magnitude of fall of blood pressure in the pulmonary artery and that in the brachial artery in the same patient after use of sublingual nitroglycerin. In 3 patients in whom it was possible to obtain pulmonary wedge pressure before and after nitroglycerin administration, prompt fall was shown in pulmonary wedge pressure and in pulmonary artery pressure. This observation suggests that in patients with failure of the left ventricle use of nitroglycerin results in decreased pressure in the left atrium and in the pulmonary artery.

The mechanism by which nitroglycerin reduces pulmonary hypertension of left ventricle failure is not fully clarified by the data presented.

► [If nitroglycerin effects a pooling of blood in the splanchnic area, as we know it does, would this not automatically relieve pulmonary hypertension through reducing the return flow to the heart from the major circulation; and indirectly would this not effect myocardial improvement in a handicapped heart? Or perhaps the thing is not this simple.—Ed.]

Diuretic Action of Two Carbonic Anhydrase Inhibitors in Congestive Failure was studied by Harry Gold, Theodore H. Greiner, Leon Warshaw, Nathaniel T. Kwit and Aaron Ganz[2] (New York). The diuretic potency of two carbonic anhydrase inhibitors, acetazolamide (Diamox®) and a new compound, ethoxzolamide (Cardrase®), in over 25 ambulant cardiac patients with congestive failure was determined by comparison with a standard, intramuscularly given meral-

(1) New England J. Med. 257:1114-1117, Dec. 5, 1957.
(2) J.A.M.A. 167:814-818, June 14, 1958.

luride (Mercuhydrin®). The drugs were evaluated by the following bioassay:

METHOD.—The criterion of response is body weight loss in the first 24 hours after the dose. This closely parallels the curve of clinical improvement in patients with congestive failure. Patients are accurately weighed, receive a dose of the drug, either meralluride given intramuscularly or the particular test drug, and are weighed again 24 hours later. They return weekly for a dose of the drug and are instructed to remain on their usual diet, with free water intake and salt restriction. Most of them also receive a daily dose of a digitalis glycoside. This regimen remains unchanged during the assay. In every group of patients, several dose levels of the standard and of the test drug are administered in random fashion. The average weight loss for the group with the various doses provides data for dosage response curves for both the standard and test drug in the same patients. Potency of the test drug is expressed in terms of the standard. Differences in response are tested for significance by standard statistical methods. In the assay of orally given diuretics which may produce disagreeable symptoms from their local actions, an inert placebo tablet indistinguishable from the test drug is included in the study, using the double-blind technic.

The average maximum diuretic response with orally given acetazolamide was obtained from a dose of about 125 mg. The average maximum diuretic effect of this drug (ceiling effect) is equivalent to somewhat less than that with 0.5 cc. intramuscularly administered meralluride. An average maximally effective oral dose of acetazolamide given with an intramuscular injection of meralluride did not enhance the diuretic response to the latter. Ethoxzolamide is a somewhat more potent diuretic agent than is acetazolamide both on a weight basis of the compounds and from the standpoint of maximum obtainable diuretic response. It is suggested that an action in addition to anhydrase inhibition may explain the difference. The average maximally effective dose of ethoxzolamide produced a diuretic effect similar to that with about 0.7 cc. intramuscularly given meralluride.

Osmotic Diuretic Treatment of Refractory Edema. Osmotic diuretics have a physical rather than a cellular metabolic effect and depend on the presence of nonabsorbable particles within the iso-osmotic proximal tubule. These retain water within the tubule to maintain a constant total osmolar concentration of 310 mOsm./L. This retained water progressively dilutes the sodium in the fluid as it traverses the proximal tubule, and the cell surface area for sodium resorption is exposed to a fluid of progressively lesser sodium concentration. Fewer sodium particles are absorbed and more pass on distally. The additional nonabsorbed sodium and accompanying anions behave as osmotic diuretic particles to retain water that is also passed on distally.

Mannitol, an almost inert, nontoxic hexose, is excreted by glomerular filtration alone. It is an osmotic diuretic that can be given parenterally. Lionel M. Bernstein, Bernard Blumberg and Murray C. Arkin[3] (VA Hosp., Hines, Ill.) administered mannitol intravenously in large doses—up to 475 Gm. in 8 hours—to 6 patients who had edema refractory to mercurial diuretics, aminophylline, ammonium chloride and Diamox®. Dietary sodium was constant for several weeks before, during and after mannitol. Water was given ad lib. Thiomerin®, a mercurial diuretic, was given intravenously as a single 2-ml. dose or as two 1-ml. doses 3-5 hours apart.

Whatever the previous excretion of sodium, chloride and water, administration of mannitol markedly increased the levels. Mannitol combined with a mercurial diuretic was much more effective than either alone in increasing excretion of sodium (up to 660 mEq./day) and water (up to 8,685 ml./day) and causing edema losses, whether the edema was of renal, cardiac or hepatic origin. Diuresis was not necessarily accompanied by clinical benefit. Serum electrolyte concentration did not change significantly.

In 1 patient with nephrotic edema, mannitol with Thiomerin was effective and without adverse reactions. In 2 with cardiac edema, mannitol infusion caused pulmonary edema during the diuresis. In 1 patient with cirrhotic edema, marked diuresis was followed by early signs of central nervous system symptoms of hepatic insufficiency. In 2 other patients, 1 with cirrhosis and 1 with lupus nephritis, diuresis did not occur, probably because dose was inadequate and filtration rates markedly reduced.

The data conclusively demonstrate the ability of mannitol, an osmotic diuretic, to increase markedly urinary excretion of water, sodium and chloride in refractory edema, apparently by shifting toward greater tubular rejection of sodium and water. When edema states are refractory to all other diuretic

(3) Circulation 17:1013-1020, June, 1958.

therapy, osmotic diuretics in adequate doses combined with a mercurial diuretic should be considered.

Urea, the Forgotten Diuretic. A new assessment of the diuretic properties of urea was made by Cornelio Papp and K. Shirley Smith[4] (London Chest Hosp.), who conclude that when integrated in action with mercurial diuretics, urea has a special place in therapy of chronic heart failure with edema. Study was made of 17 patients with obstinate and prolonged right ventricular failure. Fourteen had chronic rheumatic valvular heart disease, and some of these had cardiac hepatic cirrhosis with ascites; 6 underwent mitral valvotomy. Two of the other patients had coronary heart disease and the third had hypertensive cardiac disease. Urea was administered in doses of 15 Gm., dissolved in 57 ml. water or grapefruit juice 3 times daily. Treatment was maintained for 2½ weeks to 7 years.

In about half the patients a negative fluid balance was changed to positive on urea alone. In cases in which it remained negative, fluid retention became less. Urea produced such effects even after mercurial diuretics had become useless. In several patients mercurial diuretics were greatly augmented in their effect when urea was given concurrently.

At worst urea administration is never harmful, but it may have to be discontinued on account of the patient's distaste or because of nausea and vomiting. At best it may be the means of maintaining in a quiet occupation for several years a patient with grave valvular heart disease in whom this result is unattainable by other medicaments singly or in combination. Between such extremes are patients in chronic congestive failure who may receive many months of benefit, at first by prolongation of quiet acitivity free from edema and later by mitigation or abolition of distressing edema and effusions until the last days of the illness.

► [Urea has the one great advantage, shared with practically none of the other diuretics, of continuing to exert its effect as long as its administration is continued, though of course not irrespective of the advancing pathology. In the presence of reduced renal function it may contribute to the picture of nitrogen retention.—Ed.]

► ↓ The current impression that the mercurial diuretics are "out the window" since the advent of chlorothiazide is shown not to be justified in the following article, which reveals them still the most potent for parenteral use.—Ed.

(4) Brit. M. J. 2:906-911, Oct. 19, 1957.

Choice of Diuretic Agent Based on Pharmacologic Principles. Ralph V. Ford, Jethro B. Rochelle III, Carroll A. Handley, John H. Moyer and Charles L. Spurr[5] (Baylor Univ.) studied urinary excretion of sodium, chloride, potassium, ammonium, bicarbonate and phosphate ions by a method of fractional urine collections in a series of patients receiving a diet constant as to water, sodium and calories. The

RELATIVE MERITS OF FIVE GROUPS OF DIURETICS

	Mercurials, Meralluride and Chlormerodrin	Carbonic Anhydrase Inhibitors, Acetazolamide	Aminouracils, Amisometradine and Aminometradine	Chlorothiazide	Chlorazanil*
Parenteral efficacy	++++	+	+	++	
Oral efficacy	+++	+	+	++++	+
Toxicity	++	+	+	0†	++
Drug tolerance	0	+++	+++	0	0
Biochemical alterations					
Hypochloremia	++	0	+	++	0
Acidosis	0	++	0	0	0
Azotemia	0	0	0	0	++
Usefulness in various syndromes					
Cardiac	++++	+	+	+++	++
Pregnancy	++	+	+	+++	+
Hepatic	+++	+	+	+++	++
Renal	+++	0	+	+++	0
Steroid	++++	0	+	+++	+

*No parenteral preparation available.
†Gastrointestinal upset orally or pain on parenteral injection.

effects of 5 different diuretics were compared (table). Each gave a distinct pattern of electrolyte excretion. They differed in potency when given in clinically tolerated doses to patients in comparable states of edema.

The mercurials are the most potent diuretic agents currently available in parenteral form. Acetazolamide and chlorothiazide are available for injection, but their duration of action is short and the total 24-hour loss of sodium after their use is less than that observed after administration of meralluride. Aminometradine and chlorazanil are not commercially available in parenteral form.

(5) J.A.M.A. 166:129-136, Jan. 11, 1958.

Among the orally active diuretics, chlorothiazide is the most potent, followed by chlormerodrin and chlorazanil. The aminouracils (aminometradine and amisometradine) are almost as potent acutely but are not continuously effective on daily administration. The same is true of the carbonic anhydrase inhibitors.

The development of drug tolerance or "compensation" on consecutive daily administration was not observed with mercurials, chlorothiazide or chlorazanil, but it seriously limits the usefulness of aminouracils and carbonic anhydrase inhibitors in chronic states of edema.

Nephrotic Syndrome Complicating Mercurial Diuretic Therapy was observed in 5 patients by Margaret Riddle, Frances Gardner, Isobel Beswick and Ian Filshie[6] (Royal Free Hosp., London). The following were the reasons for attributing renal damage in these patients to long-term mercurial diuretic therapy. (1) No patient had a previous history of kidney disease, and 3 were known to have had normal urine when treatment with mercurials was begun. (2) Pathologic changes were similar in all 3 patients who died, resembling those in acute mercuric chloride poisoning. (3) Excessive amounts of mercury were found at autospy in the renal tubules in 2 patients. (4) No cause other than mercurial damage to the kidneys was found.

The significant pathologic finding was necrosis, degeneration and regeneration of renal tubules. The glomeruli were normal.

The principal warning signs of the nephrotic syndrome complicating mercurial diuretic therapy are: (1) Failure of albuminuria to decrease after satisfactory diuresis, (2) increasing edema, especially of arms and face, in the absence of other signs of cardiac failure and (3) absence of diuresis after mercurial therapy.

Treatment of the fully developed syndrome is unsatisfactory. BAL (dimercaprol), corticotropin, ion exchange resins and decapsulation of kidneys have all been tried without benefit. The survival of 1 patient who received no specific therapy indicates that in some instances the condition is reversible.

---

(6) Brit. M. J. 1:1274-1277, May 31, 1958.

► ↓ I sing the clarion sweet praises of Diuril® in the next 5 articles before the croaking voices of discontent boom into the chorus. There are other articles on the drug in the sections on hypertension and the liver disorders and elsewhere.—Ed.

Clinical and Laboratory Observations on Chlorothiazide (Diuril®): Orally Effective Nonmercurial Diuretic Agent. Chlorothiazide increases elimination of sodium, chloride and water. It is a nonmercurial, orally effective agent with diuretic effects equal to or greater than any other oral diuretic.

Ralph V. Ford, John H. Moyer and Charles L. Spurr[7] (Baylor Univ.) studied effects of the drug in 10 men who were in compensated congestive heart failure and in unhydrated and hydrated dogs. The effective dose lay between 1 and 2 Gm.; 4 Gm. produced no toxicity but also showed no additional diuretic effect. The drug is a potent inhibitor of renal tubular reabsorption of sodium and causes minimal excretion of bicarbonate but considerable excretion of chloride. An oral dose has rapid effect, within 2 hours, and duration of action of less than 12 hours. When given in repeated daily doses, chlorothiazide is recurrently effective. It produces no metabolic acidosis and has a high therapeutic index. Oral administration is more effective than intravenous. Administration at 12-hour intervals results in greater increase in sodium excretion than the same total dose given as a single dose/24 hours.

The predominant electrolyte excretion after chlorothiazide is in sodium and chloride. The effect on potassium and bicarbonate is smaller in the presence of an alkaline urine. A dose of about 500 mg. chlorothiazide is roughly equivalent to 40 mg. Neohydrin® (4 tablets) and about twice as potent as Diamox®. A dose of slightly more than 1 Gm. is equivalent to 1 cc. Mercuhydrin® given intramuscularly.

An average dose of chlorothiazide effective in controlling chronic congestive heart failure is 500 mg. given twice daily. Clinical experience over 3 months indicates that this drug is effective in replacing current oral and parenteral diuretic agents in managing chronic congestive heart failure.

Clinical Observations on Chlorothiazide: Orally Effective Nonmercurial Diuretic Agent. Ray P. Landes and Michael Peters[8] (Grand View Hosp., Sellersville, Pa.)used chloro-

(7) A.M.A. Arch. Int. Med. 100:582-596, October, 1957.
(8) Postgrad. Med. 23:648-654, June, 1958.

thiazide (Diuril®) in 60 patients with edema, due in 32 to primary heart disease with congestive heart failure. It was administered almost entirely by the oral route. The average dose was 1,000-2,000 mg. and most patients, especially those with more severe edema states, received 2 doses daily. Others with less severe edema were placed on one of several intermittent dosage schedules. Up to the limits of the dosage used, there appeared to be a direct relation between size of dose and amount of diuresis.

Chlorothiazide proved to be a potent diuretic agent causing excretion of large amounts of sodium and chloride along with large quantities of urine. Symptoms of dyspnea, orthopnea, cough and restlessness were simultaneously improved. In most instances, the diuresis began in about 2 hours and reached a maximum in 4-6 hours. Duration of the action rarely extended beyond 8-12 hours.

Initial therapy differed little from maintenance therapy with respect to dosage. Of 32 patients with cardiac edema treated, 14 were successfully maintained on chlorothiazide as the only diuretic agent. It was especially effective in edema of pregnancy in the presence or absence of toxemia. Remarkable relief of the edema associated with premenstrual tension was noted. No significant toxicity was noted though several patients received 2,000 mg. daily for up to 9 months. Although there was markedly increased sodium chloride excretion and a slight increase in potassium excretion with chronic administration of the drug, plasma studies consistently revealed a normal electrolyte balance. Gastrointestinal symptoms were absent except for nausea, diarrhea and abdominal cramps in 2 patients. Mild paresthesias were observed occasionally.

Chlorothiazide: New Approach to Therapy of Edematous States is discussed by Stanley I. Fishman, Robert J. Jaffe, George Schwartz, George H. Stechel, Arthur Fankhauser, Donald J. Behr and Jacob J. Yarvis.[9] (Kings County Hosp. Center, Brooklyn). An effective oral diuretic must (1) be a potent inhibitor of renal reabsorption of sodium, (2) cause minimal excretion of bicarbonate and, therefore, reciprocally, considerable excretion of chloride, (3) have brief action after a single dose and (4) be recurrently effective when admin-

(9) New York J. Med. 58:1679-1683, May 15, 1958.

istered repeatedly over a long period. It should not produce metabolic acidosis or other physiologic or pharmacodynamic side effects and should have a high therapeutic index and low inherent toxicity.

Chlorothiazide (Diuril®) appears to be such an agent. It was given to 125 patients with evidence of peripheral edema demonstrable on physical examination who responded incompletely or not at all to the usual therapeutic regimen. Initial dosage was 2 Gm./24 hours. In most instances this dosage was continued as maintenance therapy. Most patients were instructed to take 1 Gm. after breakfast and 1 Gm. before supper. All medications other than diuretics (digitalis, antihypertensive agents) were continued as before.

Weight loss in the 1st week of therapy was 1-13 lb. Most patients lost their total amount within the first 4 weeks and had little or no further weight loss after that. Almost all reported improvement in exertional ability with decrease in breathlessness, cough, orthopnea and paroxysmal nocturnal dyspnea. Nausea was the commonest side effect. No adverse hematologic, dermatologic or neurologic effects were noted. Hypokalemia developed in 2 patients and was reversed with potassium chloride. The daily ingestion of oranges or bananas was uniformly effective as prophylaxis against hypokalemia. The cause for 11 failures was not obvious.

Effect of Chlorothiazide on Edema of Cirrhosis, Nephrosis, Congestive Heart Failure and Chronic Renal Insufficiency was studied by George E. Schreiner and H. Allan Bloomer[1] (Georgetown Univ.) in 36 patients. The drug was given orally every 6 hours in doses of 5, 10 or 15 mg./kg. estimated dry body weight throughout the study period. Salt and water excretion studies were made on 20 patients.

A dose of 5 mg./kg. produced significantly negative balances of sodium, chloride and water in edematous patients with cirrhosis, nephrotic syndrome and congestive heart failure. Significant potassium loss was also shown and was fairly marked in an occasional patient with hyponatremia or on a high-potassium diet. The diuretic response was prompt and began a few hours after ingestion. In many cases there appeared to be an increase in salt excretion on the 2d and 3d days of administration, suggesting that intermittent dosage

(1) New England J. Med. 257:1016-1022, Nov. 21, 1957.

might be more effective in 3-day blocks than on an interrupted 1-day schedule. No apparent further benefit was derived from higher doses. In patients with normal or only moderately reduced filtration rates, chlorothiazide was able to counteract the salt retention of therapeutic levels of adrenal steroids. This is particularly valuable for management of the nephrotic syndrome. Chlorothiazide effected massive diuresis in nephrotic patients not receiving ACTH or steroids and produced significant weight losses even in the presence of a steroid-induced antidiuresis. A patient with amyloid nephrosis who originally had anasarca and did not respond to chlorothiazide when receiving ACTH had subsequent diuresis with steroids and albumin.

No urines became alkaline, and there was no evidence of significant carbonic anhydrase inhibition as the mechanism of action of chlorothiazide. In some patients, chloruresis seemed to dominate the response, suggesting that chlorothiazide might be ideal for management of renal hyperchloremic acidosis. This was tested in 1 patient with ureterosigmoid anastomoses who had diuresis on the 1st day of treatment but whose clinical course was too complicated to permit analysis of the data. After the reported studies, several patients were given short courses of acetazolamide combined with chlorothiazide. There was enhancement of natruresis without an increment of chloruresis, suggesting separate mechanisms for these drugs. A few patients were given mercurial diuretics, with an apparent additive effect. Chlorothiazide was unable to produce significant diuresis in the presence of marked reduction of glomerular filtration. In some patients the concentration of salt in the urine did increase, suggesting a possible value in long-term administration.

Effect of Chlorothiazide on Electrolyte Transport in Man. Its Use in Treatment of Edema of Congestive Heart Failure, Nephrosis and Cirrhosis was studied by John H. Laragh, Henry O. Heinemann and Felix E. Demartini[2] (Columbia Univ.) in 32 patients. All were in advanced states of fluid retention and were given the drug orally in a dosage of 2 Gm./day.

Results indicated that chlorothiazide is a useful diuretic. It

(2) J.A.M.A. 166:145-152, Jan. 11, 1958.

seems to be as potent as a mercurial diuretic given intramuscularly and can act to remove edema when other measures fail.

Chlorothiazide increases the renal excretion of chloride, sodium and potassium without apparent effect on glomerular filtration. The mode of action of chlorothiazide seems different from that of other known diuretics. Its effects are additive to those of an organic mercurial or a carbonic anhydrase inhibitor and appear to be independent of plasma chloride concentration. Moreover, the drug may be effective in conditions resistant to mercurial diuretics. In short-term studies in 2 normal persons, chlorothiazide and meralluride were shown to have qualitatively different effects on the clearance of "free" water.

Refractoriness does not develop readily, and no significant toxicity was observed in this series. The continued daily use of the compound usually leads to hypokalemic alkalosis. This effect is readily reversed by administration of potassium chloride. The data suggest that the compound should be given either on an intermittent dosage schedule or should be supplemented by potassium chloride therapy. Alternation with a carbonic anhydrase inhibitor may also be advantageous. In certain instances a combination of chlorothiazide with an organic mercurial has lead to striking diuresis after other measures had failed.

The fact that the compound was effective in all types of edema studied supports the hypothesis that similar mechanisms operate in the abnormal renal retention of sodium in heart failure, hepatic cirrhosis and nephrosis.

A patient who had been receiving chlorothiazide therapy intermittently for about 6 months, in addition to a number of other drugs, died of renal failure. Although it does not seem likely that renal failure resulted from chlorothiazide therapy, the case is reported to alert others to this possibility.

Dichlorphenamide as Diuretic Agent is a relatively simple disulfamyl compound (1,3-disulfamyl-4,5-dichlorobenzene), commercially named Daranide, that has some unusual, striking differences from the carbonic anhydrase inhibitors. J. B. Rochelle, III, John H. Moyer and Ralph V. Ford[3] (Houston) studied its action in 32 dogs and 20 men who had

(3) Am. J. M. Sc. 235:168-178, February, 1958.

well-controlled congestive heart failure. Within 30 minutes after administration of 0.5 mg./kg. dichlorphenamide, urine volume and sodium excretion increased significantly, then returned to normal within 1½-2 hours. With doses of 2 mg. and 10 mg./kg., the diuresis continued for 4 hours. Potassium excretion also increased, but not to the same extent.

The patients were maintained on a balanced diet of 50 mEq. sodium daily. After 50 mg. dichlorphenamide orally twice daily, excretion of sodium, potassium and bicarbonate increased slightly and urinary pH remained elevated throughout 24 hours. With doses of 500 mg. twice daily, sodium excretion was about the same, potassium and bicarbonate excretion less, but chloride excretion was greatly increased, as compared with the smaller dose. Average increase in 24-hour urinary sodium was 15 mEq. after the 50 mg. dose and 61 mEq. after 100 mg.

Dichlorphenamide acts as a carbonic anhydrase inhibitor but differs from acetazolamide (Diamox®) in that chloride excretion is increased; therefore metabolic acidosis is less of a problem and activity of the compound is retained even with chronic administration. The effective clinical dose is 50-100 mg. as a single dose; with doses in excess of 200 mg., anorexia, nausea, vomiting, dizziness, ataxia, tremor and tinnitus tend to appear. The potency of dichlorphenamide is about twice that of acetazolamide at its maximal effective dose. An oral dose of 100 mg. dichlorphenamide produces increase in sodium excretion comparable to that from 1 ml. meralluride intramuscularly.

Dichlorphenamide is a useful oral diuretic, but only moderately potent. It is indicated in treating patients with mild heart failure or for prolonging the period between injections of the organomercurials in patients with moderately severe to severe heart failure. This agent remains effective on repeated, chronic administration, and systemic acidosis is not as prone to develop, as with use of other carbonic anhydrase inhibitors. At optimal clinical doses, there are no significant side effects.

► [Perhaps it would be better to say "significant side effects were not seen by us"?—Ed.]

Diuretic Effect of Chlorpromazine in Patients with Congestive Heart Failure varies according to whether the condition is due to cor pulmonale, hypertension or aortic insufficiency, reports A. M. Cohen[4] (Hebrew Univ., Jerusalem). Seven patients without cardiac or renal disease confirmed the reported effect of continuous intravenous infusion of 5% glucose containing 11.9 mg./100 ml. chlorpromazine at a rate of 30 cc./hour. Excretion of sodium, chloride, potassium and water was measured before, during and after infusion. Glomerular filtration rate was determined by creatinine or inulin clearance. Similar studies were carried out in 3 patients with congestive heart failure due to hypertensive cardiovascular disease, in 2 with failure due to aortic insufficiency and in 10 in whom congestive failure was due to chronic cor pulmonale.

Normal subjects showed an increased urinary flow, averaging 4 times the original volume during the third 45 minutes of infusion, without marked change in the rate of excretion of electrolytes or in the glomerular filtration rate. Patients with congestive failure due to hypertension or aortic insufficiency showed no significant diuresis, change in electrolyte excretion or change in filtration rate. In those with cor pulmonale, water excretion was increased approximately sixfold by the end of the infusion period, potassium excretion was constant, but excretion of sodium chloride was doubled. The glomerular filtration rate also increased, accounting for the increased excretion of sodium and chloride in contrast to potassium, which is more closely related to tubular function.

Further Clinical Trials of Oral Diuretics of Aminouracil Group (Mictine®, Rolicton®) Compared with Diuretic Effect of Theophylline are reported by N. I. Nissen and B. Zachau-Christiansen[5] (Copenhagen). Previous studies showed that 800 mg. Mictine (aminometradine) orally on 3 successive days/week effected a total increase in diuresis in cardiac decompensation comparable with that after injection of 1 ml. Thiomerin®. Of 62 patients treated, 15 acquired gastrointestinal symptoms—5 nausea, 4 nausea and vomiting, 5 diarrhea, 2 heartburn and 1 anorexia—and 2 had fatigue. None had albuminuria.

Ten patients with similar degrees of decompensation re-

(4) Am. Heart J. 54:907-914, December, 1957.
(5) Acta med. scandinav. 160:385-395, 1958.

ceived theophylline, 2 tablets 3 times daily, corresponding to 600 mg. theophyllamine, for 3 days. No increase in diuresis occurred in 3, but 5 had results comparable to those which occurred with Mictine. Of 55 others who received 800 mg. daily for 3 days, 6 showed no increased diuresis, but 43 had diureses similar to those from Mictine. Six could not complete therapy, because of gastrointestinal symptoms, and 5 others were inconvenienced by nausea, vomiting or heartburn.

Twelve patients with edema were treated with Rolicton, 1,600 mg. daily for 3 days. The diuretic effect was as potent as with Mictine, but the incidence of side effects was only one-third as great.

Mictine has a significantly greater diuretic effect than theophylline. The maximum effect of Mictine is attained on the 2d day of therapy, similarly to that of theophylline. Rolicton given in twice the dose of Mictine has as much potency, but side effects are much less frequent. Both Mictine and Rolicton presumably inhibit resorption of sodium and chloride in the renal tubules.

► [The agents of this group apparently specifically inhibit, by unknown means, the tubular reabsorption of sodium and chloride without alteration in acid-base regulation; there seems to be no effect on glomerular filtration.

In dosage of 400 mg. 3 times daily for 2 days, Rolicton was found by A. D. Jose and P. Wood (Brit. M. J. 1:9, Jan. 4, 1958) to have 40% of the diuretic potency of 2 ml. mersalyl intramuscularly; the 20 patients had congestive heart failure.—Ed.]

Clinical Experience with Amisometradine (Rolicton®) on Ambulatory Patients is reported by Martin S. Belle[6] (Univ. of Miami). The drug, an aminouracil derivative, was given to 25 ambulatory patients with edema of congestive heart failure originating in various forms of heart disease. Dosage was 800-1,600 mg. daily and the patients were followed 3-9 months from initiation of the study. A definite diuretic response was obtained in all but 1. Satisfactory response was obtained in 23 patients, all of whom were able to discontinue other oral diuretics, some of which were not as well tolerated or as effective as Rolicton. In 17 patients Rolicton replaced other diuretic therapy entirely and in 6 it permitted a decrease in the frequency of mercurial therapy.

Side effects attributable to the drug were minimal. Twenty-

(6) Am. Heart J. 55:114-119, January, 1958.

one patients had no side effects and 3 had nausea on higher dosages but were able to continue therapy on a daily dose of 800 mg.; only 1 patient had to discontinue use of the drug because of nausea or vomiting.

Considering these results, the author feels Rolicton has a definite place in maintenance therapy of mild and moderate congestive heart failure. Being a nonmercurial, nonsulfonamide diuretic, this drug avoids the limitations of those classes of compounds. Its significant reduction of side actions, lack of toxicity and failure to cause resistance permits its continuous use and makes it a preferable oral diuretic. Since it is compatible with other medication, does not cause electrolyte imbalance and appears safe even in the presence of kidney or liver impairment, Rolicton may be used also in severe congestive heart failure as an adjunct to parenteral mercurial therapy.

Sodium and Potassium Dehydrocholate as Diuretic Agents should be considered in the management of edematous states in view of the observations of Alfred Vogl and Miltiades Kaizer[7] (New York). The reported potentiating effect of sodium dehydrocholate (Decholin® sodium) on mercurial diuresis was confirmed in studies on 19 patients with enlargement of the liver and marked peripheral edema. Three also had ascites, 11 arteriosclerotic heart disease, 2 cor pulmonale and 6 Laennec's cirrhosis.

After a control period, 9 were given 2 intramuscular injections of 2 cc. Mercuhydrin® at 3-4 day intervals. A week later the course was repeated, and the mercurial was followed by intravenous injection of 10 cc. of 20% Decholin sodium after 1 hour. The other 10 patients were similarly treated, except that the combined therapy was given first, followed a week later by the mercurial alone. All received a low-salt diet.

In the first group there was a significant increase in diuresis and a corresponding weight loss in 5 patients when the drugs were used in combination in comparison with the control period with the mercurial alone; 3 showed only a fair response and 1 none at all. In the second group the response significantly favored the combination in 6 cases, only slightly so in 3 and not at all in 1.

Injection of Decholin sodium slowly over 5 minutes avoids

(7) Angiology 8:145-155, April, 1957.

the bad taste and nausea accompanying rapid injection. Sodium chloride and potassium excretion were normal despite diuresis. Liver function in the patients with cirrhosis showed little change except that elevated icterus indexes returned to normal after 2 or 3 weeks of treatment. Blood urea also returned to normal in 4 patients with mild nitrogen retention.

Two studies were carried out with Decholin potassium administered intravenously in doses of 5-10 cc. of 20% solution. In the first study, 10 patients, aged 65-85, with inoperable cancer or advanced senility, most of whom had arteriosclerotic heart disease and coronary sclerosis but none of whom were in frank failure, were examined by ECG during and after the injection. No arrhythmias or changes in the T wave or QRS complex were seen in 3 patients receiving a 5-cc. injection. Similar results, except for one extrasystole during injection which was not repeated despite continued administration, were obtained in 7 patients receiving 10 cc.

The second study, identical with that using Decholin sodium, was performed on 12 patients—5 with arteriosclerotic heart disease, 2 hypertensive heart disease, 1 rheumatic heart disease, 1 beriberi heart disease, and 3 Laennec's cirrhosis. Six showed a good response, 1 a fair response and 5 no potentiating effect. Thus potassium dehydrocholate does not appear to offer an advantage over the sodium compound.

Woman, 60, in congestive heart failure for about 2 years, was hospitalized with severe respiratory distress, pulmonary congestion, large bilateral pleural effusion, ascites, greatly enlarged liver and anasarca of the entire body surface. There had been a loss of 20 lb. with considerable relief during the previous week on 2 cc. Thiomerin® every other day, 0.5 Gm. aminophylline intravenously twice a day and 250 mg. Diamox® daily. Nausea prevented continuation of the aminophylline, even when given in suppositories. During 26 days on Thiomerin twice a week and Diamox intermittently, weight remained constant, daily urine was 800-1,200 cc. and there was a 2+ edema of the legs. The liver reached the iliac crest. Thereafter, over a 10-day period she received 2 cc. Thiomerin subcutaneously on the 1st, 4th, 7th and 9th days; 10 cc. Decholin potassium on the 1st and 9th, and 10 cc. Decholin sodium intravenously on the 4th. On days when Decholin was injected, diuresis rose to 1,850-2,100 cc. Weight dropped 6½ lb. during the 10 days, and peripheral edema completely disappeared. The liver was 4 fingerbreadths below the costal margin.

A study was made of oral Decholin combined with Diamox.

The results were somewhat erratic, but it appeared that there was no potentiating effect on diuresis.

Coronary Disease

L-Norepinephrine in Myocardial Infarction should be used with ECG supervision according to T. R. Littler and C. S. McKendrick[8] (Liverpool). Despite the widespread view that the drug is free from central effects on the myocardium, they observed serious arrhythmias in healthy rhesus monkeys and dogs given norepinephrine. A dosage of 0.5 μg./kg. often produced ventricular extrasystoles. As dosage increased, nodal rhythm, auriculoventricular dissociation, multifocal ventricular extrasystoles and paroxysms of ventricular tachycardia were observed. Epinephrine and norepinephrine [Levophed®] were essentially similar in this respect. Despite the tendency of l-norepinephrine to produce arrhythmias, its pressor effect was strikingly superior to that of mephentermine, methoxamine and methylamphetamine.

Results Obtained with l-Norepinephrine

Reference	No. of patients	No. who gave a pressor response	No. of survivors	Comments
Gazes et al. (1953) ..	7	7	6	Arrhythmias observed in 4 cases
Smith and Guz (1953)	6	6	4	No arrhythmias noted
Moyer et al. (1953) .	14	12	6	No arrhythmias noted
Miller et al. (1953) ..	9	8	5	No arrhythmias noted
Kurland and Malach (1952)	14	10	4	No arrhythmias noted
Calenda et al. (1953) ..	13	9	2	No arrhythmias noted
Sampson and Zipser (1954)	30	20	16	Arrhythmia observed in 1 case
Binder et al. (1955) ..	25	23	8	No arrhythmias noted
Present series .. .	22	10	..	Arrhythmias observed in 4 cases

Slow intravenous infusion of 4-64 ml. l-norepinephrine in 540 ml. saline or glucose solution was given 22 patients with myocardial infarction in an attempt to control severe shock. Only 10 showed a pressor response and none lived. Cardiac arrhythmias were observed in 4. The reported experiences of others is shown in the table.

(8) Lancet 2:825-827, Oct. 26, 1957.

The possibility of cardiac arrhythmia from l-norepinephrine should be more widely considered, especially when dealing with myocardial infarction.

► [It is the fact that 1-norepinephrine has a lower tendency than epinephrine to induce arrhythmias which justifies its use in the cardiogenic shock of myocardial infarction, but one must remember that in contradistinction to epinephrine it strikingly increases cerebrovascular resistance and decreases cerebal blood flow despite the incease in mean systemic arterial pressure. The principal damage, therefore, in association with its use is cerebral hemorrhage, which should be avoidable, by proper care in adjustment of dosage. The patient should be under constant surveillance with frequent blood pressure readings.—Ed.]

Use of Pressor Agents in Shock in Myocardial Infarction is outlined by Oliver Garai and K. Shirley Smith[9] (Charing Cross Hosp., London). Hitherto myocardial infarction accompanied by severe shock has carried a mortality of 80%. Of the authors' 25 patients, only 12 died. Early recognition of shock and its prompt treatment may save many patients.

The authors used two pressor agents: l-norepinephrine (Levophed®) mephentermine sulfate (Mephine). The former is the most powerful pressor and general vasoconstrictor agent known. It differs from epinephrine in its effects on the cardiovascular system in some important respects. Unlike epinephrine, l-norepinephrine does not increase the rate or output of the heart. Whereas the total oxygen consumption is raised by 20-30% by epinephrine, it is virtually unaltered by l-norepinephrine. The latter, being an over-all vasoconstrictor, increases both systolic and diastolic pressure. Mephentermine has little or no direct action on the heart muscle and causes no alteration in the heart rate or changes in the ECG. Although the blood pressure rises owing to an increase in peripheral resistance, cardiac output is not significantly altered. Mephentermine is metabolized rapidly, and there is no danger of cumulative action. The intravenous dosage varies from 10 to 30 mg. and intramuscularly up to 70 mg., whereas 15-30 mg. can be given at half-hour intervals if necessary.

Initial treatment of lesser grades of shock should be by intramuscular mephentermine; l-norepinephrine should be used for severe shock and in less severe illness when mephentermine is not effective. Whereas mephentermine is readily administered as emergency treatment when the patient is first seen, l-norepinephrine requires careful attention to its

(9) Brit. M. J. 1:247-251, Feb. 1, 1958.

continuous intravenous administration, thus generally necessitating hospitalization.

For good results, the duration of shock before treatment is started should be less than 2 hours. Shock present for over 5 hours, raised jugular venous pressure, a history of previous infarction and a persistent tachycardia are poor prognostic signs.

Effect of ACTH and Cortisone on Inflammatory Reactions in Myocardial Infarction is negligible, according to Gustaf Myhrman[1] (Örebro, Sweden). Fifteen men received 15 mg. ACTH 3 times a day (in some cases reduced to 10 mg. 3 times daily after about a week) during the 2 weeks immediately after typical myocardial infarction. Injections of 100 mg. cortisone daily, usually reduced to 50 mg. after a week, were given to 10 others. Case records provided controls.

Temperature changes, fasting blood sugar, normochromic anemia, serum iron levels and sedimentation rates showed essentially identical trends in the treated and control groups. Higher white blood cell counts were observed in the treated groups, and the typical drop in cell count was followed in the treated patients by a secondary rise after about a week. Otherwise, the hormone treatment did not seem to modify the volley of inflammatory reactions after myocardial infarction.

► [And if it had? These things are certainly only secondary manifestations of the primary insult, and perhaps it might even be harmful from the standpoint of over-all care to alter them independently of effect on the process which they reflect. Of course the study is of value as a contribution to academic knowledge.—Ed.]

Symmetrical Hemorrhagic Necrosis of Adrenal Glands Complicating Coronary Thrombosis: Case Report with Discussion of Possible Role of Corticotropin and Heparin is presented by Sylvan E. Moolten[2] (New Brunswick, N. J.). Adrenal hemorrhage may cause pain in the abdomen, tenderness and spasm. Pallor, prostration, drop in blood pressure, cyanosis, nausea and vomiting, and finally shock develop. Fever and leukocytosis are common. In acute infections, adrenal cortical damage may occur and, if extensive, may lead to peripheral circulatory collapse. Large doses of corticotropin given to experimental animals has duplicated these lesions.

(1) Acta med. scandinav. 159:239-242, 1957.
(2) J. Mt. Sinai Hosp. New York 24:1042-1046, Nov.-Dec., 1957.

Caution is advised in giving large doses of corticotropin for treating conditions associated with extreme grades of stress. Adrenal apoplexy is probably just a sequel to other severe degenerative changes in the adrenal cortex due to stress.

Man, 52, had typical myocardial infarction proved by ECG. Blood pressure intermittently dropped to as low as 60/50, but responded each time to injections of Wyamine®. Intramuscular heparin was given 50 mg. every 4 hours. Chest pain persisted for 1 week, and the patient complained at times of upper abdominal pain. His face was gray and he sweated profusely, but blood pressure was maintained at 130/100 without vasopressors. Heparin dosage was increased to 75 mg. every 4 hours, but after the second dose, bloody diarrhea developed, the patient's condition worsened and the pressure dropped to 82/60. He was given Wyamine, adrenochrome and a whole-blood transfusion. Heparin was stopped and protamine sulfate (5 cc.) was given intravenously. As an added measure to control hemorrhage, corticotropin was begun on the 11th hospital day, 20 mg. every 12 hours for 3 days, then 15 mg. every 12 hours for 3 days. Heparin was started again. Two days after resuming heparin and while the patient was still receiving corticotropin, abdominal cramps and tenderness recurred in the left costovertebral angle. On the 22d day, he had an embolus from the mural thrombus to the right popliteal artery. Embolectomy was elected, but while general anesthesia was being induced, he suddenly died.

Autopsy revealed pulmonary congestion, pericarditis, a recent myocardial infarction with a mural thrombus, and anemic infarcts due to emboli in the kidneys and spleen. The most striking finding was massive symmetrical, bilateral hemorrhage in the adrenals. The residual cortex was reduced to a thin remnant of necrobiotic tissue with only a narrow layer of viable cells in the extreme outer margin.

This unusual complication of myocardial infarction centers attention on the risk of corticotropin therapy in provoking changes in the adrenal cortex, predisposing to hemorrhage when heparin is given simultaneously.

Nitroglycerin and Other Nitrites in Treatment of Angina Pectoris: Comparison of Six Preparations and Four Routes of Administration was made by Joseph E. F. Riseman, George E. Altman and Sidney Koretsky[3] (Boston) in 34 patients by measuring the amount of work that could be performed under standardized conditions without inducing angina and also by observing the clinical response and the exercise ECG.

Glyceryl trinitrate (nitroglycerin), erythrol tetranitrate, mannitol hexanitrate (Maxitate®; Nitranitol®) and tri-

(3) Circulation 17:22-39, January, 1958.

ethanolamine trinitrate biphosphate (Metamine) were all much more effective sublingually than when swallowed (Fig. 4). Nitroglycerin and erythrol tetranitrate administered sublingually are among the most effective of all prophylactic agents available for treatment of patients with angina pectoris. The comparatively prolonged action of erythrol tetranitrate given sublingually is of clinical value, but the

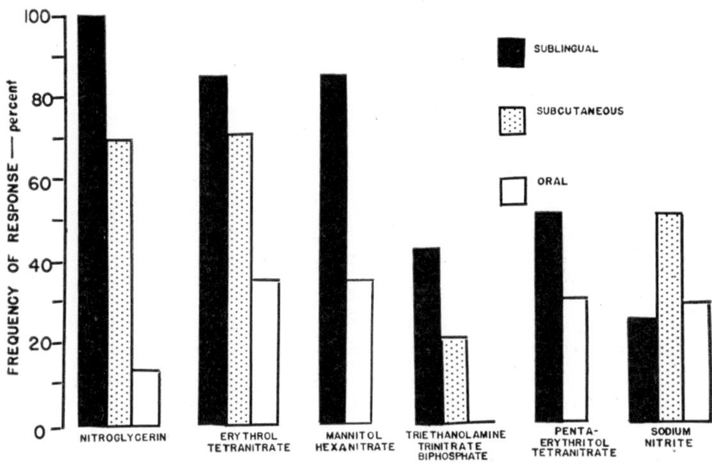

Fig. 4.—Frequency of moderate or marked response to 6 nitrites administered sublingually, subcutaneously and when swallowed among subjects who showed marked response to nitroglycerin administered sublingually. (Courtesy of Riseman, J. E. F., *et al.*: Circulation 17:22-39, January, 1958.)

onset is too slow. Because the solubility of this compound in water is less than that of nitroglycerin, it is unlikely to replace the latter in treating individual attacks.

Nitroglycerin and erythrol tetranitrate were also effective administered parenterally or by inunction, but their value was markedly limited when they were swallowed, suggesting that these nitrites are inactivated in the gastrointestinal tract. Mannitol hexanitrate also was more effective sublingually than when swallowed, but was of limited clinical value because of the large size of the tablets available. Triethanolamine trinitrate was moderately effective administered sublingually, but was of no demonstrable value when swallowed. Sublingual therapy with this drug is limited, because of the frequent glossitis that follows its use.

Pentaerythritol tetranitrate showed little difference in the frequency of response when administered sublingually or when swallowed, but the increase in exercise tolerance was somewhat greater with sublingual administration. This drug was only of moderate value in the treatment of patients with angina pectoris. Sodium nitrite was more effective given subcutaneously than given sublingually or swallowed, but its usefulness was slight and the frequency of untoward reactions too high to indicate clinical value.

► [Tolerance for the vasodilating action of the nitrites, that practically always occurs in time, usually reverts if the drug is omitted for 10-14 days. Alcohol appears to accentuate nitrite action.—Ed.]

Therapeutic Effectiveness of Elixophyllin as Compared with Aminophylline in Severe Angina Pectoris was studied by Alexander Oscharoff[4] (Long Island City, N.Y.), on the basis of the number of attacks per week, severity and nitroglycerin requirement. The study group consisted of 20 men and 10 women selected from 140 patients previously treated with other long-acting coronary vasodilators. These 30 had little or no response to the drugs used. Elixophyllin is a 20% hydroalcoholic solution of theophylline, a tablespoonful of which contains 80 mg. free theophylline and 3 ml. ethyl alcohol and is equivalent to 100 mg. aminophylline.

After a month of study on nitroglycerin alone to establish a base line, the patients were divided into two groups as similar as possible with respect to severity and duration of disease, age, sex and amount of nitroglycerin needed. One group was then given elixophyllin and the other aminophylline in doses equivalent to 80 mg. theophylline 3 times a day for 4 weeks. The two groups were then interchanged for a 2d month. The experiment was repeated twice more with dosages double and triple the original. Seven patients dropped out during this study, leaving 23, of whom 11 showed a satisfactory response to elixophyllin, whereas none responded to aminophylline. No reduction of the number of attacks, severity of pain or nitroglycerin consumption was seen at the 1-tablespoon elixophyllin dosage level, but there was about a one-third reduction in the number of attacks and number of nitroglycerin pills required at the dosage (2 tablespoonfuls) equivalent to 160 mg. theophylline 3 times a day,

(4) New York J. Med. 57:2975-2979, Sept. 15, 1957.

and slightly more reduction at 240 mg. (3 tablespoonfuls). Pain was considered less than average a little more frequently at these levels. At the higher levels some patients receiving aminophylline had nausea with epigastric pain, vomiting and diarrhea.

Studies of the blood level of theophylline in 3 patients responding to elixophyllin were made, with the patients receiving the equivalent of 160-mg. and later 240-mg. doses over 7 days. Blood samples were taken the 7th day, one 14 hours after the previous dose, another ½ hour after the morning dose and a third 2½ hours after the noon dose. The results (table) suggest that the greater efficacy of elixophyllin

MEAN BLOOD THEOPHYLLINE LEVELS FOLLOWING ADMINISTRATION OF ELIXOPHYLLINE AND AMINOPHYLLINE

Drug and doses	Theophylline Equivalent (Mg.)	Micrograms of Theophylline per Ml. of Blood: 1st Specimen	2nd Specimen	3rd Specimen
Elixophyllin 2 tablespoons*	160	3.3	7.4	4.9
Aminophylline 200 mg.*	160	2.4	4.3	4.2
Elixophyllin 3 tablespoons*	240	5.7	6.1	9.6
Aminophylline 300 mg.*	240	3.7	4.4	5.8

*Three times a day

may be attributed to more rapid absorption of the alcoholic solution and perhaps some tranquillizing effect of the alcohol.

► [In a study of theophylline blood levels after oral administration of three different preparations, Joseph Schluger *et al.* (1957-58 YEAR BOOK, p. 15) found patient response differing markedly, but comparison of mean values indicated that theophylline appeared in the blood stream significantly earlier when administered as elixophyllin than as Choledyl® or as aminophylline. Likewise, the blood levels were higher at all times after elixophyllin than after Choledyl.—Ed.]

Modification of Anxiety State Associated with Myocardial Infarction by Meprobamate: Preliminary Notes. Samuel Waldman and Louis Pelner[5] (Brooklyn) used meprobamate in 20 patients with acute myocardial infarction as an adjuvant to other established therapy. When the patient's condition was being affected in some way by the emotional state,

(5) New York J. Med. 58:1285-1288, Apr. 15, 1958.

recovery from an acute episode of coronary thrombosis was favored by inclusion of meprobamate.

Man, 55, was hospitalized with acute coronary insufficiency. He was extremely apprehensive, but barbiturates, in addition to aminophylline and papaverine, failed to quiet him. Four days later, with progression of the anterior infarct, anxiety increased, so that he constantly turned, fidgeted and moved about in bed, and occasional extrasystoles were heard. Twice dyspnea developed, probably due to overbreathing. To allay the patient's anxiety, meprobamate (200 mg. or ½ tablet) was given 3 times a day. Thereafter, he remained tranquil. There was no more dyspnea, and premature auricular beats became rare. Meprobamate did not interfere with the maintenance of therapeutic levels of prothrombin time.

In most patients meprobamate was used only during the acute cardiac episode. After recovery, it was necessary to continue the drug in but 2 patients. All 20 patients manifested anxiety, such as restlessness, irritability, restless sleep or insomnia, palpitation, increased physical tension and a fear of the outcome. Some had palpitation, sighing dyspnea and sticking precordial pains thought to be noncardiac in origin. The anxiety-tension state was definitely ameliorated in all patients in 1-4 days. All survived. The premature contractions diminished markedly in frequency; in 1 patient they disappeared completely.

Reduction in Elevated Blood Cholesterol Levels by Large Doses of Nicotinic Acid: Preliminary Report. William B. Parsons Jr. and John H. Flinn[6] (Jackson Clinic, Madison, Wis.) found that administration of nicotinic acid (niacin) orally in large doses (3-6 Gm. daily) to 24 patients with hypercholesteremia resulted in significant reduction in blood cholesterol levels in 16 (66.7%). Normal levels were attained in 6 of 8 patients followed 30 weeks or longer and in 7 of 16 other patients followed at least 12 weeks.

Doses higher than 3 Gm. nicotinic acid daily were required in more than 50% of patients. Significant reduction in blood cholesterol occurred with doses of 6 Gm. daily in 4 of 5 patients whose levels had remained above normal after smaller doses, suggesting the possibility of future improvement in 7 other patients who thus far have failed to respond to a daily dose of 4.5 Gm. Substitution of nicotinamide in equal dosage after 30 weeks of therapy with nicotinic acid in

(6) J.A.M.A. 165:234-238, Sept. 21, 1957.

8 patients was followed by prompt return of blood cholesterol to pretreatment levels in all.

Figure 5 shows the prompt reduction to normal cholesterol levels in 1 patient on the initial dose of 3 Gm. nicotinic acid daily. When the dose was reduced to 1.5 Gm. daily, the cholesterol levels again rose. Resumption of the original dose

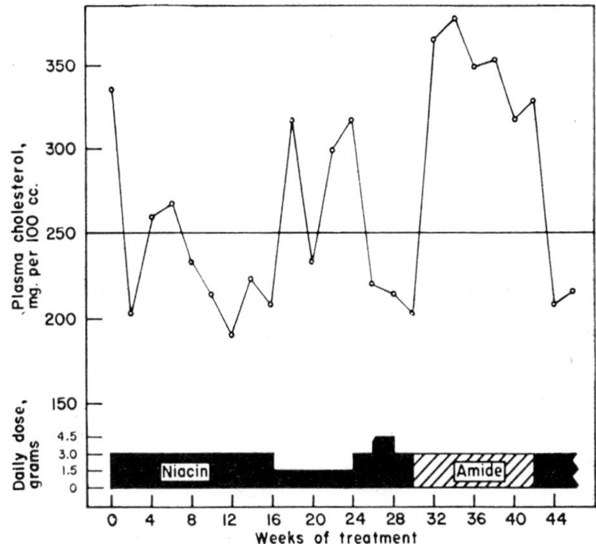

Fig. 5.—Reduction of blood cholesterol by administration of 3 Gm. nicotinic acid (niacin) daily, return to elevated levels during use of 1.5 Gm. nicotinic acid daily, reduction to normal levels when daily dose of 3 Gm. was resumed, return to elevated levels when nicotinamide (niacinamide) was substituted and reduction to normal levels when use of nicotinic acid was again resumed. (Courtesy of Parsons, W. B., Jr., and Flinn, J. H.: J.A.M.A. 165:234-238, Sept. 21, 1957.)

resulted in reduction to normal levels again. When nicotinamide was substituted at the end of 30 weeks, blood cholesterol levels rose to values as high as those observed before treatment. After 12 weeks of administration of nicotinamide, nicotinic acid was again given in the original dose, followed by prompt reduction of blood cholesterol level to normal.

Flushing and pruritus, which occur after ingestion of nicotinic acid, subsided within the 1st week of therapy in nearly all cases. No serious reactions or toxic effects have been observed which could be attributed to nicotinic acid. Nicotinic acid proved effective in lowering cholesterol levels, despite continuation of the patients' customary diets. The mechanism by which nicotinic acid produced the observed changes in blood lipids remains obscure.

Treatment of Hypercholesteremia with Nicotinic Acid was studied by Richard W. P. Achor, Kenneth G. Berge, Nelson W. Barker and Bernard F. McKenzie[7] (Mayo Clinic and Found.) in 33 patients. The drug was given orally in doses of 1.5-6 Gm./day for 3 months to 1½ years.

In most instances large doses of nicotinic acid decrease the concentration of plasma cholesterol, total lipids and serum beta lipoprotein cholesterol. This decrease can be maintained for periods exceeding 1 year, but disappears when treatment is stopped. The degree of response to treatment varies widely but is reasonably reproducible for each person.

A distinct relation between dose and effect was demonstrated for individual patients as well as for those in whom changes in dose were studied. Increasing the daily dose of nicotinic acid resulted in further lowering of concentration of the blood lipids from those values obtained after administration of a lesser dose. This result was reversed when the amount of nicotinic acid was decreased. By using nicotinic acid in doses of 3 Gm./day and by increasing this dose as needed, three fourths or more of patients with hypercholesteremia obtained a satisfactory decrease of their blood lipids.

Patients with higher initial concentrations of cholesterol in the plasma usually respond better to treatment than did those whose values were lower before treatment. As a group, women showed better results than men.

Severe cutaneous flushing and pruritus occurred in nearly all patients when treatment with nicotinic acid was started, but this usually subsided rapidly. Many persons experienced mild flushing subsequently, but this did not constitute an appreciable limitation to therapy. Anorexia and nausea occurred less often than did the cutaneous effects.

Nearly all patients experienced subjective improvement in well-being that seemed unrelated to any objective findings. No increase in severity of angina pectoris was noted by patients with this symptom, and many experienced less angina during treatment.

(7) Circulation 17:497-504, April, 1958.

Hypertension

Evaluation of "Medical" Therapy in Essential Hypertension was undertaken by J. W. Woods, J. D. Dorsett, Jr., K. L. White, H. Smith, Jr., R. Hill and June Watson[8] (Univ. of North Carolina). In an attempt to control some of the so-

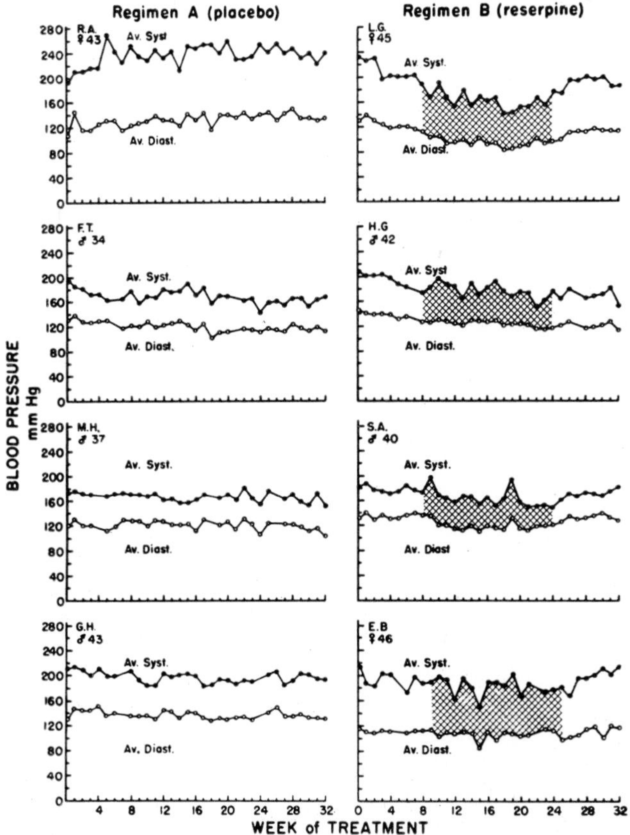

Fig. 6.—Individual blood pressure graphs for patients receiving regimens *A* and *B*. Regimen *A* consisted of placebo only for 32 weeks. Regimen *B* consisted of 8 weeks of placebo, 16 weeks of reserpine (cross-hatched area) and 8 weeks of placebo. First measurements in each graph were taken under standard conditions before starting placebo therapy. Each value plotted is average of 3 recumbent measurements. (Courtesy of Woods, J. W., *et al.*: J. Psychosom. Res. 2:274-284, 1958.)

(8) J. Psychosom. Res. 2:274-284, 1958.

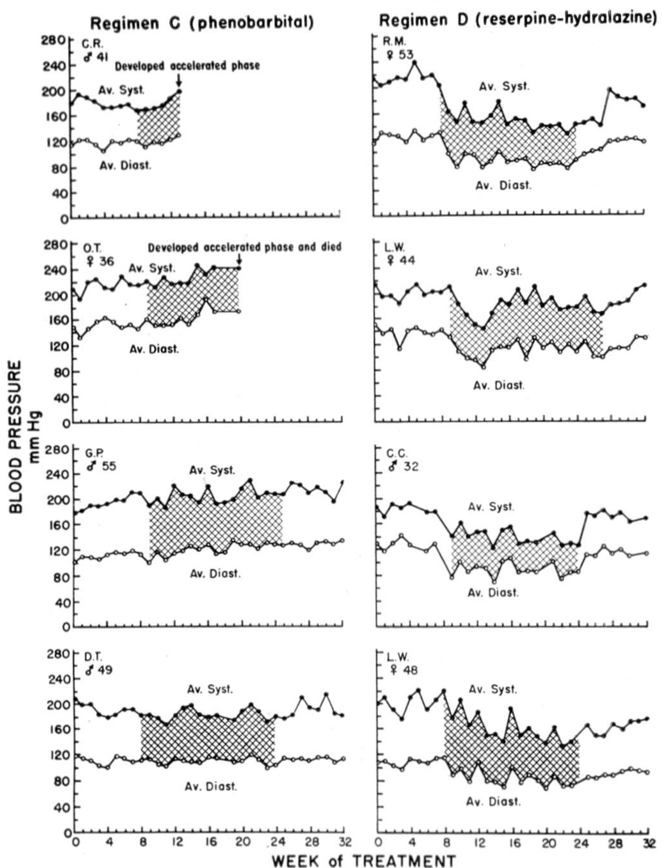

Fig. 7.—Graphs for patients receiving regimen *C* (8 weeks of placebo, 16 weeks of phenobarbital, 8 weeks of placebo) and regimen *D* (8 weeks of placebo, 16 weeks of reserpine-hydralazine combination, 8 weeks of placebo) (Courtesy of Woods, J. W., *et al.*: J. Psychosom. Res. 2:274-284, 1958.)

cial and emotional factors known to influence blood pressure, the following study plan was used: meticulous selection of patients with moderately severe, unequivocal essential hypertension; weekly clinic visits; "social stress" index based on questionnaires and interview data obtained by sociologists; double-blind technic for treatment regimens insofar as physician, nurse and patients were concerned; double-blind technic as to knowledge of the blood pressure readings insofar as the physician and patients were concerned; and random assignments to treatment regimens by a biostatistician.

Of four regimens (placebo, phenobarbital, reserpine and reserpine combined with hydralazine), evaluated within 32 weeks and including two 8-week placebo periods before and after 16 weeks of treatment, only one (reserpine combined with hydralazine) had significant hypotensive properties (Figs. 6 and 7).

To be an effective hypotensive agent, a drug should be capable of lowering blood pressure in properly selected patients to levels well below those occurring during two control periods in the face of over-all upward trends in the blood pressure and despite negative patient-physician relationships, fundamental deleterious emotional conflicts and high degrees of social stress. In a controlled clinical evaluation of pharmacologic agents, many variables may be partially controlled, but the subtleties of the patients' life situations, the intensities of the transference and counter-transference between physicians, nurses and patients, and the degrees of realistic and unrealistic anxiety by the investigators are factors which cannot be controlled by present technics. All these influences, especially the elements of human variability, combined with the specific and nonspecific side effects of the drugs used, impose serious limitations on the double-blind technic.

Long-Term Combined Drug Therapy in Nonmalignant Hypertension. In hypertensive disease, the final proof of improvement is a decided decrease in the mortality, but patients survive untreated for so long that this criterion is not applicable until after 5-10 years of treatment. In severe hypertensive disease or in the malignant phase, the organic complications progress and ultimately decide the prognosis. Regressive changes in these complications can be used as a guide.

H. Stürup and Alice Grüner[9] (Copenhagen) treated 51 patients for 6-30 months with combinations of reserpine (Serpasil®), hydralazine (Apresoline®) and pentapyrrolidinium (Ansolysen®) designed to bring the blood pressure as near to normal as possible. All had about the same degree

(9) Acta med. scandinav. 160:251-260, 1958.

of hypertension. None had choked disks. Pretreatment diastolic pressure in each averaged at least 110 mm. Hg, and objective changes had occurred in the heart, eyes, kidney, brain or some combination of these organs. All were controlled for some time before treatment was started. Serpasil was started alone, 1-2 mg. daily. If after 1-3 months the response was unsatisfactory, Apresoline was added and the dose slowly increased to 400 mg. daily. If necessary, Ansolysen was added in the required and tolerated doses. Blood pressures were measured with the patient sitting down after a short rest. These measurements were made in the same room, at the same time of day, by the authors. In Ansolysen-treated patients, pressures were also measured in the erect position about 2-4 hours after the last dose.

A sustained, unequivocal and satisfactory drop in blood pressure occurred in 26 patients. This was obtained with Serpasil alone in 10, with Serpasil plus Apresoline in 7 and with combinations including Ansolysen in 9. The average decline in mean blood pressure was 35 mm. Hg, corresponding to a drop from 220/127 to 175/97. In the other 25 patients, the response was unsatisfactory; the mean blood pressure fell only 17 mm. Hg, or from 219/129 to 202/112.

Heart size changed in only a few patients, but the change was only minor. After the blood pressure responded to treatment, t wave alterations in the ECG became upright in 6 of the 9 patients in whom the waves had been inverted. In 14 patients who did not respond to therapy, the t waves remained inverted. Retinal hemorrhages and exudates disappeared in 13 of 14 patients in both response groups together, regardless of the blood pressure response. The number of patients with albuminuria was reduced from 11 to 2 in the satisfactory response group and from 10 to 8 in the unsatisfactory group.

Antihypertensive treatment is indicated in most or all patients with diastolic hypertension associated with organic changes. Blood pressure should preferably be brought as near normal as practicable in such cases.

Drug Therapy in Primary Hypertension in Relation to Severity of the Disease. Milton Mendlowitz, Albert D. Parets, Theodore Gold and Stanley R. Drachman[1] (Mt. Sinai Hosp., New York) evaluated response to therapy in 116 patients observed over a mean of 9.3 months. The patients were divided into three groups according to severity of disease: a mild group with persistent hypertension but no organic involvement; a severe group with greater hypertension and involvement of two or more organs, such as the kidney, heart or brain, and with grade 2-4 retinopathy; and a moderate group, between mild and severe. Response to therapy was considered good if pressure dropped substantially to normal or near normal with regression of organic involvement if present. Response was poor if changes were absent or only equivocal. Intermediate responses were considered fair.

A good response was observed in 42% of the patients; the other 58% showed only a fair to poor response. The effect was better in the initial or mild stages than in the moderate or severe stages, hence early treatment is advocated.

The various rauwolfia preparations were similar in effect, provided equivalent doses were used. The usual side effects of diarrhea, nasal stuffiness and drowsiness were encountered. The most serious side action, requiring stoppage of the drug, was psychic depression. The veratrum drugs were used sparingly and seemed to add little to the effect obtained by the rauwolfia agents. Tolerance developed frequently. Anorexia, nausea and vomiting were often problems as dose was increased. Hydralazine was chiefly valuable in advanced cases. The daily dose was limited to 300 mg., and no lupus-like reaction was noted. Other side actions such as angina, tachycardia, skin eruption, dyspnea, edema, diarrhea, nausea and vomiting occasionally necessitated cessation of therapy.

The ganglion-blocking drugs all had similar actions. Pentolinium seemed more readily absorbed from the intestinal tract than hexamethonium. The most important side action was collapse, in part due to postural hypotension. Most annoying was constipation, combated in part by pilocarpine and neostigmine cathartics and enemas. Blurred vision, dry mouth, impotence and bladder dysfunction also occurred. Tolerance to all preparations developed within several weeks; dosage was increased to maintain the desired effect.

(1) J. Chron. Dis. 7:484-492, June, 1958.

Antihypertensive Therapy for the Elderly Patient. In the malignant phase of hypertension antihypertensive therapy relieves serious signs and symptoms and prolongs life. In the nonaccelerated form of hypertension, improved prognosis has not been definitely proved, but accumulating evidence indicates the desirability of antihypertensive therapy for patients with sustained and greatly elevated diastolic blood pressure. John R. Beem and John H. Moyer[2] (Hahnemann Med. College) studied 443 patients, of whom 346 were under and 97 above age 60.

The mean arterial blood pressure was reduced 20 mm. Hg or more in 41% of the elderly group by rauwolfia alone and in 90% of those treated with rauwolfia and mecamylamine. Blood pressure became less than 150/100 mm. Hg in one fourth to one half of these patients. From one-third to one-half showed improvement in headache, angina pectoris, congestive failure, reduced pulse rate and smaller hearts. They felt well. Eyegrounds, renal function and ECG's were rarely improved, perhaps because their defects were due to advanced arteriosclerosis.

Side effects were similar to those previously reported. Nasal congestion tended to be slightly more pronounced. Palpitation, headache and angina pectoris were somewhat more frequent during hydralazine therapy. Weakness and dizziness accompanying rauwolfia and a ganglion-blocking agent were slightly more common. Nevertheless, antihypertensive therapy proved as safe in patients above 60 as in younger ones.

Large individual differences exist in reactivity and tolerance to the available drugs. A drug regimen must be designed for each patient. Therapy is initiated with the less rigorous drugs and other agents added if needed. If the diastolic pressure is less than 100 mm. Hg, no therapy is given. If it is 100-120 mm. Hg, initial therapy is with chlorothiazide, with rauwolfia or rauwolfia plus hydralazine as adjunctive therapy. If diastolic pressure is above 120 mm. Hg, initial therapy is with chlorothiazide plus rauwolfia, with hydralazine or ganglion-blocking agents as adjunctive therapy. Potent antihypertensive drugs are usually not given to patients who

(2) Geriatrics 13:378-390, June, 1958.

have severe nitrogen retention (blood urea nitrogen above 60 mg./100 ml.) after recent myocardial infarction or recent cerebrovascular accident, unless it is urgent that blood pressure be reduced.

Chlorothiazide alone is mildly antihypertensive in some patients. It markedly augments other agents. It increases excretion of sodium, chloride and water and obviates the need for a rigidly restricted sodium diet. This is particularly valuable in elderly patients who tend to eat poorly and who find a low-salt diet most unpalatable. It is given first alone, 0.5 Gm. twice daily. In some, after a few days or weeks, rauwolfia and sometimes other drugs are added if needed. Patients treated with ganglion blockade or sympathectomy are highly responsive to chlorothiazide, and the initial dose should be 0.125-0.25 Gm. once or twice daily, cautiously increased by increments of 0.125-0.25 Gm. at intervals of 3-7 days. With chlorothiazide as basic therapy, it is seldom necessary to exceed daily maximums of 0.25 mg. reserpine, 100 mg. rauwolfia root, 300 mg. hydralazine or 15-20 mg. mecamylamine.

Effect of Treatment on Vascular Deterioration Associated with Hypertension, with Particular Emphasis on Renal Function. John H. Moyer, Charles Heider (Hahnemann Med. College), Keith Pevey and Ralph V. Ford[3] (Baylor Univ.) studied renal clearance in 133 patients with hypertensive vascular disease, 116 of whom were followed for 2-5 years. In 64 of these patients serial renal function studies were made; 45 of the 64 patients were treated and 19 were untreated.

Comparison of treated and untreated patients showed that effective reduction in blood pressure arrested the renal vascular deterioration in patients with severe and moderately severe hypertension. Untreated patients with mild and moderately severe hypertension did not show the rapid renal deterioration that occurs in patients with more marked elevation of blood pressure.

Mortality was significantly lower in treated than in untreated patients. Of the patients who died, 75% were untreated. In none of the treated patients was uremia the sole

(3) Am. J. Med. 24:177-192, February, 1958.

cause of death, whereas 15 untreated patients died of uremia. Five of the 9 treated patients who died of cerebrovascular accidents had had effective treatment and control of blood pressure but voluntarily discontinued treatment. All 5 died in less than 3 months after discontinuing medication. These results emphasize not only the value of antihypertensive therapy but also the importance of maintaining treatment.

TABLE 1.—COMPARISON OF FOLLOW-UP RENAL STATUS IN 21 TREATED AND UNTREATED PATIENTS WITH MALIGNANT HYPERTENSION

Data	Treated		Untreated	
	No.	%	No.	%
Patients	12	57	9	43
Mortality	2	17	9	100
Survival time or follow-up period if living	29 mo.	...	12 mo.	...
Average	C	D_1	C	D_1
Blood urea nitrogen (mg. %)	31	27	29	106
Glomerular filtration rate (cc./min.)	66	68	70	44
Renal blood flow (cc./min.)	513	579	628	351
Mean blood pressure (mm. Hg)	175	122	184	197
Duration ($C - D_1$)	28 mo.	...	10 mo.	...
Improved (%)	...	...	...	...
Urinalysis	36	...	0	...
Electrocardiogram	54	...	0	...
X-ray	54	...	0	...

NOTE: C indicates control period; D_1 follow-up period.

Comparison of the renal status of 12 treated and 9 untreated patients with malignant hypertension is presented in Table 1. Only 2 of the 12 treated patients died; average follow-up for the entire group was 29 months. All 9 untreated patients died; average survival time was 12 months. The status of renal function in the 12 treated patients did not change during an average follow-up of 28 months, although the mean blood pressure was effectively reduced from 175 to 122 mm. Hg. In contrast, renal function in the 9 untreated patients was reduced to approximately 60% of control values during only 10 months. The mean blood pressure in the untreated group increased from 184 to 197 mm. Hg. The clinical status and results of therapy in 31 patients with malignant hypertension, including the 21 in Table 1, are given in Table 2.

Five patients with hypertension due to unilateral renal artery occlusion were studied. Glomerular filtration rate and renal blood flow were reduced significantly in the contralateral kidney as a result of the severe hypertension. This vascular deterioration in the unoccluded kidney was arrested and became partly reversible when the blood pressure was reduced effectively.

TABLE 2.—FOLLOW-UP IN 31 PATIENTS WITH MALIGNANT HYPERTENSION

Cause of Death	Treated Patients*	Untreated Patients†
No. of patients observed.......	13	18
Cerebrovascular accident......	1	3
Cerebrovascular accident + uremia.................	1	1
Uremia...................	0	11
Cardiac..................	0	2
Average survival time (mo.) or follow-up period if living..	30	14

*Thirteen patients treated; 11 living, 2 dead.
†Eighteen patients untreated; 1 living, 17 dead.

These results indicate that renal deterioration can be arrested by effective treatment of hypertension and thereby the lives of hypertensive patients can be prolonged. It is recommended, therefore, that hypertensive vascular disease be treated early and vigorously in the hope that morbidity and mortality can be reduced.

New Drugs for Hypertension, with Special Reference to Chlorothiazide, are discussed by Robert W. Wilkins[4] (Boston Univ.). There is a difference in the so-called emetic-hypotensive ratio of the pure veratrum alkaloids (protoveratrine A and protoveratrine B), but for clinical purposes it can be said that the hypotensive dose of all available veratrum preparations is uncomfortably close to the nauseating dose. Clinically, there are no important differences among the various well-standardized preparations of veratrum,

(4) New England J. Med. 257:1026-1030, Nov. 21, 1957.

whether they are extracts, alkaloidal mixtures or pure substances. The starting doses of the commonly used preparations are: Veriloid®, 2 mg., Vergitryl®, 1 unit, Provell®, 0.25 mg., Veralba®, 0.25 mg., and Protalba, 0.1 mg., given at least 4 hours apart, 3 or 4 times a day. These doses should be increased gradually until either the desired hypotension or nausea is produced.

Standardized preparations of the crude root of Rauwolfia serpentina, or alkaloidal extracts of this root, are as useful clinically in hypertension as the pure alkaloids or their analogues. Of the pure alkaloids, reserpine is the most effective. Daily oral doses of reserpine over 1 mg. are not more effective for chronic antihypertensive treatment than doses up to 1 mg., although increasing the dose up to 1 mg. a day may increase the hypotensive effect of this drug. Two or 3 months of continuous treatment may be necessary in certain patients to arrive at the full hypotensive effect of 1 mg. reserpine orally a day; after this time the dose usually should be decreased to prevent mental depression without loss of the hypotensive effect. The suggested starting doses for rauwolfia preparations are: Raudixin®, 50 mg., Rauwiloid®, 2 mg., and reserpine, rescinnamine or deserpidine, 0.1 mg. 1-4 times a day. These may be increased gradually to 100 mg., 4 mg. or 0.25 mg., respectively, 4 or 5 times a day. However, after 1-3 months dosages should be reduced to the minimal effective hypotensive dose to prevent mental depression, nightmares or insomnia.

Hydralazine remains the sole clinically useful representative of the direct renal vasodilators. If used with rauwolfia or reserpine and in low, gradually increasing doses, hydralazine is usually well tolerated. It is also frequently used in combination with various ganglion-blocking agents. The starting dose of hydralazine (Apresoline®) is 10 mg. 4 times a day, increased gradually as necessary to 50 or 100 mg. 4 times a day. On this regimen the late lupus-like "hydralazine syndrome" has rarely been encountered.

The various ganglion-blocking agents cause troublesome side effects in many patients, such as faulty accommodation of the eye, dry mouth and throat, sluggish intestinal motility, incomplete emptying of the bladder, sexual impotence and particularly orthostatic arterial hypotension. Wilkins suggests reserving these drugs for only the most urgent and resistant phases of malignant hypertension. Starting doses are hexamethonium (Bistrium®), 62.5 mg., pentolinium (Ansolysen®), 20 mg., chlorisondamine (Ecolid®), 10 mg., and mecamylamine (Inversine®), 2.5 mg., 2-4 times a day. The individual successive doses of each drug should be carefully increased by no more than the amount of the initial dose until the desired effect on blood pressure (taken in the upright position) is obtained. Since blood pressure is more responsive to blocking agents after sleep, the first dose on awakening usually should be smaller than subsequent doses.

It has been observed that reserpine markedly depletes the body of its natural stores of serotonin. Furthermore, its action as a tranquilizing or sedative agent in animals was found to be related directly to its depleting the brain of serotonins and not to its own presence (or absence) in the brain. Various synthetic analogues of serotonin, particularly the benzyl analogue of serotonin (BAS), have been found to have antiserotonin activity. Of various preparations tried, only BAS was suitable for long-term oral use in hypertensive patients. The starting dose of BAS is 12.5 mg. 1-4 times a day, average dose 25 mg. 4 times a day and maximum dose 50 mg. 4 times a day. Higher doses usually cause intolerable sedation.

A new oral diuretic, chlorothiazide (Diuril®), was found to have hypotensive properties. It is more effective as a hypotensive agent when given with other drugs than it is alone. However, some of the less desirable hypotensive agents can be reduced or even omitted when chlorothiazide is used as an adjunct.

Chlorothiazide alone had a definite hypotensive effect in 9 of 17 hypertensive patients. Reductions in blood pressure ranged from 20 systolic 10 diastolic to 60 systolic 30 diastolic (average, 21 systolic 12 diastolic). Chlorothiazide added to other antihypertensive drugs reduced the blood pressure in 19 of 23 patients, with reductions ranging from 20 systolic 10 diastolic to 60 systolic 30 diastolic (averaged, 32 systolic 21 diastolic). Most patients who responded to chlorothiazide were not in congestive heart failure, did not lose weight and were taking a regular salt diet. However, restriction of salt appeared to increase markedly the antihypertensive effect of chlorothiazide in some patients. On the other hand, chlorothiazide added to a regimen of other antihypertensive agents was more hypotensive than simple salt restriction added to the same regimen.

The starting hypotensive dose of chlorothiazide is 125 mg., average dose 250 mg. and maximum dose 500 mg. 3 times a day. The drug has few side effects but in larger doses can cause weakness, dizziness or lassitude and in large single doses can produce gastric irritation associated with epigastric and substernal burning. Occasionally, it lowers serum potassium and rarely, serum sodium content.

► [Elsewhere, Wilkins (J.A.M.A. 167:803, June 14, 1958) has stated that a lowering of the serum potassium level occurs in about 40% of patients taking chlorothiazide continuously without supplementary potassium for more than a week and that in about half these patients the level will fall below the 3.5 mEq. L. lower limit of normal. This may be corrected in time by the body itself, but restriction of dietary sodium lessens the likelihood of this, presumably because potassium is excreted more actively if sodium is not freely available. Therefore, patients on a low-sodium diet should relax it when chlorothiazide is started. In a new patient with coronary disease, or one who is taking digitalis, Wilkins begins chlorothiazide therapy very cautiously and gives supplementary potassium as indicated by weekly determinations of the potassium level as well as by clinical and ECG assessments of myocardial irritability and digitalis intoxication.—Ed.]

Treatment of Essential Hypertension with Chlorothiazide (Diuril®): Its Use Alone and Combined with Other Antihypertensive Agents is described by Edward D. Freis, Annemarie Wanko, Ilse M. Wilson and Alvin E. Parrish[5] (Georgetown Univ.). Pharmacologic studies in animals and man have shown marked increase in urinary excretion of sodium, potassium and chloride after oral administration of chlorothiazide. Ten patients, previously untreated, were hospitalized, placed on a diet containing 1.25 Gm. salt daily and 3 Gm. sodium chloride in tablets. After the blood pressure had stabilized, they were given orally 0.5 Gm. chlorothiazide 3 times daily for 6 days. The blood pressure fell in each patient, the systolic an average of 18.7% and the diastolic, 13.9%. When chlorothiazide was withdrawn in 5 patients, the pressure gradually returned to pretreatment levels.

Chlorothiazide, 0.5 Gm. twice daily, was added to the regi-

(5) J.A.M.A. 166:137-140, Jan. 11, 1958.

men of 73 patients with hypertension; 33 were being treated with ganglionic-blocking agents with or without reserpine and/or hydralazine, 19 were receiving veratrum alkaloids with or without other medication and 21 were taking reserpine alone or combined with hydralazine. In each patient, the blood pressure fell further. In 32 of the 73, all antihypertensive medications except chlorothiazide were withdrawn and the patients were maintained on chlorothiazide alone. In 10 of these, the blood pressure level over 1½ months did not rise, but in 22, it rose 10% or more in the diastolic. In 6 of the 22, the elevation approached pretreatment or control levels. Five patients who had lumbodorsal splanchnicectomy 6 months to 3 years earlier responded to chlorothiazide alone with significant additional reductions of blood pressure, averaging —21%. Fifteen hospitalized normotensive patients under the same controlled salt intake regimen showed no change in blood pressure when chlorothiazide was given. No other antihypertensive agent has shown such specificity for hypertension.

Most patients noted diuresis the first 1-2 days after chlorothiazide treatment. Six complained of nausea and 4 of weakness during the 1st month of treatment, but stopping the drug for 1 day promptly cleared these symptoms. Chlorothiazide exaggerated postural hypotension when it was present but did not produce it. To prevent postural collapse, the dose of ganglionic-blocking agents had to be reduced when chlorothiazide was begun. No sign of electrolyte depletion was observed, but injudicious elevation of doses or continued administration of the drug in combination with diets severely restricted in sodium or when significant extrarenal salt loss occurs might lead to severe electrolyte imbalance.

Enhanced Effectiveness of Ganglion-Blocking Agents in Hypertensive Patients during Administration of Saluretic Agent (Chlorothiazide). Fernando A. Tapia, Harriet P. Dustan, R. A. Schneckloth, A. C. Corcoran and Irvine H. Page[6] (Cleveland Clinic) made observations on 9 patients with severe hypertension under treatment with ganglion-blocking drugs (3 on mecamylamine, 1 on pentolinium tartrate and 5 on chlorisondamine chloride). After a control

(6) Lancet 2:831-833, Oct. 26, 1957.

period, chlorothiazide was given in doses of 2 Gm. daily (1 Gm./day in patients weighing less than 100 lb.) for 3 days. Then during a 4-day recovery period, sodium chloride was given by mouth in amounts equivalent to from one-half to the total sodium output during the diuretic period.

In all 9 patients chlorothiazide caused diuresis with excess excretion of sodium, chloride and potassium. Increments of sodium and chloride output were proportionally greater than that of potassium. Losses of body weight and decreases in plasma volume with hemoconcentration also occurred. These changes were associated with sharp decreases in ganglion-blocker requirements and reductions in systolic and diastolic pressure averages, lying and, to a greater degree, standing. All these changes were consistently greater in patients who had maintained sodium restriction before and during administration of the diuretic than in those on unrestricted sodium intake. Blood pressure, body weight, plasma volume and drug requirement tended to return to control levels after sodium repletion. No significant changes were observed in plasma electrolyte concentrations, which varied only slightly and within normal limits.

Observations were continued 1-5 months after the patients left the hospital. Weekly courses of chlorothiazide led to similar responses in blood pressure, body weight and ganglion-blocking requirement, though weight loss was usually not as great as it had been during hospitalization.

These observations must be extended to establish the possible therapeutic value of the regimen. Seven patients who were under observation during the 1-5 months showed progressive decreases in ganglion-blocking requirements and better control of hypertension than formerly. Symptoms of parasympathetic blockade (constipation, dryness of the mouth, blurring of vision) were abated or eliminated. Most patients reported improvement in general well-being and capacity for work. There was no evidence of intolerance, toxic effects or irresponsiveness to chlorothiazide.

Though other mechanisms such as depletion of sodium from ganglions or vessel walls may enter into the antihypertensive effect of intermittent courses of chlorothiazide, the authors believe the effect is primarily hemodynamic. Presumably decreased plasma volume decreases venous return and lowers blood pressure, particularly when the patient is standing.

Effect of Rauwolfia Serpentina and Reserpine on Blood Pressure in Essential Hypertension: Long-Term Double-Blind Study (2-year) of 18 ambulatory patients treated with these drugs is presented by Murray B. Sheldon and J. Harold Kotte[7] (Univ. of Cincinnati). A statistical study, using analysis of variance, revealed a significant depressor effect by Rauwolfia serpentina and its derivatives over placebo on the systolic pressure in 7 of 18 patients and on the diastolic pressure in 10 of 18 patients. A significant placebo effect on the systolic and diastolic pressures occurred in 2 and 4 of the 18 patients, respectively. Statistically significant responses were in the range of 9-21 mm. Hg systolic and 7-15 mm. Hg diastolic. Therefore, they were not necessarily significant clinically. In no case was there any serious reaction during therapy. The dose of Rauwolfia serpentina used was 50 mg. 4 times daily; the dose of reserpine, 0.2-0.25 mg. 4 times daily.

► [This is the kind of article that really tells us something about a drug —a protracted, double-blind study of a small number of intensively observed cases. Unfortunately, many drugs do not lend themselves easily to such studies because something in their action or toxicity betrays their use and confounds the double-blind approach. The necessity to individualize dosage is often a handicap also. Nevertheless, this sort of experiment is the thing to strive for.—Ed.]

Rauwolfia Toxicity in Treatment of Hypertension: Comparative Toxicity of Reserpine and Alseroxylon. Ralph V. Ford (Baylor Univ.) and John H. Moyer[8] (Hahnemann Med. College) found on analysis of the clinical records of 120 patients receiving reserpine [Serpasil®] and of 332 receiving alseroxylon [Rauwiloid®] for hypertension that there were significantly more frequent and severe reactions to reserpine. Of the patients receiving reserpine, 43% noted a mild to moderate sedative effect, 27% for more than 3 months. A sense of well-being was observed in 11%, which persisted for more than 3 months in only 8%. Of the patients receiving alseroxylon, 81% exhibited a moderate sedative effect, 41% for more than 3 months. A sense of well-being

(7) Circulation 16:200-206, August, 1957.
(8) Postgrad. Med. 23:41-48, January, 1958.

was noted by 85%; 75% experienced this effect for more than 3 months.

Of the patients receiving reserpine, 86% had weakness and fatigue, 73% malaise and 52% dizziness. In most patients these symptoms persisted for more than 3 months. Moderate reactions were less frequent. Nightmares occurred in 53% and frequent insomnia in 51%; both symptoms persisted as long as the drug was taken. Severe reactions were noted in a smaller group. Agitation was observed in 31% and persisted for more than 3 months in 26%. Depression occurred in 15% and lasted more than 3 months in 10%. Serious agitated depression was observed in 15%; 10% experienced this reaction for more than 3 months.

The incidence of weakness and fatigue among the patients receiving alseroxylon for hypertension was 84%. Malaise was noted in 65% and dizziness in 29%. About one fifth of the group had these symptoms for more than 3 months. Moderate reactions consisted of nightmares in 18% and insomnia in 7%, continuing in most instances throughout therapy (average 2.1 years). Severe reactions were less frequent with alseroxylon than with reserpine. Thirteen patients (4%) had agitation, and in 9 it persisted for more than 3 months. Five patients (2%) had a severe depressive reaction, in 2 lasting more than 3 months. A disabling agitated depression occurred in 3 patients (0.9%) and lasted more than 3 months in 2.

Predisposing factors to adverse reactions due to reserpine include previous neuropsychiatric diagnoses and a daily dosage of 1 mg. reserpine or more, but the severity of the hypertensive disease apparently did not influence the toxicity.

A useful procedure in the initial treatment of hypertension is to start with reserpine, giving 0.25 mg. twice daily concurrently with alseroxylon, 2 mg. 4 times daily. The response to reserpine begins in 3-5 days, whereas the maximal response to alseroxylon is not obtained for 14-21 days. After 2 or 3 weeks reserpine may be discontinued, since the alseroxylon effect has become established, and the dose of the latter may be reduced to 2 mg. twice daily. Ancillary antihypertensive therapy may be added as indicated.

Mecamylamine: Ganglion-Blocking Drug for Treating Hypertension. Arthur Kitchin, Clifton P. Lowther and Richard W. D. Turner[9] (Edinburgh) report that in 14 of 20 patients treated with mecamylamine [Inversine®] the results were good in that the standing diastolic pressure was reduced to normal or nearly normal levels. In 6 patients the pressure was considerably lowered, but remained well above normal, and hence the results were considered fairly good. The dose of mecamylamine required for stabilization was 30-120 mg. (average 60 mg.) daily. Patients were followed for periods up to 18 months.

Reasons for failure to achieve a good result included resistance to mecamylamine and intolerance of parasympathetic side effects or occasionally secondary effects from hypertension. An appreciable degree of tolerance developed initially in many of the patients, but persisted in only a few. Side effects were troublesome in most cases, particularly impairment of accommodation, dryness of the mouth and constipation. In some patients diarrhea was severe but did not persist.

In 9 of 13 cases a combination of mecamylamine with Serpasil® (0.5-1 mg. daily) or Rauwiloid® (4-8 mg. daily) produced better results than mecamylamine alone. Either a smaller dose of the latter drug was needed or a lower level of blood pressure was reached.

The authors conclude that though mecamylamine is probably the best of the ganglion-blocking drugs presently available, it is not ideal.

Effective Combination in Treatment of Hypertensive Patient. Harvey E. Nussbaum, William A. Leff, Virginius D. Mattia, Jr., and Ernest Hillman[1] (St. Barnabas Med. Center, Newark, N. J.) report that of 37 patients treated with a combination of mecamylamine [Inversine®] and meprobamate [Miltown®] for 6 months, 35 showed good response. A reduction in the mean blood pressure of 20 mm. Hg or more or a return to normotensive levels was the criterion for response. During 18 months of therapy with mecamylamine alone, 28 of 37 patients treated showed a response that was significant.

Meprobamate alone had no effect on the blood pressure of the same group. Though significant further reduction in

(9) Lancet 2:605-609, Sept. 28, 1957.
(1) Am. J. M. Sc. 234:150-154, August, 1957.

blood pressure did not occur with meprobamate, management of the patients was aided considerably. A general sense of well-being, loss of many mild, chronic symptoms and loss of apprehension were all evident in most patients. Most patients required at least 10 mg. mecamylamine/day, others up to 90 mg./day. The meprobamate dosage was 400 mg. 4 times a day.

Meprobamate has distinct advantages over phenobarbital and reserpine for adjunctive therapy, since it has none of the habituating liabilities of phenobarbital and is free from the threat of severe mental depression, water retention and nasal stuffiness present with reserpine.

Mecamylamine (Inversine®) in Treatment of Hypertension. John Moyer, Charles Heider and Edward Dennis[2] (Baylor Univ.) tested the effectiveness of combining reserpine with mecamylamine in treating hypertension in 75 patients, all of whom had sustained blood pressure levels above 150/100 mm. Hg before treatment. A comparison was made between one group of 17 patients receiving mecamylamine alone and another group of 58 receiving mecamylamine with reserpine.

Reserpine was given as 1 mg. daily by mouth in 4 equally divided doses. The optimal dosage of macamylamine was determined by a set dose titration procedure for each patient, beginning with 2.5 mg. twice a day; the average dose of mecamylamine for those patients who did respond to the drug alone during prolonged treatment was 34 mg. daily. There were some patients who did not respond satisfactorily to double this dose. The data include the average of all blood pressure levels and pulse rates obtained weekly or biweekly for 3 months about 1 year after therapy with mecamylamine was begun.

A patient was described as responding to treatment if it brought about a fall of 20 mm. Hg or more in the mean blood pressure or a reduction to the normotensive level, taken as below 150/100 mm. Hg. The over-all response rate for the group receiving mecamylamine alone was 57%; the corresponding figure for the group receiving the combination of drugs was 92%.

Comparison of results with mecamylamine, hexamethoni-

(2) J.A.M.A. 164:1879-1886, Aug. 24, 1957.

um, chlorisondamine (Ecolid®) chloride and pentolinium (Ansolysen®) tartrate indicates that mecamylamine is a much more potent ganglion-blocking agent than the other drugs. Also, the response is less variable due to the complete absorption of this agent. Side effects are primarily those of ganglion blockade, which are present to a lesser degree with mecamylamine than with the other blocking agents and are decreased when mecamylamine is used in combination with reserpine.

Clinical Study of Hydergine in Essential Hypertension was carried out by R. P. Malhotra and S. P. Gupta[3] (Amritsar Med. College). Hydergine, a combination of three hydrogenated ergot alkaloids, has been reported to exert a purely sympatholytic action. Observations on 30 ambulatory and 10 hospitalized patients supported the expectation that it might prove relatively free from the atropine type of side action troublesome with other drugs used in ganglion blockade.

Placebos were administered for varying periods, then one of three programs of drug administration was begun without the patients' knowledge. One group was started on 4 sublingual tablets daily; the number was gradually increased to 7 or 8 tablets a day and treatment continued until no further drop in blood pressure was observed. Injections of 1 cc. hydergine 2-3 times/week, increasing to daily injections, were then given in addition to the tablets. In the second group this procedure was reversed, beginning with the injections and later adding the tablets. The third group had the combined forms of therapy from the start and received the most benefit.

A drop in blood pressure of more than 20 mm. systolic and 10 mm. diastolic was considered a fair response and was experienced by 52.5% of the patients, with an average reduction of 30.7 mm. systolic and 14.7 mm. diastolic. In 5 patients this resulted in normal pressures, and 7 more were considered to have reached satisfactory levels. Of the 19 patients who did not respond well, 5 showed higher pressures after therapy than before, possibly due to excessive doses.

The degree of fundus change provided the best index to the probability of satisfactory response: patients with grade

(3) Indian Heart J. 9:9-23, January, 1957.

II or III changes were less likely to benefit than those with grade I.

Subjectively, 84% of the patients reported complete or partial relief from general symptoms. Half of those with cerebral symptoms were improved in this respect. Side effects were infrequent and not serious: nasal block and dryness of mouth in 10, mild abdominal distention in 4, nausea and vomiting in 5, constipation in 3, loss of appetite in 3 and blurring of vision in 2. One man reported tender enlargement of the breasts and 1 diminished libido. In general, these effects responded to symptomatic treatment and did not necessitate reduction of dosage. In only 2 cases was it necessary to discontinue therapy. Myocardial infarction in 1 patient during therapy may possibly have been due to exacerbation of existing coronary insufficiency. Hydergine should be used with caution when coronary arterial disease is known to exist.

Polyneuritis Occurring during Hydralazine Therapy: Report of Two Cases and Discussion of Adverse Reactions to Hydralazine. A syndrome resembling lupus erythematosus is a well-known and dramatic complication of hydralazine [Apresoline®] therapy. Hydralazine can also form a stable chelate with certain trace minerals and is an antienzyme for several biologic systems. Like isoniazid, it may cause peripheral neuritis, possibly by interference with pyridoxine metabolism. In the 2 cases reported by Walter M. Kirkendall and Elisabeth B. Page[4] (State Univ. of Iowa), pyridoxine intake was probably at the lower limit of estimated daily requirements. This was a likely factor in development of the polyneuritis.

Toxic reactions to hydralazine can be grouped into three general categories: acute or cardiovascular effects; connective tissue, blood and skin reactions; and polyneuritis syndrome. Tachycardia, nasal stuffiness, occipital headache, dyspnea, malaise, anxiety, nervousness, retrosternal distress, peripheral edema and angina pectoris reflect cardiovascular disturbances, perhaps related to release of histamine-like substances. The lupus-like reaction is a connective tissue reaction which may be due to depletion of a trace metal rather than to a hypersensitivity state. The polyneuritis syndrome, possibly due to interference with pyridoxine metabo-

(4) J.A.M.A. 167:427-432, May 24, 1958.

lism, is readily reversed by withdrawing the drug and, perhaps, by supplementing the diet with pyridoxine. The incidence of polyneuritis is low, only 2 cases having been noted among 700 patients treated with hydralazine.

Man, 62, had hypertension and a long history of drinking 2 or 3 bottles of beer daily and 1/5 gal. whisky a week. Kidney studies revealed chronic pyelonephritis, and he had left ventricular hypertrophy. He was treated with a 500-mg. sodium diet, hexamethonium chloride subcutaneously in increasing doses from 5 to 40 mg. twice daily and hydralazine orally, the dose being increased slowly from 10 mg. 4 times daily to 700 mg. daily. By the 25th day blood pressure had fallen to 160/110 mm. Hg, and proteinuria, papilledema and many of the fundus exudates and hemorrhages had disappeared. On the 83d day the patient complained of soreness and numbness of the right ankle, and 5 days later the left ankle was affected. Perception of pinprick and cotton was decreased. Five days after symptoms appeared, oral therapy with 100 mg. pyridoxine daily was started. Within 2 weeks, the numbness and tingling had decreased. Hydralazine administration was stopped. Eleven weeks later all symptoms had disappeared. The diagnosis was peripheral neuritis due to hydralazine.

Antihypertensive Drugs as Cause of Acute Abdomen was observed by Wesley Furste, Darwin Phelps and Philip Taylor[5] (Ohio State Univ.) in 3 men and 1 woman, aged 46-67, who had been on various antihypertensive drugs from a few days to several months. In all, the clinical picture suggested an acute abdominal condition. They were eventually diagnosed as having paralytic ileus and/or vomiting from antihypertensive drugs.

Man, 49, was hospitalized because of shortness of breath and pedal edema. Blood pressure was 260/160 mm. Hg. Moist râles were heard posteriorly at both lung bases. The heart was enlarged to the left. A 2+ pitting edema was present over both lower extremities. On cardiac management, the hypertension persisted. Administration of 2.5 mg. mecamylamine hydrochloride (Inversine®) and 25 mg. hydralazine hydrochloride 4 times daily was started. The dosages were slowly increased, and later 0.25 mg. reserpine (Serpasil®) 4 times daily was begun. The dosage of mecamylamine had been increased to 15 mg. and hydralazine to 100 mg. 4 times daily. About 3 weeks after antihypertensive treatment was begun, the patient began to complain of constipation and to become moderately lethargic; the abdomen became distended and the blood pressure gradually fell to 150/100 mm. Hg. All drugs except gitalin were withdrawn and administration of 5 mg. pilocarpine nitrate 3 times daily was started. Abdominal x-rays indicated numerous loops of dilated small intestine. On conservative management, the paralytic ileus slowly subsided and the patient recovered.

(5) J.A.M.A. 166:2111-2114, Apr. 26, 1958.

Thrombosis, Thrombophlebitis and the Anticoagulant Drugs

Long-Term Anticoagulant Therapy, as applied at the Mayo Clinic, is described by J. Earle Estes.[6] Prolonged administration of coumarin compounds may be needed if there is sufficient danger of thromboembolism to warrant the attendant risk of hemorrhage, the inconvenience and the cost. The various factors should be explained to the patient, and he should have a voice in the decision.

Conditions in which long-term anticoagulant therapy has been used are listed in Table 1, but the decision in a given case rests finally on the judgment and experience of the physician. Thus, myocardial infarction may be treated if (1) there is rapid recurrence, (2) thromboembolism and (3) cardiac failure or arrhythmia in certain cases. Treatment is indicated in auricular fibrillation with intractable cardiac decompensation or recurrent arterial embolism.

It is not practicable to give treatment to all patients with arteriosclerosis obliterans; it is given only when thrombotic occlusions occur frequently. If a source of embolism is a continuing threat, treatment is indicated, though when that source is an aneurysm the possibility of hemorrhage is prohibitively great. In cerebrovascular disease, focal weakness of an extremity suggested localized ischemia or infarction, and long-term therapy is justified in an attempt to limit further damage. This is not the case in chronic hemiplegia. Therapy is contraindicated in intracranial hemorrhage. It may be difficult to distinguish hemorrhage from thrombosis.

In venous disease, long-term anticoagulant therapy is used if thrombophlebitis recurs in less than 4 months. No tests to measure the threat of future embolism exist. The danger of hemorrhage with properly controlled anticoagulant therapy is not great but must be weighed against knowledge of the clinical condition.

Dicumarol® is equal or superior to similar compounds, though Tromexan® has a more rapid and transient effect. The coumarin drugs exert their effect by limiting hepatic production of prothrombin and its stable conversion factor, so that the drugs cannot be assayed at the therapeutic level

(6) Postgrad. Med. 22:323-329, October, 1957.

by bleeding or coagulation time. Quick's one-stage prothrombin assay (coagulation time of recalcified plasma at 37 C. with excess thromboplastin) must be used to control dosage. Correct performance of the test is essential, and the technician must understand that the percentage of normal refers to prothrombin activity rather than to coagulation

TABLE 1.—SOME CONDITIONS IN WHICH LONG-TERM ANTICOAGULANT THERAPY WAS USED

Cardiac diseases
- Myocardial infarction
- Cardiac decompensation
- Auricular fibrillation

Arterial diseases
- Arteriosclerosis obliterans
- Thromboangiitis obliterans (active stage)
- Simple thrombosis (thrombophilia, polycythemia vera)
- Arterial occlusion due to embolism
- Cerebrovascular thrombosis
- Occlusion of central retinal artery

Venous diseases
- Recurrent thrombophlebitis (idiopathic or secondary)
- Recurrent pulmonary embolism (idiopathic or secondary)
- Occlusion of central retinal vein

TABLE 2.—CONTRAINDICATIONS TO ANTICOAGULANT THERAPY WITH COUMARIN DRUGS

Absolute
- Purpura of any type
- Blood dyscrasia with bleeding tendency
- Recent operation on brain or spinal cord
- Subacute bacterial endocarditis
- Inadequate facilities for determining prothrombin time

Relative
- Hepatic insufficiency
- Renal insufficiency
- Indwelling gastrointestinal tube e.g., Miller-Abbott tube
- Malnutrition

time, otherwise a fatal mistake is possible. Adequate testing facilities are therefore essential to therapy. Other restrictions on therapy with coumarin drugs are shown in Table 2. Relative contraindications are factors which do not prohibit use of the method but must be considered against the possible benefits.

On the 1st day of therapy, 300 mg. Dicumarol is administered. Thereafter, daily doses are determined after the prothrombin time for that day has been reported. The aim is to maintain prothrombin activity between 10 and 30% of normal. Dosages vary from 0 to 200 mg., until the level is established; 25-50 mg. usually maintains the level, though there are individual differences in response and there may be differences from time to time in one patient. When the maintenance dose is known, blood assay may be performed once a week or every 2 weeks—no longer.

Rapid reduction of the prothrombin level may be achieved by an initial dose of 200 mg. Dicumarol plus 900 mg. Tromexan. Immediate reduction is obtained by parenteral administration of 50 mg. heparin, which may be repeated every 4 hours and does not interfere with oral administration of Dicumarol-Tromexan the same day.

Normal prothrombin levels are reached a few days after cessation of treatment. This may be hastened with 250 mg. vitamin K_1 orally or, when contraindicated as in biliary fistula, 100 mg. intravenously. These doses may be repeated every 4-6 hours. Stored blood will serve for transfusion, as the prothrombin elevation from fresh blood is transitory.

Patients undergoing prolonged anticoagulant therapy should understand their condition and carry vitamin K_1 and an explanatory card. With proper precautions, the treatment may be considered safe and effective.

Long-Term Anticoagulant Therapy in Coronary Atherosclerosis. Results of a pooled clinical investigation in 1,091 patients are presented by E. Sterling Nichol, John N. Keyes, Joseph F. Borg, Thomas J. Coogan, John J. Boehrer, William L. Mullins, Thornton Scott, Robert Page, George C. Griffith and Edward Massie.[7] The treatment period varied from 3 to 100 months (average 22.4 months). Dicumarol was given to 924 patients, Cumopyran® to 100 and Hedulin® to 60. A few patients were treated with Tromexan®, Coumadin®, Sintrom® or Marcumar®. Daily doses of Dicumarol ranged from 25 to 200 mg. (average, 60 mg.). Dosage for other anticoagulants was proportionately almost as variable. Other treatment included coronary vasodilators, hypotensive reagents, when needed, weight reduction and, in some cases, restriction of foods high in fat and cholesterol. Reasonably limited activity was imposed when indicated.

(7) Am. Heart J. 55:142-152, January, 1958.

Nonfatal thromboembolic complications occurred in 4.4% patients under treatment. Of these, 24 had subendocardial infarction, 16 transmural myocardial infarction and 8 peripheral or pulmonary thromboembolic episodes. Over-all mortality was 12%. Mortality was 6.2% in 96 patients with impending infarction, 10% in 735 patients with single infarctions and 20% in 260 patients with multiple infarctions (Fig. 8).

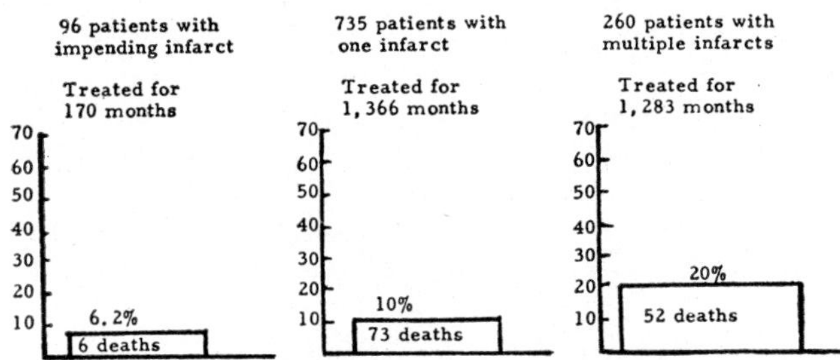

Fig. 8.—Deaths in 1,091 treated patients while on anticoagulants. (Courtesy of Nichol, E. S., *et al.*: Am. Heart J. 55:142-152, January, 1958.)

The regimen was abandoned by 319 patients (29.2%). An average 18.4 months' follow-up showed that 28.2% died within 4 years, mainly of cardiac disease. These 319 patients served as "controls." Comparison of this group with that remaining on treatment offers clear-cut evidence that survival rates are much higher in patients receiving anticoagulants (Fig. 9).

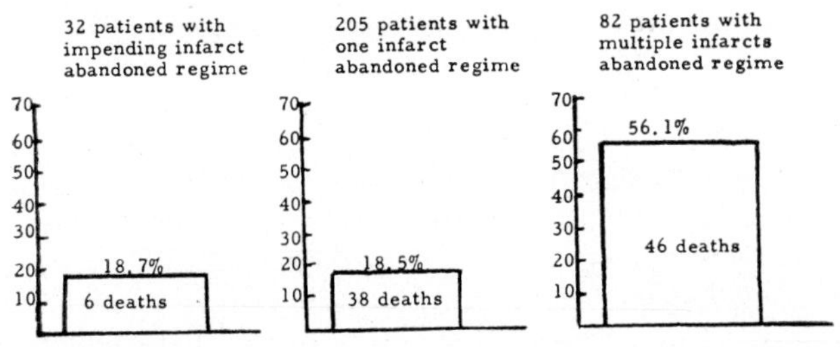

Fig. 9.—Deaths in patients who abandoned anticoagulants. (Courtesy of Nichol, E. S., *et al.*: Am. Heart J. 55:142-152, January, 1958.)

Hemorrhage occurred in 20.1% of patients and appeared more often in those who had used anticoagulants for years. Hematuria was the commonest type of hemorrhage; the second most frequent type was hematoma or ecchymosis. In only 6 patients was death attributable to use of anticoagulants; 4 had cerebral hemorrhage and 2 had subendocardial hemorrhage.

A group of 417 patients not given anticoagulants were used as additional "controls" and followed for an average of 38.1 months. Of these, 37.4% died (Fig. 10), most of cardiovascular disease.

The data, though not amenable to statistical analysis, warrant the conclusion that long-term anticoagulant therapy

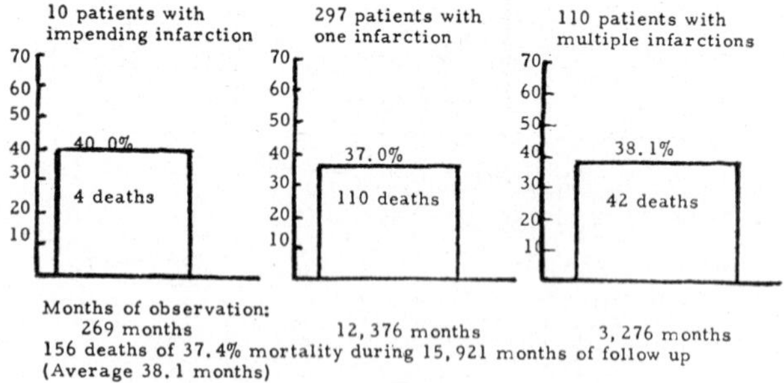

Fig. 10.—Deaths in 417 patients without anticoagulant therapy. (Courtesy of Nichol, E. S., *et al.*: Am. Heart J. 55:142-152, January, 1958.)

prevents recurrent attacks of myocardial infarction. The most significant control study is afforded by the 319 patients who abandoned anticoagulant regimen and had a mortality of 28.2%, due mainly to cardiac disease, during the follow-up period. The mortality of 12% in the whole group maintained on anticoagulant therapy is exceedingly favorable. Furthermore, the fact that generally the more seriously ill patients stayed on the regimen and those who abandoned treatment did well tended to "weight" survival data against the anticoagulant group. The possibility that abrupt abandonment of long-term anticoagulants strengthens the tendency to vascular thrombosis is suggested by the fact that 20 deaths, mainly due to recurrent myocardial infarction, occurred within 1 month after treatment was stopped.

Value of Continuous (1-10 Years) Long-Term Anticoagulant Therapy was studied by Benjamin Manchester[8] (George Washington Univ.) in 712 patients with one or more myocardial infarctions. The incidence of infarction, mortality, congestive heart failure, angina pectoris, thromboembolic complications and survival by patient-years was observed in the control and anticoagulant groups.

Alternate patients received an oral anticoagulant and ascorbic acid, and the controls received a placebo of ascorbic acid, 250 mg. daily. Except for oral anticoagulants—Dicumarol® or Sintrom®—both groups received the same medical care, dietary regimen, digitalis, diuretics and/or sedatives as required. All patients were asked to have blood prothrombin determinations by the author's capillary blood prothrombin test every 1-4 weeks. After 10 years there were 404 patients who had co-operated and continued this medical program uninterruptedly.

The incidence of subsequent infarction was three times greater in the control group and the mortality rate was eight times greater. Thromboembolic complications exclusive of myocardial infarction also were less in the anticoagulant group.

The incidence of bleeding in this series was 2.9%. Administration of vitamin K_1 oxide intravenously corrected the hypoprothrombinemia without hospitalization. The danger from bleeding is thus far less than the danger associated with the inherent hazard of subsequent myocardial infarction.

Anticoagulants in Myocardial Infarction. As a result of an analysis of patients at Radcliffe Infirmary, Honey and Truelove concluded that anticoagulants have but little value in the treatment of acute myocardial infarction. M. Toohey[9] (London), using all the bad-risk factors mentioned by Honey and Truelove, classified 326 patients treated at New End Hospital from 1951 to 1957. In the Radcliffe Infirmary group of 110 untreated patients there were 24.5% good risks, and the mortality rate, excluding deaths in the first 48 hours, was 28.3%. In the New End Hospital series of treated patients the percentage of good risks was 25.7, but the mortality rate was only 13.6% (table). These findings confirm the view,

(8) Ann. Int. Med. 47:1202-1209, December, 1957.
(9) Brit. M. J. 1:252-255, Feb. 1, 1958.

widely accepted by most authorities, that anticoagulants are of real value in acute myocardial infarction.

It is suggested that all bad-risk patients should be treated with anticoagulant therapy. Bad-risk factors include a history of infarction, intractable pain, cardiac failure, arrhythmia, significant cardiac enlargement, diabetic acidosis, and severe shock and hypotension.

For short-term treatment of the acute illness, as opposed to long-term preventive treatment, the quick-acting coumarin drugs such as phenindione and warfarin sodium are much

COMPARISON OF NEW END HOSPITAL AND RADCLIFFE INFIRMARY SERIES

	NEW END	RADCLIFFE
Total no. of patients	326 (treated)	110 (untreated)
Early deaths in first 48 hours	26	18
Late deaths	41	26
Late mortality rate	13.6%	28.3%
Good-risk patients	25.7%	24.5%

easier to control than long-acting drugs such as Dicumarol® and Marcumar®. (For long-term therapy, the opposite holds true.)

With experienced control, serious hemorrhage is very rare, and minor hemorrhage, though not infrequently seen with adequate therapy, does not call for cessation of treatment.

Oral antibiotics, particularly the broad-spectrum drugs such as the tetracyclines and to a less extent penicillin, may call for a reduction in the dose of the anticoagulant drug. Aspirin, phenylbutazone and probably quinine should not be given at the same time as anticoagulant therapy, and liquid paraffin is also best avoided.

Emergency surgical procedures, including major operations, can be carried out on patients still receiving adequate anticoagulant cover without necessity for the treatment to be stopped altogether. This is particularly important in relation to long-term therapy.

Analysis of Factors Affecting Recurrence of Thromboembolism off and on Anticoagulant Therapy was made in 90 patients by Stefan A. Carter, Ellen McDevitt, Barbara W. Gatje and Irving S. Wright[1] (Cornell Univ.). Statistical analysis revealed that the recurrence rate of thromboembolism was significantly reduced by anticoagulant therapy. Al-

(1) Am. J. Med. 25:43-51, July, 1958.

though in individual patients a statistically significant effect from treatment, using the chi-square test, was usually not brought out until they received anticoagulants for at least 2 years and/or exhibited a strong tendency to recurrent thromboembolism, in about 80% of patients benefit was apparent when the less rigid sign test was applied. This indicates that longer observation of patients on treatment is necessary before a long-term effect may be shown by the chi-square test for individual patients. Patients who did have thromboembolism during anticoagulant therapy appeared to

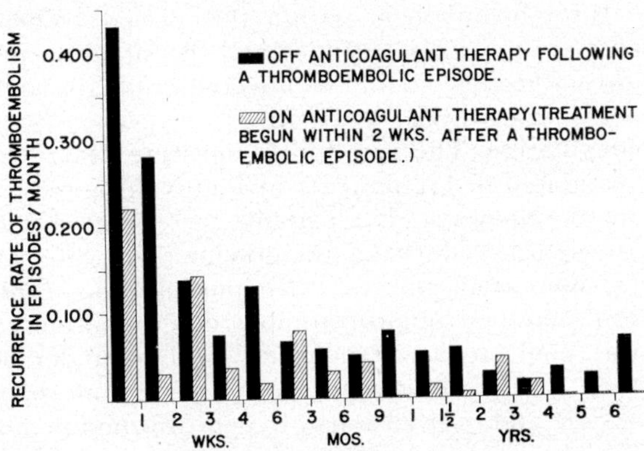

Fig. 11.—Time course of recurrence rate of thromboembolism in patients off and on anticoagulant therapy in relation to previous thromboembolic episode. Based on records of 90 patients. (Courtesy of Carter, S. A., *et al.*: Am. J. Med. 25:43-51, July, 1958.)

have more advanced disease, as indicated by a high incidence of congestive heart failure, atrial fibrillation, myocardial infarction, double mitral lesion and involvement of other valves. Although the rate of recurrence of thromboembolism was equal in patients with and without congestive heart failure during the periods they were off therapy, those with failure had reduced but relatively higher rates during anticoagulant treatment than did those without failure.

Figure 11 shows that the rate during periods the patients were off anticoagulant treatment was highest during the 1st week after a previous episode and declined with time, though it reached a comparative plateau after the first 6 weeks. The differences between the recurrence rates during the first and the second 3 weeks and between the second 3 weeks and the period from 6 weeks to 6 years were statistically significant at the 1% level (chi-square test). No striking decline in the recurrence rate could be shown following the first 6 weeks after a thromboembolic episode. The recurrence rate during anticoagulant treatment followed roughly a similar pattern, though at a much lower level during most intervals, as would be expected.

Patients with thromboembolism, whether on long-term therapy or not, should be given 6 weeks of anticoagulants after a thromboembolic episode because of an increased tendency to thromboembolism within this period. When anticoagulants are to be discontinued and the situation permits, the prothrombin time should be lowered gradually and carefully over a few weeks.

Anticoagulation Therapy for Congestive Heart Failure was investigated in 122 patients in Ragnvald Konow Thorsen[2] (Gjøvik, Norway). The patients were treated with bed rest, a low-salt diet, digitalis, theophylline and, after at least 3-5 days, mercurial diuretics. Dicumarol® was controlled by Owren's method of prothrombin determination; an attempt was made to maintain p—p% values under 30 and higher than 10%. Two patients had values within this range on admission, and over 23% had hypoprothrombinemia (under 70%). The most severe forms of congestive heart failure were usually found in this group.

Nine patients had hemorrhages, 3 severe. In each of the severe cases p—p% was zero; 5 of the other 6 had values below 10%. Not all zero values were attended by hemorrhage.

Eight thromboembolic episodes were diagnosed in the 122 patients, an incidence sufficiently below that seen in a control group of 65 patients, in which 10 such episodes occurred, and below the control figures reported by others to warrant anticoagulation therapy in congestive heart failure.

The author suggests that the initial hypoprothrombinemia present in a fourth of the patients diminishes during treatment and may complicate the problem of estimating the Dicumarol requirement.

Critical Evaluation of Anticoagulant Therapy in Peripheral Venous Thrombosis and Pulmonary Embolism. According-

(2) Acta med. scandinav. 158:203-212, 1957.

ing to W. W. Coon, J. W. Mackenzie and P. E. Hodgson[3] (Univ. of Michigan), who studied 511 patients, anticoagulants prevented death in 7 of every 10 in whom venous thrombosis or nonfatal pulmonary embolus was recognized and treated as compared with the expected mortality attending use of conservative measures alone. Anticoagulants were of additional value in reducing morbidity during the early course of the disease and in achieving appreciable reduction in postphlebitic complications and a three- to fourfold decrease in hospital stay.

Age distribution of the patients was similar to that noted in other studies of thromboembolism. Mean age fell between 50 and 60 years. No difference in age was found in comparison between patients with an initial manifestation of venous thrombosis alone and those with pulmonary embolism, or between those with complications as compared to those free from complications.

These patients presented a wide range of diseases in association with thromboembolism. Of the 511 patients, 42 had fracture of the femur or tibia; the common association of thromboembolic disease with trauma to the lower extremity has been recognized by others. Incidence of complications of the thromboembolic disease was no higher in this group than in the group as a whole. Eighty-eight patients had some form of heart disease. The higher incidence of associated heart disease in pulmonary embolism represents a highly significant statistical difference ($P =$ less than 0.005). The larger percentage of patients with heart disease in the group with pulmonary embolism in whom complications developed subsequent to start of anticoagulant treatment approaches significance ($P =$ less than 0.1 and greater than 0.05).

There was no valid difference in duration of disease before anticoagulant therapy between patients who showed complications and those who did not.

In a significant fraction of the patients thromboembolic disease developed postoperatively: 43% had onset of venous thrombosis or pulmonary embolism within 7 days and 77% within 14 days after operation. Occurrence of complications was not significantly influenced by the interval between operation and onset of the disease. There was no significant

(3) Surg., Gynec. & Obst. 106:129-136, February, 1958.

difference in the complication rate between the 175 patients who did not receive initial heparin treatment and 326 patients who did.

The level of reduction of prothrombin activity as a result of anticoagulant therapy did not appear to be important in treatment of thromboembolic disease. There was also striking similarity in duration of treatment between patients treated successfully and those in whom complications developed during or after anticoagulant therapy. No significant difference in the rate of complications was noted between patients with a well-controlled early course of therapy and those who escaped frequently to 30% prothrombin activity or above.

Of 20 patients who died during or within 12 weeks of therapy, in 5 deaths was due to metastatic neoplasm and in 7 the cause of death was in doubt. Bleeding occurred in 14.8% of the 540 courses of anticoagulant treatment, but no patient died of hemorrhage.

An appreciable reduction in morbidity and mortality from thromboembolism must await more accurate clinical or laboratory diagnosis of this process, or a rational, economically feasible program for mass prophylaxis.

Anticoagulant Therapy in Cerebral Vascular Disease: Current Status. Clark H. Millikan, Robert G. Siekert and Jack P. Whisnant[4] (Mayo Clinic and Found.) treated 317 patients with manifestations of cerebral vascular disease with anticoagulant drugs. All were carefully chosen and had intermittent insufficiency in the vertebral-basilar system, intermittent insufficiency in the carotid system, thrombosis in the vertebral-basilar system with infarction or actively advancing occlusion of the carotid system. Diagnosis was established by analysis of detailed histories and neurologic examinations.

Heparin was given intravenously in doses of 50 mg. every 4 hours when rapid anticoagulant action was desired. Ethyl biscoumacetate [Tromexan®] and bishydroxycoumarin [Dicumarol®] were administered together. No patient received more than 1 dose of ethyl biscoumacetate. Bishydroxycoumarin was given whenever long-term therapy was de-

(4) J.A.M.A. 166:587-592, Feb. 8, 1958.

sired. The quantity of drug used was carefully regulated from day to day.

In 90 of 94 patients who had intermittent insufficiency in the vertebral-basilar system, attacks stopped completely soon after effective anticoagulant action was obtained. The other 4 patients had less severe and less frequent attacks. Thrombosis and infarction did not develop. Of 85 patients who had intermittent insufficiency of the carotid system, 82 ceased to have attacks.

A group of 107 patients with irreversible vertebral-basilar thrombosis had a mortality rate of only 8% on anticoagulant therapy as compared with a rate of 58% reported in 31 similar patients who did not receive anticoagulants. Among 31 patients actively advancing carotid thrombosis went on to hemiplegia in only 6% as compared with 35% in a reported series of 17 similar patients who did not receive anticoagulants.

Anticoagulant treatment is preventive rather than reconstructive, but it does alter favorably the natural history of cerebral vascular disease in patients of the four types treated by the authors. Much further study with long-term follow-up data will be needed to determine the optimal duration of anticoagulant treatment in each category. At present ingestion of the anticoagulant for 6-12 months is advised, with re-evaluation of the problem at the end of that period.

Use of Anticoagulants in Treatment of Cerebral Vascular Disease: 10-Year Experience in Treatment of Thromboembolism. Ellen McDevitt, Stefan A. Carter, Barbara W. Gatje, William T. Foley and Irving S. Wright[5] (Cornell Univ.) studied the long-term effects of anticoagulant therapy in 100 patients with evidence of cerebral vascular thrombosis or embolism. Included were 51 patients with rheumatic heart disease, 28 with arteriosclerotic and/or hypertensive heart disease, 10 with recurrent focal cerebral ischemia and 11 with various diagnoses.

The incidence of thromboembolism on and off anticoagulant therapy in 90 patients (excluding the 10 with cerebral insufficiency) is shown in the table. If the first episode which marked the beginning of the period of observation is excluded, 229 thromboembolic episodes, of which 67 were cere-

(5) J.A.M.A. 166:592-597, Feb. 8, 1958.

bral, occurred during a total of 2,842 patient-months off therapy. During 2,291 patient-months on anticoagulants there were 72 episodes, of which 16 were cerebral. Of these, 20, including 5 cerebral episodes, occurred when the nearest prothrombin time was below 20 seconds. A decrease in incidence of thromboembolic episodes was present in all three diagnostic groups during periods of therapy.

A total of 48 thromboembolic episodes occurred in 18 of 36 patients on interrupted therapy during 1,311 patient-months, whereas 15 occurred in 8 of 28 patients on continuous treatment during 957 patient-months. There was no striking difference in the incidence of cerebral episodes, which were few in both groups.

The dosages of anticoagulant (usually bishydroxycoumarin) were aimed to keep the prothrombin time for the undiluted plasma between 20 and 40 seconds. There was a total of 51 hemorrhagic complications in 30 patients; 40 were minor and 11 of these occurred in 1 patient. Of 11 major complications, 5 were due to cerebral hemorrhage and only 3 of the 11, all cerebral, were fatal. These complications occurred during 2,532 patient-months.

OCCURRENCE OF THROMBOEMBOLISM ON AND OFF ANTICOAGULANT THERAPY

Group	No. Patients	Anticoagulant Therapy	Total Patient-Mo.	No Patients with Recurrent Episodes	Thromboembolic Episodes	
					Total	Cerebral
Rheumatic heart disease	51	Off	1,747	43	197 (146*)	70 (37†)
		On	1,515	20	55 (16‡)	10 (3‡)
Arteriosclerotic and/or hypertensive heart disease	28	Off	648	21	74 (46*)	32 (17†)
		On	501	8	11 (4‡)	4 (2‡)
Miscellaneous	11	Off	447	10	48 (37*)	20 (13†)
		On	275	5	6 (0‡)	2 (0‡)
Total	90	Off	2,842	74	319 (229*)	122 (67†)
		On	2,291	33	72 (20‡)	16 (5‡)

*Excluding the first thromboembolic episode.
†Excluding cerebral episodes which were the first thromboembolic episodes.
‡Nearest prothrombin time less than 20 seconds.

On the basis of this and other studies, it is concluded that long-term anticoagulant therapy can be considered to be indicated in a number of types of cerebral vascular disease such as embolic conditions which include fibrillating heart, myocardial infarction with mural thrombus and chronic rheumatic heart disease with normal sinus rhythm; intermittent insufficiency or thrombosis in the vertebral basilar or carotid systems; thrombosis in cerebral artery branches; and multiple strokes involving several areas of the brain. The physician should consider each case singly and assess the possible contraindications. There must be weighed against the urgency of the indication for anticoagulants, and if the treatment is decided on special caution must be exercised. Diagnosis of the cerebral lesion must be established as exactly as possible before anticoagulant therapy is started, because of the risk inherent in administration of anticoagulants to patients with cerebral hemorrhage.

Treatment of Thromboembolism with Aqueous Heparin. Harold W. Harrower, Alfred Hurwitz and Raymond Yesner[6] gave concentrated aqueous heparin (200 mg./cc.) by deep subcutaneous injection to 15 healthy adults and 75 patients with thromboembolism. Clotting time determinations and blood viscosity profiles were made.

In 44 of 47 patients who received subcutaneous heparin as definitive therapy, results were satisfactory. Thrombophlebitis recurred or pulmonary emboli occurred during or after treatment in the other 3 patients.

A 12-hour interval between heparin injections was generally preferred. Body weight was a helpful but not reliable guide to heparin dosage. Because of variations in heparin requirements among different patients and in the same patient from time to time, frequent clotting time determinations were necessary for control of therapy.

Repeated subcutaneous injections of heparin were well tolerated and could be continued in the nonhospitalized patient No sensitivity reactions were encountered.

With subcutaneous heparin administration, hemorrhagic complications seemed to be more frequent than with intermittent intravenous therapy The concomitant administration of subcutaneous heparin and oral Dicumarol® was found to be contraindicated.

In the normal subjects and in the patients with thromboembolism, the changes in blood viscosity profiles after sub-

(6) Surg., Gynec. & Obst. 106:293-305, March, 1958.

cutaneous heparin administration were similar to those produced by intravenous administration but were more prolonged. The degree and duration of alteration of viscosity profiles tended to, but frequently did not, parallel changes in clotting times. Pretreatment blood viscosity profiles were abnormal in about half the patients with thromboembolism.

The authors believe that in acute thromboembolic conditions, after recent surgery, and in patients who present more than the usual risk of hemorrhage, heparin treatment should consist of intermittent intravenous injections. Subcutaneous heparin administration may be substituted after heparin requirements have been stabilized, provided the clinical course is satisfactory.

In those rare instances in which thromboses progress or pulmonary emboli occur during therapy, ligation of the inferior vena cava is performed as an emergency. Heparin therapy is reinstituted postoperatively to preserve collateral venous channels.

Subcutaneous Heparin with and without Hyaluronidase. Arthur Hollman and R. E. Nagle[7] (Univ. College Hosp., London) compared the clotting time after subcutaneous injection of heparin mixed with hyaluronidase, with that of subcutaneous heparin alone and with that of heparin given intravenously. Hyaluronidase hastened the absorption of heparin from the skin to a significant extent in only 15% of cases and did not diminish local bruising. Eight-hourly subcutaneous injections of heparin, with or without hyaluronidase, satisfactorily maintained the clotting time at 2-3 times normal after an initial delay averaging 14 hours. Severe local bruising occurred in 25% of cases.

Heparin Neutralization with Polybrene Administered Intravenously is discussed by William A. Weiss, Janet S. Gilman, Alfred J. Catenacci and Arnold E. Osterberg.[8] Polybrene neutralizes the anticoagulant action of heparin in vivo and in vitro. It is a quaternary ammonium salt with an empiric formula of $(C_{13}H_{30}Br_2N_2)x$. It is a polymer, probably linear, with the chemical name of 1,5-dimethyl-1,5-diazaundecamethylene polymethobromide.

Heparin neutralizers—protamine, toluidine blue and Poly-

(7) Brit. M. J. 2:182-185, July 27, 1957.
(8) J.A.M.A. 166:603-607, Feb. 8, 1958.

brene—were compared as to efficacy in 23 heparinized dogs. Polybrene was also studied in 30 patients, most with cardiac or respiratory disease, who had been heparinized by intravenous injection of 1.5 mg./kg. heparin. Dosage of Polybrene was 1.5 mg./kg. intravenously in half the patients, and 1.1 mg./kg. in the others. The smaller dose was adequate.

Polybrene was further compared with protamine in observations on 107 patients who had open-heart surgery with extracorporeal circulation. Heparin neutralization was accomplished with intravenously injected Polybrene. The postneutralization Lee-White coagulation time averaged 5 minutes 48 seconds.

Polybrene, protamine and toluidine blue all cause disagreeable side effects in some patients, but Polybrene injected intravenously did not cause the methemoglobinemia and hypoxia seen after toluidine blue or the dangerous degrees of hypotension seen after protamine. Given in the dose of 0.7 mg. Polybrene to 1 mg. heparin, the former promptly and completely neutralized the anticoagulant action of heparin. Dilution of the total dose of Polybrene to a concentration of 1 mg. in each cubic centimeter of 5% dextrose in distilled water is recommended. The intravenous flow rate should be adjusted for a total administration time of 10 minutes.

Coagulation times were improved to within accepted limits by intravenous Polybrene in 2 patients who presented a heparin-like syndrome after open-heart surgery under hypothermia; in 2 patients with mitral stenosis who had prolonged Lee-White coagulation times preoperatively; and in 2 patients on heparin therapy for 3 and 5 days postoperatively and in whom bleeding developed at the operative site.

Arterial Embolism Occurring during Systemic Heparin Therapy. In recent years, concomitant with more aggressive medical and surgical management of various vascular disorders, Rodger E. Weismann and Richard W. Tobin[9] (Hanover, N. H.) have observed and treated an increasing number of patients who have had major arterial embolism while on an active systemic heparin therapy program. Among 10 patients, aged 46-86, with clearcut arterial embolisms, these were multiple in 9 and single in 1. Rapid propagation of aortic mural thrombi with aortic occlusion, besides distal em-

(9) A.M.A. Arch. Surg. 76:219-227, February, 1958.

Summary of Data in 10 Cases of Arterial Embolism Occurring during Herapin Therapy

Indication for Heparin	Day Rx	L. W. C.*, Min.	Complication
Thrombophlebitis: (?) allergic vasulitis	15	65	Rt. femoral embolus; lt. popliteal embolus
Thrombophlebitis (?) arteritis	10 12 12	23 15 15	Rt. femoral embolus; saddle embolus; rt. popliteal embolus
Lt. femoral thromboendarterectomy	8 11 11	27 13 13	Rt. femoral embolus; rt. popliteal embolus; saddle embolus
Lt. femoral thromboendarterectomy	11	58	Lt. femoral embolus; propagating aortic thrombus
Thrombophlebitis	13 13 13	66 66 66	Acute myocardial infarct; lt. popliteal embolus; cerebral embolus
Pulmonary infarct (postabdominal perineal resection)	11 12 14	31 16 15	Rt. popliteal embolus; lt. common iliac embolus; saddle embolus
Rt. femoral artery thrombosis	8 12 15	30 79 34	Lt. femoral embolus; lt. external iliac embolus; rt., common iliac embolus
Rt. femoral artery embolism	7 9	37 53	Cerebral embolus; bilateral iliac embolism; renal emboli
Lt. popliteal artery thrombosis	9 ..	43 ..	Propagating aortic thrombus; rt. renal embolus; inferior mesenteric embolus
Acute femoral occlusion, bilateral; (?) allergic arteritis	10 13	41 16	Rt. cerebral embolus; multiple emboli (superior mesenteric, rt. iliac, lt. common femoral)

*L. W. C. refers to Lee-White clotting time on day embolism occurred.

bolization, was suspected in 3 patients. The source of the emboli was thought to be aortic mural platelet-fibrin thrombi in all instances. All patients showed some clinical evidence of predisposing cardiovascular disease. Heparin therapy, preceding the first complication, lasted 7-15 days. Data correlating excessive depression of the Lee-White clotting time with occurrence of embolization were suggestive but inconclusive (table).

There were 6 deaths. Two patients survived unilateral midthigh amputation: 1 later required contralateral thigh amputation, the other, transmetatarsal amputation. Two patients lived without loss of limbs. Antemortem aortic mu-

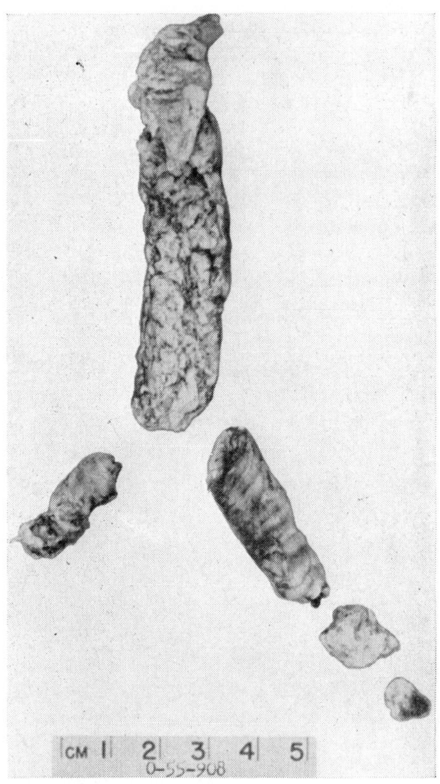

Fig. 12.—Emboli removed from aorta and iliac arteries. Note unusual length and cylindric shape, suggesting origin in proximal aorta. (Courtesy of Weismann, R. E., and Tobin, R. W.: A.M.A. Arch. Surg. 76:219-227, February, 1958.)

ral platelet thrombi were recovered from 3 patients who came to autopsy.

Woman, 62, recovering from eye surgery, presented signs and symptoms of left iliofemoral thrombophlebitis, for which systemic heparinization was begun. She received heparin sodium in divided subcutaneous doses, totaling 150-300 mg./day. After 10 days' anticoagulation therapy, sudden signs of right common femoral arterial embolism developed. Successful femoral embolectomy was carried out. She was kept on adequate heparin and made a satisfactory initial recovery, then signs of sudden occlusion of the distal aorta appeared. After intravenous administration of protamine sulfate, prompt transperitoneal distal aortic and bilateral iliac embolectomies were performed (Fig. 12). In the next 24 hours, because unsatisfactory distal circulation persisted, the patient underwent left femoral exploration, with no abnormal findings, and right popliteal exploration, which revealed an embolus. She subsequently had a favorable course, surviving prolonged ileus and never showing ischemic changes more serious than a small area of superficial gangrene of the right great toe and several small areas of skin infarction of the right leg. Heparin was discontinued 12 days after the final surgical procedure. Angiography excluded paradoxical embolism. At follow-up 6 months later, the edema had disappeared, pedal pulses were palpable and symptoms of arterial insufficiency were absent. All embolic material recovered was nearly devoid of red cells.

Experience with Anticoagulant, Marcumar®, in the treatment of 1,729 patients during 2 years is recorded by Robert E. Ensor and H. Raymond Peters[1] (Univ. of Maryland). Cases were classed as coronary disease, phlebitis and postoperative and postpartum prophylaxis. Each type of case presented its own difficulties and therapeutic problems, and dosage schedules used in each are cited.

Of 56 consecutive patients with acute myocardial infarction, 29 had excellent levels of 25-35 seconds at all times while under treatment with Marcumar. Good levels of 20-30 seconds were maintained in 7 patients. Twelve were sensitive (excellent levels most of the time, but occasional levels of 40-50 or 60 seconds). Eight patients were classed as resistant (occasional drop below 20 seconds).

Of 24 patients with acute phlebitis excellent levels were maintained in 19, 1 was sensitive and 4 resistant. Of 397 patients given postoperative prophylaxis, 304 had excellent prothrombin records, 29 were sensitive and 64 resistant. Of 91 patients given postoperative prophylaxis in bowel, stomach or gallbladder surgery, 56 had excellent levels, 10 were sensitive, 18 resistant and 7 showed fluctuation. There was no instance of thromboembolism in these patients. Of 1,000 patients given Marcumar post partum, 716 showed excellent control.

A comparison of Marcumar with Dicumarol® and Cumopyran® in 288 long-term out-patients with coronary disease demonstrated the superiority of Marcumar, even in the most

(1) Ann. Int. Med. 47:731-743, October, 1957.

difficult cases. Another spot check of 161 out-patients with phlebitis and coronary disease verified the satisfactory levels obtained with Marcumar. Marcumar by its prolonged action gives a more stable and satisfactory type of curve. Its advantages far overshadow its initial delayed action. In this respect it is stressed that any case requiring urgent anticoagulation requires heparin rather than the short-acting anticoagulants.

In the entire series there was no death due to hemorrhage. There was no incidence of bleeding in 1,080 coronary, phlebitis and postpartum cases and only 3 of minimal bleeding in 400 routine postoperative cases. In the 91 postoperative bowel, stomach and gallbladder cases, despite their known liability to anticoagulant hemorrhage, only 1 case of moderate gastrointestinal hemorrhage occurred.

► [The experience of I. Prior (New Zealand M. J. 46:545, 1957), who compared Dicumarol with Marcumar, is somewhat at variance, for while the control achieved was better with Marcumar than with Dicumarol, the incidence of hemorrhage was also higher. J. F. Fairbairn and J. E. Estes (1957-58 YEAR BOOK, p. 130) did not feel that Marcumar had significant advantages over Dicumarol. Both drugs are coumarin derivatives and hence are antidoted by vitamin K_1.—Ed.]

Clinical Experience with G-23350 (Sintrom®). Sintrom is a synthetic anticoagulant of the coumarin group, thus resembling chemically Dicumarol® and ethyl biscoumacetate (Tromexan®) and having the same action in inhibiting synthesis by the liver of prothrombin and factor VII (convertin). R. Johnson, A. David and Y. Chartier[2] (Notre Dame Hosp., Montreal) administered Sintrom to 50 patients. A therapeutic level was reached within 48 hours in 35 cases (70%). The initial dose was inadequate in 9 cases at the beginning of the study in the light of further experience. Therefore, the authors believe that with adequate dosage a therapeutic prothrombin level can be achieved in 85-90% of cases within 48 hours. Initial doses of 20-28 mg. were used, and in most cases the prothrombin level fell to 20-40%. Subsequent doses for maintenance were unpredictable and required daily adjustment.

In no case did the prothrombin time reach a dangerous level with the initial dose used. Eight patients were considered sensitive to the drug. One patient was markedly re-

(2) Canad. M. A. J. 77:756-761, Oct. 15, 1957.

sistant, requiring large doses to reach the therapeutic level and maintenance doses about twice the usual level. Six patients were slightly resistant, requiring in general 2-4 mg. above the usual dosage.

Sintrom has no cumulative effect. Response to it disappears within 72 hours after the last dose is administered. As with other anticoagulants, there is a synergistic action with certain drugs such as salicylates and its effect is inhibited by vitamin K.

In the present group 2 patients had macroscopic hematuria, 1 with a prothrombin level of 14% and the other with a level of 20%. In these 2 cases the hemorrhagic accidents had no serious consequences. In a third patient, massive hemoptysis occurred with a prothrombin level of 8%. The patient had had acute pulmonary edema for 12 hours and was dying. These accidents were attributed to the inherent risk of all anticoagulant therapy. No untoward or toxic effect of the drug on any system or organ was observed. Gastrointestinal tolerance was excellent.

Sintrom is easier to give (1 daily dose only) than Tromexan and its action is more predictable. Since it does not have the cumulative effect of Dicumarol, the danger of prolonged hemorrhagic accidents is lessened. Though the response to Sintrom, as with other anticoagulants, is an individual one, when the personal response is well known, the drug can be given over a long period with weekly or twice monthly control of prothrombin time.

► [Last year, W. S. Wilson *et al.* (1957-58 Year Book, p. 133) concluded that Sintrom probably acts more rapidly than Dicumarol but not as rapidly as Tromexan. Maintenance dosage was found difficult to establish, and escape from therapeutic levels occurred frequently.—Ed.]

Comparative Clinical Study of Coumadin® Sodium and Dicumarol® in Patients with Thromboembolic Diseases is reported by Charles M. Shapiro, Ruben Lisker, Alvin M. Lichtman and Aaron M. Josephson[3] (Michael Reese Hosp.). Coumadin sodium (warfarin) was given to 100 patients and Dicumarol to 100 others. The initial dose of Coumadin sodium was arbitrarily fixed at 50 or 60 mg. From 5 to 30 mg. was given on the 2d day. Average daily maintenance dose was 5-10 mg. Dicumarol was given initially in successive

(3) Am. Heart J. 55:66-72, January, 1958.

daily doses of 300, 200 and 100 mg. As patients receiving this drug showed poor stability, maintenance dosage was quite variable.

A therapeutic anticoagulant range was considered to be reached when the prothrombin time was between 24 and 36 seconds (11-26% prothrombin activity). Prothrombin times within this range were found in 70.8% of daily determinations in patients taking Coumadin sodium and in 70.3% of daily determinations in those taking Dicumarol.

Patients receiving Coumadin sodium were within the therapeutic range in an average of 43.4 hours. Administration of heparin had no definite effect in shortening the time.

TABLE 1.—Latent Period with and without Heparin

	Coumadin Sodium		Dicumarol	
	Number of Cases	Average Time (Hours)	Number of Cases	Average Time (Hours)
No Heparin	43	42.0	37	87.0
Heparin	50	44.7	55	74.9
Total number of cases*	93	43.4	92	80.3

*Data not available for all patients due to interchange of anticoagulants; in a few instances patients entered hospital on anticoagulant therapy.

The latent period in the Dicumarol group averaged 80.3 hours, heparin shortening the period by about 12 hours (Table 1). Escape from the effect of the anticoagulant occurred 27 times in the Coumadin sodium group and 42 times in the Dicumarol group. Average interval until the therapeutic range was attained again was 2.7 days for the Coumadin sodium and 3.6 days for the Dicumarol group (Table 2). Hypersensitivity occurred 9 times in the former and 7 times in the latter group.

Seven patients on Coumadin sodium and 6 receiving Dicumarol were given vitamins K or K_1. One patient in each group failed to respond. Hemorrhagic phenomena were seen in 11 patients taking Coumadin sodium and in 8 taking Dicumarol. Only 1 death, that of a patient on Dicumarol, was attributable to anticoagulant therapy.

The mode of action of Coumadin sodium and Dicumarol

TABLE 2.—ESCAPE FROM ANTICOAGULANT EFFECT

DRUG	TOTAL DAYS OF THERAPY	NUMBER OF ESCAPES	TOTAL DAYS UNTIL WITHIN THERAPEUTIC RANGE	AVERAGE NUMBER DAYS RETURN TO THERAPEUTIC RANGE	ESCAPE DAYS (% OF TOTAL DAYS)
Coumadin Sodium	1,842	27	73	2.7	3.95
Dicumarol	2,211	42	151	3.6	6.83

Hypersensitivity to Anticoagulant

DRUG	TOTAL DAYS OF THERAPY	NUMBER OF HYPERSENSITIVE EPISODES	TOTAL DAYS UNTIL WITHIN THERAPEUTIC RANGE	AVERAGE NUMBER DAYS RETURN TO THERAPEUTIC RANGE	HYPERSENSITIVE DAYS (% OF TOTAL DAYS)
Coumadin Sodium	1,842	9	20	2.2	1.08
Dicumarol	2,211	7	16	2.3	0.72

is not solely through depression of the prothrombin activity of the blood. Stable factor, required for normal coagulation, is more significantly affected. Preliminary experiments indicate that depression of stable factor activity accounts for most of the "hypoprothrombinemic" state, as measured by routine prothrombin time determinations.

Clinical Experiences with Warfarin (Coumadin®) Sodium as Anticoagulant. Samuel Baer, M. William Yarrow, Charles Kravitz and Victor Markson[4] (Philadelphia) used Coumadin sodium and bishydroxycoumarin (Dicumarol®) in a study of the effects of anticoagulant therapy on 200 patients, most of them with acute myocardial infarction or severe coronary insufficiency. Coumadin sodium was given orally to 164, prothrombin times being determined daily. An initial dose of 60-75 mg. was given, depending on the estimated size of the patient. Individual dosages were adjusted until the daily dose (usually 5-7.5 mg.) needed to maintain the prothrombin level between 15% and 30% was found. Patients treated with bishydroxycoumarin (36) were begun on 200-300 mg. and then given maintenance doses varying between 20 and 100 mg. daily.

Coumadin solution was found to be far superior to bishy-

(4) J.A.M.A. 167:704-708, June 7, 1958.

droxycoumarin. It had the advantages of quicker effect, producing the desired prothrombin levels within 48 hours in 87% of patients. A disturbing aspect of bishydroxycoumarin therapy was the frequency and unpredictability with which patients receiving this drug escaped from therapeutic range.

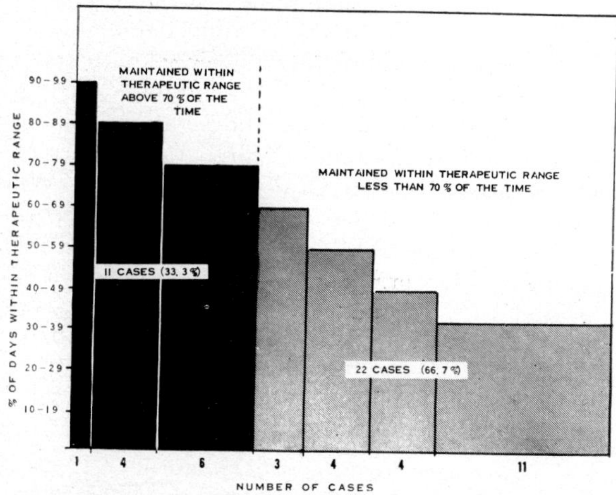

Fig. 13.—Days within therapeutic range with bishydroxycoumarin (33 patients). (Courtesy of Baer, S., *et al.*: J.A.M.A. 167:704-708, June 7, 1958.)

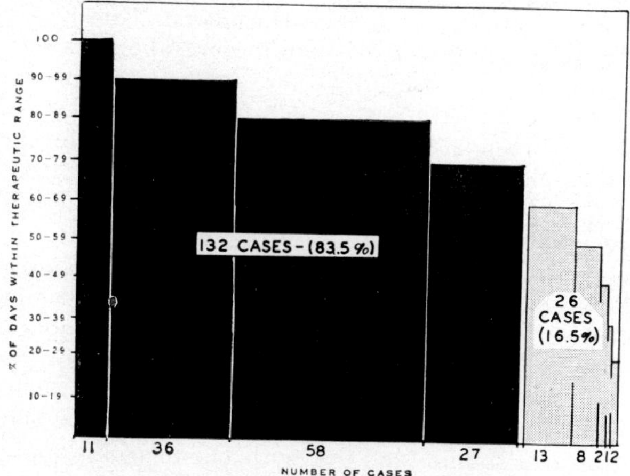

Fig. 14.—Days within therapeutic range with warfarin sodium (158 patients). (Courtesy of Baer, S., *et al.*: J.A.M.A. 167:704-708, June 7, 1958.)

Only one third of the 36 patients were within therapeutic range 70-100% of the time; 22 patients (66.7%) were within therapeutic range less than 70% of the time (Fig. 13). In contrast, 132 (83.5%) of the 158 patients receiving Coumadin sodium for more than 4 days were within therapeutic range 70% or more of the time (Fig. 14).

The frequency of side effects (mainly hemorrhagic) was slightly, though not significantly, lower in patients treated with Coumadin sodium. Nine who exhibited bleeding phenomena promptly responded to withdrawal of Coumadin sodium or treatment with vitamin K preparations.

Clinical Experience with Orally Administered Warfarin Sodium in 170 hospitalized patients requiring anticoagulant therapy is reported by Harold G. Danford, John L. Juergens and Nelson W. Barker.[5] For comparison, 100 similar patients treated with Dicumarol® were observed.

METHOD.—The initial dose was usually given in the afternoon or evening. Each subsequent daily maintenance dose was given in the early afternoon 4-5 hours after blood samples had been obtained to determine the prothrombin time and following receipt of the results of that test. Initial dose of warfarin sodium was 40-60 mg. and daily maintenance dose ranged from 0 to 20 mg., usually 5-10 mg. In the patients receiving Dicumarol, an initial dose of 300 mg. of this drug was combined with 1,200 mg. ethyl biscoumacetate (Tromexan®) to produce a more rapid therapeutic effect. Thereafter, 0-200 mg. Dicumarol alone was given daily. The one-stage (Quick) method was used to determine the prothrombin time.

Initial doses of warfarin sodium were about as effective as initial combined doses of Tromexan® and Dicumarol with respect to the rapidity with which therapeutic levels of hypoprothrombinemia were attained. About 45% of the patients in each group had prothrombin activities of 30% or less in 12-24 hours. At the end of 36-48 hours of therapy, the effectiveness of the two programs again was comparable.

The relative efficiency of the two coumarin compounds may be shown by comparing the incidence of so-called escape periods during which a shift in the prothrombin activity above or below the therapeutic range occurs after the daily doses of the anticoagulant have been relatively stabilized for the individual patient. This incidence was 5% with warfarin sodium and 9% with Dicumarol.

There was a small incidence of bleeding, mostly of minor

(5) Proc. Staff Meet. Mayo Clin. 33:359-363, July 9, 1958.

degree, which could be considered similar to that observed in corresponding types of patients treated for comparable periods with Dicumarol. No other untoward effects attributable to warfarin sodium were observed and vitamin K_1 proved to be an effective antagonist.

It appears that warfarin sodium possesses modest advantanges over Dicumarol as an anticoagulant.

► [Warfarin does have this distinction, however, of being the first synthetic anticoagulant that can be administered by other than the oral route. Its intramuscular use is the subject of the succeeding article.—Ed.]

Intramuscular Administration of Anticoagulant Warfarin (Coumadin®) Sodium, the first synthetic anticoagulant that is effective orally, intravenously and rectally, is discussed by Shepard Shapiro and Flavio E. Ciferri[6] (New York). They used two forms of the drug. The first preparation consisted of 75 mg. in 2 cc. of a 3.5% solution of povidone (polyvinylpyrrolidone); the second, and the presently preferred form, is an injection unit consisting of a vial containing 75 mg. warfarin in powder form with an accompanying 3-cc. am-

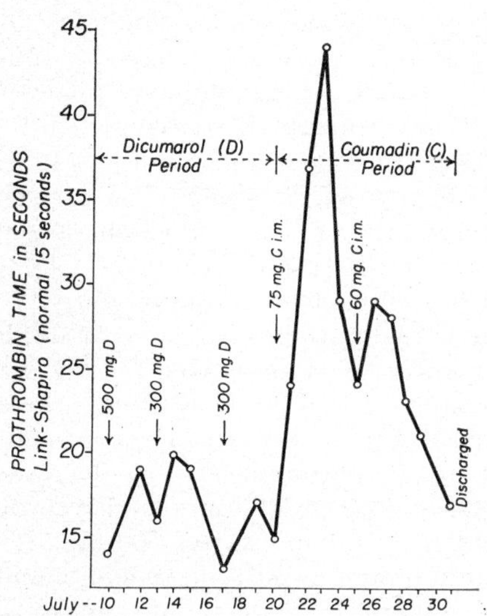

Fig. 15.—Course of patient with pulmonary infarction who was first given Dicumarol®, with no ensuing prothrombin depression, and then was given Coumadin intramuscularly, with resulting prothrombin depression. (Courtesy of Shapiro, S., and Ciferri, F. E.: J.A.M.A. 165:1377-1380, Nov. 16, 1957.)

(6) J.A.M.A. 165:1377-1380, Nov. 16, 1957.

pule of water for injection. The solution can be prepared immediately before intramuscular (or intravenous) administration. Responses with the two forms were similar.

Injections were made in the upper outer quadrant of the buttocks, or, in a few instances, in the deltoid region. The drug was well tolerated, and serial blood pressure readings showed no significant change. None of the patients received heparin. Usual initial warfarin dosage was 75 mg., regardless of body weight; the peak effect was observed on the 2d and 3d days. Subsequent dosing was mostly oral.

The usefulness of intramuscularly administered warfarin is shown in Figure 15. The patient represented did not respond to 500, 300 and 300 mg. bishydroxycoumarin given during 6 days. Intramuscular administration of 75 mg. warfarin was followed by a therapeutic degree of hypoprothrombinemia and uneventful recovery.

The prompt absorption after intramuscular administration may well make this the parenteral route of choice.

Anisindione: New Anticoagulant with Unusual Properties. Anisindione (2-p-anisyl-1,3-indandione) an anticoagulant of the inandione type, has displayed an unusual freedom from toxic effects on the hepatobiliary apparatus and on the blood in animal experiments. Kurt Lange, Eli Perchuk, Murray Mahl, Josef Enzinger and George Mouratoff[7] (New York Med. College), with the technical assistance of Peter Demoleas, studied the effects of anisindione given to 52 patients with vascular disease for a total of 1,198 days.

The initial decrease in prothrombin activity after 1 dose of anisindione varied with dosage. After a single dose of 200 mg., prothrombin activity decreased to 75% within 6 hours and to a maximum of 40% after 30 hours; the effect was no longer present (in 4 patients) after 110 hours (Fig. 16). After a dose of 400 mg., prothrombin activity decreased to 50-60% within 6 hours, to 30% in 50 hours, and returned to normal (in 4 patients) in 150 hours. After 500 mg., it decreased to 45-55% within 6 hours, to 30% in 32 hours, and reverted to normal (in 4 patients) between 110 and 150 hours. After 600 mg., the activity fell to 35-45% within 6 hours, to 25-30% in 36 hours, and returned to normal (in 3 patients) in 158 hours. The response was usually uniform.

(7) Am. Heart J. 55:73-79, January, 1958.

Through trial and error, a dosage was determined for initiation of a satisfactory reduction in prothrombin activity. The schedule consisted of 500 mg. the 1st day, 300 mg. the 2d, nothing the 3d and 300 mg. the 4th day. When this dosage was used in 23 patients, everyone had a therapeutic level of 15-30% within 72 hours. After this level was reached, it was maintained by giving 250 mg. anisindione every 3d day.

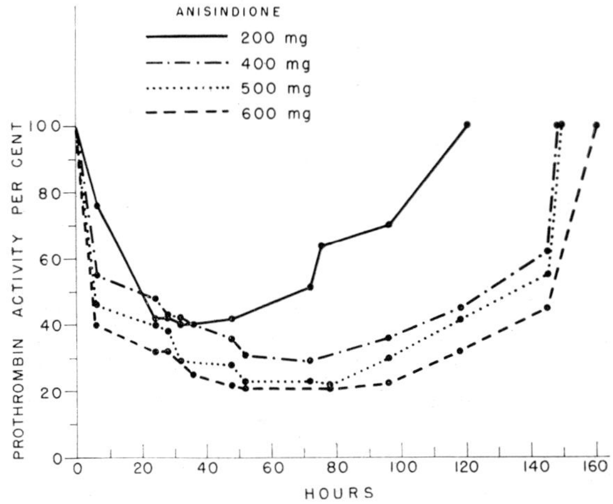

Fig. 16.—Response to 1 dose of anisindione of varying amounts in different patients. (Courtesy of Lange, K., *et al.*: Am. Heart J. 55:73-79, January, 1958.)

It was found that maintenance doses helped to retain the anticoagulant effect previously established with Dicumarol®. The effect of anisindione can be interrupted rapidly by use of phytonadione. The anticoagulant effect can be restored rapidly by remedication. When phytonadione was given in the course of Dicumarol treatment, a period of resistance to remedication after return to normal, prothrombin activity was regularly noted.

Side effects of anisindione were noticeably absent. Three instances of hematuria were noted, 1 occurring at a therapeutically desirable level, 1 in a patient with renal calculus and 1 at a purposely induced, extremely low prothrombin activity. No chromaturia, petechiae, agranulocytosis or liver damage occurred.

Orally Administered Phytonadione in Bishydroxycoumarin-Induced Hypoprothrombinemia was investigated by Milton Shoshkes, Bernard Robins and Gabriel Yelin[8] (Beth Israel Hosp., Newark, N.J.). Thirty adults, 28 hospitalized for acute myocardial infarction and 2 for acute thrombophlebitis of an extremity, had been maintained at 10-40% of the normal prothrombin level with Dicumarol. On the last day of such therapy, 10 were given 2 phytonadione (Mephyton®) tablets containing 5 mg. vitamin K_1 each, 10 were given 25 mg. and 10, 50 mg. Prothrombin times were determined just before administration of the vitamin and at intervals for 24 hours after. There was an appreciable response within 2 hours, increasing to about an equal extent at the 3 dosage levels during the first 8 hours. Thereafter, the mean prothrombin time was reduced more rapidly in those with the higher doses, though the distinction was not statistically significant. In general the response was the same as that seen with 100 mg. phytonadione injected intravenously.

Personal differences in response were extreme. The authors previously recommended a level of 50% of normal as an index to the normal coagulation mechanism. Of the 10 patients given 25 mg. of the vitamin, 9 reached this level in 24 hours, but only half the patients in the larger and smaller dosage groups did so. Though oral administration is effective, it is essential that the response be followed by actual assay, rather than by reliance on an early test showing immediate response. Further oral or intravenous administration of phytonadione may be needed to establish safe levels after overdosage of anticoagulant or in emergencies requiring termination of hypoprothrombinemia

► ↓ It must be admitted by even the most ardent enthusiasts for anticoagulant therapy that however effective these agents may be in preventing the extension of existing thromboses, or their recurrence, they are not active in promoting dissolution of the original thrombosis itself. For this purpose a fibrinolytic agent is required. The drug streptokinase-streptodornase (Varidase), used in debridement procedures in surgery, is a fibrinolytic agent but it is suitable only for local and topical employment. The fibrinolytic action of this mixture resides in the streptokinase portion and it is only an indirect one since the enzyme activates a plasma constituent called plasminogen, the product of this activation being the active lytic enzyme, plasmin, which very quickly splits the fibrin molecule into large polypeptides. In the succeeding article the feasibility of using this plasmin itself in the treatment of thomboembolism is explored.—Ed.

(8) J.A.M.A. 165:330-333, Sept. 28, 1957.

Thrombolysis with Fibrinolysin (Plasmin)—New Therapeutic Approach to Thromboembolism. Kenneth M. Moser[9] (Georgetown Univ.) studied the effects of intravenously given fibrinolysin (plasmin) in 52 patients with various forms of thromboembolic disease. The resulting increase in fibrinolytic activity of the patient's plasma was demonstrated by laboratory determinations of the rate of dissolution of a standard fibrinogen-thrombin clot. When the dosages were 40,000-50,000 fibrinolytic units, 92% of the recipients manifested an enhanced plasma fibrinolytic activity at some time after the infusion. No hemorrhagic phenomena were encountered in any patient, including 29 who were simultaneously receiving anticoagulant drugs. Disturbances of blood-coagulating factors were minimal.

Although individual patients showed moderate variation in rapidity and degree of response, the over-all experience with fibrinolysin infusion in deep venous thrombophlebitis included (1) loss of heat, tenderness and muscle turgidity and significant decrease in leg size within 24 hours; (2) return of the involved area to its prephlebitic state within 72 hours after infusion; and (3) no recurrence of signs of phlebitis when ambulation was allowed.

Eight patients with pulmonary embolism in whom no definite thrombotic source could be incriminated received fibrinolysin infusion within 72 hours of the embolic event. In 4 patients, fibrinolysin therapy exerted some beneficial effect, as suggested by rapid resolution of ECG abnormalities; rapid relief of chest discomfort, tachypnea and other symptoms and signs induced by embolization; and interruption of a course of recurrent embolization which had not responded to anticoagulant therapy.

Animal studies suggest that rethrombosis after successful clot dissolution may occur if fibrinolysin is used alone but can be prevented if heparin is used concurrently. Therefore, it appears that anticoagulant drugs should be used to avoid rethrombosis in all patients unless circumstances clearly indicate that the factors which led to thrombosis have subsided.

Use of Adenylic Acid Suppositories in Subacute Thrombophlebitis and Varicose Ulcers is reported by Elias D. Lawrence[1] (Paterson, N. J.). Adenosine-5-monophosphate, also

(9) J.A.M.A. 167:1695-1704, Aug. 2, 1958.
(1) Am. J. Surg. 95:434-437, March, 1958.

known as muscle adenylic acid, has been successfully used intramuscularly in pruritus and varicose vein complications. It provides marked relief from itching and decrease in the inflammatory process associated with thrombophlebitis and rapidly clears varicose ulcers.

The author tried suppositories of muscle adenylic acid, each containing 100 mg. adenosine-5-monophosphate, in 51 patients, 23 with subacute thrombophlebitis and 28 with varicose ulcers. In those with varicose veins, use of the drug was limited to treatment of the various complications, i.e., acute, subacute and chronic thrombophlebitis, varicose eczema, stasis cellulitis, epidermitis and varicose ulcers. Varicose veins, per se, without any of these complications do not constitute an indication for this treatment. The objectives of the evaluation were to determine (1) any sensitivity or irritating effects of the suppository itself, (2) any objection of the patient to use of suppositories and (3) the efficacy of treatment as compared with parenteral adenylic acid therapy.

Most patients improved markedly, often within 48-72 hours. No irritation or significant side effects were attributable to use of the suppositories and no objections were made to this form of medication.

Suppositories containing adenosine-5-monophosphate and marketed as My-B-Den® suppositories should be considered an integral part of the therapy for complications of varicose veins and thrombophlebitis.

DERMATOLOGIC MALADIES

Dermatologic Uses of Urea. Albert M. Kligman[2] (Univ. of Pennsylvania) states that, owing to its lack of toxicity, concentrations of urea of 40% or more may be used topically. At these strengths the antibacterial effects of urea are similar to those of the antibiotics, with the further advantage that all the common organisms are susceptible and the possibility of resistant strains need not be seriously considered. Urea also has a strong proteolytic action and is mildly

(2) Acta dermat.-venereol. 37:155-159, 1957.

keratolytic. It is an effective deodorizer, chiefly because it suppresses bacterial overgrowth.

Compresses and soaks of 40% urea may be used advantageously for inflammatory skin lesions which present elements of exudation, suppuration and crusting, especially when there is evidence of secondary infection. It is the "dirty" lesion, regardless of origin, for which urea is suited. Conditions for which urea can be advised, provided the specifications of a "complicated" dermatitis are met, include contact dermatitis pre-eminently, burns, impetiginized eruptions, nummular eczema, various kinds of hand and foot dermatitis and any eczematous process in which suppression of bacteria and debridement appear desirable. If the lesion is of the kind which will not heal spontaneously when it has been "cleaned up" by soaking and compresses the underlying process must be treated by other measures after the superimposed infection has been removed. For the primary pyodermas, impetigo, ecthyma and the like, antibiotic ointments are clearly superior.

Urea is of value for initial local treatment of suppurating wounds, necrotic malignancies, foul ulcers with a purulent slough and similar lesions. The crystals may be liberally sprinkled into the lesion, which is then covered with a wet compress to effect solution, or a 40% compress may be applied directly. If treatment is maintained for 20-30 minutes and repeated several times daily, striking deodorization may be achieved and variable reduction in the accumulated discharge and slough. Streptodornase-streptokinase combinations or trypsin may achieve more debridement in a shorter period, but often the final result is not much more striking. Since these agents are not antibacterial, their deodorizing abilities are far less notable.

Treatment of Chilblains by Phenoxybenzamine: Clinical Trial in General Practice by Southeast Scotland Faculty of the College of General Practitioners is reported by the Faculty Research Committee.[3] The double-blind method was used. Phenoxybenzamine (Dibenzyline®) was administered to some patients and lactose as a control to others. During the 1st week the dosage was 10 mg. once daily. If no undesirable effects occurred and if cure was not achieved at the

(3) Brit. M. J. 2:1521-1522, Dec. 28, 1957.

end of this period, the dose was increased to 10 mg. twice daily during the 2d week. Similarly, during the 3d and 4th weeks of treatment, 10 mg. phenoxybenzamine was administered 3 times daily.

Complete remission of chilblains was observed in 24 of 28 patients who took phenoxybenzamine for 4 weeks and in 17 of 34 who took lactose. The difference is statistically significant. In a group under treatment for less than 4 weeks, results were also better in those taking phenoxybenzamine than in those taking lactose.

Phenoxybenzamine opposes the vasoconstrictor action of the sympathetic nervous system. Undesirable effects are not rare. In 9 of 59 patients given the drug these effects were so severe that administration had to be stopped. In 13 others side effects of lesser degree occurred. These include dizziness, paresthesia, tachycardia, swollen eyelids, lethargy, dryness of the mouth and nasal congestion.

► [Many persons feel excessively fatigued while taking this drug. One should remember also that the condition of a patient with pre-existing cardiovascular disease may be jeopardized by its use since the pressure-sustaining reflexes are eliminated.—Ed.]

Evaluation of Meprobamate in Management of Selected Dermatoses. F. T. Becker, M. G. Fredricks, J. F. Schmid and J. L. Tuura[4] (Duluth, Minn.) gave meprobamate, 400-2,400 mg./day in divided doses, to 260 patients with various dermatoses as an adjunctive to local therapy. Most patients had chronic eruptions or repeated exacerbations of their cutaneous disease and were emotionally disturbed.

An excellent to good effect in all types of disseminated neurodermatitis occurred in nearly 50%. This favorable outcome could be explained by the fact that the drug was only prescribed when tension was a predominant symptom. The reason for the good results in seborrheic dermatitis and psoriasis is unknown. Meprobamate alone gave little relief from pruritus. It was not as efficient as the anticholinergic drugs in reducing hyperhidrosis. Allergic reactions were encountered in nearly 4% of the patients treated, and undesirable side effects occurred in 10%. Except for 1 suicide, there were no serious sequelae.

Meprobamate is a satisfactory sedative in therapy of se-

(4) A.M.A. Arch. Dermat. 77:406-411, April, 1958.

lected patients with dermatoses when relief from emotional tension is important.

Therapeutic Effectivenesss of Raudixin® in Psoriasis: Impression Type Study. Using the double-blind technic, Samuel J. Zakon, Malcolm Spencer and J. Harvey Johnston[5] studied the effectiveness of Raudixin in 95 patients with psoriasis and 24 with other dermatologic conditions. Since Raudixin was used as adjunctive therapy, the usual modalities of treatment were continued: topical applications, nonspecific parenteral injections, autohemotherapy, dietary restrictions, ultraviolet light and x-ray therapy. However, no other tranquilizing drugs were prescribed. Initial Raudixin dosage consisted of 2 tablets at bedtime; after tolerance was established, this was increased to 3 or 4 tablets daily.

About one fourth of the patients were resistant to all therapy, one fourth showed minimal response and half achieved 50-100% improvement. This was true whether they received Raudixin or placebo. No significant untoward reactions to the medication were noted. Many patients commented that they slept better and were less nervous. Among patients with psoriasis the better results occurred in the summer months. Although the consensus among those who participated in the study was that Raudixin had no specific effect on psoriasis per se, those who received the drug were more calm about being afflicted with psoriasis and were easier to manage.

Sulfonylurea Derivatives in Treatment of Psoriasis Vulgaris: Preliminary Report. G. Kabelitz and W. Kappel[6] switched 2 diabetic patients with psoriasis from insulin to Artosin, a benzolsulfonylurea derivative. After 3-4 weeks' treatment with 0.5-1 Gm. Artosin daily, the psoriasis improved considerably. Trial of Artosin in 25 more psoriatic patients without diabetes led to healing or great improvement in 17 during a follow-up of 6-12 months. Only far-advanced and extensive psoriasis responded to Artosin. Response was independent of age, sex or age at onset of the disease. A hypoglycemic reaction which required discontinuance of the medication occurred only once. In mild reactions, temporary reduction of the dose sufficed.

(5) Quart. Bull. Northwestern Univ. M. School 32:131-134, Summer, 1958.
(6) Deutsche med. Wchnschr. 83:1167, July 4, 1958.

The effective daily dose of Artosin is 0.5-1 Gm., given in 2 divided doses. Improvement can be expected in 15-20 days. Medication must be continued until cure or great improvement. A smaller maintenance dose is advisable afterward. A relapse calls for a new course of Artosin. The mode of action of the drug in psoriasis is unknown.

Three-Way Therapeutic Effectiveness of Tar-Steroid Cream. Ashton L. Welsh and Mitchell Ede[7] (Cincinnati), who studied 367 patients for 20 months, report that in certain selected dermatoses the tar-steroid combination, Tarcortin, is more effective than the alcoholic extract of crude coal tar in cream form or hydrocortisone alone. Tarcortin contains 5% refined alcoholic extract of crude coal tar, lanolin and methol, incorporated in a nongreasy vanishing-cream base, combined with 0.5% hydrocortisone (free alcohol).

Prompt, satisfactory response was obtained when the tar-steroid cream was prescribed for patients presenting acute episodes of atopic dermatitis, contact dermatitis, psoriasis, chronic infectious eczematoid dermatitis and other eczematous dermatoses. From past experience it was known that in such conditions an ointment containing the plain alcoholic extract of crude coal tar would not be tolerated. Formerly, the authors had to wait for the cooling down of such dermatoses by use of wet dressings, bland lotions or ointments. With the tar-steroid cream, however, prompt remission of the acute phase was achieved and the patient could be tided over until the anti-pruritic and anti-eczematic effects of tar therapy could be exerted. Thereafter, appropriate coal-tar therapy alone could be used, with consequent reduction in cost to the patient. Dermatoses deemed to be so acute that they could not be controlled by tar-steroid cream were not included in this study.

Of the 367 patients, 165 were 100% cleared, 173 were 75-100% improved, 19 were 50-74% improved, 7 showed no improvement and 3 had suggestive but unconfirmed reaction. These results were considerably better than those obtained in 150 controls who had received therapy with alcoholic extract of crude coal-tar cream before start of therapy with the tar-steroid combination. Folliculitis developed in only 1 pa-

(7) J.A.M.A. 166:158-159, Jan. 11, 1958.

tient during therapy. No instance of sun sensitization was noted.

Use of Relaxin in Treatment of Scleroderma. Animal studies have shown that relaxin [Releasin®] increases elasticity of the skin. Gus G. Casten and Robert J. Boucek[8] (Univ. of Miami) treated 23 patients who had different stages of scleroderma with relaxin for 6-30 months. For 2 weeks before start of therapy or simultaneously with it, all were given 1.25 mg. conjugated estrogenic substances (Premarin®) for priming purposes. A saline solution of relaxin was given subcutaneously or intramuscularly in amounts of 20 mg. twice daily for 1-2 weeks, then a gelatin preparation was substituted in amounts of about 10 mg. intramuscularly daily. To maintain the effects of relaxin, it was necessary to administer the hormone daily or every other day. Beneficial effects from the hormone injections usually were not evident until the patient had been receiving therapy for 3-5 weeks.

Of 21 patients with a significant degree of Raynaud's phenomenon, 18 noted improvement after treatment. The improvement, which was transitory in nature, began 2-3 hours after injection of 20 mg. of the saline solution of relaxin and persisted for 7-8 hours. When relaxin in the slowly absorbed gelatin base was given, reduction of the vasospastic phenomenon was maintained for 24 hours or longer. With some of the even more slowly absorbed agents, the effect persisted for 2-3 days. In only 2 patients was Raynaud's phenomenon completely ameliorated while the patients received relaxin.

Of 18 patients with trophic ulcers, 14 noted great improvement; most observed complete healing of the ulcers. Generalized skin tightness was observed in 22 patients, but after treatment, 16 noted softening and loosening of the skin, particularly of the face and upper extremities. Withdrawal of relaxin caused return within 3-10 days of Raynaud's phenomenon and the skin tightness. Side effects were minor: in 3 female patients, menorrhagia occurred during the first few menstrual periods after start of therapy; 1 patient noted distressing local reactions; 1 noted gynecomastia that disappeared after the hormone dose was reduced; and 3 had weakness, sufficient in 1 patient to discontinue therapy.

(8) J.A.M.A. 166:319-324, Jan. 25, 1958.

Other manifestations of scleroderma, such as renal, pulmonary or myocardial failure, were unaltered by relaxin.

Since no consistently successful therapy has been reported for scleroderma, relaxin represents a therapeutic advance because it significantly influences certain distressing features of the disease.

► [There are articles on relaxin in the Obstetrics and Gynecology section of the book.—Ed.]

Efficacy of Tetracycline-Nystatin in Therapy of Pustular Dermatoses. Charles R. Rein, Leonard A. Lewis and Lionel A. Dick[9] (New York) divided 350 patients with various pustular dermatoses (mainly acne vulgaris) into 4 groups and placed them on the following regimens: (1) 250 mg. tetracycline 4 times a day; (2) 250 mg. tetracycline and 250,000 units of nystatin (an antifungus antibiotic) 4 times a day; (3) 500 mg. tetracycline 4 times a day; and (4) 500 mg. tetracycline and 500,000 units of nystatin 4 times a day. Treatment was continued 4 weeks, unless earlier complete involution of skin lesions or serious drug toxicity occurred.

Therapeutic response in the 312 patients who completed therapy was similarly excellent with any of these regimens. Concentrations of tetracycline in the serum were the same whether tetracycline-nystatin or tetracycline alone was administered, indicating that nystatin neither enhances nor interferes with the absorption of tetracycline.

The over-all incidence of gastrointestinal and other side effects was similar with tetracycline-nystatin and tetracycline alone, though nausea and vomiting were more frequent with the former (at a 2-Gm. daily dosage schedule but not with 1 Gm.), and frequent bowel movements and frank diarrhea with the latter. Though the frequency of side effects of tetracycline therapy possibly due to monilial overgrowth was somewhat higher in those exhibiting a positive candida complement fixation test before treatment, this finding cannot be considered to be of practical significance.

The tetracycline-nystatin combination need not be used routinely in instances in which tetracycline therapy is required. However, its use is indicated in selected patients in whom the possibility of monilial superinfection is relatively great. These include debilitated and/or geriatric patients,

(9) Antibiotic Med. & Clin. Therap. 4:771-780, December, 1957.

infants and those who require prolonged tetracycline therapy.

Sulfapyridine in Dermatitis Herpetiformis: Report of Case under 11 Years of Continuous Treatment is presented by Merril M. Cooper[1] (New York Univ. Post-Grad. Med. School). The response of dermatitis herpetiformis to sulfapyridine is difficult to interpret, as neither the mechanism of action in this disease nor the etiology of the disease itself are known. The mechanism is unlikely to be an antibacterial action against the disease or against a focus of infection, since as little as 0.5 Gm. daily may control symptoms and clinical manifestations for prolonged periods. Sulfapyridine generally induces a good therapeutic response in dermatitis herpetiformis, but some patients cannot tolerate the drug because of side effects which include nausea, malaise, vertigo, mental depression, rash and agranulocytosis. In these patients, the sulfones often prove beneficial.

Woman, 56, had an itching, crusting eruption that began on the arms and legs and then became generalized. She had up to palm-sized patches of grouped, excoriated, papulovesicular lesions, widely distributed over the entire body except on the face, neck, hands, feet and genitalia. Some hyperpigmentation was present in the subsiding and healed areas. She had coin-shaped eczematous plaques on the medial surface of one ankle.

She was started on sulfapyridine 3 Gm. daily with sodium bicarbonate orally. Within a week the eruption was 80% improved, pruritus was less and no new lesions developed. When the dose was reduced to 2 Gm. daily, pruritus reappeared, and it again subsided when the dose was increased to 3 Gm. One month later the drug had to be discontinued because of neutropenia, but 7 days later pruritus again recurred and did not respond to 2 Gm. but did to 3 Gm. daily. The patient was adequately maintained on 1-2 Gm. daily. Five years after the drug was started it was again discontinued but had to be resumed because of increased pruritus. For 2 years control was adequate with only 0.5 Gm. daily, but later this had to be increased to 1 Gm. because of increased crusting. Since then she has been maintained on 0.5 Gm. daily and is doing well. If she neglects to take 1 tablet, pruritus develops within 24 hours. Regular blood studies have shown no abnormality, since the neutropenia which developed during the 3d month of therapy.

Use of Polyvinylpyrrolidone Iodine in Eczematoid Ringworm is favored by Theodore Cornbleet, Sidney Barsky and Ben Firestein[2] (Univ. of Illinois), because of its observed effectiveness in 50 patients. Povicone, containing 10% aque-

(1) U. S. Armed Forces M. J. 9:907-910, June, 1958.
(2) A.M.A. Arch. Dermat. 77:335-336, March, 1958.

ous polyvinylpyrrolidone, equivalent to 1% available iodine, 0.5% sodium iodide, 1% glycerin and a wetting agent, gave excellent results in 24 patients, some improvement in 17 and had no effect in 8. Topical application twice daily gave better results than daily applications, but more frequent use offered no advantage. No irritation or other untoward effects were seen, and no patient had a relapse during therapy. Polyvinylpyrrolidone iodine is therefore suitable for prolonged use and as a preventive.

Reactions to Chloroquine Observed during Treatment of Various Dermatologic Disorders. Chloroquine [Aralen®] as used commonly in dermatologic practice has relatively low toxicity, even in a prolonged course of therapy extending over weeks, months or years. Leon Goldman and Robert H. Preston[3] (Univ. of Cincinnati) found the most frequent reactions are anorexia, weight loss, nervousness, nausea and difficulty in visual accommodation. Many of these symptoms disappear with reduction in dosage without interruption of medication. Maculopapular cutaneous eruptions occasionally occur. Such eruptions recur in some patients if chloroquine is administered again after being discontinued but not in others. Lichenoid and exfoliative eruptions are uncommon results of chloroquine sensitivity. Liver damage and leukopenia are also rare.

Attention to minor reactions to chloroquine will often prevent more serious reactions later. Hydroxychloroquine (Plaquenil®) is usually, but not always, more easily tolerated than chloroquine.

► [Reasoning that the efficacy of antimalarial agents in certain dermatoses may be explained on the basis of their ability to screen out ultraviolet light, Cornbleet (1957-58 Year Book, p. 151) used these drugs in psoriasis, a malady that is benefited by exposure to ultraviolet light. The eruption became more acute and spreading in all the patients and in one instance developed into exfoliative dermatitis.—Ed.]

Cadmium Shampoo Treatment of Seborrheic Dermatitis. J. Fred Mullins and James R. Barnett[4] (Univ. of Texas) report results of treatment in 200 patients with seborrheic dermatitis of the scalp. The patients were instructed to use their regular shampoos to cleanse the scalp every 3-7 days. This was followed by 2 latherings with a shampoo containing 1% cadmium sulfide. The last application was left on the scalp

---

(3) Am. J. Trop. Med. 6:654-657, July, 1957.
(4) Texas J. Med. 53:640-642, August, 1957.

about 10 minutes. Criteria for good results included absence of scaliness, lack of pruritus and patient acceptance. Results were considered good in 77.5%, fair in 10.5% and poor in 12%. In 60, results were compared with those achieved with selenium disulfide. Cadmium sulfide was considered equally as effective by 27 patients, but over-all patient acceptance favored cadmium; 6 felt that cadmium was superior, and 25 felt that selenium was superior. In 2 patients, neither shampoo was beneficial.

The only untoward reactions to cadmium shampoo were 2 possible cases of contact dermatitis. The hair did not become oily after its use, and gray hair was not discolored. Cadmium sulfide is not a definitive cure, but it is useful in control of chronic or recurrent seborrheic dermatitis of the scalp.

Treatment of Aphthous Ulceration of Mouth. This common minor malady usually appears as a single ulcer or small crop of ulcers on the buccal mucous membrane several times a year. Most often they are on the inside of the cheeks, opposite the molar teeth, inside the lips and occasionally on the tongue. They are painful, interfere with speech and eating, but normally run a short course and heal in about a week without scarring. The major form is more severe. Ulcers are multiple and the patient may be seldom, if ever, free from them over the course of years. Illness may be incapacitating.

The ulcers may be only one feature of a disease involving several mucous membranes and skin, such as erythema multiforme (Stevens-Johnson syndrome) and Behçet's syndrome, or they may be a symptom of some underlying disease such as tropical sprue, idiopathic steatorrhea or ulcerative colitis. Since the etiology is unknown, treatment has been empiric. Simple mouth washes and paints yield little benefit. Cautery with a silver nitrate stick or chromic acid solution enlarges the ulcers and is likely to cause residual scarring. Folic acid, nicotinamide, riboflavin, vitamin B mixture, small doses of cortisone orally, ethisterone and local radiotherapy are all ineffective. S. C. Truelove and R. M. Morris-Owen[5] (Oxford, England) devised a tablet especially for use in the mouth which contained 2.5 mg. hydrocortisone in its hemisuccinate sodium form, a compound freely soluble in water and dissolving slowly.

(5) Brit. M. J. 1:603-607, Mar. 15, 1958.

In 23 patients with the minor form of aphthous ulceration, 1 tablet placed near the ulcer to dissolve (which takes about ¾ hour) usually completely relieves pain. This is repeated up to 4 times daily until the ulcer disappears. When the ulcer is fully developed before treatment, healing takes 36-48 hours. If treatment is given early, while the ulcer is 1-2 mm. in diameter, healing is commonly complete by the next day.

Girl, 16, had recurrent aphthous ulcers. An unusually severe ulcer developed and was treated by placing a tablet in the mouth in contact with it. The next morning it appeared to be healing and was not painful. By the 2d day it was gone. Four recurrences since then were treated while the aphthous ulcers were still small, and in none of these instances did a full ulcer develop. A conspicuous feature was prompt relief of pain.

In 22 cases of the major form, treatment was started with 1 tablet 4 times daily and continued until ulceration had ceased. Maintenance therapy of 2-4 tablets daily has kept 5 patients completely free from ulceration for months, but most of the others have continued to get sporadic sore spots, though without ulceration. Only one showed a tendency to relapse during treatment. Seven special cases associated with Behçet's syndrome, erythema multiforme, idiopathic steatorrhea and ulcerative colitis also responded well. Since the maximum dose has been 4 tablets daily, this represents only 10 mg. hydrocortisone, which is unlikely to have any harmful systemic effects. None was noted in these patients.

Dermatitis of Diaper Region: New Remedy for an Old Affliction. Because of good results achieved by others in prophylaxis and management of diaper dermatitis with an emulsion containing silicones, glyoxyl diureide and hexachlorophene, Henry W. Kaessler[6] (Mt. Vernon, N. Y.) investigated the efficacy of a similar combination in a fine talc base (Baby Silicare Powder). Complete clearing of severe dermatitis of the diaper region occurred in all of 84 infants on whom the test powder was used. Time required for clearing was 6-28 days. During the same period, 8 of 42 infants treated with preparations normally used in routine hospital care failed to respond.

The test powder was used in prevention of diaper rash in 127 infants. Among 51 infants whose diapers were changed day and night whenever necessary, diaper rash occurred in

(6) Arch. Pediat. 74:47-50, February, 1957.

6. Among 76 whose diapers were changed only 3 times a day and after a bowel movement, dermatitis occurred in 16.

Tolerance of the test powder was entirely satisfactory in all infants. Patch tests in more than 200 were all negative. The rationale for the efficacy of the test powder lies in the ability of silicone to repel moisture, the stability and nonirritant keratolytic qualities of diureide of glyoxilic acid which stimulates epithelial healing and the nonsensitizing bacteriostatic attributes of hexachlorophene.

Thyroid-Iodine Therapy of Blastomycosis. Use of iodides has been standard therapy for the deep mycoses during the past half century. It has withstood well the test of time, not because it was remarkably effective, but because there was no remedy quite as good. In view of the relative innocuousness of iodide directly for deep mycotic organisms in vitro and the pre-eminent position of it in the thyroid alone of the organs of the body, it was felt that approach to treatment of blastomycosis through that gland might be fruitful.

Theodore Cornbleet[7] (Univ. of Illinois) first tried blocking the thyroid by use of antithyroid agents (propylthiouracil). Bad results, as described in a patient, led to the use of glandular products instead.

Man, 34, had a solid raised verrucous patch of dermatitis, 5 cm. at its greatest diameter, below the right scapula and a smaller lesion above the right clavicle from which blastomycetes were cultivated and shown directly. He was given 9.71 Gm. potassium iodide 3 times a day and 50 mg. propylthiouracil twice a day. Within 5 days the lesions enlarged and became more inflamed. Propylthiouracil was stopped and 0.065 Gm. thyroid substituted. Five days later the thyroid dose was raised to 0.130 Gm. and the potassium iodide to 1.746 Gm. a day. Two weeks later there was noticeable improvement in the lesions. The dose was increased progressively during the first 6 weeks to 0.389 Gm. thyroid and 90 drops of iodide solution. The lesions became dry, pale and flat, and 2 weeks later the crusts separated, leaving slightly depigmented atrophic areas somewhat smaller than the original lesions. Active treatment was continued 2 weeks longer, a total of 10 weeks. There has been no recurrence in 7 years nor any new formation of papules or pustules in the healed scars, as often is noted in blastomycosis.

Subsequently combined thyroid and iodide was used in 9 patients with blastomycosis: 7 had cutaneous and 2 had systemic types of infections. All were clinically cured. Two others with blastomycosis and 1 with systemic sporotrichosis

(7) A.M.A. Arch. Dermat. 76:545-548, November, 1957.

treated with thyroid and iodide by colleagues were reported to be favorably influenced.

Clinical results, therefore, would seem to show that thyroid administration enhances the effects of iodide in blastomycosis. There are insufficient data to clarify how this is accomplished.

Evaluation of Steroids in Systemic Lupus Erythematosus with Particular Emphasis on Triamcinolone and Methylprednisolone is presented by Edmund L. Dubois[8] (Univ. of Southern California). Methylprednisolone (Medrol®) was tried in 16 patients with systemic lupus erythematosus. The average duration of therapy was 2.9 (maximum 7) months. The potency of this hormone is equal to prednisone milligram for milligram. Clinical results and side effects closely paralleled those observed with prednisone. No distinct advantages of this steroid over the older ones were noted. In 1 patient in whom muscular weakness developed on triamcinolone, this disappeared after transfer to hydrocortisone. Within 2 months after she was placed on methylprednisolone, 32 mg./day, she had an identical recurrence of muscle weakness; 2 weeks after transfer back to hydrocortisone, strength again began to improve.

Triamcinolone (Aristocort®), a new synthetic unsaturated prednisolone derivative, was given to 31 patients with systemic lupus erythematosus for up to 14½ months. This hormone is 1.3 times as powerful as prednisone and 4.4 times more potent than hydrocortisone as an anti-inflammatory agent.

Fourteen patients had received prior steroid therapy with all the older anti-inflammatory hormones, and 7 were better controlled and felt better with triamcinolone than with previous steroids. The average initial dose in mild systemic lupus erythematosus was 20.6 mg./day. The average maintenance dose used to control mild exacerbations was 26 mg./day. There was no evidence of sodium retention or potassium loss. Routine sodium restriction, potassium supplement or prophylactic ulcer diet were not used.

Sixteen patients had upper gastrointestinal series before and every 1-2 months after start of triamcinolone therapy. There was evidence of peptic ulceration in only 1 patient

(8) Metabolism 7 (pt. 2):509-525, July, 1958.

who was receiving 96 mg. triamcinolone/day. Gastric analyses after histamine (9 patients) and 24-hour urine uropepsin determinations (13 patients) were done before and about every 2 months during triamcinolone therapy. No significant changes were found, even in the patient with the new ulcer.

The pattern of clinical improvement closely paralleled that obtained by previous treatment with older steroids. All clinical and laboratory abnormalities produced by the disease, except long-standing renal involvement, disappeared. A major difference between triamcinolone and other steroids was a tendency noted in 18 patients toward progressive, gradual weight loss, averaging 7.8% of initial body weight. Some of this was due to fluid loss; however, Cushing appearance caused by prior therapy with other steroids did not disappear. Cutaneous side effects, particularly Cushing appearance, hirsutism and striae, were more marked than with older steroids. The most serious side effect was muscle weakness, which appeared in 6 patients 4-32 weeks after start of triamcinolone. There seemed to be no relation between the dose and this symptom. Male patients showed no Cushing features on this steroid, even in doses as high as 48 mg./day for 6 weeks. In men this may be the steroid of choice.

► [Regarding the two agents employed in the studies described in this and the 3 succeeding articles, Medrol and Aristocort, one should still have tongue in cheek. These corticosteroids, prednisolone substitutes, have only their newness so far established; superiority and lower toxicity remain to be determined. Smaller dosage is in itself no advantage unless it means a lower cost to the patient.—Ed.]

Treatment of Psoriasis and other Dermatoses with Triamcinolone (Aristocort®). Walter B. Shelley, Joseph S. Harun and Donald M. Pillsbury[9] (Univ. of Pennsylvania) treated 60 patients who had all forms, types and degrees of psoriasis with triamcinolone, a corticosteroid, in doses of 12-16 mg. daily by mouth. In 36 patients, response was prompt and unquestionable; within a week the scaling and erythema diminished significantly, and within 2-4 weeks of continued adequate dosage the psoriasis was, in some, completely erased. This group presented the distinctive finding of local involution of psoriasis at the site of injection of triamcinolone intradermally. Relapses invariably occurred

(9) J.A.M.A. 167:959-964, June 21, 1958.

when triamcinolone was withheld. Topical triamcinolone was without effect.

A wide variety of reversible side effects was observed. Some were favorable, such as stimulation of hair growth in alopecia areata, and many were unfavorable, such as flushing, hyperhidrosis, facial hirsutism and facial contour changes. Triamcinolone proved remarkably effective in treatment of alopecia areata. This compound seems to have a specific stimulant effect on hair growth. In view of the rapid relapse which invariably followed suspension of triamcinolone therapy for psoriasis, reduction of the dose to zero will probably offer great difficulty in many patients.

Triamcinolone was highly antiallergic, anti-rheumatic and anti-inflammatory and, therefore, useful in various dermatitides. Its use in psoriasis should probably be limited to acute extending cases not controllable by other means or to extensive, severe chronic forms.

Use of New Corticosteroid (Aristocort® Diacetate) in Dermatology. Charles R. Rein, Raul Fleischmajer and Albert L. Rosenthal[1] (New York) treated 26 patients who had severe dermatoses, often generalized, with marked inflammatory changes and uncontrollable pruritus. Most of them had previously received prolonged courses of prednisolone, with satisfactory results, but many had side effects. Aristocort (triamcinolone diacetate) was given in initial dosage ranging from 10 to 32 mg. daily. Maintenance levels required for complete control of symptoms varied from 4 to 16 mg. daily. No dietary limitations, such as sodium restriction, were imposed, and no supplemental potassium was prescribed.

Marked improvement was noted in 16 patients with generalized incapacitating atopic dermatitis. Some patients were controlled on maintenance doses as low as 4-6 mg. daily. Similar results were obtained in 2 patients with dermatitis herpetiformis. In 2 patients with exfoliative dermatitis of long duration, who had relapsed while receiving 20 mg. prednisolone daily, the condition was controlled with 20 mg. Aristocort and then maintained satisfactorily on 10-12 mg. daily. A third patient who relapsed while receiving 15 mg. prednisolone was controlled with 12 mg. Aristocort daily. The condition of 1 patient with severe generalized angio-

(1) J.A.M.A. 165:1821-1823, Dec. 7, 1957.

neurotic edema was completely under control 48 hours after initiation of therapy with 32 mg. Aristocort daily. A patient with alopecia totalis showed considerable regrowth of hair 2 weeks after initiation of therapy with 32 mg. daily.

Aristocort was more active than prednisolone, in that similar therapeutic efficacy was obtained with two-thirds to three-fourths the equivalent dosage. The incidence of side effects due to Aristocort was low, and in no instance was it necessary to interrupt therapy. Some patients with moon facies due to previous prednisolone therapy showed an improvement in this condition while taking Aristocort. Two patients had gastrointestinal symptoms (1 had transient nausea and the other mild abdominal cramps). One patient had headaches and tremors. Two patients exhibited a mild acneiform eruption on the face after 2 weeks of therapy. One patient with pemphigus erythematosus had received previous therapy with prednisolone with an initial dosage of 60 mg. daily. Glycosuria developed after 7 weeks and persisted when therapy was continued with Aristocort.

Clinical Response of Dermatoses to 6-Methylprednisolone. Lawrence C. Goldberg[2] gave 6-methylprednisolone to 201 patients with 17 dermatoses. Average starting dosage was 8-12 mg. daily; this was reduced as soon as individual response warranted. Treatment was usually continued 10 or more days after the patient was well. Rebound reactions did not appear as frequent when the drug was suddenly stopped as they had with other corticosteroids. Though this series included patients with cardiac disease, diabetes and previous peptic ulcer, only 11 patients had side actions; 3 had gastric symptoms, 2 depression, 1 excitation, 3 mild acne and 2 cramping pains in the legs. Most reactions were seen in the first 7 days of treatment.

When 6-methylprednisolone is used systemically as adjunctive therapy, it enhances the effectiveness of local treatment and helps shorten the disease. Dermatoses with allergic backgrounds give the best response. Ointments of 6-methylprednisolone in 0.25 and 0.5% concentrations are of value when applied locally in indicated cutaneous diseases.

Of the 201 patients, 159 had a better than 70% improvement within a relatively short time while receiving the drug

(2) Metabolism 7 (pt. 2):530-533, July, 1958.

RESPONSE OF VARIOUS DERMATOSES TO 6-METHYLPREDNISOLONE

Dermatoses	*No. of Cases*	*Dosage per day*	*Less than 50% improvement*	*Better than 70% Improvement*	*Reactions*
1. Psoriasis vulgaris					
Acute	4	8–12 mg.		4	
Chronic	14	8–12 mg.	8	6	(1)* cramping pains in legs
2. Seborrheic dermatitis	20	8 mg.	4	16	(2) gastric complaints
3. Dermatitis venenata (vegetation)	20	8 mg.	2	18	(1) depression
4. Contact dermatitis	22	8 mg.	7	15	(1) gastric complaints
5. Infectious eczematoid dermatitis	21	8–12 mg.	4	17	(2) development of acne
6. Dermatitis medicamentosa	5	8–12 mg.	1	4	
7. Urticaria	17	8–12 mg.	3	14	
8. Atopic dermatitis	13	6–8 mg.	5	8	(1) development of acne
9. Erythema multiforme	9	8–12 mg.	1	8	(1) excitation
10. Alopecia areata	6	8–12 mg.		6	(1) cramping pains in legs
11. Hodgkin's disease	3	12 mg.		3	
12. Pyoderma gangrenosum	2	12–24 mg.		2	
13. Herpes zoster	9	8–12 mg.	4	5	
14. "Id" reactions	28	8–12 mg.	3	25	
15. Subacute lupus erythematosus	2	8–12 mg.		2	
16. Sarcoidosis	1	8–12 mg.		1	
17. Actinic dermatitis	5	8–12 mg.		5	(1) depression
Total	201		42	159	11

*Numbers in parentheses indicate number of times each reaction was observed in this study.

(table). This justifies the use of 6-methylprednisolone, an improved and superior corticosteroid, as adjunctive therapy in dermatologic problems, many of which have resisted conventional treatment.

Topical Hydrocortisone Therapy in Acne Rosacea and Acne Vulgaris is discussed by Stuart C. Way, George C. Andrews (San Francisco) and Anthony N. Domonkos[3] (New York). Hydrocortisone (alcohol) is thought to prevent hyperkeratosis at the follicular orifices and subsequent occlusion and irritation and to mitigate perifollicular inflammation and hyperemia. These functions could prove to be valuable adjuncts, particularly in treatment of rosacea with extensive flush areas. Topical application would achieve

(3) New York J. Med. 57:3463-3465, Nov. 1, 1957.

concentration of dosage at the site of desired action without subjecting the patient to undesirable side effects through the systemic circulation.

The authors tried 2% resorcin, 5% colloidal sulfur, 8.5% N-sulfanilyl-acetamide and 0.25% hydrocortisone (alcohol) in a flesh-colored lotion containing zinc oxide, talc, iron oxides, propylene glycol, alcohol and water. The pH of the lotion was 5.9. Concomitantly other hygienic and therapeutic measures, including frequent removal of comedones, incision and drainage of pustules, proper cleansing of the skin, frequent shampoos and dietary measures were instituted. In severe cases internal medication with sulfonamides or antibiotics was prescribed. The lotion was tried on 170 patients with acne vulgaris and 32 with acne rosacea. The results could be evaluated in 156 patients who had a long enough follow-up. Excellent to good results were achieved in 75.1% of those with acne vulgaris and in 70.3% with acne rosacea.

Treatment of Ophthalmic Zoster with Prednisone. A. Barham Carter and J. E. Royds[4] treated 15 consecutive patients with prednisone and antibiotics and compared the results with those achieved without prednisone in a similar group treated in 1951. Prednisone was given in doses of 10 mg. every 6 hours for 4 days, followed by 10 mg. every 8 hours for 3 days. The dose was then reduced by 5 mg. each day until it was discontinued on the 15th day. Tetracycline was given in doses of 250 mg. every 6 hours for 7 days. Vitamin B complex was also given for 7 days. Locally, oxytetracycline cream 1% was applied to the rash; and atropine 1%, sulfacetamide 30% and hydrocortisone 1% were applied as drops in the eye.

Edema was less and the eruption dried quicker in the treated group. The lesions were more hemorrhagic than in the control group and pustule formation in early treated cases was minimal. Fresh lesions did not appear after 24 hours of treatment, and scarring was considerably reduced. Herpetic pain was much less severe in the treated group, but no effect on postherpetic neuralgia was observed.

All patients in both groups showed conjunctivitis, and in the treated group 6 patients had keratitis with some evidence of iridocyclitis. In 1 patient it was severe enough to require

(4) Brit. M. J. 2:746-748, Sept. 28, 1957.

tarsorrhaphy, and 1 patient had a panophthalmitis with complete loss of vision. This patient was not admitted until the 16th day of illness and the tarsorrhaphy patient was first treated on the 7th day. In the control group, 8 patients had keratitis and iridocyclitis; 2 required tarsorrhaphy and 2 had corneal scarring sufficient to impair vision severely. Prednisone treatment seemed to have no effect on the incidence of ophthalmic complications, but seemed beneficial for such complications when they occurred.

The earlier prednisone is started the better will be the result, and such treatment is probably useless after the first 10 days, except locally for the eye. By using prednisone rather than cortisone and restricting treatment to 2 weeks, complications were avoided. The use of antibiotics with prednisone is considered essential to prevent septicemia as a complication of the secondary skin infection.

► [Warning! see the next article.—Ed.]

Injudicious Use of Steroid-Containing Eye Drops may exacerbate herpes simplex keratitis, leading to loss of vision or even loss of the eye, according to Donald P. Tucker[5] (Massachusetts Eye and Ear Infirm.). Attention of the general practitioner is called to reports in ophthalmic literature indicating that rare complications of herpetic infection have become more frequent and severe since the advent of topical steroid preparations. Without the aid of the slit lamp, irritation may be diagnosed as simple conjunctivitis and be treated with an antibiotic-steroid combination. A week or two later, the patient may have a deep stromal ulcer, resulting in permanent scars in the pupillary area. Fungus keratitis has also been reported on the increase since the use of topical steroids in eye therapy.

Contact Dermatitis Treated with Fludrocortisone: Steroid-Antibiotic Combination in Inflammatory Dermatoses. Sigmund J. Clayman[6] (Perth Amboy) treated 60 patients who had various inflammatory dermatoses with lotion or ointment (Florinef-S®) containing 0.1% fludrocortisone combined with 0.25% neomycin sulfate and 0.25% Gramicidin®. In 28 of 36 patients with contact dermatitis, improvement was obtained rapidly, and in the other 8 the effect was

(5) New England J. Med. 258:946-947, May 8, 1958.
(6) J. M. Soc. New Jersey 55:168-169, April, 1958.

satisfactory. Of 24 patients with various inflammatory skin conditions, 17 showed marked and prompt improvement, and 7 had satisfactory results. In only 1 case (pityriasis rosea) was no relief from itching obtained.

Transient local irritation was observed in 2 cases, but it was not necessary to discontinue therapy. There was no evidence of percutaneous absorption of the steroid.

Lotion or ointment containing 0.1% Florinef-S® is regarded as among the most effective medications available for treatment of contact dermatitis and other inflammatory dermatoses, especially for relief of pruritus.

Topically Applied Prednisone and Prednisolone in Treatment of Selected Dermatoses. Gerald R. Frolow, Victor H. Witten and Marion B. Sulzberger[7] (New York) treated a small group of patients with various skin diseases generally responsive to topical hydrocortisone therapy with 2 different lots of prednisone, 2 different lots of prednisolone, with 1% hydrocortisone and with the blank vehicle. In most cases the method of symmetical paired comparison was used.

The results indicated no essential difference in the therapeutic effectiveness of topically applied prednisone and prednisolone. Neither 0.5% of the first prednisone or 0.5% of the first prednisolone was as effective as 1% hydrocortisone. However, 0.5% concentrations of the second batches of prednisone and prednisolone were as effective as the hydrocortisone ointment. The second batches of prednisone and prednisolone were said by the manufacturer to be more purified, but they appeared to be chemically and physically identical with the original product.

There was a high incidence of worsening of the dermatoses following use of the first lots of prednisone and prednisolone ointments (4 of 13 patients made worse). Such worsening is rare with hydrocortisone and with the hydrocortisone derivatives previously tested in topical therapy. This untoward effect did not occur in any cases treated with later lots of these compounds. The number of patients treated in this study is too small to permit definite conclusions.

Treatment of Pemphigus with Corticosteroids: Study of 52 Patients treated in the dermatologic wards of Bellevue Hospital is presented by Maurice J. Costello, Leon Jaimo-

(7) A.M.A. Arch. Dermat. 76:185-188, August, 1957.

vich and Marvin Dannenberg.[8] Of 50 whites, 60% were Jews. Of the total patients, 42 (81%)had pemphigus vulgaris, 5 pemphigus foliaceus, 4 pemphigus erythematosus and 1 pemphigus vegetans. The sex incidence was about equal.

The initial site of the pemphigus bullae was the mucous membranes of the mouth in nearly 55% of the patients. The high incidence of this site is important in early diagnosis of pemphigus vulgaris. Unruptured bullae are rarely seen on the oral mucosa because their thin walls are immediately ruptured by mastication and deglutition. Persistent, eroded patches of the oral mucous membranes, especially in adults, should prompt a thorough skin examination. After exclusion of Vincent's infection, desquamative gingivitis, gangrenous stomatitis, syphilis, vitamin deficiency and drug eruptions, a patient with mucosal bullae should be considered as having pemphigus until proved otherwise. Early diagnosis and treatment may not only save the patient's life but also prevent the distressing side effects of prolonged steroid therapy.

To bring pemphigus under control as rapidly as possible, it was found efficacious to administer initial high doses of corticosteroids. If the urgency was great, 25 units of corticotropin dissolved in 500-1,000 cc. of 5% dextrose was administered intravenously daily, or 40 units of repository corticotropin was given twice daily. In less urgent but moderately extensive eruptions, 20 (5-mg.) tablets of prednisone were given daily until the disease was controlled. The dose was then gradually reduced to maintenance level, which was usually 20-40 mg. daily for several weeks or longer. Most patients eventually required only 15-20 mg. daily. It was advantageous to augment this routine with 40 units of repository corticotropin intramuscularly once or twice a week. Several patients showed complications of steroid therapy and the disease recurred promptly after discontinuation of the drug. In these cases, it was usually decided to re-treat the patient with corticosteroids in view of the hopeless prognosis with other forms of therapy.

Pemphigus was treated in 270 patients at the Bellevue Hospital during the 40 years before introduction of steroid

(8) J.A.M.A. 165:1249-1255, Nov. 9, 1957.

therapy. The mortality was more than 90% in this group, but in the steroid-treated group it was 33%. This is probably a higher figure than that of other series reported because of the older age groups represented (78% were past age 50), the severity and extensiveness of the disease and the inadequate but prolonged corticosteroid therapy given many of the patients before hospitalization. Two of the steroid-treated patients died of gastrointestinal hemorrhages, a complication which was not observed in the presteroid series.

Corticosteroids were of greatest value in treating pemphigus vulgaris, of less value in pemphigus erythematosus and of little permanent benefit in pemphigus foliaceus. Few patients with pemphigus have been free from symptoms for 1-2 years or more without treatment.

Scleroderma (Acrosclerosis): I. Treatment of Three Cases of Noncalcific Variety by Chelation (EDTA) is discussed by John G. Rukavina, Charles Mendelson, J. M. Price, R. R. Brown and S. A. M. Johnson[9] (Univ. of Wisconsin). Chelate compounds are essentially co-ordinate compounds, with the co-ordinate bonds arising from sharing an electron pair between the ion or atom of a metal and an ion or atom in the complex-forming structure (ligand). The most common electron-donating or electron-sharing atoms in ligand molecules are nitrogen, oxygen and sulfur, although others are known. When two bonding groups are present with proper spatial orientation in a single molecule, a heterocyclic ring involving the metal ion may be formed in contrast to a "complex" which exists in a nonring form.

One classification of chelate compounds is based on the number of ligands tied together in a single or multiple claw, i.e., monodentate, bidentate (a single ring being formed) etc. Generally, the most stable chelate rings consist of five and six members. They are among those most frequently encountered, although others have been described. The formation of these rings is of utmost biologic importance, in that they confer behavior properties on both the chelated metal and the ligands not previously characteristic of either alone.

It has been found that chelating agents (EDTA) serve as an aid in delineation of calcium metabolism. Furthermore, when EDTA is introduced into a physiologic environment

(9) J. Invest. Dermat. 29:273-288, October, 1957.

its primary gross action is on the bivalent cation present in greatest concentration, namely, calcium.

The authors treated 3 patients with noncalcific scleroderma (acrosclerosis) with disodium ethylenediamine tetraacetic acid (Na_2+EDTA).

Woman, 31, was hospitalized for treatment of "scleroderma," present for 4 years. Symptoms included pain, swelling and stiffness of the hands, especially in winter; recurrent "ulcers" of the fingertips and elbow; recent "gangrene" of the middle finger of the right hand; "arthritis" of the wrists, elbows, shoulders, back, hips and knees; "tightness" and "hardness" of the skin of the face, neck and especially the upper extremities. During pregnancy, she noticed a diminution of pain and healing of the ulcers on the hands. After pregnancy, the condition worsened.

Pertinent physical findings were those of the cutaneous system. The skin of the face, neck, upper chest and extremities was indurated, shiny and bound down. Increased pigmentation was noted in the neck and upper extremities. The tip of the right finger had a small painful ulceration, together with redness, swelling, tenderness of the distal phalanx and an accompanying nail deformity. The fingers were thin, elongated and fixed in a position of flexion. Movement of the shoulders, elbows, wrists, fingers, back, hips and knees was accompanied by pain. There were erythema, warmth and extreme tenderness over the wrist area. The right elbow was fixed in a moderately flexed position. Except for a blood pressure of 90/70, physical findings were noncontributory. Skin biopsy and x-ray changes in the terminal phalanges of the fingers were consistent with scleroderma.

Therapy consisted of 3 Gm. Na_2EDTA (Endrate) given intravenously over a 4-hour period daily for 5 days. Three consecutive weekly courses (45 Gm.) constituted the treatment program. Significant changes were noted during the 2d week of therapy. The previous inability to wrinkle the forehead, smile and open the mouth were profoundly altered. The skin of the face, neck and upper extremities appeared to be less tense and indurated. The skin over the hands, although less bound down, seemed to be least affected by therapy. While clinical range of motion was not remarkably changed, absence of pain on motion was striking. The extreme tenderness of the wrists was unchanged, but the fingers appeared to be warmer. Temperature challenge (cold) of the digits caused only slight pain.

Biopsy study of the skin (dorsum, hand) showed an increased prominence of rete ridges, less dense fibrous tissue in the corium, adnexal structure increased and an increase in subcutaneous fatty tissue. At no time during or after therapy was there any adverse change in the complete laboratory evaluation of the patient. Even though serum calcium levels, determined shortly after infusion, decreased to 5.8 mg./100 ml., no clinical evidence of tetany was found. Generally, except for pain near the intravenous site, the patient tolerated the procedure well. The 24-hour urinary copper and zinc excretion progressively increased, especially in the zinc fraction (9.97 mg./L.).

After hospitalization, general improvement was maintained with 1.5 Gm. oral Na_2EDTA daily. However, wrist tenderness and pain remained unchanged.

The patient had a second course of intravenous therapy (3 weeks, 45 Gm.) about 6 weeks later. Clinical reassessment appeared to indicate a progressive, though moderate, decrease in skin induration. Residual joint pain seemed to diminish further, but wrist pain remained totally resistant to the drug.

DIABETES MELLITUS

Further Experience with Lente Insulins. W. M. Lancaster and Ian Murray[1] (Victoria Infirm., Glasgow) treated 335 diabetics with insulin zinc suspension (I.Z.S.) for at least 6 months. Of these, 134 were "new" patients who had never previously taken insulin, and 201 were "old" patients who had been treated with some other insulin before receiving I.Z.S. None was obese; all were of the insulin-deficient type liable to ketosis, and 60% of the old patients had been instructed in a prescribed diet with carbohydrate adjusted to personal requirements.

Highly satisfactory results were obtained in 82.5% of the new patients. A single daily injection of unmodified I.Z.S. proved adequate in 121 (90%); 9 (7%) required relatively more I.Z.S. amorphous and 4 (3%) relatively less. There was much variation in the size of dose required. In 107 new patients (80%) this did not exceed 40 units, but 22 (16%) needed 40-80 units and 5 (4%) had up to 120 units daily. No correlation was found among the degree of control obtained and the personal variations in the proportions of I.Z.S. amorphous (semilente) and I.Z.S. crystalline (ultralente), the size of the dose or age of the patient.

Among the old patients, those with excellent or good control was increased from 68 to 130 (64.7%). Improvement was noted in 94 patients (46.8%), and in about the same number the degree of control was unaltered, although in 8 of these control had been so excellent that further improvement could

(1) Brit. M. J. 1:1331-1333, June 7, 1958.

not be expected. Six patients, previously poorly controlled, continued so with I.Z.S. These were unstable diabetics who eventually had to resume multiple injections and were regarded as failures with I.Z.S. In 12 patients, control deteriorated after change to the newer insulin. For the 189 patients with equally good or better control, the dose of I.Z.S. was greater than that of the former insulin in 86, but in 40 a smaller dose sufficed. When the dose had to be raised, the increase was commonly about 50%. Some patients, however, required as much as double the former dose. In 68% of patients I.Z.S. alone was suitable; the rest obtained best results on a regimen varying from I.Z.S. crystalline alone, through various combinations to I.Z.S. amorphous alone. Such variations in dosage and in the amorphous and crystalline proportions occurred irrespective of the degree of control exerted by the previous insulin and were noted in patients of all groups. Neither the age of the patient nor the duration of the diabetes appeared to affect the nature of the response to transfer to I.Z.S.

Some patients stated that insulin reactions became altered in character, tending to come on with little or no premonitory symptom, and this led to reversion to their previous type of insulin. Local allergy at the site of injection was much less. It was on this account that 27 of the old patients previously treated with protamine zinc insulin, alone or combined with soluble insulin, were changed to I.Z.S.; 23 obtained complete relief and improvement was noted in the rest. Three patients had fat atrophy at the site of injection.

In the presence of intercurrent infection, lapse from diabetic control with I.Z.S. appeared to occur more readily than with some other insulins. It is suggested that in such circumstances it is I.Z.S. crystalline which becomes relatively ineffective, since transfer temporarily to 2 injections a day of I.Z.S. amorphous re-establishes control.

► [Last year A. Marble (1957-58 YEAR BOOK, p. 179) concluded that if a patient is well controlled on NPH, globin or other insulin, with or without accompanying crystalline insulin, there is no advantage in shifting to lente. He would consider using lente (1) when insulin treatment is first instituted, (2) in cases difficult to regulate with other types of insulin and (3) in patients with allergies to other types.—Ed.]

Rapid Treatment of Severe Diabetic Ketosis Associated

with Severe Insulin Allergy is reported by Harvey Poliakoff[2] (Rockville Centre, N. Y.).

Man, 52, had giant urticaria with swelling of the feet, ankle and knee joints, hands and lips and temperature of 101 F., starting a few days after taking 30 units of NPH insulin daily. He had taken insulin for a few months about a year before, but had discontinued treatment because the urine still showed sugar and the insulin often caused hives. Insulin was stopped and he was given 1 dose of 40 units of ACTH gel and 50 mg. Pyribenzamine® 3 times daily. The urticaria promptly receded. Three days later he was hospitalized because of disorientation, hyperpnea, dehydration, vomiting and acetone breath.

At 7:55 a.m. the blood sugar was 1,042 and CO_2-combining power 10 vol%. He was given 100 mg. Benadryl® intravenously. Five minutes later he was given 0.5 cc. epinephrine intravenously followed in 2 minutes by 5 units of crystalline insulin intravenously. Ten minutes later 10 units of crystalline insulin was given. In 30 minutes, 30 more units was given intramuscularly, followed in 10 minutes by 50 units intravenously. At 9:30 a.m. blood sugar was 1,242 and Co_2-combining power 14 vol.%. The patient was given 100 mg. Benadryl intravenously, followed by 50 units of insulin intravenously and 50 units intramuscularly. An intravenous dose of 750 cc. of 1/6 m lactate was started. Insulin was given in increasing doses. At 1:30 p.m. his condition was still critical. He had received 1,095 units of insulin and 3,000 cc. fluids. He was still disoriented, and the blood chemistry had not improved. Insulin, 100 units intravenously and 100 units intramuscularly, was continued about every hour. Moderate generalized hives appeared about 2 p.m. but were controlled by 100 mg. Benadryl and 20 units of ACTH intravenously. By 3:30 p.m. the blood sugar was 660 and CO_2-combining power was 15. At 9:30 p.m. blood sugar was 322, and at 10 the next morning it was 100. At this time there was still acetone in the urine. Subsequently an all-beef insulin was used. In the hospital and at home the patient was controlled on a 1,500-calorie carbohydrate diet. At discharge he was receiving all-beef crystalline insulin, 65 units before breakfast and 40 units before supper. Fasting blood sugar was normal and the urine showed 0-0.25% sugar. He had an occasional hive at the injection site but no generalized reactions. Four months later, on the same diet, he was controlled on 40 units of all-beef crystalline insulin before breakfast and 20 units before supper.

Generalized reactions to insulin occur in approximately 1 of 1,000 cases. No case of fatal anaphylactic reaction to insulin has been described. The allergy may be due to insulin protein, modifying protein or species protein. In the present case the possible anti-insulin effect of ACTH was a calculated risk. The emergency management and follow-up treat-

(2) New York J. Med. 58:243-244, Jan. 15, 1958.

ment with insulin caused desensitization, so that the patient could continue to take insulin without untoward reaction.

Treatment of Sympathotonia in Labile Diabetes Mellitus is discussed by Julius Pomeranze[3] (New York Med. College). Juvenile diabetic patients often have rapid, unaccountable metabolic fluctuations unrelated to infection, trauma, unusual exertion, insulin changes or dietary indiscretions. The relation of emotional influences to this irregular control is pertinent. Acute anxiety can upset the diabetic status even to the extent of ketonemia and ketonuria. Anxiety may be present with or without somatic manifestations of sympathetic preponderance.

In the management of the young, labile diabetic, control of anxiety is important. The first effort is to avoid "stepladder" therapy, using increasing doses of insulin which lead to hypoglycemia and hypoglycemic-induced anxiety. When severe ketonemia is not impending, insulin dosage should be increased slowly, care being exerted to avoid hypoglycemia. Control of emotional disturbances, especially anxiety, depends on a careful program of reassurance and emotional support aided by a carefully considered dosage of Raudixin®. Treatment with this drug requires that the physician be aware of its cumulative effects, the wide dose-patient ratio and the lack of side effects when the dose is maintained at the proper level. There is evidence of wide variations in therapeutic dose level, and side effects are always controlled when the dose is kept at the lowest level of efficacy. The author treated 16 young variably labile diabetic patients successfully with requisite doses of Raudixin.

Man, 29, had had diabetes for several years. Weight decreased from 180 to 118 lb. and he had been having frequent attacks of ketosis, during which more regular insulin was given. These were followed by severe hypoglycemic episodes treated with large amounts of readily available carbohydrates. This recurring cycle of acidosis and hypoglycemia was the inevitable result of increasing and irregular doses of insulin and intake of increasing and irregular amounts of carbohydrate foods.

Although the patient was withdrawn and appeared calm, he had constant tachycardia and labile hypertension, perspired easily and showed other evidence of hypermetabolism. The BMR was +15% and the serum protein-bound iodine level was normal. With 100 mg. Raudixin 3 times daily and a constant, lower level of insulin, better

(3) New York J. Med. 57:3326-3328, Oct. 15, 1957.

control was maintained despite occasional ketosis. In a short time he came under good diabetic control by using 55 units of NPH insulin and 15 units of regular insulin daily. Weight was 137 lb., pulse 82 and blood pressure 120/82. He had no hypoglycemic episodes and infrequent ketonuria.

Glucagon Treatment of Insulin Reactions. Studies on the treatment of 41 induced and spontaneous insulin reactions in 18 diabetic patients with crystalline glucagon are presented by Harold Elrick, Thomas A. Witten and Yoshiaki Arai[4] (VA Hosp., Denver). In 24 of 27 spontaneous insulin attacks, complete recovery occurred 5-30 minutes after a single intramuscular injection of 1 mg. glucagon. In the other 3 attacks (all in the same patient), there was no clinical response in 2 and partial response in the third which was associated with a blood sugar rise from 44 to 96 mg./100 ml.

Blood samples were obtained before glucagon administration in 8 attacks, and all were in the hypoglycemic range. In 6 of these, 1-5 blood samples were obtained during the 1st hour after glucagon administration. The blood sugar rose, and the rise was maintained during the test period in all patients. On 3 occasions in 1 case complete relief from symptoms occurred before the blood sugar rose appreciably. In no case did blood sugar rise above 116 mg./100 ml. after glucagon.

Insulin reactions were induced in 14 patients. Of these, 13 exhibited the characteristic clinical picture of hypoglycemia before glucagon administration, attained complete relief 5-30 minutes after administration and had no relapse during the test period of 1 or 2 hours. Among these 13 were 3 who had such severe signs as unconsciousness, convulsions and cardiac arrhythmia. One patient showed no signs or symptoms of hypoglycemia, though his arterial blood sugar fell to hypoglycemic levels.

After glucagon injection, blood sugar rose in all patients, but in 3 it did not rise above hypoglycemic levels. Among the other 11 patients who attained normal glucose levels, the blood sugar returned to hypoglycemic levels during the test period in 3. One patient had a mild recurrence of hypoglycemic symptoms 2 hours after glucagon. Some patients began to recover (after glucagon) before an appreciable rise

(4) New England J. Med. 258:476-480, Mar. 6, 1958.

in arterial blood sugar occurred or while hypoglycemia was still present. The maximum blood sugar after glucagon was 153 mg./100 ml.

Since glucagon makes use of endogenous glucose, it is less likely than glucose to upset diabetic control in the patient with severe or "brittle" diabetes. Also subcutaneous or intramuscular injection of glucagon is easier and more convenient than intravenous administration of glucose in the unconscious or un-co-operative patient with a severe insulin reaction. These considerations suggest that glucagon might also prove useful for management of insulin reactions outside the hospital. Since it can be administered like insulin, mild or moderate attacks could be treated by the patient himself without disturbing diabetic control. Severe attacks could be treated more promptly by the patient's family, thereby avoiding the dangers entailed by delay in obtaining the services of a physician. No harmful effects would result from administration of glucagon to patients with symptomatology mimicking hypoglycemic reactions. Indeed, failure to respond to glucagon would suggest that causes other than an insulin reaction should be sought.

► ↓ The following 7 articles are chosen not only because they are representative of what is being done with tolbutamide (Orinase®) in the oral therapy of diabetes mellitus but also because they originate in 6 distinctly different geographic areas and are thus indicative of the world-wide experience.

In the first, an American article, there is substantiation of the earlier impression that best results are usually to be expected in patients whose diabetes was detected after age 40 and whose insulin requirement is below 20 units.

In the second, also an American article, it is shown that the result obtained in the early trial of the drug in an individual case may not be reliably indicative of the ultimate responsiveness of the patient since an early resistance may be overcome or, contrariwise, an early favorable response may fail to be sustained.

In the third, or Scandinavian article, evidence is presented that the development of resistance to the drug in patients who had responded initially does not imply that insulin requirements will be increased when therapy with the hormone is resumed.

In the fourth, or Indian article, the necessity for accompanying dietary restrictions is shown, and it is made apparent that the drug becomes less effective as the patient's weight is allowed to increase.

In the fifth article, the one from England, there is evidence that tolbutamide action is independent of the patient's age, weight and heredity and of the symptoms and duration of the disease, but depends entirely on the severity as revealed in the insulin requirement.

In the sixth, or South African article, it is shown that the optimal tolbutamide effect is often delayed and that even greatly increased dosage cannot control the hyperglycemia and ketosis associated with intercurrent infection, injury, major surgical procedures, etc.

Finally, in the seventh, or French article, the attempt is made to classify cases of diabetes on the basis of response to tolbutamide.

The total number of cases involved in the combined studies was 1,618, and the incidence of untoward side actions or toxicities was strikingly low: very little significant hypoglycemia; a few instances of urticaria or skin rashes; some minor gastrointestinal disturbances; an instance of activation of duodenal ulcer with melena; headache, muscular weakness, tingling, hemiparesis associated with hypoglycemia; transient alterations in the platelet count; temporary reversal of the neutrophil-lymphocyte ratio (in 37 of the 105 South African cases); an instance of severe leukopenia which resolved without alteration in dosage. Still, there is considerable variety here, and I should say that we are not yet able to delineate fully the potential toxicity of this drug. At 2 autopsies on patients whose deaths were unrelated to administration of tolbutamide there was no pancreatic or hepatic damage attributable to it.

In articles not included in this YEAR BOOK, C. Schnall and J. S. Wiener (J.A.M.A. 167:214, May 10, 1958) reported an instance of nephrosis occurring during tolbutamide administration but not conclusively ascribable to it, and W. W. Engstrom *et al.* (GP 17:96, 1958) recorded 2 instances in which diabetic acidosis promptly developed when tolbutamide was substituted for insulin.—Ed.

Results of Long-Term Use of Tolbutamide (Orinase®) in Diabetes Mellitus are discussed by Hellmut Mehnert, Rafael Camerini-Davalos and Alexander Marble[5] (Boston). Tolbutamide was given to 1,030 patients, in 772 of whom maintenance studies were begun with this drug alone. At the time of completion of the study, treatment had been carried out for 1-20 months in 594 patients.

BLOOD SUGAR LEVELS AND AMOUNTS OF SUGAR IN URINE USED AS STANDARDS OF CONTROL*

	Degree of Control†			
	Good		Fair	
Relation to Food	Blood Sugar, Mg./100 Cc.‡	Urine Sugar, %	Blood Sugar, Mg./100 Cc.‡	Urine Sugar, %
Fasting	110	Trace	130	0.1
1 hr. p.c........	150	0.3	180	0.5
2 hr. p.c........	130	0.1	150	0.3
2 hr. p.c........	110	Trace	130	0.1
Urine sugar in 24 hr.	2 Gm. or less		5 Gm. or less	

*For purposes of classification as to degree of control, the majority of values must conform with the standards listed in the table. All others are considered poor.
†These standard values are the highest acceptable.
‡"True" glucose as determined by the Somogyi-Nelson procedure.

Various methods of establishing the dosage were used. At

(5) J.A.M.A. 167:818-827, June 14, 1958.

first many patients were given 3 Gm. daily for 1 or 2 days, then 2 Gm. daily for 1 or 2 days and finally a maintenance dose of usually 1 Gm. daily. More recently, some patients were started immediately on 1 Gm. daily, with success. In general, the entire dose was given daily before breakfast.

Standards of control were arbitrarily chosen (table). Good control of hyperglycemia and glycosuria was obtained in 407

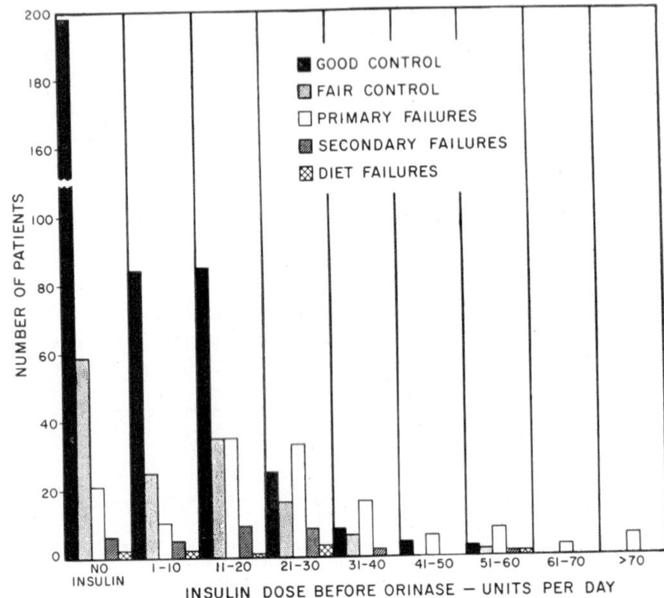

Fig. 17.—Correlation of insulin dosage before using tolbutamide, with outcome of treatment. (Courtesy of Mehnert, H., *et al.*: J.A.M.A. 167:818-827, June 14, 1958.)

(52.6%)and fair control in 143 (18.5%) of the 772 patients. The incidence of failures was as follows: "primary," i.e., within the 1st month of treatment, 136 patients (17.6%), "secondary," 31 patients (4%); failures due to disregard of diet, 9 patients (1.2%). In 33 patients (4.3%) the drug had been used for less than 1 month; in 8 (1.1%) treatment with tolbutamide was stopped because of toxic side effects; and in 5 (0.6%) treatment was discontinued for nonmedical reasons.

Factors favoring success with tolbutamide were primarily maturity-onset type of diabetes (onset usually above age 40) and a low insulin requirement (less than 20 units daily). A single-dose, 4-hour sulfonylurea response test was found to be of value in pointing out those patients in whom primary failure with tolbutamide therapy is likely to occur.

The influence of the prior insulin dosage on the outcome of treatment with tolbutamide is shown in Figure 17. As might have been anticipated, successes were much more common in patients whose insulin dosage was smallest, and the relative number of failures rose as insulin dosage increased. It is important to make a distinction between insulin dosage and insulin requirement. One knows what the patient's insulin dose was, but it is not easy in retrospect to state accurately what the true insulin requirement or deficit was.

Among those patients tabulated in Figure 17 as receiving no insulin were many with newly discovered diabetes who had never taken insulin and yet actually had an insulin requirement. As is evident from the figure, some responded satisfactorily to tolbutamide, and others, presumably those with larger insulin requirements, proved to have primary failures.

Untoward effects were low in incidence and in general consisted chiefly of urticaria and minor digestive disturbances. In one patient with cirrhosis of the liver, jaundice occurred 3 months after starting treatment with tolbutamide; the relation of jaundice to the drug is uncertain. In 2 patients dying of causes unrelated to tolbutamide administration, histologic examination revealed no evidence of damage to the pancreas or liver attributable to the drug.

In addition to convenience, treatment with tolbutamide has the added advantage of almost complete freedom from significant hypoglycemia. In only a few instances was symptomatic hypoglycemia recognized, despite the fact that most adult patients at the start were given a full dose of 3 Gm. in the fasting state, with food withheld for 4 hours to carry out the tolbutamide response test.

In selecting patients for tolbutamide treatment, care should be taken to avoid, on the one hand, unnecessary use in those in whom dietary restriction will suffice and, on the other hand, unwise use in those requiring insulin for maintenance of control of diabetes.

Use of Orinase® as Basic Adjuvant in Management of Insulin-Dependent Diabetes. Maximilian Fabrykant[6] (New York Univ.) carried out a long-term evaluation of Orinase as a supplement to insulin therapy for up to 20 months with 38 stable and 12 labile diabetics. Orinase therapy was begun in the hospital with 8 stable diabetics who had cardiovascular complications and with 10 of the labile diabetics. Combined Orinase-insulin therapy was started on an ambulatory basis in the rest. Both stable and labile diabetics can begin on combined therapy without hospitalization, but initial hospitalization is recommended for patients with cardiovascular disease.

The data obtained showed that in most insulin-dependent diabetics use of Orinase combined with insulin provides benefits unobtainable with insulin alone. Beneficial effects were obtained in 28 stable and 9 labile diabetics: decrease in insulin requirement, easier regulation and stabilization of diabetes and increased feeling of well-being.

The results demonstrated that the short-term effects of Orinase may not reflect the effects to be obtained by its prolonged administration. In some patients with stable, mild diabetes, an early favorable response to Orinase, which seemed to indicate that it might serve as a complete replacement for insulin, proved to be only temporary within 2-3 months of the start of treatment. In patients with stable diabetes and a high insulin requirement and in those with labile diabetes, an initial resistance to therapy with Orinase was followed by remarkable improvement with its continuous use. In the light of present experience it appears that forecasts of responsiveness based on Orinase-loading tests or on short-term experiments may be misleading. The use of Orinase is an individual experiment in each case.

In 6 patients with angina pectoris, striking relief from anginal pain coincided with institution of Orinase therapy and persisted for the entire period of observation (7-19 months). More extensive studies are necessary, however, to corroborate the existence of a relationship between the use of Orinase and the observed relief from anginal pain.

Secondary Resistance in Oral Treatment of Diabetes is discussed by Gerhard Dotevall[7] (Varberg, Sweden). Oral

(6) Metabolism 7:213-221, May, 1958.
(7) Acta med. scandinav. 161:251-256, 1958.

antidiabetic drugs have been used in active therapy for over 2 years. The types in use are BZ- 55 and D- 860. The latter is more widely used because of its lower toxicity and because it is not a sulfonamide.

The author treated 65 diabetics with BZ- 55 or D- 860. Secondary resistance occurred in 15 after an observation period of 2-18 months. Secondary resistance means that patients who have responded well to oral antidiabetic medication for 2 months or more become resistant to the drug.

This resistance appeared mainly in the first 6 months, and particularly in patients previously treated with insulin. Nine had had insulin treatment earlier. Most patients with secondary resistance did not require a larger quantity of insulin after discontinuing oral treatment than before commencing it.

The mean duration of the diabetes was 6.7 years in patients with secondary resistance and 2.5 years in the others.

It is suggested that secondary resistance is due to a reversible collapse of the beta cells in the pancreas.

Oral Treatment of Diabetes with Tolbutamide. Inder Singh[8] treated 136 patients with "adult-onset" diabetes mellitus and a child, aged 4, with congenital diabetes. The patients were given a high-carbohydrate, low-fat diet adjusted to individual needs. Initially, 1 Gm. tolbutamide was given twice daily for 2 days; the dose was then reduced to 0.5 Gm. twice daily. When an adequate response was obtained, maintenance dosage was worked out in each case. If the response was inadequate, the morning dose was increased to 1 Gm. In patients subject to ketosis the previous insulin treatment was continued until the oral drug had had a hypoglycemic effect. In all other patients insulin treatment was discontinued at once.

Results were considered very satisfactory in 94 (68%) patients and satisfactory in 32 (23%). There were 11 failures (9%). In the very satisfactory group, the time required for a complete response was 2 weeks in 58 patients, 4 weeks in 24 and 6 weeks in 12. Generally the more complete the response the lower the maintenance dose. The result was very satisfactory in 80% of patients who had been treated with insulin for 1 year or less, in 56% of those treated with insulin for 2-5

(8) Brit. M. J. 2:1345-1347, Dec. 7, 1957.

years and in only 6% of those treated with insulin for more than 5 years. It was very satisfactory in all patients who had received 10-20 units of insulin daily, in 75% of those who had had 20-40 units, in 66% of those who had had 40-60 units, in 31% of those who had had 60-80 units and in none of those who had had more than 80 units daily. Results did not appear to have been influenced by the age of the patient, body weight, heredity, duration of the disease or presence or absence of symptoms.

The incidence of adverse effects due to tolbutamide was low. Transitory headache occurred in 6 patients, muscular weakness due to low blood sugar in 7, tingling of the finger tips, toes and lips in 2 and skin rash in 2. Two elderly patients became hypoglycemic during the 1st week of treatment, and temporary hemiparesis developed without warning. Two patients had an initial fall in the platelet count, but subsequently the count rose to normal. In another patient platelet counts showed a progressive increase before stabilization.

Clinical Experience with Tolbutamide. G. Walker, J. D. H. Slater, E. K. Westlake and J. D. N. Nabarro[9] (Middlesex Hosp., London) report results of a tolbutamide trial in 72 patients observed up to 1 year. The trial was conducted on an outpatient basis. Patients were selected who were not grossly obese and had "mild" diabetes that could not be satisfactorily controlled by calorie and carbohydrate restriction alone. All patients taking carbutamide and a few taking insulin were transferred to tolbutamide. Those transferred from carbutamide were initially given the same dose of tolbutamide. Those who had been taking insulin were given reduced doses for a few days; the injections were then stopped and tolbutamide was started the next day. Patients who had had neither carbutamide nor insulin were observed on a strict low-carbohydrate diet for at least a month. If the midmorning blood sugar remained above 200 mg./100 ml., they were given tolbutamide. The starting dose for these patients and for those transferred from insulin was 0.5 Gm. 2 or 3 times daily, taken with the main meals. The dose was subsequently adjusted to a maximum of 4 Gm. daily, according to the blood sugar response.

Of the 72 patients, 41 had previously been treated by diet

(9) Brit. M. J. 2:323-325, Aug. 10, 1957.

alone, 19 were transferred from carbutamide and 12 were transferred from insulin (12-60 units, mean 26 units daily); 12 other patients, including 4 in the carbutamide group, had taken insulin previously.

Age at diagnosis varied between 22 and 78 years (mean 53) and duration of diabetes between 1 and 30 years (mean 6.6). Thirty-five patients were within 10% of their "expected"

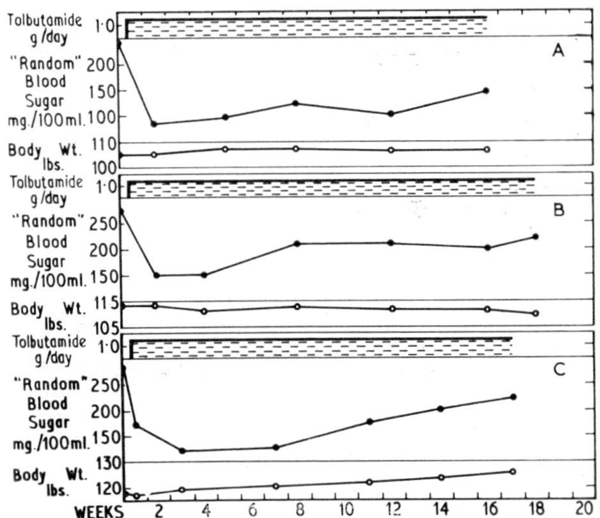

Fig. 18.—Immediate type of response to tolbutamide. *A*, woman, 56, with diabetes for 4 years; no insulin; expected weight 131 lb. *B*, woman, 73, with diabetes for 26 years, transferred from protamine zinc insulin, 16 units; expected weight 127 lb. *C*, woman, 62, with diabetes for 4 years; previous insulin, expected weight, 130 lb. (Courtesy of Walker, G., *et al.*: Brit. M. J. 2:323-325, Aug. 10, 1957.)

weight when treatment was started, 20 were more than 10% overweight and 17 were more than 10% underweight. Seven patients are known to have been mildly ketotic and 5 had diabetic retinopathy.

The necessity for following a strict diet was stressed. The diets prescribed varied from 1,000 calories with 80 Gm. carbohydrate, to 2,200 calories with 220 Gm. carbohydrate.

Treatment was stopped by 19 patients for the following reasons: resistance (requiring insulin), 2; failure to respond, 6; rash, 2; abdominal symptoms, 4; not required, 1 irregular attendance, 2; returned to insulin at own request, 2.

Of the 53 patients who had not been treated with carbutamide, 7 showed no response, 33 showed an "immediate" response, the blood sugar falling during the 1st week of treatment, and 13 showed a "delayed" response, the blood sugar falling to a minimum in 12-16 weeks, irrespective of changes in weight. Twenty patients (61%)who showed an "immediate" response and 9 (69%) who showed a "delayed" response appeared to be satisfactorily controlled by tolbuta-

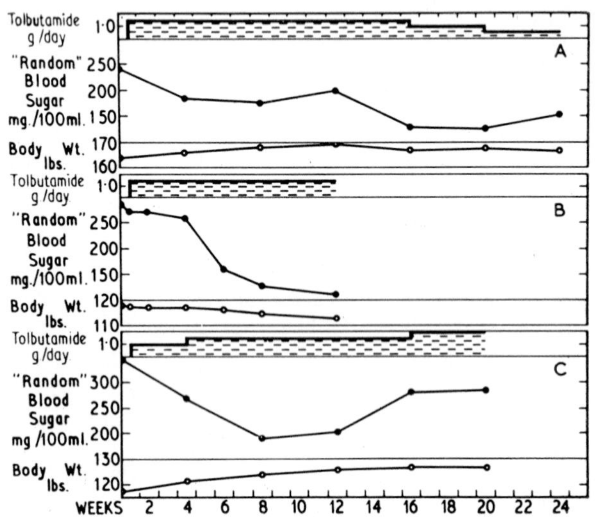

Fig. 19.—Delayed type of response. *A,* man, 81, with diabetes for 30 years; no insulin; expected weight 145 lb. *B,* woman, 67, with diabetes for 1 year; no insulin; expected weight 119 lb. *C,* woman, 76, with diabetes for 2 years; no insulin; expected weight 130 lb. (Courtesy of Walker, G., *et al.*: Brit. M. J. 2:323-325, Aug. 10, 1957.)

mide. Examples of the two types of response are shown in Figures 18 and 19. All patients who had responded to carbutamide did so to tolbutamide, but 1 became resistant to it.

Side effects were: rash in 2 patients, abdominal pain in 4, vomiting in 1 and activation of duodenal ulcer with melena in 1.

Two patients who had a good initial response failed to maintain a satisfactory blood sugar level despite increasing doses of tolbutamide, strict adherence to a suitable diet and failure to gain weight. They were both transferred to insulin treatment. It seems that 4 others are becoming resistant to the drug.

Seven patients showed unequivocal failure to respond to tolbutamide. These include 2 who had been transferred from insulin treatment and 4 of 7 known to have been mildly ketotic at some time.

This study suggests that about 50% of patients with "mild" diabetes that cannot be controlled by diet alone will benefit from tolbutamide. Patients who respond usually gain weight and must follow a diet restricted in calories and carbohydrates. Increasing weight is often associated with decreasing effectiveness of the drug.

Further Experiences in Use of Tolbutamide (D-860) in Diabetes Mellitus are reported by T. Schneider, S. Lopis and W. M. Politzer[1] (Johannesburg). All the 105 diabetic outpatients treated were over age 43 and most over 60. A dose of 3 Gm. tolbutamide was given the 1st day and decreased by 0.5 Gm. daily until a maintenance dose of 1-1.5 Gm. daily was reached. If the previous dose of insulin did not exceed 20 units, insulin was discontinued on the day tolbutamide therapy was begun. If the dosage exceeded 20 units, insulin was gradually withdrawn by reducing the dose by 5-10 units daily.

Good control was obtained in 42.9% of patients, fair control in 23.8% and poor control in 33.3%. Side effects were minimal. The drug was discontinued in 2 patients because of nausea and in 1 because of angioneurotic edema. Temporary reversal of the neutrophil-lymphocyte ratio occurred in 37 cases. Severe leukopenia was observed in 1 patient, but this disappeared despite continued tolbutamide in unchanged dosage. Deterioration in control occurred in 8 patients after several months of tolbutamide therapy. A gain in weight often accompanied loss of control, and deterioration perhaps resulted from less strict adherence to diet.

Although effective control is often achieved within the 1st week of tolbutamide administration, it is advisable to persist for at least 3 weeks because the optimal effect may be delayed. Infections, injuries and operations may disorganize diabetic control, and it has been found that tolbutamide, even in increased dosage, cannot control the resulting hypergly-

(1) South African M. J. 32:149-153, Feb. 8, 1958.

cemia and ketosis. Insulin is then required as an emergency measure. Ketosis definitely contraindicates use of tolbutamide, and it is dangerous to continue with the drug in its presence.

Mechanism of Action of Hypoglycemic Sulfonamides: Concept Based on Investigations in Animals and in Man is presented by Auguste Loubatières[2] (Montpellier, France). Two types of substances have been studied, the thiodiazole derivatives (2254-RP, IPTD) and the urea series (carbutamide, tolbutamide). The pancreas is indispensable to the hypoglycemic action of these drugs; the effect does not occur in the totally depancreatized animal. Other endocrine glands are not essential. The beta cells of the islets seem to be the preferential site of action of the sulfonamides.

Acute administration of the drugs apparently acts on the beta cells to cause liberation of endogenous insulin. This insulin is secreted into the portal vein and reaches the liver cells directly. Large doses of the sulfonamides potentiate the effects of exogenous insulin. This phenomenon may be due to an anti-insulinase action in the liver, but this has not yet been specifically demonstrated. Chronic administration of the sulfonamides can cause new formation of beta cells, as well as liberation of insulin from them. The metabolic benefit produced by these substances depends on the number of beta cells that are not damaged or that can be regenerated.

The action of these drugs on enzymatic mechanisms in the liver concerned with insulin destruction or with sugar metabolism is not completely explained. These enzymatic inhibitions are manifest only after large doses of the drugs, and they may or may not be specific. A stimulatory action of the sulfonamides on the adrenals may explain in some fashion the responses shown by treated animals to hypoglycemic convulsions.

In normal persons and in some diabetic patients the hypoglycemic action of the sulfonamides is easily observed. The hypoglycemia may require intravenous injections of glucose. The degree and rapidity of the hypoglycemia obtained by a test dose of one of the drugs seem to be in accord with present knowledge of the insulin contained in the normal and diabetic pancreas.

(2) Diabetes 6:408-417, Sept.-Oct., 1957.

Contradictory results have been obtained concerning the effects of the drugs on glucose tolerance. Some patients respond rapidly and favorably, others only after many weeks. A potentiating effect on exogenous insulin has been observed in the diabetic, but the phenomenon is not constant. The response may depend on the type of diabetes and on the manner in which insulin and the drugs have been used.

The antidiabetic action observed in human diabetics consists of a temporary remission or apparent cure of the diabetes for several weeks after cessation of treatment with restoration of a normal glucose balance. This phenomenon is relatively frequent in diabetics over age 50, but it has been seen in younger patients, particularly those with diabetes of recent onset. Such remissions are apparently due to beta cell regeneration which permits the patient to enter a phase similar to the prediabetic state.

Diabetics may be divided into three groups on the basis of their response to sulfonamides. The first group comprises patients who have reacted favorably to the sulfonamide regimen; this group consists in general of patients of the lipoplethoric type over age 45. They tolerate the diabetic state well but need insulin because of glycosuria and complications. In this group the sulfonamides generally can replace 20-30 units of insulin, sometimes more. Patients in this group correspond clinically to those with a pancreas containing many beta cells and an insulin content about 50% of normal.

The second clinical group consists of patients who have not benefited from therapy. They are mainly young persons, but some older diabetics are also included. Insulin treatment is obligatory because ketosis appears when the hormone is withdrawn. The patients belong to the group completely deficient in insulin. The pancreas in such patients has few intact beta cells and the insulin content is close to 10% of normal.

The third group comprises those patients who have benefited partially. It is possible to reduce, but not completely eliminate, insulin in these patients. The partial benefit may be due to some liberation of endogenous insulin, to the potentiation effect or perhaps to new formation of cellular elements in the pancreas.

When sulfonamides are used for chronic therapy of diabetes there is the possibility that a decompensation and weakening of the beta cell system may occur. With judicious administration and good clinical indications, this would probably be uncommon.

As a chemical group, the hypoglycemic sulfonamides are probably not devoid of toxicity. They may provoke sensitization, accumulate in various organs and tissues and block some enzyme systems in the course of long-term administration. Some persons originally sensitive to their action may later become refractory, though this is extremely rare.

Clinical Trials with DBI, a New Nonsulfonylurea Oral Hypoglycemic Agent, are reported by Leo P. Krall and Rafael Camerini-Davalos[3] (Boston). Oral hypoglycemic agents in clinical use thus far have been sulfonylurea derivatives with blood sugar-lowering ability in certain types of diabetes. Recently, a new group of compounds classified as formamidinyliminoureas have been introduced. These drugs are biguanides, not to be confused with the diguanidines, which include Synthalin (guanidine-deca-methylene-guanidine). They also have no structural relationship to either carbutamide or tolbutamide and have no sulfonyl radical in their formulas. One of these agents, phenethyl-formamidinyliminourea hydrochloride, has been reported to be effective orally in both normal and alloxan diabetic animals. The mechanism of action is not definitely known.

The authors tried N^1-β-phenethyl-formamidinyliminourea hydrochloride (DBI), a new nonsulfonylurea compound with blood sugar-lowering ability in 121 patients with a restricted diet. The average dosage was 200 mg. (50-450 mg.) daily in divided doses; the average maintenance dose was 150 mg. (25-400 mg.). Side-effects, involving the gastrointestinal tract, were observed in about one third of the patients, because of which 19 had to discontinue the medication.

A blood sugar-lowering effect was seen in 90 patients (86%). It occurred in every age group and type of patient, including juvenile diabetics. "Good" or "fair" control was achieved in 66 of the 88 evaluated in this manner. Sixty patients are still maintained with DBI. Only 6 of these take supplemental insulin, and these take less than 50% of their

(3) A.M.A. Arch. Int. Med. 102:25-31, July, 1958.

previous daily dose. Frequent liver function, blood and other studies revealed no toxicity.

► [Last year, J. Pomeranze *et al.* published the first description of a trial of this new antidiabetic compound for oral use (1957-58 YEAR BOOK, p. 177); the present article may be looked on as a follow-up of that study, though performed by another group of workers. The British, too, have been busy in this field, G. H. Hall *et al.* (Brit. M. J. 2:71, July 12, 1958) having administered the agent to 40 patients with diabetes of all grades of severity. A significant fall of blood sugar occurred in about two thirds of them, but ketosis was not rectified, and occasionally developed, in patients under treatment; in 5 patients, however, DBI was effective when tolbutamide (Orinase®) had failed. It was felt that the gastrointestinal effects that developed in 25 of the 40 patients preclude the general use of the drug.—Ed.]

GASTROENTEROLOGIC DISORDERS

Role of ACTH and Adrenal Steroids in Perforation of Colon in Ulcerative Colitis: Clinical-Pathologic Study is presented by Moshe B. Goldgraber, Joseph B. Kirsner and Walter L. Palmer[4] (Univ. of Chicago). The records of 10 patients with active colitis who died of perforation of the bowel were reviewed. Eight died in the presteroid era, and the histologic findings in these cases were compared with those of 2 patients who had received steroids.

ACTH and corticoids depress tissue reactivity and, therefore, may be beneficial in diseases in which this type of reactivity is increased. However, the inhibitory effect on mesenchymal elements would prevent or retard the processes of healing and repair. In this study there were no discernible, significant differences in the cellularity of the colonic mucosa, in fibroblastic proliferation or in leukocyte accumulation in the inflamed serosa in patients with colonic perforation treated with or without steroids. The peritoneal reaction was not marked in either group.

Cases with masked symptoms were encountered both in the presteroid era and after steroid therapy. The incidence of perforation was 2.5% in the presteroid era (10 of 400 patients) and 1% among those treated with ACTH and/or corticoids (2 of 200 patients). Giant perforations were observed in both periods.

(4) Gastroenterology 33:434-456, September, 1957.

Ileostomy was performed in 3 patients before the acute illness. This operation did not prove to be a safety valve for preventing perforation. The hydraulic stress factor must have been of secondary importance in these cases and the ulcerative process the more important.

Organized thrombi were found in small venules in 7 of the 10 cases. Thrombosis, in the general circulation or in the portal system, and its complications were the principal causes of death in 9 patients with ulcerative colitis examined at autopsy. The high incidence indicates a need for a separate and careful study of the interrelation of ulcerative colitis and thromboembolic phenomena.

No cases of inflammation of arteries were observed in the present group. There were occasional foci of perivascular infiltration but these were not impressive. Arterioles with thickened walls and slitlike vascular lumens were repeatedly observed. Whether or not this vascular appearance implies an impairment of blood supply which, with venous thrombosis might favor the unusual depth of ulceration, is difficult to state.

Diagnosis of pericolitis and peritonitis is often made during the course of ulcerative colitis. The incidence of such cases, improving and surviving, is difficult to determine, because of lack of conclusive evidence of the perforative event in most of them. Some patients with clinical evidence of peritoneal irritation received ACTH and corticoids and showed dramatic improvement. These observations do not agree with the view of withholding ACTH in the possible presence of peritoneal irritation. The authors conclude that the hazard of perforation of the colon in chronic ulcerative colitis is no greater during administration of ACTH and steroids than in their absence.

► [Last year Fierst and his group (1957-58 YEAR BOOK, p. 184) concluded that the corticosteroids suppress the constitutional manifestations but do not alter the natural history of the disease. In their series, regression of symptoms occurred more promptly with than without steroids, but there was no evidence of an increased number of remissions resulting from their use. Though these agents may not increase the likelihood of perforation of the colon, as suggested in the present article, their penchant for masking the signs of intercurrent infection is well known and should always put the prescriber on his guard. Other facets of steroid therapy in this baffling malady are presented in the 3 following articles.—Ed.]

Present Status of Treatment of Chronic Ulcerative Colitis with Steroid Hormones was analyzed from questionnaires to 157 physicians and by examination of 60 patients by Bernard D. Rosenak, Robert D. Pickett, Helen D. Van Vactor, James B. Hammond, Robert J. Healey and Rollin H. Moser[5] (Indiana Univ.). Less than half the physicians queried use steroid hormones in treating most patients. Sixty-five per cent consider adequate initial doses to be: intramuscular cortisone, 200-300 mg./day intravenous, 20-30 mg.; ACTHAR® gel, intramuscular, 40-80 units/day. Only a third report increased complications resulting from use of hormone therapy.

Among the 60 patients studied, half received corticotropin plus cortisone or prednisone, 14 received cortisone only, 10 corticotropin only, 5 prednisone and 1 hydrocortisone. Treatment ranged from 5 to 520 days. Remission was obtained in 32 patients; 6 showed no improvement and 7 died.

This study indicates that hormone treatment should be terminated shortly after acute symptoms have been controlled and may be resumed with onset of a new exacerbation. Long-term therapy may lead to dependence and mask symptoms without exerting curative effect.

Certain complications such as peptic ulcer, psychoses, adrenal insufficiency and electrolyte disturbances are more common in ulcerative colitis now than before steroid therapy was introduced. Administration of penicillin and streptomycin is considered essential during hormone therapy, to minimize the danger of secondary infection.

It is recommended that steroid preparations not be used routinely but be reserved for patients with acute fulminating ulcerative colitis, for those who do not respond to routine medical management and those who must undergo surgery or who experience complications such as arthritis or uveitis.

Preliminary Observations on Use of Medrol® in Ulcerative Colitis are presented by Joseph B. Kirsner and Jean A. Spencer[6] (Univ. of Chicago). Ulcerative colitis often undergoes spontaneous, albeit temporary, remission. Thus, evaluation of therapy is difficult; there is no specific treatment. The usual program consists of rest, bland diet, sedation and antispasmodics. Various sulfonamide preparations and intramuscularly administered penicillin and streptomycin may be helpful in the control of secondary infection. However, opin-

(5) Gastroenterology 34:879-891, May, 1958.
(6) Metabolism 7 (pt. 2):537-542, July, 1958.

ions vary as to the value of oral antibiotics, corticotropin, adrenal steroids and surgery.

In many instances the improvement following corticotropin or steroid therapy is dramatic. In almost every instance of improvement the patient passes through a period (varying greatly in duration) during which a threshold level of steroid dosage is established. Below this level, active disease is manifest; above it, the disease is controlled. Many instances of failure with steroids are attributable to lack of recognition of this threshold level and unwillingness to prescribe sufficiently large doses to control the disease.

The authors tried Medrol in 11 patients with recurrent ulcerative colitis. Preliminary observations suggest a varying individual response to this drug, as has been found with other steroids. Slight to excellent improvement was achieved in 7 patients. One patient responded well to Medrol enemas. Failures were probably due to several causes, such as too small doses, too early cessation of treatment, increasing severity of the disease or, quite often, emotional problems interfering with treatment in general. In 1 patient, adequate steroid therapy was prevented by 4+ glycosuria on relatively small amounts of Medrol.

Treatment of Ulcerative Colitis with Local Hydrocortisone was studied by S. C. Truelove[7] (Oxford, England), using various methods. The first study involved 21 courses of treatment using hydrocortisone. Because hydrocortisone has a low solubility in water, it was dissolved in 50% ethyl alcohol. This was diluted with 10 times its volume of saline for actual use in the colon and was dripped into the rectum from a modified blood transfusion set. In 14 instances, rapid clinical remission was achieved within a few days. Histologic examination, however, showed no corresponding improvement. This raised the possibility that the alcohol which formed part of the diluent for the hydrocortisone might itself have a bad effect on the inflamed colonic mucosa and prevent it from healing.

The second study involved 18 courses given with hydrocortisone hemisuccinate sodium, which is highly soluble in water. There were 11 rapid remissions. The sigmoidoscopic appearances improved in proportion to the clinical response,

(7) Proc. Roy. Soc. Med. 51:429-431, June, 1958.

accompanied by a definite improvement in the colonic mucosa, as judged from biopsy specimens.

In a planned therapeutic trial, 40 courses were involved. First, hydrocortisone hemisuccinate or a similar-looking inert preparation was used. One or the other was allotted the patients at random for 1 week. In each patient, this was followed by 2 weeks of treatment with known hydrocortisone hemisuccinate sodium, together with penicillin and streptomycin added to the rectal drip. At the end of the 1st week, of 20 courses of treatment given with the inert preparation only 1 resulted in clinical remission, whereas of 20 courses of treatment with real hydrocortisone hemisuccinate 11 resulted in remission. A fortnight later, after known treatment with hydrocortisone and antibiotics, the two groups were closely similar. Thus, it may be assumed that hydrocortisone hemisuccinate dripped into the rectum has a real effect in bringing about clinical remission in many patients.

Results of local treatment were highly favorable also in severe attacks. In 2 pregnant patients a nightly rectal drip of hydrocortisone was continued until after delivery. The results were excellent in both.

Of 15 patients treated during 1955-56, 6 remained in perfect remission; 7 had 1 or more recurrences but responded swiftly to further courses of local treatment; 2 had recurrences which did not respond to a further course.

Clinical Observations with Cantil®, New Anticholinergic for Colon Disorders, have led Jacob A. Riese[8] (Med. Center, Jersey City, N. J.) to consider it singularly free from side effects and successful in reducing diarrhea, distention and pain in functional and organic colon disorders. This piperidol anticholinergic, N-methyl-3-piperidyl-diphenyl-glycolate methobromide, was used in 79 patients, 44 of whom had diarrhea, pain and distention due to spastic or irritable colon, 16 ulcerative colitis, 3 ileitis, 15 infectious gastroenteritis and 1 gastrogenous diarrhea. Cantil was given alone or with phenobarbital when patients were tense and anxious. Dosage was initially 25-50 mg. 4 times daily, with 12.5 mg. 3 or 4 times a day as the usual maintenance dose.

Diarrhea was the principal symptom in 26 patients with functional disorders. They were maintained on Cantil with

(8) Am. J. Gastroenterol. 28:541-547, November, 1957.

phenobarbital 3 times daily for 3-12 months. Most were symptom free during this period. Rectal bleeding was controlled in 2 with ACTH, prednisone or both during acute attacks. Pain and distention were chief symptoms in the other 18 with functional disorders. Four did not respond to therapy, 8 were partially controlled and 6 completely so.

The 1 patient with diarrhea due to achlorhydria was treated with ACTH and Cantil, followed by Cantil alone, which kept the diarrhea completely under control. In ulcerative colitis, frequency was reduced, resulting in formed stools and checking hemorrhage. Used with adrenal cortical hormones, Cantil often led to normal bowel function. Cramps, rectal lesions and weight and spirits improved, but x-ray studies failed to show definite changes. Bacterial gastroenteritis was treated with the appropriate antibiotic when feasible. Cantil was administered after the acute stage subsided and was generally successful in controlling symptoms.

Patients with ileitis did not respond to Cantil, as might be expected in view of the selective action on the colon. The same property leads to fewer side effects than experienced with other anticholinergic agents. Patients with ulcerative colitis had some blurring of vision and dryness of the mouth which disappeared when dosage was reduced. Two had retention of urine, 1 being able to continue with Cantil at a lower dosage.

Management of Peptic Ulcer with Unrestricted Diet and New Combination of Therapeutic Agents was investigated by Louis A. Rosenblum[9] (Forest Hills, N. Y.). Restricted ulcer diets probably interfere with and delay the healing of ulcers and also produce vitamin and protein deficiencies. Relief of symptoms and healing of peptic ulcer, as evidenced by x-rays, was achieved in 97% of 145 private patients with an unrestricted and unlimited diet combined with antacid-antispasmodic medication. All but 3 were managed on an ambulatory basis and were permitted to continue their usual occupations. Treatment was continued without interruption 4-20 months.

The antacid-antispasmodic preparation (Pepulcin®), in tablet form, consisted of aluminum hydroxide, 200 mg.; magnesium oxide, 50 mg.; scopolamine methylbromide or methyl-

(9) Am. J. Gastroenterol. 28:507-517, November, 1957.

nitrate, 2 mg.; and ascorbic acid, 10 mg. Treatment was begun with 2 tablets 4 times daily after meals and at bedtime. This dose produced considerable constipation, dryness of mouth and blurred vision. Reducing the dose to 1 tablet produced the same therapeutic results, with significant lessening of side effects.

The tremendous psychologic benefit provided by allowing the patient to live and eat as a normal person, without interference with his occupation (which would introduce an element of insecurity), is a potent force in treating peptic ulcer, which probably is a basically psychosomatic disease.

Doxinate® in Treatment of Constipation. Doxinate (dioctyl sodium sulfosuccinate) differs from all other substances used in treatment of constipation in that its sole action is fecal softening. This action of the drug depends on reduction of the surface tension at the oil-water interface in the heterogeneous fecal material. Leo J. Cass and Willem S. Frederik[1] (Harvard Univ.) studied the action of dioctyl sodium sulfosuccinate in 74 patients with long histories of chronic functional constipation. Use of the agent resulted in easier passage of the softened stools, increased frequency of bowel movements and increased patient satisfaction. Side effects of both laxation and constipation were markedly reduced. The need for enemas and laxatives became negligible. Administration of the drug for 20 days or more is desirable.

Clinical observations were made on 40 patients who received dioctyl sodium sulfosuccinate for constipation due to or accompanying various conditions (redundant bowel, Hirschsprung's disease, multiple sclerosis, cerebral accident, cardiac conditions, hemorrhoids, use of narcotics or psychodynamic drugs). In most of these patients loss of tonus or suppression of the anal reflex made frequent laxation necessary to avoid impaction. Routine continuing administration of dioctyl sodium sulfosuccinate maintained the feces in a soft, normal form, so laxation could be decreased to 4 or 5-day intervals without tenesmus at passage and with no danger of impaction.

An outstanding advantage of the use of dioctyl sodium sulfosuccinate is that the full daily dosage of 1 or 2 small capsules can be given at one time, with no necessity for ad-

(1) Am. J. Gastroenterol. 26:691-698, December, 1956.

ministration several times a day. No evidence of toxicity has been observed.

Timed Integration of Stool Hydration and Peristaltic Stimulation in Constipation Correction provides what Alvin D. Yasuna and Alfred Halpern[2] (New York) describe as a new dimension in laxative therapy. The necessary dosage of dioctyl sodium sulfosuccinate and the time needed after administration to soften a fecal mass were judged by determining the amount needed to lower the surface tension of artificial intestinal juice below 35 dynes/sq. cm., the time needed to disintegrate dry, hard fecal samples of various weights and the time required after administration to produce the needed reduction in the surface tension of colostomy exudates.

The effective wetting concentration in the juice, in which bile salts abet the action, was reached at 0.015% and no further reduction of surface tension resulted from concentrations in excess of 0.05%. It was concluded that ineffective therapy could not be corrected by the use of doses larger than 50 mg.

The effective wetting level was found in colostomy exudates from 3 patients on uniform, fat-free diets in 6½-7 hours after administration of this dose. The time needed to disintegrate fecal masses was added to this interval, since it had been observed that the size of the mass was not a factor in the time required. To be effective, stimulation of Auerbach's plexus should occur 7½-10 hours after administration of the softening agent when constipation is due to neuron deficit.

Standardized senna pod glycosides, a preparation known as Senokot®, stimulates 8 hours after ingestion, acts solely on the colon and is free from irritation and rebound constipation. Capsules containing 50 mg. dioctyl sodium sulfosuccinate and 225 mg. Senokot, called Senokaps®, were given to 32 patients with refractory constipation who had not had success with wetting agents alone. Evacuation was produced in 10-24 hours. Six patients with hemorrhoids and constipation had similar results and experienced less pain and trauma when Senokaps were used. The capsules were administered 3 or 4 days after hemorrhoidectomy in 8 pa-

(2) Am. J. Gastroenterol. 28:530-540, November, 1957.

tients and in 4 with fissurectomy. All had uneventful convalescence. In none was treatment effective in less than 10 hours and in only 4 was it delayed more than 16. There were no observable side effects. The combined, co-ordinated treatment is effective and the results predictable.

New Evacuant Suppository: Results in Treatment of Rectal Dyschezia of Chronic Sick and Geriatric Patients. Recently a new laxative, dulcolax, (4,4′-diacetoxy-diphenyl)-(pyridyl-2)-methane, has been reported to be orally effective, nontoxic and not absorbent systemically. A. N. G. Clark[3] (St. James's Hosp., Leeds, England) reports results of a clinical trial of a suppository containing this laxative.

In the first part of the investigation, 289 suppositories were administered to 84 patients who were having regular enemas or who had had no bowel action for 3 or more days. Patients were aged 32-92, and more than three-fourths were over 70. The suppositories, each containing 10 mg. of the active ingredient, were inserted as high as possible into the rectum with the gloved finger. In 216 (75%) instances results with only 1 suppository were thought to be as good as after a successful enema. In 39 (13%) instances results were moderately good; in 34 (12%), little or no feces were passed. Stools were loose and unformed in only 9 instances. In 256 (88%) instances the result was a single stool; in the others, 2 or more stools were passed.

In the second part of the investigation, suppositories were administered to 48 patients on 155 occasions when an enema would ordinarily have been given. In 131 (84%) instances results were excellent after using only 1 suppository. In 12 (8%), a satisfactory result was obtained after a second suppository; in the other 12, a satisfactory result was produced after an aperient at night and a suppository the next morning. In no patient was an enema necessary, and none was given in the wards during the study.

The incidence of reactions was negligible. During administration of 480 suppositories, 3 patients had slight abdominal pain and 1 had a feeling of nausea; vomiting in another may have been unrelated to use of a suppository. Among 100 consecutive patients, bowel action occurred within 30 minutes after insertion of a suppository in 5, between 30 and 60

(3) Brit. M. J. 2:866-868, Oct. 12, 1957.

minutes after insertion in 56 and more than an hour after insertion in 39.

This trial indicates that the use of dulcolax suppositories in chronically sick and aged patients is safer and more convenient than enemas.

Treatment of Nausea Following Therapeutic Irradiation. One of the distressing complications of irradiation therapy is the nausea and vomiting which follow it in many patients and is thought to be related to absorption of the protein split-products from damaged tissues. Because antiemetic drugs have been reported to be successful in varying degrees, J. E. Lofstrom, Samuel Balotsky, Nicholas Jackiw and A. J. Spanjers[4] (Wayne State Univ.) studied the effectiveness of a combination of meclizine and pyridoxine (Bonadoxin®).

Of 91 patients with a variety of malignancies, 9 were excluded because of central nervous system metastases which made determination of effectiveness of the drug or cause of vomiting difficult or because of carcinoma of the stomach in which application of irradiation directly to the tumor area could well cause profound gastrointestinal disturbances. Of the 82 other patients, 45 (55%) showed some nausea or vomiting. Bonadoxin was given to 40 of the 45. At some time in the study, 15 received a placebo; 3 received no medication. Of 4 who received only placebo, none was benefited.

Of 40 who received Bonadoxin, 35 (87%) had dramatic and complete relief from nausea and vomiting or were definitely improved. Of 11 who received Bonadoxin and placebo alternately, only 2 (13%) reported benefit from the placebo. No side effects were noted. Bonadoxin appears to be of definite value in control of radiation sickness in many patients.

Prochlorperazine for Treatment of Nausea and Vomiting of Early Pregnancy was tried in 80 cases by Charles Leavitt Sullivan[5] (St. Elizabeth's Hosp., Boston), who administered 30 mg. of the drug daily. Relief was obtained in 90% of cases and side effects were observed in only 8.7%. The drug was equally effective in daily divided doses or in one daily administration at 9 p.m. in Spansule® form. In 40% of cases therapy was started by the 6th menstrual week, and few patients required drug therapy after the 12th to the 15th men-

(4) West. J. Surg. 65:306-307, Sept.-Oct., 1957.
(5) New England J. Med. 258:232-234, Jan. 30, 1958.

strual week. In certain cases, the earlier it was necessary to initiate treatment, the longer it had to be continued.

With the use of chlorpromazine, augmentation of the natural lethargy of early pregnancy was noted to the point of distress in 25% of cases. With 30 mg. prochlorperazine daily incidence of this untoward effect was reduced to 6%. The rate of occurrence of spontaneous abortion in patients requiring definitive drug therapy for control of nausea and vomiting of pregnancy was roughly 5%, whereas in 3,467 consecutive pregnancies it was 13.2%.

Buclizine Hydrochloride for Nausea and Vomiting of Pregnancy. F. J. Conklin and Robert E. L. Nesbitt, Jr.[6] (Johns Hopkins Hosp.) treated 58 pregnant women complaining of nausea and vomiting with a variety of drugs, including the recently developed antihistamine, buclizine hydrochloride. This drug, given in dosages of 50 and 25 mg. twice daily, constituted effective treatment, superior to that noted for the combination of meclizine dihydrochloride, 25 mg., and pyridoxine hydrochloride, 50 mg., and other compounds administered under similar conditions.

Thirty-one of 32 patients treated with buclizine had complete relief from symptoms or marked improvement. Treatment was effective, regardless of the patient's attitude and the duration and severity of symptoms before therapy. Buclizine was effective within 24 hours in most patients and within 48 hours in all but 1. Beneficial effect lasted longer than the time between doses, namely, 10-12 hours.

Drowsiness, the only significant side effect, necessitated stopping treatment in only 1 patient, and only after complete relief from primary symptoms had been achieved. Administration of a relatively large dose of buclizine over a long period to 30 women in the 3d trimester was unassociated with maternal or fetal complications.

Vomiting in Infancy and Early Childhood: Treatment with Prochlorperazine. Persistent vomiting often impedes prompt treatment in children and may lead to dehydration. Various phenothiazine derivatives have been shown to have antiemetic activity, and among the newest of these is prochlorperazine (Compazine®). C. E. Hopkins and T. V. Geppert[7] (Univ. of Wisconsin) studied the effect of syrup of

(6) Obst. & Gynec. 11:214-219, February, 1958.
(7) J. Pediat. 52:687-689, June, 1958.

prochlorperazine in 44 children, aged 4 months to 9 years, who had had 3 or more vomiting episodes daily. In 36, symptoms of acute gastroenteritis, measles, mumps encephalitis, diarrhea, acute pharyngitis, acute nasopharyngitis, pertussis, acute glomerular nephritis, acute tonsillitis, streptococcic pharyngitis or atherostomatitis were present. Vomiting had persisted 18 hours to 3 days. In the other 8 children, further symptoms were nervousness, overactivity, insomnia, abdominal pain, eye blinking and facial grimacing. Vomiting had persisted sporadically for 7-10 days.

Doses of prochlorperazine were graduated from 2.5 mg. (½ teaspoon) 3 times daily for the youngest patients to 5 mg. 4 times daily for the oldest. Therapy for the underlying condition—diet restriction, antibiotics and intravenous fluids—was given to 18 patients.

Of the 36 whose vomiting was associated with organic disease, 14 had an excellent response; vomiting abated after the second dose. In 19 others the response was good, 1 was only fair and 2 did not respond. Thus 92% were free from vomiting and could retain fluids and medication within 12 hours after 3 or, in a few cases, 4 doses. Those whose vomiting had persisted less than 36 hours before treatment had a higher percentage of excellent responses. The drug was as effective in infants as in older children. Of the 8 children whose vomiting was associated with psychic disturbance, 3 had a good response, 1 fair and 4 did not improve.

No side effects were observed. No patient manifested jaundice, abnormal urinary findings or changes in white or red blood cell counts. The fruit-flavored syrup was acceptable to the children. Resistance to the second and third doses was less than to the initial dose or was absent.

► [H. H. Berman *et al.* (J. Dis. Child. 95:146, 1958) found this drug fairly effective in combating the vomiting associated with psychic phenomena in severely retarded children.—Ed.]

Promethazine Suppositories for Management of Nausea and Vomiting in Children. Thomas E. Cone Jr.[8] (US Naval Hosp., Bethesda, Md.) tried promethazine (10-[2-dimethylaminopropyl] phenothiazine hydrochloride) suppositories in 150 children for control of vomiting due to acute nonspecific gastroenteritis, infections, motion sickness and deep abdominal irradiation.

(8) A.M.A. J. Dis. Child. 95:397-400, April, 1958.

Suppositories containing 12.5 mg. promethazine were administered to children under age 5; for older children, 25 mg. suppositories were used. The suppository was inserted digitally beyond the sphincter, the buttocks being held firmly together for 5 minutes to prevent expulsion.

Results were evaluated as good if there was no further emesis after treatment with 1 promethazine suppository and fair if 1-4 episodes occurred after use of the suppository. Treatment was considered a failure if the patient vomited over 4 times after being given 1 suppository.

Control of vomiting was good to fair in 90%. One suppository sufficed to control vomiting in 77% (good result). For 13% (fair result), a second suppository was required and for a few, a third. Ten per cent were not relieved. The use of promethazine suppositories was extremely valuable, representing a real advance in treating nausea and vomiting in acute nonspecific gastroenteritis. On prompt control of emesis, an oral electrolyte nutritive solution was retained; hence serious complications were prevented. Emesis was controlled by 1 suppository in 4 patients undergoing mechlorethamine therapy and in 5 of 6 receiving deep irradiation of abdominal malignant tumors. The sixth patient had a fair result. As these patients experienced only slight nausea, their appetites remained good.

The quiescent effect produced by promethazine was advantageous. Almost all children slept 4-6 hours after insertion of suppositories. However, none showed evidence of lethargy or depression of the sensorium. All could be aroused easily for nursing attentions. There were no toxic effects and no clinical signs of rectal irritation. None of the patients complained of discomfort after insertion of the suppository.

Perphenazine as Antiemetic Agent in Cancer and Other Chronic Diseases. Freddy Homburger[9] (Tufts Univ.) gave 5 mg. perphenazine intramuscularly 4 times a day or 8 mg. orally 2-4 times a day to 37 patients who had had repeated vomiting for several days. Treatment was continued until they stopped vomiting or until side effects or intermittent events prevented further medication. In some instances, a medicament given orally was given parenterally after arrest of vomiting. Eight patients had previously received

(9) J.A.M.A. 167:1240-1241, July 5, 1958.

varying doses of chlorpromazine or prochlorperazine. In several others, placebos of lactose were given 6-14 days before the start of perphenazine therapy and occasionally after vomiting had stopped under medication. Most patients had metastasizing cancer.

Nausea and vomiting were controlled in 27 patients, partly controlled in 6 and 4 had no apparent benefit. In 21, one or more side effects were observed, whereas 16 had none. Undesirable side effects in descending order of frequency were drowsiness, dryness of the mouth, nervousness and lethargy. Nervousness occurred in 3 patients as severe anxiety and apprehension, insomnia, tremulousness and agitation with threats of suicide.

Perphenazine may not be the drug of choice with which to begin therapy, because of the relative frequency of side effects observed in these debilitated patients, but occasionally it affords relief where other drugs have failed and does so quickly in instances in which it is effective.

Adrenal Steroids in Treatment of Malabsorption Syndrome. Tropical sprue, nontropical sprue, often called idiopathic steatorrhea syndrome, and celiac disease of childhood are thought to be clinical varieties of the same metabolic disorder, primary or idiopathic malabsorption syndrome. Standard treatment is empiric. Low-fat, high-protein diets with moderate amounts of carbohydrates and, more recently, gluten free diets have had variable results. David Adlersberg[1] (Mt. Sinai Hosp., New York) reports results of steroid therapy in 33 patients who had sprue refractory to standard therapy. Thirty patients were observed for 6 months to 6½ years.

During the acute phase, intravenous corticotropin, 20-30 units, or hydrocortisone, 50-120 mg., produced striking improvement. The usual therapy consisted of relatively large doses—100 mg. cortisone, 80 mg. hydrocortisone or 50-60 mg. prednisone—orally in divided doses and ACTH gel intramuscularly, 80-100 mg. in 2 doses 12 hours apart. The initial dose was maintained for 8-10 days, then reduced by weekly decrements of 10-20 mg. until the maintenance dose was reached, as indicated by the number of stools, appetite, weight and well-being.

(1) M. Clin. North America 41:1597-1602, November, 1957.

During the initial period, the diet was the standard for sprue. It was gradually liberalized to a bland mixed diet limiting fats, coarse vegetables and fruits, supplemented by calcium and potassium salts, liver extract, folic acid and vitamin B_{12}.

In 28 patients, clinical remissions were obtained, with increased well-being, better appetite—often ravenous—subsided diarrhea and diminished steatorrhea. Serum albumin and calcium increased; also fasting carotene and vitamin A levels. Oral dextrose tolerance and vitamin A tolerance tests improved, and symptoms related to hypoalbuminemia and hypocalcemia disappeared. In some, the sprue pattern improved, as evidenced by x-ray. At times drug administration was interrupted for several weeks, but signs of relapse necessitated resumption of steroid therapy.

Complications attributable to steroid therapy were infrequent, probably because of low doses during the long-term management, often as low as 15 mg. cortisone or 5 mg. prednisone daily.

HEMATOLOGIC DISORDERS

Comparison of Hematologic Responses Following Routine Prenatal Administration of Intramuscular and Oral Iron. Low hemoglobin concentration is common in pregnancy, and large volumes of blood are often administered in attempts to correct it. In 1 year, 31% of the patients on one obstetric service received 1 pt. blood or more. Jack A. Pritchard and Charles F. Hunt[2] (Univ. of Texas) selected patients who were late in the 2d trimester of pregnancy and assigned them at random to one of three groups before any other clinical or laboratory evaluation. One group was given 1,000 mg. iron intramuscularly as iron-dextran; 5 ml. (250 mg. iron) was injected deep into each buttock at the first visit and again 1-3 weeks later. Another group received tablets of ferrous gluconate, 0.3 Gm. 3 times daily for the rest of pregnancy. The third group received lactose tablets 3 times daily.

(2) Surg., Gynec. & Obst. 106:516-518, May, 1958.

In the 49 subjects who received only a placebo, the initial mean hemoglobin level was 11 Gm. (8.8-12.8) and the final concentration averaged 11.3 Gm. (8.8-13.7). In the 49 patients who received 1,000 mg. iron intramuscularly, the initial mean hemoglobin level was 10.9 Gm. (8.8-13) and the final concentration averaged 12.5 Gm. (10.7-15). In the 74 who were given ferrous gluconate, the initial hemoglobin averaged 11.1 Gm. (8.2-13.9) and the final mean was 12.5 Gm. (10.3-14.5). The average increase in hemoglobin thus was 0.3, 1.6 and 1.4 Gm., respectively, in the three groups. This demonstrates again the value of routine iron supplements during pregnancy. No advantage was obtained by intramuscular over simple oral administration.

► [In a comparable study last year, E. Cope *et al.* (1957-58 YEAR BOOK, p. 196) found the orally administered salt as effective as the intramuscular or intravenous doses in all but a few refractory patients, and the latter responded satisfactorily to intramuscular doses.—Ed.]

► ↓ The indications for intramuscular iron and the contraindications to its use, as well as the reasons why intravenous iron should be abandoned, are all well presented in the following article.—Ed.

Parenteral Use of Iron in Treatment of Anemia has been unsuccessful in the past because of marked local and systemic toxic reactions and because of the small content of iron in preparations used for this purpose. Saccharated iron oxide was introduced in 1947 for intravenous use. It is hematologically effective and relatively safe but causes local inflammation. In 1954 a low molecular iron-dextran complex, Imferon®, containing 50 mg./ml. elemental iron, became available. Albert B. Hagedorn[3] reviews experience in 50 patients treated with Imferon.

The first prerequisite for parenteral iron therapy, i.e., that iron is indicated, is fulfilled only in the presence of iron deficiency. In any other type of anemia, iron is probably contraindicated, because all iron which enters the body is essentially quantitatively retained. Severe iron deficiency is usually not difficult to detect, because of the hypochromic and microcytic changes in the peripheral blood. In less advanced cases, diagnosis may be difficult. No test is reliable for iron depletion. Serum iron content, number of sideroblasts and qualitative estimation of stainable iron granules in bone marrow are unreliable. The only ultimate proof of iron-deficiency anemia is adequate response to therapy.

(3) Proc. Staff Meet. Mayo Clin. 32:705-711, Dec. 11, 1957.

For intramuscular administration, 1,000, 1,500 or 2,000 mg. iron is given to adult patients, depending on clinical evaluation and degree of hemoglobin deficit. Most patients have had hemoglobin values of less than 9 Gm./100 ml. Imferon, 5 cc., or 250 mg. iron can be given simultaneously into each gluteal region daily up to the desired amount.

A total of 400 injections were given to 50 patients without significant local or systemic reaction. Imferon is nonirritating and free from general systemic actions when given deep into the muscle. Staining of the skin has been reported when there has been leakage beneath the skin. Imferon is apparently highly toxic given intravenously.

Many patients had impressive therapeutic responses, equal to or better than those observed after intravenous therapy. Iron intramuscularly should essentially supplant the further use of intravenous iron, because of its relative safety. Fewer injections are necessary and the over-all cost of equal doses is less. Total iron content equivalent to that in 2 units of whole blood can be administered safely and comfortably to a patient at a single sitting; that equivalent to 6 units is easily given within 24 hours. The danger of transfusion reaction, possibility of initiating antibody response and transmission of homologous serum jaundice are circumvented by intramuscular administration of iron-dextran complex when the sole need is iron.

Oral iron is effective and is the treatment of choice in most iron-deficiency anemias. However, in some patients with regional enteritis, active chronic ulcerative colitis or extensive resection of bowel and in those intolerant of or sensitive to oral iron, Imferon given intramuscularly is probably the drug preferred. If a maximal rate of hemoglobin regeneration is needed and in patients with massive hemorrhage who will not take transfusions because of religious belief and those unresponsive to oral iron after adequate trial, intramuscular Imferon is probably also indicated. Intramuscular iron is reportedly ineffective in immobile bed patients, markedly obese patients and those with significant chronic infections.

Hemopoietic Effect of Iron in Small Doses on Repeatedly Phlebotomized Volunteers: With Note on Addition of Ascorbic Acid is reported by R. Philip Custer, James Butcher,

Raymond Conover and Walter Cervoni[4] (Univ. of Pennsylvania). Ten healthy men, aged 22-26, were bled of 500 ml. at 0, 1, 2, 3 and 5 weeks. Before each bleeding and for 3 weeks after the last, these medical students were questioned and examined for symptoms related to anemia, and laboratory studies were made.

Treatment began after the third bleeding, at which time hemoglobin and serum iron levels indicated a depleted iron reserve. Exsiccated ferrous sulfate in pellets selectively coated to give release throughout the stomach and small intestine were placed in a capsule to make a total dose of 47 mg. elemental iron. Five subjects received 1 capsule daily; the other 5 were given similar doses in capsules also containing 75 mg. ascorbic acid. All received normal diets containing 10-15 mg. iron daily, with vitamin C restricted by elimination of citrus and tomato juices.

No alarming symptoms occurred. Several subjects engaged in athletics without difficulty. There were no digestive troubles and the feces were but slightly discolored; no undissolved pellets were found. The fall in hemoglobin, red cell count and hematocrit during the 3 weeks without treatment agreed with reports of similar experiments in other laboratories and was checked by the treatment given.

When iron is administered in this way, protected by the coating until located appropriately for quick absorption, ascorbic acid does not appear to be needed to promote absorption. The small dose is adequate to control anemia caused by chronic bleeding and the greater intestinal disturbance attendant on larger doses may be avoided.

► [Ascorbic acid (vitamin C) is present in some commercially available preparations of iron for oral use because it is an unobnoxious reducing agent that is calculated to hold the iron in ferrous form for maximum absorption. Actually, some years ago J. Groen showed (Biochim. et biophys. acta 1:315, 1947) that ferrous sulfate would not be taken up from isolated loops of rat intestine unless reducing substances were added, of which ascorbic acid was best. However, the amounts required to effect a pronounced upswing in absorption were out of all proportion to those available in the tablets offered for human use. This was the experience also of C. V. Moore and R. Dubach (Tr. A. Am. Physicians 64:245, 1951): ascorbic acid would enhance the uptake of radioiron in several series of individuals, but the greater assimilation was significant only when 1 Gm. ascorbic acid was added to the test meal. It is difficult to avoid the conclusion that the amount of the vitamin present in the proprietary tablets has only token value.—Ed.]

(4) Am. J. M. Sc. 235:309-316, March, 1958.

Chelate Iron Therapy is discussed by Murray Franklin, Wayne G. Rohse, Jesus de la Huerga (Chicago) and Cecil R. Kemp[5] (Decatur, Ill.). Administration of effective doses of iron in treating iron deficiency anemia is complicated by the fact that iron compounds are not innocuous. Toxicity experiments on dogs and rabbits showed that the concentration of iron attained in the animal's serum determined the severity of the acute symptoms. Iron in the form of ferrous sulfate or ferrous gluconate raised the serum iron level higher and caused more intense symptoms of intoxication than did equivalent doses of iron choline citrate. Presenting the iron to the system as a chelate complex caused less adverse effects than the use of ionized or readily ionizable preparations.

Chelation is a chemical process wherein metallic ions are sequestered and bound into clawlike rings within the chelating molecule. Metals thus bound lose their ordinary properties when they enter into the chelate union. The amount of a given metal which can be taken into solution may be greatly altered, and the metal may resist forces which would precipitate it from solution were it present in an ionic form. One gram of iron choline citrate will dissolve in 0.2 ml. water, a solubility of 500 Gm./100 ml. Moreover, the iron of this chelate will remain in solution at pH values up to 10.2 and in the presence of such natural iron precipitants as protein, phosphates and carbonates. Dialysis studies reveal that the diffusibility of iron from iron choline citrate is low compared with the iron of ferrous sulfate and ferrous gluconate. These properties may account in part for the effectiveness of the chelate as a therapeutic agent, for its iron may be maintained in solution over a greater area of the gastrointestinal tract, thus permitting an optimal physiologic uptake by union with iron acceptors. At the same time, direct diffusion into the circulation may be minimized even if high concentrations of iron are ingested.

Hemoglobin has long been recognized to be a chelate complex of iron, but only recently has chelation been associated with other phases of iron metabolism.

Test doses containing 120 mg. iron were given orally to 5 volunteers, first as ferrous sulfate solution, then 2 weeks

(5) J.A.M.A. 166:1685-1693, Apr. 5, 1958.

later as iron choline solution; determinations of serum iron before and after each administration showed that the sulfate caused a higher and less sustained rise in serum iron than did the complex. Given orally in tablet form [Ferrolip®] thrice daily to 131 patients in doses of 120-240 mg./day for a total of 3,303 treatment days, iron choline citrate caused gastrointestinal symptoms in only 6 patients, and in these it was possible to continue the medication since all symptoms presently disappeared. The clinical responses, both symptomatically and from a laboratory viewpoint, were entirely satisfactory, comparable to those previously attained from other iron preparations used under similar circumstances.

► [This confirms the findings of J. Pomeranze and R. J. Gadek last year (1957-58 YEAR BOOK, p. 201) in a much smaller series of cases.—Ed.]

Oral Maintenance Therapy in Pernicious Anemia with Vitamin B_{12} and Hog Intrinsic Factor was studied by Poul Bastrup-Madsen[6] (Aarhus, Denmark) because of many reports of patients who ceased to respond to oral treatment after initial remission. Twenty-five patients with pernicious anemia demonstrated by macrocytic anemia, megaloblastic marrow, histamine-fast achlorhydria, typical reticulocyte and red cell response to therapy, exclusion of other forms by study of diet, examination for steatorrhea and x-rays of the gastrointestinal tract were studied. Three preparations were used: (1) a tablet with 7.5 μg. vitamin B_{12} and 100 mg. hog pyloric mucosa, (2) a tablet with 20,000 coli units of intrinsic factor plus 10 μg. vitamin B_{12} and (3) a capsule with 50 mg. desiccated mucosa and 5 μg. vitamin B_{12}. Dosage was varied to suit personal needs; the dose was increased when red blood cell counts or hematocrit readings decreased. If no beneficial effects were derived from 30 μg. vitamin B_{12}/day, oral treatment was considered useless. After remission and release from the hospital, patients were examined every 2-4 months. Maintenance therapy at home was given as 1 daily dose. This was continued for 18 months to 2 years.

A satisfactory response (complete remission during maintenance) was obtained in 17 patients. Of these, 8 showed subnormal serum vitamin B_{12} levels on bioassay and 1 was not tested. In 8 patients response was unsatisfactory. Initial hematologic improvement was not maintained in 6 on oral

(6) Acta med. scandinav. 159:323-337, 1957.

therapy, 5 of whom responded promptly thereafter to parenteral vitamin administration. Two had neurologic difficulties.

Prolonged administration of hog gastric mucosa may in some way lead to decreased absorption of vitamin B_{12}. Serum assays were not available until late in the study and it was concluded that, in the absence of such a guide to the success of therapy, oral vitamin and intrinsic factor is not sufficiently reliable as a maintenance procedure.

► [A few other isolated observations in recent years have cast doubt on the reliability of B_{12}-intrinsic factor preparations, the most recent perhaps being that of R. Berlin *et al.* (Acta med. scandinav. 161:143, 1958); in 22 of his 66 patients refractoriness to the treatment developed on the average after 12 months. Parenteral B_{12} therapy is still certain and sure and in most instances not excessively inconvenient for the patient, and with its use the physician retains full control of the situation.—Ed.]

Folinic Acid in Megaloblastic Anemia of Pregnancy was investigated by Jean M. Scott[7] (Glasgow). Varying doses of folinic acid were given 19 patients, 17 diagnosed ante partum. The optimum dose, given to 10, was 12 mg. intramuscularly the 1st day, followed by daily injections of 6 mg. until a reticulocyte peak (between 8 and 19%) was reached, usually in 8 days. No further treatment was given, yet all continued to improve. Initially hemoglobin levels ranged from 3.6 to 9.3 Gm./100 ml. and red blood cell counts from 1,800,000 to 3,260,000/cu. mm. At term, the antepartum patients had an average hemoglobin of 10.4 and a red blood cell count of 3,350,000. Two months later the hemoglobin was 12.7 and the count 4,430,000. Seven patients seen 6 months after delivery were well and had normal counts. When calcium leucovorin became available, 3 patients were given folinic acid orally in this form at the same dosage and showed equal benefit.

Folinic acid [Leucovorin] has to be given in sufficiently large amounts initially to produce satisfactory response. Once a satisfactory reticulocyte response is obtained, folinic acid may be discontinued. Since maintenance treatment is not required, the existence of an absolute deficiency is improbable.

► [The megaloblastic anemia of pregnancy frequently responds very slowly if at all to liver extract or cyanocobalamin (vitamin B_{12}), but folic acid is effective. Since folic acid is converted in the body, through the catalytic action of vitamin C, into folinic acid (citrovorum factor) the use of folinic acid in the first place is logical.

(7) Brit. M. J. 2:270-272, Aug. 3, 1957.

The megaloblastic anemia of infancy always responds to folic acid and hence might be expected to respond to folinic acid also, but it also sometimes responds to liver extract or cyanocobalamin; it may be a syndrome rather than a single entity.

The nutritional megaloblastic anemia syndrome, of which tropical macrocytic anemia is a geographic type only, responds best to the combined use of cyanocobalamin, folic acid and large doses of thiamine.

The anemias of sprue, fish tapeworm infestation, celiac disease, gastrointestinal disease and surgery (when macrocytic) respond best to cyanocobalamin and folic acid used together.—Ed.]

Cobalt Folliculitis, acneform eruption or aggravation of pre-existing acne were observed in 60 patients receiving cobalt chloride, according to Chester M. Sidell, J. Gordon Erickson and Jack E. McCleary[8] (Univ. of Southern California). The reactions were observed in patients aged 10-58, predominantly in females. In 20 patients, classed as having primary disease, the eruption developed in essentially normal skin. In 40 patients, classed as having secondary disease, the eruption constituted aggravation of existing acne or reactivation of pre-existing acne. The period of ingestion of cobalt before the reactions appeared varied from 1 to 10 weeks. The most severe manifestations appeared in patients taking cobalt-iron preparations, but others occurred in those taking various vitamin-mineral combinations that contained cobalt. Vitamin B_{12} preparations containing cobalt given parenterally also produced similar skin manifestations in some instances.

In the primary group, after elimination of cobalt, the lesions tended to clear spontaneously. Disappearance of the folliculitis usually occurred gradually in 4-6 weeks. The period of involvement could be greatly shortened by use of antibiotics of the tetracycline and the erythromycin groups. In the secondary group, aggravation of the acneform eruption was more persistent but again was shortened by use of antibiotics in addition to routine acne therapy. The mechanism by which cobalt produces the abovementioned reactions is obscure.

Active acne contraindicates use of vitamin-iron-mineral supplements containing cobalt.

► [Other reactions to cobalt that have been reported are gastrointestinal disturbances, precordial pain, renal injury, tinnitus and temporary deafness, thyroid hyperplasia with hypofunction and thrombocytosis.—Ed.]

---

(8) California Med. 88:20-21, January, 1958.

Treatment of Symptomatic Hemolytic Anemia with Prednisone. Herbert C. Lichtman, S. Fred Rabiner, George S. Shields, Nathan Plotkin and Richard Levere[9] treated 9 patients with hemolytic anemia secondary to malignant, mesenchymal, proliferative disorders. Five had chronic lymphocytic leukemia, 2 lymphosarcoma and 2 multiple myeloma. Diagnosis of hemolytic anemia was established mainly by clinical observation of a fall in circulating hemoglobin levels or a loss of transfused blood in excess of 1%/day. Gross or occult blood loss was excluded in each case.

In all but 1 patient the hemolytic state was brought under control. As much as 80 mg. prednisone/day was necessary for therapeutic benefit in several patients. After the anemia was controlled, it was usually possible to decrease the daily dose slowly, but in most cases a level was reached below which relapse occurred. In no case could therapy be stopped completely without relapse. The 1 patient who was not benefited was refractory to 100 mg. prednisone daily and died of bronchopneumonia.

Rise in hemoglobin after institution of adequate steroid therapy was frequently dramatic. In no case did the hemolytic process relapse during observation periods of 7-110 weeks, unless the steroid was reduced or discontinued. The steroid did not appear to have a direct effect on the underlying disease. Rather, the effectiveness of this therapy in raising the hemoglobin and red blood cell count seemed to be due to a reduction in the rate of hemolysis and to augmentation of bone marrow erythropoiesis.

Because of the relatively large doses of prednisone used, all patients manifested varying degrees of obesity suggesting Cushing's syndrome. Glycosuria occurred in several. One patient had a Staphylococcus aureus bacteremia which could be controlled only by reducing the dose of prednisone to low levels. Another had an overwhelming septicemia after more than 2 years of treatment.

Four patients had been treated initially with cortisone. In 2 of these, side effects were so severe that cortisone was discontinued and prednisone substituted. Another did not benefit from cortisone but later responded to 60 mg. prednisone daily. The 4th patient received a maximum of 350 mg. corti-

(9) New England J. Med. 257:631-637, Oct. 3, 1957.

sone daily without improvement but responded dramatically to 90 mg. prednisone daily.

► [There has been pretty general satisfaction with the response of acquired hemolytic anemia to ACTH and the adrenal corticoids, so much so indeed that this malady is included in all listings of the entities that can usually be counted on to be benefited by use of these agents. However, there are instances in which the cortisone or hydrocortisone dosage required is so high that a prohibitive degree of side actions results. It is in such recalcitrant cases that the superiority of prednisone seems to have been demonstrated in the present article.—Ed.]

Influence of Method of Administration on Cortisone Effect in Thrombocytopenia. P. Weller[1] (Martin Luther Univ.) reports 2 cases of idiopathic thrombocytopenia in which 100 mg. cortisone by mouth daily significantly increased thrombocytes, though neither patient responded to cortisone given parenterally. This difference in effect was demonstrated on several occasions. Results were similar with cortisone acetate.

Girl, 16, had had frequent nasal and dental bleeding and hematomas in the skin on the slightest injury for 2 years. For some weeks she had also had spontaneous cutaneous hemorrhages. Petechiae were especially prominent on the extremities. The spleen was not enlarged. The thrombocyte count was 36,000. The blood picture was not remarkable; bleeding and clotting times were normal. Rumpel-Leede and Coombs tests, both direct and indirect, were negative. Sternal puncture revealed no abnormality. A therapeutic test with ACTH, 100 units daily for 6 days, had no effect, nor did 200 mg. cortisone parenterally daily for 6 days. After oral administration of cortisone, thrombocytes definitely increased from the 3d day to 120,000; after reduction of the dose, the count fell and then was constant around 60,000-70,000 without medication. After repeated oral administration of cortisone, similar results were obtained.

When the suspension of cortisone acetate usually given by injection was given by mouth, a less striking increase in thrombocytes was obtained with about double the dose given in the tablets. After substitution of cortisone tablets, thrombocytes again reached a high level; with parenteral administration, it again sank after the 3d day to pretherapeutic levels. The leukocyte curve followed a course similar to that of the thrombocytes.

The patient reacted to 125 and 250 mg. Diamox® with Quincke edema of the face. Diamox appeared to be indicated to combat a Cushing syndrome which appeared after a parenteral course of cortisone (which did not affect the thrombocytes). This offered proof of the activity of the preparation used for parenteral injection.

Clinical Use of Methylprednisolone in Certain Hematologic Disorders was studied in 58 patients by Adel A. Yunis

(1) Deutsche med. Wchnschr. 82:1340-1342, Aug. 16, 1957.

and William J. Harrington[2] (Washington Univ.). Dosages were selected according to the patient's disease and history of previous steroid therapy. When feasible, in patients previously treated with prednisone, 4 mg. methylprednisolone was given for every 5 mg. prednisone previously used. Average duration of treatment was about 4 weeks, depending on the patient's course and response and the side effects of corticosteroid therapy.

Acute lymphocytic leukemia was treated in 5 patients; of these, 1 died of bacteremia 1 day after initiation of treatment, 2 had no significant response to continued therapy with methylprednisolone and amethopterin, 1 obtained a partial remission and the other a complete remission lasting 1½ months. Chronic lymphocytic leukemia was treated in 13 patients, 1 of whom manifested severe exfoliative dermatitis as his main problem. He had been treated elsewhere with nitrogen mustard, irradiation and prednisone. At a time when his skin condition was improving after a course of nitrogen mustard and a daily prednisone dose of 10 mg., methylprednisolone was started, 16 mg. daily. There was further improvement and a significant rise in hemoglobin. Subsequently the dermatitis was kept under control wth 8 mg. methylprednisolone daily. In the other 12 patients, methylprednisolone was used initially at 60-160 mg. daily. All patients improved clinically and most of them showed a significant rise in hemoglobin. The total white cell count tended to rise initially and then fall.

Of 5 patients with monocytic leukemia, only 1 improved definitely and did well on a maintenance dose of 60 mg. methylprednisolone. Other patients, including a child, did not benefit from daily doses of 16 mg.

Two patients in the blastic phase of chronic granulocytic leukemia were treated. The first, a man aged 28, had associated severe hemolytic anemia and marked splenomegaly. Methylprednisolone, 160 mg. daily, resulted in striking subjective improvement, reduction in transfusion requirement and moderate regression in splenic size. Treatment of the other patient possibly accelerated the leukemic process.

Lymphosarcoma was treated in 3 patients; 1 achieved marked symptomatic improvement and mild regression of

(2) Metabolism 7 (pt. 2):543-568, July, 1958.

lymph nodes and hepatosplenomegaly. Of 4 patients with hypoplastic anemia, 1 obtained a well-defined clinical and hematologic response. Anerythrocytogenic anemia was successfully treated in 2 patients. Among 10 cases of thrombocytopenia, 8 were of the idiopathic variety; 7 of the patients showed a satisfactory response. Two patients with symptomatic thrombocytopenia and adequate megakaryocytes in the bone marrow showed no response to therapy. There were 5 patients with acquired hemolytic anemia. In 2, hemolysis had been controlled with prednisone, and when methylprednisolone was substituted, improvement was maintained; the other 3 obtained a satisfactory response to initial therapy with this corticosteroid.

One patient who had systemic lupus erythematosus with circulating anticoagulant, maintained free from symptoms with 15 mg. prednisone daily, remained asymptomatic when given 12 mg. methylprednisolone daily instead. One man who had pancytopenia, refractory anemia and dysproteinemia was unaffected by methylprednisolone, 100 mg. daily for 10 days and 60 mg. for 15 days. A young woman with post-streptococcic purpura fulminans made a good recovery while receiving the drug. However, she also received heparin, antibiotics and other treatments, which made evaluation difficult. One instance of allergic purpura did not respond to methylprednisolone, 16 mg. daily for 15 days. A patient with pseudohemophilia and one with normocytic normochromic anemia and a Cr^{51}-red cell half-life of 17 days obtained no benefit from methylprednisolone. Another with advanced scleroderma showed some subjective improvement and slight improvement in finger movements after a total dose of 130 mg.; however, he also received physiotherapy in the interval. In 1 patient with nephrosis and massive edema, diuresis did not follow methylprednisolone in daily doses of 40 mg. for 10 days.

HYPOTHYROIDISM

► ↓ It is pertinent to remark that with the use of the drug Cytomel®, the subject of the next 3 articles, there may be wide variations in the metabolic status of the patient since the agent has a short duration of action in comparison wih thyroid substance. Its omission, or spacing of the doses too widely, may cause distressing withdrawal symptoms.—Ed.

Sodium Liothyronine in Metabolic Insufficiency Syndrome and Associated Disorders: Preliminary Report is presented by Joseph H. Morton[3] (New York). The syndrome of metabolic insufficiency is characterized by a low-normal or subnormal basal metabolic rate (usually —15 to —30%), by clinical signs and symptoms of deficient metabolism and by normal thyroid function, as indicated by the serum protein-bound iodine, cholesterol and I^{131}-uptake tests. It appears that thyroxin must be deiodinated to liothyronine in the peripheral tissues before it becomes active. In patients with metabolic insufficiency this conversion may be incomplete. Signs and symptoms include chronic fatigue, somnolence or lethargy, dry hair and skin, infertility, dysmenorrhea, menstrual irregularity, sensitivity to cold, joint and muscle aches and stiffness, obesity, irritability, emotional instability and constipation. These are similar to changes in hypothyroidism but less severe.

Good to excellent responses to treatment with sodium liothyronine [Cytomel®] were elicited in 46 of 51 patients with metabolic insufficiency. Only 3 had previously shown good to excellent responses to desiccated thyroid, thyroglobulin or thyroxin. Of 29 patients with specific metabolic disorders (female sterility, male infertility, obesity, gynecologic disorders or intractable salt and water imbalance) 25 showed good to excellent response to sodium liothyronine. Thus the relation of such disorders to insufficient metabolism is suggested. It appears that the basic defect causing metabolic insufficiency is severe in certain organ systems in patients with specific metabolic disorders.

Side actions of nervousness, insomnia and tachycardia were noted in 4 of the total of 80 patients treated. No signs of acquired intolerance were observed. It is concluded that so-

(3) J.A.M.A. 165:124-129, Sept. 14, 1957.

dium liothyronine is highly effective and safe for treating patients with metabolic insufficiency and other nonmyxedematous metabolic disorders. A case illustrating excellent response is described here.

Woman, 32, sought treatment because of chronic fatigue, vague muscle pains, obesity and inability to conceive for 7 months. Her hair was thick and coarse. The protein-bound iodine level was 3.6 μg./100 ml. serum, and the BMR was −21% after many months of treatment with desiccated thyroid. Premenstrual smears showed a late secretory phase and increased estrogenic stimulation. Other findings were normal.

After taking 5 μg. sodium liothyronine daily for 1 week, the patient had marked improvement in outlook and energy. The dose was gradually increased to 25 μg. daily. After 6 weeks she felt fine, had more energy, no joint stiffness and "no complaints." She had lost 9.5 lb. and her hair appeared soft and oily.

Triiodothyronine: Clinical Effects in Patients with Suboptimal Response to Other Thyroid Preparations were studied by Stanley Newman and Roberto F. Escamilla[4] (Letterman Army Hosp.). Thirty patients with evidence of hypometabolism or a clinically related condition were given triiodothyronine after suboptimal response to thyroxin or desiccated thyroid. The d,l and l isomers of triiodothyronine were given in doses at least equivalent to the previously administered dose of thyroid, so that the effects could be compared.

Improvement was noted in 13 patients (43.3%); the rest were unimproved or became worse. Side effects occurred in 9 of 34 trials (26%) and could not always be eliminated by decreasing the dosage. The highest percentage of good responses occurred in 4 of 5 who received a combination of desiccated thyroid or thyroxin with supplemental triiodothyronine.

Despite careful analysis of the data, no basis of predicting which patients would benefit from the triiodothyronine was found. However, the occasional, sometimes dramatic improvement, suggested that a therapeutic trial with triiodothyronine in difficult or unresponsive cases of hypometabolism or hypothyroidism is justified.

Clinical Applications of Triiodothyronine. A. W. G. Goolden and Craig D. Burrell[5] have used triiodothyronine when hypothyroidism must be rapidly corrected, in thyroid

(4) California Med. 88:206-210, March. 1958.
(5) Brit. M. J. 2:1028-1032, Nov. 2, 1957.

carcinoma between doses of radioactive iodine, for diagnostic suppression of thyroid function, as a therapeutic test for hypothyroidism and in treatment of myxedema coma. Most of these conditions are rare in general medical practice.

Triiodothyronine is about 5 times as active as thyroxin on a molar basis and, qualitatively, the 2 compounds appear identical. The exact site of formation of triiodothyronine is unknown. Experimental studies have suggested formation in the thyroid gland and in peripheral tissues. Thyroxin is associated with a globulin fraction between $alpha_1$ and $alpha_2$. Triiodothyronine is associated with this same protein fraction, but the complex is less stable than that of thyroxin, which may account for the more rapid disappearance of triiodothyronine from the serum. Triiodothyronine is a normal constituent of human plasma and is the only substance known to have greater activity than natural thyroxin. Any clinical application must obviously depend on its rapid effect because the qualitative effect is the same as that of thyroxin. It usually is not necessary or desirable to correct myxedema rapidly, except perhaps on a rare occasion.

Man, 52, was given therapeutic I^{131} for severe angina of effort, then maintained on 0.1 mg. l-thyroxin daily. He remained free from angina and could do light work. Sixteen months later paranoid psychosis suddenly developed. He had no other sign of hypothyroidism except dry, scaly skin and slight puffiness of the eyes. Plasma cholesterol was 510 mg./100 ml. He became violent. He was given 10 µg. l-triiodothyronine intravenously followed by a maintenance dose of 0.1 mg. l-thyroxin orally. Peripheral circulation increased and cutaneous flush was noted. The daily intravenous dose was increased until he was receiving 40 µg., and 0.1 mg. thyroxin was continued orally. Signs of hyperthyroidism appeared with marked increase in peripheral circulation and sweating of the palms of the hands. The dose was reduced. During the next week he improved daily. Within 3 weeks he was mentally normal.

It later was discovered that he had been taking 0.1 mg. dl-thyroxin due to an error by the pharmacist. Rapid correction of the hypothyroidism was desirable because of the psychosis, but a delicate balance had to be maintained because of the angina condition. Triiodothyronine was eminently suitable in these rather unusual circumstances.

INFECTIOUS DISEASES

Sulfonamides and Antibiotics—General Considerations

When Can Combinations of Antibiotics Be Used? Harry F. Dowling[6] (Univ. of Illinois) points out that although many reasons have been given for administration of combinations of antibiotics and many such combinations have been recommended, there often is no clinical proof that they are effective. The combining of antibiotics resulted from the theory that such combinations broaden the spectrum of antibiotic activity. It is difficult to find an antibiotic that will increase to any extent the spectrums of the tetracyclines (Aureomycin®, Terramycin® and tetracycline) or of chloramphenicol. Only few of the pathogenic bacteria that are not inhibited by the tetracyclines or by chloramphenicol are inhibited by other antibiotics.

Antibiotic therapy cannot eliminate all the organisms in a mixed flora. By broadening the spectrum many of the strains are eliminated, thus enabling those not affected by the antibiotics used to multiply without competition and cause superinfections. Laboratory methods used to study the synergistic action of antibiotics are a poor index of what happens in the patient. The only way to prove that 2 antibiotics will act synergistically is to compare effects of the full dose of each single drug with effects of the same dose of the combination of the 2. This takes time and painstaking observation. When several diagnoses are possible, as in various kinds of bacterial or viral pneumonia, a broad-spectrum antibiotic, such as tetracycline, can be given because this will be effective in all pneumonias that are affected by any antibiotic.

Administration of 2 antibiotics actually may be harmful, e.g., if 500 mg. of antibiotic A is effective against gram-positive cocci and 500 mg. of antibiotic B is effective against gram-negative rods and the 2 drugs are given in a 500-mg.

(6) Postgrad. Med. 23:594-597, June, 1958.

capsule, only 250 mg. of each antibiotic is acting against the micro-organisms that it affects. But, if 500 mg. of each antibiotic were included in the mixture, toxic effects would be increased, often beyond tolerance. Sometimes there is actual antagonism between the 2 antibiotics so the combination

Antibiotic Combinations

Purpose	Antibiotics	Indications for Use
To diminish toxic effects	Streptomycin and dihydrostreptomycin (streptoduocin)	When streptomycin is indicated
To prevent emergence of resistant organisms	Streptomycin plus isoniazid or para-aminosalicylic acid	Tuberculosis
	Tetracycline plus nystatin	When tetracycline is indicated
	Erythromycin or novobiocin plus chloramphenicol	Staphylococcic infections
To treat mixed infections.	Penicillin plus streptomycin	Peritonitis after ruptured viscus
	Combinations of selected antibiotics (based on in vitro tests)	Mixed infections of urinary tract
To achieve better result than can be obtained with same amount of either antibiotic alone	Pencillin plus streptomycin	Enterococcic endocarditis
	Streptomycin plus a tetracycline	Brucellosis
	Rarely, penicillin plus a tetracycline or chloramphenicol	Infections caused by resistant staphylococci

does not work as well as the most effective antibiotic used alone. When 2 antibiotics are used instead of 1, the patient is subjected to the risk of becoming hypersensitive to 2 drugs instead of 1. When 2 antibiotics are used in combination, the appearance of resistant staphylococci is delayed but not prevented and when resistant forms appear, many are resistant to both antibiotics. The few proved indications for combinations of antibiotics are outlined in the table.

Antibiotic Combinations: Tetracycline, Erythromycin, Oleandomycin and Spiramycin and Combinations of Tetracycline with Each of the Other Three Agents—Comparisons of Activity in Vitro and Antibacterial Action of Blood after Oral Administration. Wilfred F. Jones, Jr., and Maxwell Finland[7] (Harvard Med. School) found erythromycin alone was clearly superior in vitro to oleandomycin alone and much more active than spiramycin alone against most strains of gram-positive cocci tested, including all strains that were normally sensitive to erythromycin. The cross-resistance among these 3 antibiotics in strains freshly isolated from patients appears to be variable as compared with the regular and essentially complete cross-resistance that develops to all 3 agents in strains repeatedly subcultured in the presence of any one of them.

Of various mixtures used in vitro, combinations containing erythromycin were clearly superior to the others, but no combination was superior to the more active of the components used alone. In particular, no combination tested was superior to the better of the 2 agents—erythromycin or tetracycline. No added activity was provided by the presence of tetracycline in any of the mixtures tested against tetracycline-resistant strains.

Normal men were given orally 1 Gm. tetracycline, erythromycin, oleandomycin or spiramycin and 0.5 Gm. each of tetracycline combined with an equal amount of the other 3 antibiotics, and the plasmas of these subjects were assayed for activity against 3 organisms: a sensitive strain of hemolytic streptococcus and a tetracycline-sensitive and a tetracycline-resistant strain of Staphylococcus aureus. Against each strain the activity of erythromycin alone was significantly superior to that of oleandomycin or spiramycin alone. The combination containing erythromycin was similarly superior, but no combination produced any greater activity than the same total dose of the more active component alone. Against the tetracycline-resistant strain, tetracycline in the combinations did not add to and may have reduced the activity of erythromycin or oleandomycin.

Controlled comparisons were also made of the antibacterial action of blood of the same subjects after ingestion of

(7) New England J. Med. 257:481-490, Sept. 12; 536-547, Sept. 19, 1957.

500 mg. tetracycline alone and with the addition of 250 mg. erythromycin, oleandomycin or spiramycin. Addition of erythromycin enhanced the activity of tetracycline, but addition of the other 2 antibiotics did not. This result was reproduced in tests using the 2 sensitive strains used in the previous experiment and a third that was more sensitive to oleandomycin than to erythromycin.

Oleandomycin and spiramycin are sufficiently inferior to erythromycin to indicate that their general use is unwarranted. If these new agents are made available at all, they should be strictly reserved for treatment of the rare infections proved to be caused by organisms highly sensitive to them and resistant to erythromycin and other active antibiotics in common use. Use of antibiotic combinations of the types studied, particularly the combination of tetracycline with oleandomycin or spiramycin, is not justified by available data.

Survey of Current Bacterial Susceptibility to Antimicrobial Agents: Comparison with Previous Surveys. In acute or fulminating infections, prompt treatment is essential and cannot be delayed until laboratory sensitivity tests can be obtained. To establish a rational basis for selection of the most promising antibiotics in such situations, S. Stanley Schneierson[8] compiled the results of a large number of antibiotic sensitivity determinations performed on different bacteria isolated from a variety of clinical sources from July 1956 to July 1957.

All sensitivity tests were in tubes. Bacterial strains were classed as sensitive if inhibited by concentrations of standard antibiotics up to 0.5 units of penicillin, 1 μg. erythromycin, 5 μg. tetracycline, 10 μg. chloramphenicol, 5 units of bacitracin, 5 μg. streptomycin, 5 μg. neomycin, 25 μg. nitrofurantoin, 20 mg./ml. sulfonamides, 5 μg. novobiocin, 2 μg. oleandomycin and 5 μg. polymyxin/ml. If larger amounts were required, they were considered resistant. The relative effectiveness of different antibiotics against particular bacteria was graded numerically (table).

The proportion of strains of Staphylococcus aureus sensitive to penicillin has remained relatively constant between 1953 and 1957. The incidence of strains resistant to erythro-

(8) J. Mt. Sinai Hosp. New York 25:52-58, Jan.-Feb., 1958.

mycin has risen. Strains of Streptococcus viridans, beta hemolytic streptococcus and pneumococcus have remained highly susceptible to both tetracycline and chloramphenicol. The percentage of strains sensitive to tetracyclines has fallen significantly in Aerobacter aerogenes, Staph. aureus and

COMPARATIVE EFFICACY OF VARIOUS ANTIBIOTICS AGAINST DIFFERENT MICRO-ORGANISMS IN VITRO

Organism	Penicillin	Erythromycin	Tetracyilne	Chloramphenicol	Bacitracin	Streptomycin	Neomycin	Nitrofurantoin	Sulfonamides	Novobiocin	Polymyxin	Oleandomycin
Staphylococcus aureus	3*	2	4	3	1	3	1	1	5	2	—†	2
Staphylococcus albus	2	2	3	2	—	1	—	—	—	2	—	—
Enterococcus	5	2	5	2	—	5	1	1	5	5	—	—
Pneumococcus	1	1	1	1	—	—	—	—	—	—	—	—
Beta Hemolytic Streptococcus	1	1	2	1	—	—	—	—	—	—	—	—
Streptococcus viridans	2	1	2	1	—	2	—	—	—	—	—	—
E. coli	—	—	3	2	—	3	1	1	5	—	1	—
Aerobacter aerogenes	—	—	4	3	—	5	1	1	5	5	2	—
B. proteus	—	—	5	3	—	4	1	1	4	4	5	—
B. pyocyaneus	—	—	5	5	—	4	2	5	5	5	2	—
Salmonella	—	—	1	1	—	—	—	1	—	—	—	—
B. Friedlander	—	—	4	3	—	—	—	1	—	—	—	—
B. alkaligenes fecalis	—	—	—	3	—	—	—	3	—	—	—	—

*Relative effectiveness of antibiotics: 1, over 90% of strains sensitive; 2, 76-90% sensitive; 3, 51-75% sensitive; 4, 25-50% sensitive; 5, less than 25% sensitive.
†Micro-organisms with fewer than 5 strains tested against a particular antibiotic are not graded.

albus and enterococcus. The percentage of strains of Friedländer's bacillus and Staph. aureus sensitive to chloramphenicol has also decreased.

Requirement for Reduction in Antibiotic Doses during Oliguria. In oliguric patients, small doses of antibiotics may produce excessive concentrations in the blood, because the principal route for excretion of many antibiotics is the urine. The finding of extremely high concentrations of several antibiotics at the time of admission of patients with oliguria prompted a study of the blood levels of streptomycin for several days after a single dose of 0.5 Gm. William H. Meroney and Robert B. W. Smith[9] (Walter Reed Army Hosp.) in a study of 10 oliguric patients found that this dose was excessive for patients who already had a significant blood level.

In a patient who was oliguric for 97 days, 0.5 Gm. strepto-

(9) U. S. Armed Forces M. J. 9:370-374, March, 1958.

mycin was excessive as a maintenance dose (Fig. 20). Given when the blood level was already in or above the therapeutic range, it drove the concentration to toxic levels. The only time the rise was limited to the high therapeutic range (25 µg./ml.) was the one occasion when the preinjection level was rather low (2.5 µg./ml.), 6 days after the last dose.

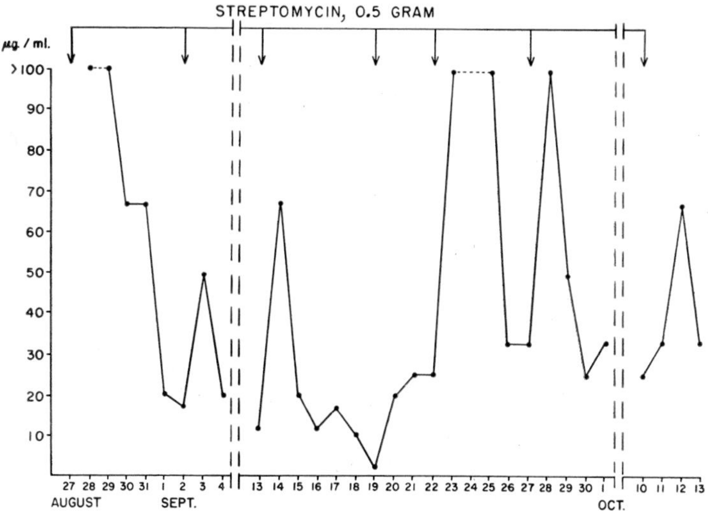

Fig. 20.—Streptomycin concentration in blood of patient with prolonged oliguria. Streptomycin, 0.5 Gm., was given at varying intervals of several days, indicated by arrows. (Courtesy of Meroney, W. H., and Smith, R. B. W.: U. S. Armed Forces M. J. 9:370-374, March, 1958.)

Another time a therapeutic concentration was still present after 6 days, the preceding levels having been extremely high.

Though the data are not adequate to establish exactly the amount or frequency of dosage required to attain and maintain but not to exceed a therapeutic level, they indicate that an initial dose of 0.5 Gm. and maintenance doses of 0.25 Gm. every 2 or 3 days would be reasonable.

Comparison of Oral Penicillin V with Injectable Procaine Penicillin. It has been shown that to equal an injection of parenteral penicillin four times as much oral penicillin G must be ingested. It is also known that the intestinal absorption of penicillin V is twice that of penicillin G. The former has been established as an effective antibiotic for the treatment of penicillin-susceptible infections. The incidence rate of allergic reactions to oral penicillin is much lower than that to parenteral penicillin.

R. S. Griffith and F. B. Peck, Jr.[1] (Indianapolis Gen'l Hosp.) compared the penicillin serum levels in 25 patients after oral penicillin V and after intramuscular penicillin G. The average serum penicillin concentration for each preparation is shown in Figure 21. It was found that a 2:1 ratio of

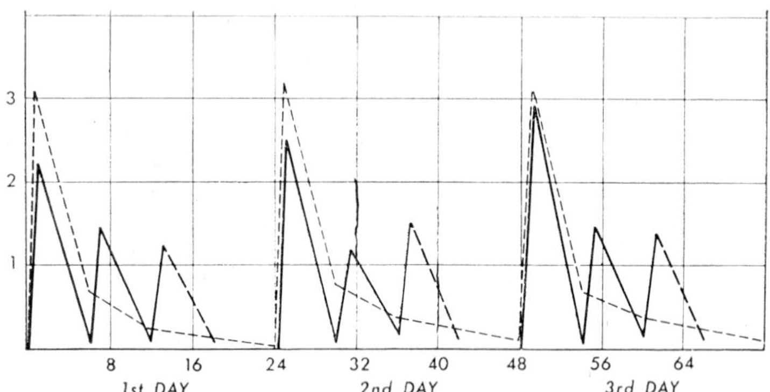

Fig. 21.—Comparison of penicillin serum levels in 25 patients. Continuous broken line represents levels of 600,000 units procaine penicillin G intramuscularly, daily; darker line, 250 mg. penicillin V orally 3 times daily. (Courtesy of Griffith, R. S., and Peck, F. B., Jr.: Antibiotics & Chemother. 8:143-148, March, 1958.)

penicillin V orally to penicillin G intramuscularly would provide equal quantities of penicillin to combat infection. The dosage schedule in this study was 250 mg. every 6 hours or 3 times daily.

Injectable penicillin did not produce more rapid therapeutic response than did adequate oral penicillin therapy. Injectable penicillin is indicated for patients who are vomiting or, for other reasons, are unable to take penicillin V by mouth.

Repeated oral administration of penicillin V, with its intermittent high bactericidal peaks, may have clinical advantages over the single initial bactericidal level obtained with procaine penicillin intramuscularly. Possibly, if clinical effectiveness rather than blood level concentrations could be used as a guide to minimal dosage, even a lower dosage of

(1) Antibiotics & Chemother. 8:143-148, March, 1958.

penicillin V could be established as well as a lower than 2:1 ratio to penicillin G.

Comparison of Penicillin Blood Levels Obtained by Inhibition of Excretion with Those Obtained by Enhancing Absorption was made by Jennie Siemienski, Robert Cade, Norman Kaplan and A. I. Braude[2] (Southwestern Med. School), using Benemid® and Remanden®. Levels obtained after oral administration of these two drugs were compared in 16 selected persons during periods of fasting and after meals.

The oral route has been used less widely for administering

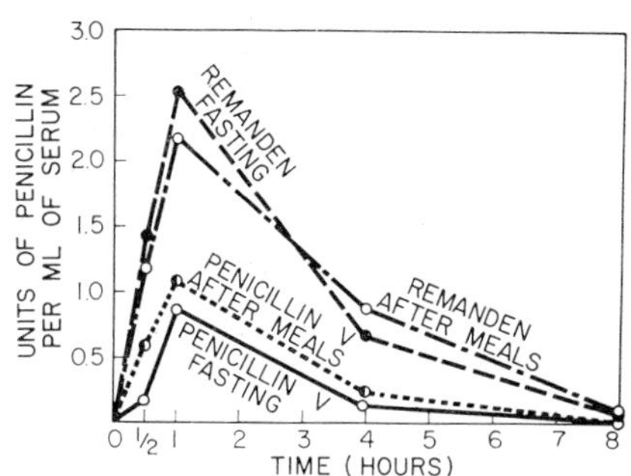

Fig. 22.—Composite curves of penicillin V and Remanden levels in sera of fasting and nonfasting persons. (Courtesy of Siemienski, J., *et al.*: Am. J. M. Sc. 235: 517-522, May, 1958.)

penicillin than for other antibiotics, because penicillin G is absorbed poorly and irregularly from the small intestine into the blood. Phenoxymethyl penicillin, or penicillin V, provides a type more suitable for oral use because of its greater stability and low solubility in acid mediums. These properties, as well as its ready solubility at the alkaline pH of intestinal secretions, seem to be the factors responsible for attaining higher blood levels after ingestion of penicillin V than after various preparations of penicillin G.

Improved intestinal absorption is not the only means, however, of providing higher blood levels of orally administered penicillin. Elevated blood levels can also be achieved by inhibiting the renal excretion of penicillins G or V with Benemid. Recently penicillin G has been combined with Benemid in Remanden.

(2) Am. J. M. Sc. 235:517-522, May, 1958.

It was found that penicillin G plus Benemid produced greater and more sustained antibacterial activity in the blood than did penicillin V in 16 subjects when these drugs were given orally. In 1, penicillin V produced a higher blood level. The average peak for penicillin activity after ingestion of penicillin G plus Benemid was more than twice that with penicillin V (Fig. 22).

Penicillin V—Clinical Assessment after One Year in 110 patients is presented by Robert Lamb and Eoin S. MacLean[3] (Greenock, Scotland). For mild and moderate infections 60 mg. was given 4 times a day in children and 120 mg. 4 times daily in adults. In some severe infections these doses were doubled.

Of 63 patients with pulmonary infection untreated before admission, 37 had lobar pneumonia, 18 had bronchopneumonia and 8 had acute bronchitis. Three deaths occurred in patients with bronchopneumonia with concurrent renal or cardiovascular disease. In 2 of these, other antibiotics were also given without resulting improvement. Of 37 patients with pulmonary infection who had had some treatment before admission (usually 1 or 2 injections of intramuscular penicillin), 11 had lobar pneumonia, 12 bronchopneumonia, 2 measles with bronchopneumonia, 1 empyema, 3 acute bronchitis, 7 chronic bronchitis and 1 bronchiectasis. Two of the patients with bronchopneumonia died. In 2 others, a change to another antibiotic was made. Two patients with chronic bronchitis and 1 with bronchiectasis were changed to another antibiotic. All others in the group responded to penicillin V.

Satisfactory response to penicillin V was observed in 2 patients with puerperal sepsis, 1 with pyemia, 2 with cutaneous anthrax, 1 with sinusitis and 1 with cellulitis. No response was noted in 1 patient with cellulitis, 1 with ulcerative endocarditis and 1 with pemphigus neonatorum.

The authors conclude that results with penicillin V given orally were as good as those achieved previously with intramuscular penicillin. There are several important advantages in the use of oral penicillin. The distress of children when subjected to injection is avoided and the possibility of sepsis is reduced. Use of compressed tablets or, better still, sealed

(3) Brit. M. J. 2:191-193, July 27, 1957.

capsules obviates the occurrence among the nursing staff of sensitization reactions. Penicillin can be given without precipitating paralysis by intramuscular injection in those with latent poliomyelitis infection.

Improved Local Tolerance to Benzathine Penicillin G. A single injection of 600,000 units generally provides adequate concentrations in the blood for 10 days, and 1,200,000 units, for 4 weeks. This usually eradicates streptococci from the

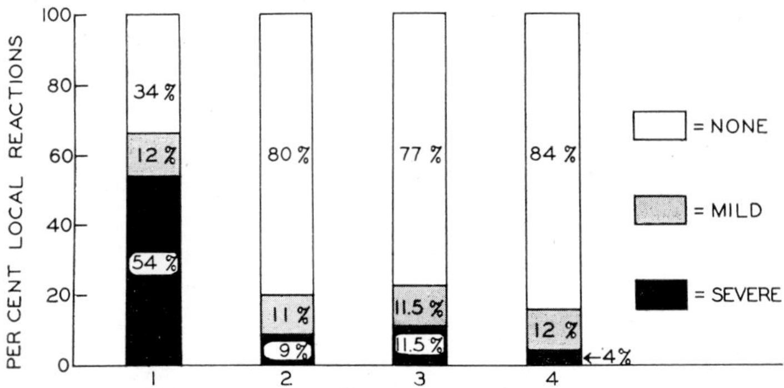

Fig. 23.—Comparative incidence of local reactions to four injectable penicillin preparations: *1,* benzathine penicillin G, 600,000 units in 1 ml.; *2,* benzathine penicillin G, 600,000 units in 1 ml. + 5 mg. prednisolone; *3,* benzathine penicillin G, 600,000 units + aqueous procaine penicillin, 600,000 units in 2 ml.; *4,* aqueous procaine penicillin, 1,200,000 units in 2 ml. (Courtesy of Krugman, S., and Ebin, E. V.: Pediatrics 21:243-247, February, 1958.)

nasopharynx and provides adequate prophylaxis against group A hemolytic streptococcic infections. Chief disadvantage is the high incidence of local reactions—painful muscle soreness and limp, which may persist for several days. Neither 5 Gm. cortisone nor 2 mg. 9α-fluorohydrocortisone alcohol has been effective in reducing the incidence. However, it was noted that a mixture of benzathine penicillin G and aqueous procaine penicillin was fairly well tolerated. Saul Krugman and Eva V. Ebin[4] (New York Univ.) evaluated four penicillin preparations in a total of 387 injections. All injections were given in the buttocks by experienced pediatric staff nurses. Every patient returned 24 hours later and was examined by the same physician (who was unaware of the type of penicillin given) for erythema, induration, tenderness, muscle spasm and pain.

(4) Pediatrics 21:243-247, February, 1958.

The incidence of severe local reactions 24 hours later (Fig. 23) was lowest in patients receiving aqueous procaine penicillin, highest in those receiving benzathine penicillin G and of about the same magnitude in those who received added prednisolone or aqueous procaine penicillin. The incidence of mild local reactions was essentially the same for all four groups.

At present, the combination of benzathine penicillin G, 600,000 units, and aqueous procaine penicillin, 600,000 units, is the best available intramuscular preparation for the one-injection treatment of streptococcic infections. It has all the advantages of ordinary benzathine suspensions as well as a significantly improved local tolerance.

Follow-up Study of Fatal Penicillin Reactions: Special Report. Abraham Rosenthal[5] presents a statistical survey of 30 authenticated fatal anaphylactic reactions to penicillin recorded in the files of the Office of Chief Medical Examiner of the City of New York. The patients' ages were 1 month to 66 years (average 33.8 years). There were 14 men and 16 women, 17 white and 13 Negro.

Six deaths occurred in the home and 12 at physicians' offices. Two patients reacted at home and 3 at physicians' offices; all 5 died shortly after hospitalization. Seven patients died at hospitals, including 2 hospital employees treated at the employees' clinic, 2 who died in an emergency room, 1 nurse treated by another nurse at the victim's request and 2 hospital patients who were being treated for other conditions.

Immediate reaction occurred in 25 and delayed reaction in 5. The time of the latter was 30 minutes for 2 patients, 20 minutes for 1 patient, 2 hours for 1 and 14 days for 1.

The amount of penicillin used was 200,000-500,000 units. In 2 instances 20 mg. chlorpheniramine maleate [Chlor-Trimeton®] was administered in the injections; 1 patient received a 10-mg. ampule of diphenhydramine hydrochloride [Benadryl®] simultaneously. These last 3 cases are the result of the warnings given by the drug houses, namely, that it is less risky, when there is doubt, to use simultaneously a dose of an antihistamine. This advice could have been misleading, since when protection against anaphylaxis is

(5) J.A.M.A. 167:1118-1121, June 28, 1958.

needed, the action of the simultaneously administered antihistamines could never be fast enough to save life. That the antihistamines might minimize a less catastrophic reaction is possible, but they probably never prevented a death.

In 14 cases no inquiry was made as to prior administration of and/or reaction to penicillin. Three patients exhibited asthmatic symptoms which should have put the physician on guard in the use of penicillin, since penicillin reactions may be more apt to occur in patients with a history of asthma. In only 1 instance was there a complete authenticated evidence of a direct inquiry having been made and a negative answer obtained.

Unknown sensitization to penicillin by ingestion of penicillin-containing milk and its products or by absorption through the skin from dermatophytes is also possible, thus paving the way for a later unpredictable reaction to the therapeutic use of the drug. Careful inquiry regarding the patient's allergic reactions in the past should precede penicillin administration. Such safety measures are important for their legal implications as well as for the patients.

Fatal Reactions to Penicillin: Evaluation of Test for Sensitivity. Deaths due to penicillin sensitivity are caused by immediate anaphylactic reactions, rather than by the delayed urticarial or serum sickness types of reaction. Lives might be saved if a reliable test procedure were routinely carried out before penicillin therapy. Vernon M. Smith[6] (US Army Hosp., Augsburg, Germany) describes a simplified procedure for testing for penicillin anaphylactic sensitivity. It consists in the application of drops of full-strength (300,000 units/ml.) procaine penicillin solution to a skin scratch and into a conjunctival sac. Patients with positive tests show erythema measuring more than 1 cm. in diameter or a wheal in the skin or itching and redness or edema of the eye. Positive test responses appear within 15 minutes.

Positive skin or eye tests were observed in 25 (1.1%) of 1,365 subjects tested. Seven patients had been brought to the hospital because of acute anaphylactic reactions to penicillin injected in nearby dispensaries and military aid stations. Each of these patients showed positive skin and eye tests 48 hours after the anaphylactic reactions, though each sub-

(6) New England J. Med. 257:447-451, Sept. 5, 1957.

ject was receiving full therapeutic doses of antihistamines.

Of 12 patients who gave a history of previous anaphylactic reactions to penicillin, 10 had positive tests. The 2 who failed to react had had anaphylactic reactions 18 and 39 months before the tests. These exceptions suggest the possibility that anaphylactic susceptibility is transient and that persons who recover from anaphylactic reactions to penicillin can, after an appropriate time, safely receive the drug again.

One subject who had a positive eye test for penicillin consulted a private physician 1 week later because of dysuria and urethral discharge. He was given an injection of penicillin and died 5 minutes later of acute anaphylactic shock.

Intramuscular injections of 600,000 units of procaine penicillin were administered to 778 patients immediately after they showed no response to the test. One had a mild anaphylactic reaction a few minutes after the injection, with tachycardia, palpitation, dyspnea and apprehension. Epinephrine, 0.3 ml. of 1:1000 solution, was given subcutaneously and recovery was prompt.

Several subjects showed positive eye tests but negative skin-scratch tests. Several others had positive skin tests but negative eye tests. Therefore, simultaneous performance of the two tests is recommended.

Penicillin Anaphylaxis Occurring in Patient on Steroid Therapy. I. Leonard Bernstein and Alfred Lustberg[7] (Jewish Hosp., Cincinnati) report a case believed to represent the first known instance in which an anaphylactic reaction was not prevented by previous steroid therapy.

Woman, 44, had had rheumatoid arthritis for 14 years. For the 4 years before the present episode she had been maintained on steroid compounds and during the last year had received 5 mg. prednisolone 3 times daily. Because of recurrent pharyngitis and acute otitis media, she had frequently received intramuscular procaine penicillin, without mishap or reaction. During childhood and in her early teens she had had attacks of mild urticaria. Once, during a blood transfusion, a severe episode of giant urticaria occurred.

Because of acute otitis media, 600,000 units of procaine penicillin was given intramuscularly. Within 30 seconds the patient experienced a severe anaphylactic reaction. Since they were immediately available, 80 units of corticotropin gel intramuscularly and 50 mg. Benadryl® intravenously were administered promptly. Intravenous administration of 4 minims of epinephrine was probably life saving. Oxygen was also given. Thirty minutes after onset of the acute reac-

(7) Ann. Int. Med. 47:1276-1279, December, 1957.

tion, 100 mg. Solu-Cortef was injected intravenously and further improvement was apparent. After several hours, the patient returned to normal physical status except for marked fatigue.

Serum obtained from the patient on the day following anaphylaxis was injected intracutaneously into the skin of a volunteer who had never received penicillin. After 48 hours, these sites were challenged with varying dilutions of procaine penicillin. Reactions were obtained with a penicillin dilution of 100 units/ml.

The authors conclude that neither corticoid compounds nor antihistamines are capable of inhibiting severe human anaphylactic reactions such as occur with penicillin administration. Judicious use of penicillin seems the only alternative. Proper emphasis should again be placed on prompt use of epinephrine in this type of anaphylactic reaction. Secondary drugs such as parenteral antihistamines and hydrocortisone hemisuccinate should be used plus routine supportive measures.

Temporary Hemorrhagic Diathesis after Penicillin Therapy was observed in an interesting case reported by P. Frick, R. Wise and R. Varco[8] (Univ. of Minnesota).

Woman, 44, had a congenital cardiac anomaly diagnosed as a septal defect by cardiac catheterization in April 1953. Before, during and after catheterization, she received 1,200,000 units of penicillin intramuscularly, which resulted in no unusual hemorrhage. She was readmitted Sept. 27, 1954 for surgical correction of the heart defect. The night before operation, she received 500,000 units of penicillin intramuscularly, and 2 hours later an ankle vein was opened to insert a catheter for administration of blood and fluid during operation. Loss of blood was so massive that the wound had to be tightly closed; severe hemorrhage continued, however, and was stopped only by the most painstaking hemostasis and application of a pressure band. The bleeding time was increased to 15 minutes, but clotting, prothrombin and thrombin times, prothrombin consumption and retraction were all normal. The platelet count was 210,000, the Rumpel-Leede test negative and fibrinogen content 410 mg./100 ml. Blood counts, sedimentation and liver function tests were normal.

Since there was no history of unusual bleeding previously, the cause of hemorrhage was presumed to be acquired. The next day all drugs (penicillin and phenobarbital) were discontinued and 2 days later the bleeding time (3 determinations) was normal. A provocative test with penicillin clarified the situation. Before injection of 300,000 units of penicillin intramuscularly, the bleeding time was 4 minutes; at ½ and 1 hour, over 15 minutes; at 3 hours, 10 minutes; at 8 hours, 7 minutes; and 12 hours after injection it had returned to 4 minutes. Throughout the test, coagulation and thrombin times, prothrombin, factors V and VII, fibrinogen, platelet count, retraction,

(8) Schweiz. med. Wchnschr. 87:1587-1588, Dec. 28, 1957.

prothrombin consumption and Rumpel-Leede test remained normal, as did leukocyte and differential counts, sedimentation and liver function tests. The provocative test was repeated with 400,000 and 500,000 units of penicillin, with the same results.

A few weeks later, a heart operation was performed under hypothermy and all penicillin was avoided. The operative result was satisfactory and the patient was in good condition 3 years later.

This case illustrates that in unexplained acquired hemorrhagic diatheses every drug administered must be considered as a possible etiologic factor and that its role can be determined by a provocative test. Statistically, penicillin is one of the last drugs to be suspected in such a situation, but in individual cases its significance must be clarified.

Reactions from Multiple Injections of Benzathine Penicillin G. Robert W. Sherwood, Christian Gronbeck and Floyd W. Denny Jr.[9] (Western Reserve Univ.) compared two dosage plans for intramuscular administration of benzathine penicillin G as prophylaxis against rheumatic fever, nephritis, and streptococcic infections in the armed forces. One group of 1,567 men received 600,000 units every 4 weeks; the other group of 1,708 men received 900,000 units every 6 weeks. A group of 214 men (6.5% of the total) gave a history of previous reaction to penicillin and were eliminated from the study.

No fatal or anaphylactic reactions occurred after injection of benzathine penicillin G, but during the 6 months of the study 16 men were hospitalized for urticaria, angioneurotic edema or joint symptoms; 11 were hospitalized after the 1st injection, 4 after the 2d and 1 after the 3d. The interval between injection and onset of reaction was not appreciably different in the two dosage schedules; 68% of reactions occurred during the 1st week and 88% by the end of the 2d. Prolonging the interval between injections (to as much as 4½ months) did not change the reaction rates.

In the 600,000-unit group the probability of reacting to the 1st injection was 3.1% and to the 2d was 1.1%. In the 900,000-unit group, the probability of reacting to the 1st injection was 3.9% and to the 2d was 1.2%. In both groups, after the first 2 injections, the probability of reacting was slightly lower and remained relatively constant for the rest of the injections. The cumulative probability of reacting to repeated in-

(9) J.A.M.A. 165:667-671, Oct. 12, 1957.

jections of benzathine penicillin G was 6.1% after 6 injections of 600,000 units and 5.8% after 4 injections of 900,000 units.

If it can be assumed that the men who gave a history of previous penicillin reactions were sensitive to benzathine penicillin G, then the data in this study indicate that most persons (85%) sensitive to the drug can be identified by an adequate history and reactions after the first injection. Because of this and since reactions in general were not serious and rates did not change when the intervals between injections were prolonged, the authors feel that routine use of repeated injections of this drug as a prophylactic agent in large groups is not only feasible, but safe.

► [A reaction rate of 1.3% was observed by R. B. McFarland (New England J. Med. 259:62, July 10, 1958) in 12,858 naval recruits receiving a single injection of this drug. Most of these were of the serum sickness type, but only about 1 in 1,000 persons required cortisone therapy. Many reactions tended to be long, and there were fairly frequent relapses. Many cleared rapidly; antihistamine therapy was only slightly helpful.—Ed.]

Penicillinase in Treatment of Penicillin Reactions. Use of penicillinase in treatment of hypersensitivity reactions to penicillin is based on the knowledge that circulating penicillinase reduces all demonstrable penicillin blood levels to zero for prolonged periods, thus rendering the penicillin nonallergenic. Alexander M. Minno and George M. Davis[1] (US Naval Hosp., Great Lakes, Ill.) treated 32 patients with moderate to severe hypersensitivity reactions to penicillin. Two principal types of reactions were treated, urticaria with generalized pruritus and serum-sickness reaction. Of 32 reactions, 14 were due to procaine penicillin and 18 to benzathine penicillin. The usual dose was 1,000,000 units of penicillinase in 2 cc. sterile distilled water, given intramuscularly. In severe cases not showing response within 48 hours, the injection was repeated. In 11 cases, more than 2 injections were given. In 6 cases, a single intramuscular injection of 2,000,000 units was used. In most cases antihistamines were also given.

Results of treatment with penicillinase were impressive. Patients were ambulatory and asymptomatic within 24 hours in 15 cases and within 48 hours in 5. In 12 cases, 4-6 days were required before all signs and symptoms disappeared.

Accurate determination of the effect of any agent in treatment of penicillin reactions is difficult, because the severity and duration of reactions are so variable. In this group some

(1) J.A.M.A. 165:222-224, Sept. 21, 1957.

patients were completely relieved in a few hours; in others symptoms became more severe for 24-48 hours after the injection. In 4 patients with moderately severe reactions, symptoms subsided within 24 hours with a placebo injection. Nevertheless, the authors believe that treatment with penicillinase rendered most patients more rapidly asymptomatic and free from relapse than other common modes of treatment. Antihistamines and penicillinase seem to be complementary and therefore combined treatment is advantageous. No toxic manifestations were encountered in the intramuscular use of penicillinase, though most patients had local pain and residual tenderness at the site of injection.

► [The successful use of penicillinase in an instance of acute renal insufficiency due to penicillin hypersensitivity, the patient having failed to respond to ACTH, prednisone and antihistaminics, has been reported by A. M. Unger and H. I. Nemuth (J.A.M.A. 167:1237, July 5, 1958.)

R. M. Becker, who introduced the antidotal use of penicillinase, has collected the records of 46 patients who were treated with the agent (Ann. Int. Med. 48:1228, June, 1958) Twenty-four received the drug alone, with uniformly good results. The other 22 had previously received concomitant antihistamine or steroid therapy; in 20 of these the favorable response seemed directly attributable to the penicillinase. Systemic toxic reactions were not noted, but there were some localized reactions at the injection site. —Ed.]

Kanamycin, an antibiotic closely related in its structure to neomycin, is discussed by Maxwell Finland[2] (Harvard Med. School). The chemical structure and physical properties of kanamycin have been almost fully elucidated and, as the sulfate, it is remarkably stable, readily soluble and suitable for intramuscular use.

In vitro, it is highly or moderately active against many common pathogenic aerobic, gram-positive and gram-negative bacteria and mycobacteria; but some pneumococci, most streptococci, and pseudomonas are moderately or highly resistant, whereas anaerobic organisms, yeasts and fungi are nearly all highly resistant. It is active against pathogenic staphylococci irrespective of their resistance to other antibiotics now in common use. Its activity parallels closely that of neomycin and paramomycin. Resistance to kanamycin can be readily induced in staphylococci and Escherichia coli. This is accompanied by complete cross-resistance to neomycin and paramomycin and partial cross-resistance to streptomycin and certain other related antibiotics, but no cross-resist-

(2) Lancet 2:209-211, July 26, 1958.

ance to any of the other antibiotics that are generally available.

Absorption and excretion from intramuscular doses in man are rapid. Peak concentrations are usually achieved in the serum in about 1 hour, which vary with, but do not exactly parallel, the size of the dose. Exact dosage regimens cannot yet be established. Oral doses are poorly absorbed.

Highly satisfactory clinical results have been reported in staphylococcic infections, including many severe cases in which the organisms were resistant to other antibiotics, particularly penicillin, streptomycin and the tetracyclines. Kanamycin appears to be highly effective in acute gonorrhea in males and is effective in most cases of severe anthrax infections. It has also proved effective in many acute and chronic infections of the urinary tract resistant to treatment with other antibiotics, but chronic infections with pseudomonas, enterococci and some proteus strains appear to be resistant, as do pneumococcic and streptococcic infections.

Kanamycin given orally, 4-8 Gm./day, proved an effective inhibitor of aerobic intestinal bacteria comparable to neomycin and useful in the preoperative preparation for large bowel surgery. In treatment of tuberculosis, some favorable effects have been reported but resistance to kanamycin is rapidly acquired.

Toxic effects observed thus far have generally been mild or moderate; serious toxicity has been encountered only rarely. Local irritation from intramuscular injections is slight and rarely interferes with continued therapy. Although sensitization, drug fever and drug rashes are uncommon, eosinophilia is common in patients treated for a week or longer. The major toxic effects are on the kidney and 8th cranial nerve.

► [This article represents a summary of the data presented at a conference on the basic and clinical research with this new antibiotic, held at the New York Academy of Sciences on July 10 and 11, 1958.—Ed.]

Hematologic Complications Arising during Ristocetin Therapy: Relation between Dose and Toxicity is discussed by Eugene J. Gangarosa, Nathaniel S. Landerman, Paul J. Rosch and E. G. Herndon, Jr.[3] (Walter Reed Army Med. Center). Ristocetin [Spontin®] is a new antimicrobial agent, a lyophilized preparation representing two antibiotics, risto-

(3) New England J. Med. 259:156-161, July 24, 1958.

Complications Arising in 8 of 10 Consecutive Cases During Ristocetin Therapy

Case No.	Age	Primary Diagnosis	Indication for Ristocetin	Total Dose	Duration of Treatment	Concomitant Medications	Complications
	yr.			*gm.*	*days*		
1	43	Rheumatic heart disease, with aortic insufficiency & bacterial endocarditis	Resistant enterococcal endocarditis	23.5	8	None	Thrombocytopenia & desquamating rash
2	36	Renal insufficiency, with uremia	Staphylococcal pneumonia	15.0	7	Hydrocortisone	Thrombocytopenia, leukopenia & acute anemia
3	50	Renal insufficiency, with uremia	Septicemia	8.0	7	None*	Thrombocytopenia & acute anemia
4	26	Hypoplastic bone marrow	Staphylococcal pneumonia	42.0	14	None	Platelet depression & neutropenia
5	27	Rheumatic heart disease, with aortic insufficiency & bacterial endocarditis	Resistant enterococcal endocarditis	22.5	9	None	Leukopenia, neutropenia, acute anemia, rash & fever
6	38	Lupus erythematosis, with uremia	Staphylococcal septicemia	57.0	11	Chloramphenicol, erythromycin & hydrocortisone	Acute anemia & rash
7	42	Rheumatic heart disease, with aortic insufficiency & bacterial endocarditis	Resistant enterococcal endocarditis	72.0	24	None	Leukopenia, neutropenia & fever
8	<1†	Periorbital cellulitis	Periorbital cellulitis	0.75	5	Hydrocortisone	Neutropenia & local thrombophlebitis

*Combined antibiotic therapy during 2d course of ristocetin.
†9 wk.

cetin A and B. These components have been isolated from the fermentation broth of the actinomycete species Nocardia lurida. In vitro and animal studies indicated marked bactericidal activity against gram-positive bacteria and mycobacteria. Advantages ascribed to ristocetin include low toxicity, lack of development of resistant organisms and absence of cross-resistance with other antibiotics.

Hematologic complications, including 3 instances of acute thrombocytopenia, were observed in 8 of 10 consecutive patients during ristocetin therapy (table). The other 2 patients were men who had staphylococcic pneumonia that responded dramatically to ristocetin with complete resolution and without laboratory or clinical evidence of complications. In addition to routine hematologic studies, the platelet count was followed carefully in 1 of these patients before, during and after therapy, and no depression was noted. The dose in both patients did not exceed 25 mg./kg./day. In the 8 who had hematologic complications ristocetin was given intravenously, diluted with glucose as recommended by the manufacturer.

Severe bleeding, which accompanied thrombocytopenia, contributed to the death of 2 patients. In the third patient with thrombocytopenia there was a prompt return of the platelet count to normal after ristocetin was reduced from 50 to 33 mg./kg.

Careful attention to the blood count, including platelet studies, is indicated in patients receiving ristocetin. Use of the agent should be limited to hospitalized patients to aid early recognition of complications and permit prompt treatment. Ristocetin therapy should be undertaken cautiously in patients with compromised renal function. The complications observed are best explained by a peripheral direct toxic effect of ristocetin. Such complications may be reversible when recognized promptly and the drug discontinued or the dose reduced. The demonstrated effectiveness of ristocetin in enterococcic and staphylococcic infections resistant to other antibiotics justifies its continued use.

Toxic Ocular Manifestation of Chloramphenicol Therapy: Report of Case of Optic Neuritis is presented by J. Gordon Cole, Helen Grady Cole and Lawrence A. Janoff[4] (New York). Two similar cases have been reported in the literature.

(4) Am. J. Ophth. 44:18-20, July, 1957.

Man, 44, had been taking chloramphenicol daily for 6 months, because of an acute exacerbation of subacute bacterial endocarditis. For 3 weeks before he was seen, he had had blurred vision. Corrected vision in each eye was 20/20, but he stated that the letters were not clear. The central field of the right eye was moderately constricted and that of the left slightly constricted. Pericentral scotomas were present in both eyes. Ophthalmoscopic examination revealed edema of the optic nervehead and dilatation of the veins.

Chloramphenicol therapy was suspended and thiamine chloride, vitamin B_{12} and Diamox® were prescribed. Two weeks later the patient could read and see more easily, but his vision was not "extremely sharp." The central field of the right eye was only slightly constricted and, in the left eye, it was normal except for the pericentral scotoma which had diminished in both eyes. A month after the first eye examination and cessation of chloramphenicol, edema of the optic nerves had decreased and dilatation of the veins was diminished. Visual fields were within normal limits and the scotoma was absent.

In the 2 other cases reported and in this one the ocular symptoms of chloramphenicol toxicity were blurred vision, pericentral scotoma and constriction of the visual field. The patient described here showed edema of the optic nerve and dilatation of the veins. One of the 2 patients reported elsewhere showed similar signs and also hemorrhages in various parts of the fundus. The other had hyperemia of the optic nerve and disk margins obscured by edema of the nerve fibers.

In long-term treatment with any antibiotic, frequent examination of the blood is standard practice. To this should be added frequent examination of the fundus, which may reveal the first signs of toxicity. Examination of the eyes by an ophthalmologist is especially important during chloramphenicol treatment if other symptoms of toxicity appear.

Respiratory Depression Due to Neomycin. Harold L. Engel and J. S. Denson[5] (Los Angeles County Hosp.) reviewed all of surgical cases (July 1953 to January 1957), whether or not neomycin was used, in which serious respiratory difficulties developed during or immediately after surgery. Among 47,000 operations, there were 225 such cases. In 4 small children, respiratory depression occurred about 15 minutes after instillation of the neomycin. No muscle relaxant, such as curare or succinylcholine, was used during the procedures. Respiration had been quite adequate before neomycin was administered.

Girl, 3, with abdominal pain and vomiting for 2 days, was prepared for appendectomy. Rectal temperature was 104 F., pulse 140, res-

(5) Surgery 42:862-864, November, 1957.

piration 36, blood pressure 100/70, hemoglobin 10 Gm. and white blood cell count 19,750. Atropine, 1/350 gr., was administered intramuscularly 30 minutes before surgery. Anesthesia was induced with open drop Vinethene® and maintained with open drop ether, with 300 cc. oxygen/minute insufflated under the mask. Respiratory rate after induction was 40/minute. Free pus was found in the abdomen, and a suppurating appendix was removed. Just before the abdomen was closed, 1 Gm. neomycin in 350 cc. saline was introduced into the peritoneal cavity. Surgery lasted 1 hour. The anesthesiologist's notes read: "Patient breathing well throughout. At about the last skin stitch she suddenly stopped breathing, although she was moving her hands. A marked bradycardia developed. The trachea was intubated and controlled breathing with oxygen begun." After 45 minutes of artificial ventilation, spontaneous respiration began to return but was not considered adequate for another hour. The child made an uneventful recovery.

This and the 3 other cases do not provide conclusive proof that intraperitoneal instillation of neomycin can produce apnea in anesthetized patients. It should be emphasized that neomycin has been used this way extensively without observed ill effect on respiration. These 4 cases seem to indicate, however, that in small children and critically ill adults, neomycin may produce severe respiratory depression.

► [Several other instances of respiratory embarrassment associated with intraperitoneal administration of neomycin are on record. The neuromuscular blocking action of the drug has been demonstrated by C. B. Pittinger and J. P. Long (Antibiotics & Chemother. 8:198, 1958) in rabbits and dogs, and the enhancement of this action by ether in the rabbit. Neostigmine (Prostigmin®) successfully antagonized the neuromuscular and respiratory depressions in the dog. The following article suggests that a similar antidotal action may occur in man.—Ed.]

Neostigmine Therapy for Apnea Occurring after Administration of Neomycin. Although only 6 cases of apnea occurring after intraperitoneal administration of neomycin have been reported, the widespread use of this antibiotic would indicate that the complication will be encountered more often. William H. Middleton, Dale D. Morgan and Jack Moyers[6] report a case in which neostigmine therapy successfully reversed the curare-like action of neomycin.

Man, 75, was hospitalized with a self-inflicted gunshot wound in the abdomen. After partial resection of the large intestine and closure of numerous perforations of the small intestine, 2 Gm. neomycin was instilled into the peritoneal cavity shortly before peritoneal closure. Succinylcholine, administered by a continuous intravenous infusion, was discontinued after peritoneal closure, when a total of 350 mg. had been given. At the time of fascial suture, he reacted well to the endotracheal

(6) J.A.M.A. 165:2186, Dec. 28, 1957.

tube, with good, spontaneous breathing. About 15 minutes after neomycin had been given and at the time of skin closure, the blood pressure fell from 100 to 70 mm. Hg systolic and he became apneic.

Artificial respiration with oxygen and levarterenol (Levophed®) drip was begun and continued for 90 minutes, when regular but feeble attempts at voluntary respiration were noted. For an additional 90 minutes, air was substituted for oxygen for short periods but no improvement was observed. During the 3-hour postoperative period, he did not react to the endotracheal tube and had no voluntary movements of limbs and face. Blood pressure remained low unless supported with levarterenol.

It was postulated that the apnea and hypotension were caused by a curare-like effect of neomycin. Although a relatively small amount of neomycin had been given (2 Gm.), it was absorbed through a peritoneal cavity which had been traumatized. Thus the drug rapidly attained a high blood level. It was decided to antagonize this curare-like effect with neostigmine. Accordingly, 0.3 mg. atropine sulfate was given intravenously, followed by 0.1-mg. doses neostigmine given intravenously every 2 minutes. After 0.5 mg. had been given, respiratory activity was definitely increased and he began to swallow. After 1 mg., respiration was essentially normal. His head moved from side to side and he attempted to remove the endotracheal tube. Soon he was transferred to the recovery room, where respiration remained normal and verbal commands were followed, but vasopressors were needed to maintain normal blood pressure. Further transfusion with whole blood was ineffective.

The patient died 23 hours after surgery. Respiration remained adequate until death. The terminal event was a shocklike state, which occurred when levarterenol infusion infiltrated and could not be started quickly. Permission for autopsy was not granted.

Renal Failure Following Administration of Intraperitoneal Neomycin for acute peritonitis demonstrates, according to Lloyd D. Mac Lean[7] (Univ. of Minnesota), that the safe dosage by this route is uncertain.

Man, 55, was hospitalized with lower right abdominal quadrant pain, rigidity and tenderness. X-rays showed small and large bowel distention and a fecolith in the region of the appendix. White blood cell count was 12,500 with 80% neutrophils, 18% lymphocytes and 2% monocytes. Hemoglobin concentration was 15.8 Gm. Urinalysis was normal with a specific gravity of 1.029. Blood urea nitrogen was 19 mg./100 ml., carbon dioxide 30 mEq./L. and chlorides 100 mEq./L.

A gangrenous, perforated appendix with a fecolith at the base was removed at laparotomy. Foul watery exudate was present in the abdominal cavity. Severe generalized peritonitis with pus in the pelvis and subphrenic spaces, yielding Escherichia coli on culture, was treated by aspiration of the purulent material, lavage with saline and placement of 100 ml. of 1% neomycin in the peritoneal cavity. Catheters

(7) Minnesota Med. 40:557-558, August, 1957.

were also placed before closure to permit introduction of more of the antibiotic postoperatively. One unit of blood was given after surgery.

Hypotension was not present during or after surgery. Rectal temperature never exceeded 101.8 F. During 36 hours after operation, 300 cc. of 1% neomycin was introduced into the peritoneum and parenteral penicillin and streptomycin were also given. Temperature and bowel activity returned to normal in 4 days. Adequate urine output existed during the illness; the urine had a fixed specific gravity of 1.010. Uremia developed rapidly, the patient became lethargic and confused and died with bronchopneumonia 4 days after operation. At autopsy the kidneys showed swelling of the proximal tubular epithelium with hydropic degeneration. The microscopic appearance was that of toxic nephropathy but not that of transfusion reaction.

Though the amount of neomycin used was believed to be less than half the dose considered safe, the normal renal function before operation and the absence of hypotension, oliguria or bacteremia suggest that the drug was the probable cause of renal failure. The vascular development due to peritonitis might have increased the absorption rate from the peritoneal surface. Neomycin may have contributed to renal failure in other cases less clearly indicated. If so, the amount of neomycin which may safely be placed in the peritoneal cavity has yet to be determined.

► [And the tendency for the drug to cause deafness without any warning vertigo must also be borne in mind when it is used parenterally; A. I. Goldner has recently reported another such instance (New York J. Med. 58:2226, July 1, 1958). Oral and topical uses are not usually accompanied by any evidences of systemic toxicity, but S. Epstein (Ann. Allergy 16: 268, 1958) observed 40 cases of contact dermatitis from neomycin during 2 years of a dermatologic practice.—Ed.]

Use of Sulfamethoxypyridazine (Kynex®) in Treatment of Infectious Diseases was investigated by Francisco Ruiz Sanchez, Amado Ruiz Sanchez, Roberto Aceves and Elba Naranjo Granda[8] (Univ. of Guadalajara). Sulfamethoxypyridazine is readily absorbed from the gastrointestinal tract and diffused to the cerebrospinal fluid. High and long-lasting blood concentrations are rapidly achieved, and acetylation is moderate. The antibacterial spectrum of sulfamethoxypyridazine is similar to that of sulfadiazine. If sulfonamide concentrations in human plasma of 10-15 mg./100 ml. are accepted as therapeutically effective, 1 Gm. sulfamethoxypyridazine daily would suffice. Urinary excretion of the drug is slow. Within the first 24 hours after ingestion, 25% is excreted.

---

(8) Antibiot. Med. & Clin. Therap. 5:437-444, July, 1958.

The authors gave sulfamethoxypyridazine to 40 patients, aged 3-69, who had carbuncles, purulent otitis media, chronic osteomyelitis, erysipelas, scarlet fever, blepharitis, acute or chronic gonococcic urethritis or abscesses. The drug was given orally, 375-3,000 mg., depending on the patient's age, daily for 3-12 days.

Results were excellent in all cases of Bacillus anthracis infection. In purulent otitis media, results were good when the causative organism was Micrococcus pyogenes. Only 50% of B. proteus infections responded. Patients with chronic osteomyelitis due to B. proteus did not respond to therapy. Patients with erysipelas, scarlet fever and streptococcic infections responded well. Results in 2 gonorrheal infections were good; 1 case did not respond. Localized infections due to M. pyogenes resolved favorably in 3 of 4 patients.

Side effects in the form of a generalized, afebrile, morbilliform exanthema occurred in 1 patient. Abdominal pain and vomiting were present in another, and in a third the erythrocyte count was lowered to under 2,000,000, with no histological lesion of the hemopoietic marrow.

► [M. Ziai and M. Finland (New England J. Med. 257:1180, Dec. 12, 1957) have found that sulfamethoxypyridazine traverses the placenta and produces levels in umbilical cord blood that approach those of the maternal blood. They feel that this may possibly be the agent of choice when a sulfonamide is desirable in the management of long and complicated labors.

There are side actions and toxicities to be aware of, however, as evidenced in the several following articles.—Ed.]

Thrombocytopenia and Leukopenia Associated with Use of Sulfamethoxypyridazine [Kynex®] were studied in 2 patients treated by Miles J. Schwartz and William S. Norton II[9] (St. Luke's Hosp., New York).

Case 1.—Woman, 36, was treated with 0.5 Gm. sulfamethoxypyridazine twice daily for 7½ days. Rash, "coffee-ground" vomitus, vaginal bleeding and blood in the stool led to hospitalization. Markedly reduced platelets in peripheral blood confirmed the diagnosis of thrombocytopenia. Treatment with ACTH gel, ascorbic acid, rutin and ferrous sulfate was successful, and the hematologic picture returned to normal.

Case 2.—Man, 64, had benign prostatic hypertrophy and nonspecific prostatitis for 5 years. He had been treated with Gantrisin® shortly before because of perineal discomfort and pus clumps in the prostatic expression. Symptoms worsened, and sulfamethoxypyridazine was administered for a 30-day period, with dosage increased to 1 Gm./day. A blood count was normal. Twelve days later he experienced chills, fe-

(9) J.A.M.A. 167:457-459, May 24, 1958.

ver and back pain relieved by aspirin. On the 44th day, thumb joints and the right shoulder became acutely painful. Petechiae were observed in axillae and groins and diffuse macular red rash covered the upper trunk. Temperature reached 104 F. Liver and spleen were enlarged. The Rumpel-Leede test was markedly positive. Platelet count was 46,000/cc. Prednisone, 10 mg. every 6 hours, was given for 4 days, then gradually reduced and withdrawn on the 10th day. On the 9th and 10th days, ACTH gel, 40 units, was given. A prompt symptomatic response followed, temperature returning to normal in 3 days, and leukopenia, maximal on the 3d day, disappeared by the 6th. Spleen, liver and lymphadenopathy were markedly reduced on discharge the 12th day.

It is interesting that both patients had had previous sulfonamide therapy without untoward reactions.

Assessment of Toxicity of New Sulfonamide, Sulfamethoxypyridazine (Kynex®) was made by John Vinnicombe[1] (St. Thomas' Hosp., London). Sulfamethoxypyridazine has been shown to have antibacterial activity equal to that of sulfadiazine, an equivalent blood level being achieved and maintained on a substantially lower dosage than with any previous preparation.

The author treated 110 patients with sulfamethoxypyridazine for nonspecific genital tract infection. A daily dose of 1.5 Gm., as 500-mg. tablets 3 times a day, was given for 5 days without a loading dose. This was deliberately higher than recommended, in view of the object of the survey. No other treatment was given.

Side effects were reported by 12 of 94 patients. Nine had headache, usually frontal, which began after 2 or 3 days' treatment and resolved within 24 hours after treatment was stopped. Four had anorexia. There was no vomiting and no serious manifestations of drug sensitivity or toxicity.

Focal Hepatitis, Fever and Skin Rash Following Therapy with Sulfamethoxypyridazine, Long-Acting Sulfonamide is reported by William A. Tisdale[2] (Yale Univ.).

Man, 68, was given sulfamethoxypyridazine [Kynex®], 1 Gm. orally each day and 2-3 weeks of nitrofurantoin therapy, 300 mg. orally daily, for pyuria. Four days after completing a 37-day course of sulfamethoxypyridazine he had severe generalized itching and noted a rapidly progressive, maculopapular eruption on the extremities and trunk. Because of the rash and a sudden rise in temperature to 102 F. on the 5th day, he was hospitalized.

Examination revealed, besides the skin eruption and fever, slight

(1) Antibiotic Med. & Clin. Therap. 5:474-476, July, 1958.
(2) New England J. Med. 258:687-690, Apr. 3, 1958.

scleral icterus, no splenomegaly or lymphadenopathy, a slightly enlarged, minimally tender liver and scattered petechial lesions of the buccal mucosa. The initial hematocrit was 40%. The total white blood cell count was 5,550 with 68% neutrophils, 28% lymphocytes, 3% monocytes and 1% eosinophils. The urine showed no albumin, and the bilirubin test was 2+. The spun sediment contained rare erythrocytes and 5-7 leukocytes/high-power field. Blood cultures were negative. Liver biopsy revealed scattered, circumscribed areas of inflammation involving not only the parenchyma and supporting stroma but also the vessels walls.

Bed rest, high fluid intake and local skin therapy produced no improvement. However, temperature subsided and the skin cleared on oral therapy with prednisone plus chloramphenicol and streptomycin for the urinary infection. A repeat liver biopsy 55 days after onset of symptoms showed complete disappearance of the focal inflammatory lesions.

The occurrence of fever, rash, leukopenia and signs of hepatic injury after chronic drug therapy strongly suggested a hypersensitivity reaction in this patient. Of the two drugs used, sulfamethoxypyridazine appeared to be the more likely offending agent, since nitrofurantoin had been discontinued at least 3 weeks before onset of symptoms. Symptoms were first noted 4 days after the last dose of sulfamethoxypyridazine, an interval consistent with previous reports of sulfonamide reactions, though these occur most commonly during the first 5-9 days of therapy.

This case illustrates the axiom that drugs known to produce any of the manifestations of hypersensitivity will be found ultimately to produce hepatitis in some persons. Previously reported reactions to sulfamethoxypyridazine have been limited to fever and cutaneous eruption.

Toxic Reaction to Sulfamethoxypyridazine (Kynex®). This new sulfonamide is supposedly effective against genitourinary infections. Some claimed advantages over other medications are high solubility in plasma and urine, low initial and maintenance doses, high diffusion rate and rapid absorption. Serious side effects are claimed to be rare and only one skin rash has been reported in a total of 52 subjects treated. Barnet M. Hershfield and Jonny J. Stern[3] (Jewish Mem'l Hosp., (New York) report 2 cases of toxic reaction: 1 patient had liver involvement, rash and pyrexia and the other a skin reaction which improved rapidly when the drug was discontinued.

(3) New York J. Med. 587:1508-1510, May 1, 1958.

Man, 63, had dysuria and pyuria which responded to Furadantin®. When symptoms recurred 1 month later, Kynex was prescribed, 0.5 Gm. 4 times for the 1st day, and 0.5 Gm. twice daily for the next 24 days. Again the infection subsided, and the drug was discontinued. Shortly thereafter, nausea, epigastric discomfort and anorexia developed and Kynex was started again for 2 days. At this time the patient was admitted to the hospital.

Examination showed a thin man with a rectal temperature of 101.6 F., icteric skin and scleras and a generalized, morbilliform rash over the trunk and extremities. The liver was down 3 fingerbreadths and the spleen edge was felt on deep inspiration. Serum pyruvic transaminase and oxaloacetic transaminase were 84 and 58 units. Alkaline phosphatase was 62 units and bilirubin 5.4 mg./100 ml. of which 3.2 mg./100 ml. was indirect.

The patient rapidly improved. Jaundice faded in about 4 days, urine became lighter and alkaline phosphatase dropped precipitously. The temperature became normal after the 3d hospital day.

This case illustrates that sulfonamides can produce hepatic injury besides the more common toxic reactions of fever and rash. Damage is both by direct toxic action and by induction of a hypersensitivity reaction. Prolonged administration may lead to focal inflammation and necrotic lesions in the liver, kidneys, myocardium and lungs. The high alkaline phosphatase in the presence of a negative cephalin flocculation test and normal thymol turbidity speaks for cholangiolitic reaction with intrahepatic obstruction.

Heinz Body Anemia Due to Salicylazosulfapyridine [Salazopyrin®]. This drug was introduced in 1942 for ulcerative colitis. Taken orally, it is absorbed from the gut and deposited in connective tissue, including the bowel, where aminosalicylic acid and sulfapyridine are gradually liberated. Free sulfapyridine can be detected in the blood. Since the drug is used extensively and its use probably will increase, its toxicity should be emphasized. About 20% of patients receiving it have nausea or vomiting. Skin rashes, drug fever and joint reactions are less common. Serious toxic reactions are said to be rare, the principal one being neutropenia going on to agranulocytosis. A. I. Spriggs, R. S. Smith, Huw Griffith and S. C. Truelove[4] (Oxford, England) describe 3 patients who acquired toxic anemia with Heinz body formation.

Almost always, the presence of many Heinz bodies indicates chemical poisoning, commonly caused by benzene derivatives with amino or nitro groups. Withdrawal of the

(4) Lancet 1:1039-1041, May 17, 1958.

Salazopyrin in these 3 cases was immediately followed by a decrease in Heinz bodies and arrest of the hemolytic anemia. The hemolytic anemia associated with Heinz bodies is mainly due to decreased life span of the affected red cells, probably aggravated by degradation of hemoglobin in such cells. The Heinz bodies are dense and contain much iron, considered to be derived from hemoglobin. They probably are formed in vivo by circulating mature red cells. Methemoglobinemia and other abnormal pigments sometimes also occur.

Woman, 65, received Salazopyrin for a malabsorption syndrome due to an ileocolic fistula with diarrhea, loose and bulky stools, macrocytic anemia and steatorrhea. The dose was 2 Gm. 3 times daily. Before Salazopyrin therapy, blood findings were normal. Two weeks after therapy was started, the hemoglobin level was 78%, reticulocyte count 4.5% and large inclusion bodies were seen in the red cells which were shown to be Heinz bodies. Plasma bilirubin was 0.9 mg./100 ml., and a little methemoglobin was found. Red cell fragility and a direct Coombs test were normal. When Salazopyrin was discontinued, the hemoglobin which had fallen to 58% rose spontaneously while the Heinz bodies fell steadily. Five weeks after discontinuance of the drug, the blood picture was normal.

Miscellaneous Infections

Penicillin in Treatment of Streptococcic Infections: Comparison of Effectiveness of Five Different Oral and One Parenteral Form. B. B. Breese and F. A. Disney[5] (Univ. of Rochester) compared the effectiveness of following penicillin preparations in children, aged 1-17, with infections due to beta hemolytic streptococcus: benzathine penicillin G (intramuscular injection), benzathine penicillin G (oral administration), a suspension of potassium penicillin G with probenecid, potassium penicillin G combined with probenecid tablets, penicillin V (oral administration) and buffered potassium penicillin G.

All forms gave uniformly good immediate results. Results after 2 months indicated that benzathine penicillin G given intramuscularly was superior to the oral preparations therapeutically and prophylactically. Among the oral drugs, no one preparation was significantly superior to the others. In addition to its therapeutic and prophylactic effectiveness, parenteral administration of penicillin is cheaper than oral

(5) New England J. Med. 259:57-62, July 10, 1958.

preparations and is not associated with their problems of administration. The allergic reaction rate was not significantly different for the two methods.

For these reasons, 1 dose of 600,000 units of benzathine penicillin G given intramuscularly is the authors' first choice in the treatment of streptococcic infections in children. Its chief disadvantage lies in frequent painful local reactions and psychologic trauma from use of a needle.

The oral preparations used were almost as effective as parenteral administration therapeutically but not prophylactically. Choice of an oral form should be based on factors other than effectiveness, since there was no evidence of the therapeutic superiority of any one product. Since cost is often the most important factor, among the oral preparations tested, 800,000 units of buffered penicillin G daily for 10 days is the authors' first choice for oral treatment of streptococcic infections in children.

Mass Prophylaxis of Epidemic Streptococcic Infections with Benzathine Penicillin G: II. Experience at a Naval Training Center during Winter of 1956-57. Robert B. McFarland, Victor G. Colvin and John R. Seal[6] (US Naval Training Center, Bainbridge, Md.) gave 12,858 men an injection of benzathine penicillin G during their 4th week of training. Those with even numbers were given 600,000 units of benzathine penicillin intramuscularly and those with odd numbers were given 1,200,000 units. Because of a history of allergy to penicillin, 237 men (1.8%) were excluded.

Throat cultures were taken immediately before penicillin injection and at about 28 and 42 days after the injection. Only 1 man acquired rheumatic fever; he had had only 1 injection of penicillin. The incidence of positive throat cultures before penicillin administration was 2.24%, in the 8th week after 0.36% and in the 10th week 1.39%. Of the 34 men who had positive cultures at sick call or at the 10th-week culture, 17 had received 600,000 units and 17 had received 1,200,000 units of benzathine penicillin at the time of the prophylactic injection. The larger dose seemed to offer no advantage over the smaller in degree or in duration of protection.

The allergic reaction rate to benzathine penicillin was 1.14% among men given 600,000 units and 1.68% among

(6) New England J. Med. 258:1277-1284, June 26, 1958.

those receiving 1,200,000 units. Most reactions were of the serum sickness type, characterized by urticaria, giant hives and edema, fever and joint symptoms. There were no anaphylactic reactions. Urticaria developed in only 2 men on the day of injection.

Benzathine Penicillin G in Prevention of Streptococcic Infections. Alton J. Morris and Charles H. Rammelkamp Jr.[7] investigated the effectiveness of benzathine penicillin G in preventing streptococcic pharyngitis during an epidemic among military personnel. Benzathine penicillin G was administered as a single intramuscular injection in doses of 1,200,000, 600,000 and 300,000 units to 246, 255 and 240 men, respectively. All 3 dosage levels were equally effective in eliminating group A streptococci from the throat of carriers. Men receiving a placebo injection continued to harbor the organism.

Duration of protection from streptococcic infection varied with the dosage. After administration of 300,000 units, infections began to occur as early as the 8th day, whereas after 600,000 and 1,200,000 units the first illnesses were observed on the 32d and 44th days.

Benzathine penicillin G was administered to a large number of patients with streptococcic infections who were subsequently observed for signs of a new infection. Among 935 patients given 1,200,000 units, the earliest time clinical illness was recognized was 44 days later. After administration of 600,000 units, the earliest infections appeared 26 days later, whereas after 300,000 units there was little protection after the 8th day.

From the present study it appears that 1,200,000 units of penicillin afforded protection for about 6 weeks. Further studies on the duration of protection provided by this dose are justified, since in the management of patients with rheumatic fever an injection every 6 weeks would have a distinct advantage over an injection every month, as is now recommended. In the protection of rheumatic patients, inapparent infections may play an important role in development of recurrences, and considerable more bacteriologic, immunologic and clinical data are required for final conclusions in relation to prophylaxis in these patients.

(7) J.A.M.A. 165:664-667, Oct. 12, 1957.

Comparison of Penicillin G and Penicillin V in Treatment of Streptococcic Sore Throat. Norbert Schalet, Bernard M. Reen and Harold B. Houser[8] treated groups of Air Force recruits with group A streptococcic sore throat. Forty-seven received 250,000 units of penicillin orally 3 times daily for 10 days and 43 received 200,000 units of penicillin V by the same schedule. The course of illness, eradication of streptococci from the nose and throat and development of streptococcic antibody, as determined by the antistreptolysin-O titer, were similar in the two groups.

Although penicillin blood levels were not determined, ample evidence has accumulated indicating that penicillin V will result in higher and more sustained levels than will equal amounts of penicillin G. That this is no advantage in treating streptococcic sore throat at the dosage level used in this study is evident from results obtained in the groups.

The dose and duration of treatment using penicillin G were those presently recommended for treatment of streptococcic tonsillitis and pharyngitis to prevent nonsuppurative complications, rheumatic fever and acute glomerulonephritis, which did not occur in the present small group. With the degree of streptococcic eradication and suppression of antistreptolysin-O equal in the groups, similar results in prevention of rheumatic fever and nephritis would be expected.

Since no attempt was made to have the patients take penicillin at least ½ hour before or more than 2 hours after meals, it was usually taken with the meal or immediately after. Thus, no practical advantage for penicillin V, with its increased resistance to destruction by stomach acid, was apparent.

It is concluded that in the dosages used penicillin V was not superior to penicillin G.

Concentration of Penicillin in Serum Following Intramuscular Administration of Benzathine Penicillin G to Children with Inactive Rheumatic Fever. Roswith I. Lade, Antoni M. Diehl, Irvin Snyder and Tom R. Hamilton[9] (Univ. of Kansas) administered 1,200,000 units of benzathine penicillin G every 28 days intramuscularly to 96 patients, aged

(8) Am. J. M. Sc. 235:183-188, February, 1958.
(9) Pediatrics 21:233-242, February, 1958.

4-20 years, with inactive rheumatic fever. The patients were studied with respect to effective and consistent concentrations of penicillin in the serum. The concentrations could be determined with certainty in 81% of the specimens and range from 0.002 to 0.125 unit/ml.

The mean concentration of penicillin in the serum of females (0.042 unit/ml.) was three times higher than that in the serum of males. The concentration in the serum of females increased with age and weight from the 10th to the 17th years. No such increase was observed in the serums of males in relation to age and weight. The differences in concentration reached in the serums of the two sexes during ages 12-17 were statistically significant (P less than 0.01). No significant difference in concentration was found between obese and thin girls aged 10-15. The explanation for the differences between the sexes is not apparent.

During the study, 491 swabs from the nose and throat yielded only 1 culture of beta hemolytic streptococcus, group A; this organism could not be typed and was not associated with an increase in the titer of antistreptolysin O. One other patient had a significant rise in antibody titer, but there was no antecedent positive culture for streptococcus. There were no recurrences of rheumatic fever.

Prevention of Rheumatic Fever by Treatment of Streptococcic Infections: II. Factors Responsible for Failures. Francis J. Catanzaro, Charles H. Rammelkamp, Jr., and Robert Chamovitz[1] studied 5,198 patients who received treatment with an antibiotic or sulfadiazine for streptococcic tonsillitis or pharyngitis to determine the factors responsible for the development of rheumatic fever after therapy. Of this group, 76 patients had acute rheumatic fever.

Analysis showed that a history of rheumatic fever and occurrence of a streptococcic infection just before the observed treated infection might contribute to a slightly increased susceptibility to rheumatic fever in this group. Likewise, patients who had an attack of rheumatic fever within the preceding 5 years also were more likely to contract rheumatic fever after a treated streptococcic infection than those who had a rheumatic attack more than 5 years previously.

When the infecting organism is not eliminated from the

(1) New England J. Med. 259:51-57, July 10, 1958.

patient by therapy, the attack rate of rheumatic fever is not reduced appreciably. Thus the most precise method for evaluation of a therapeutic regimen for streptococcic infections is determination of the presence or absence of the infecting type of streptococcus in the oropharynx after treatment. Isolation of this organism indicates failure of therapy, though failure to grow the infecting organism in any single culture does not establish that treatment was a success. It is often difficult to isolate group A streptoccocci during convalescence, so that ideally multiple cultures should be obtained in any evaluation study. Of the 76 patients in whom rheumatic fever developed, 46 (61%) showed the infecting type of streptococcus during convalescence, in contrast to 20% of the total study population who continued to carry the infecting type. Another 21% of the 76 rheumatic patients showed a new type during convalescence, compared with 10% in the total treated groups. Thus in 82% of the patients with rheumatic fever, continuing infection could be assumed. In the other 18%, group A streptococcus was probably present, but the methods used were inadequate to establish this.

If the persistence of the infecting type of streptococcus or a new infection is primarily responsible for the therapeutic failures, it is possible to improve the therapeutic regimens designed to prevent rheumatic fever. Of the various methods employed, injection of 600,000-1,200,000 units of benzathine penicillin is the least expensive; only 1 injection is required and protection is given against re-infection or new infections for 3-6 weeks. The choice of oral therapy is probably not too important, although sulfonamides should never be used, since they do not eliminate the streptococcus.

Oral Treatment of Subacute Bacterial Endocarditis with Phenoxymethyl Penicillin (Penicillin V) combined with intramuscular streptomycin and dihydrostreptomycin resulted in clinical and bacteriologic cures in 6 patients treated by Charles A. Santos-Buch, M. Glenn Koenig and David E. Rogers[2] (Cornell Univ.). Penicillin V is stable and insoluble at pH 3 and below and is readily changed to a soluble alkaline salt above pH 7. The expectation that it might achieve higher blood levels after oral administration than penicillin G was borne out by findings in normal subjects given 2,000,-

(2) New England J. Med. 257:249-257, Aug. 8, 1957.

000 units of penicillin V and G. Peak serum levels for penicillin V averaged as much as 2.1 times those of penicillin G.

In the 6 patients with streptococcic bacteremia, 2,000,000 units of penicillin V was administered orally every 4 hours for at least 4 weeks. Streptomycin was alternated with dihydrostreptomycin, 1 Gm. intramuscularly every 12 hours. In 5 patients, serum penicillin levels were maintained above 1.6 units/ml., with peaks averaging 22.3 units. In the sixth patient, probenecid was required to attain a satisfactory level.

Two patients had nausea and vomiting, and great individual differences in serum levels were noted in both normal subjects and patients. Serum levels were higher when penicillin V was taken after meals and were lower when aluminum hydroxide was taken simultaneously. There was no evidence of accumulation in the serum during therapy.

If penicillin V is used orally, regular serum assays are essential. Intramuscular penicillin G remains the preferred treatment.

Chemotherapy in Endocarditis Lenta: Two-Year Follow-up Study of 102 Cases is presented by W. J. Kaipainen and Kari Seppälä[3] (Univ. of Helsinki). At the end of 6 months, 55.2% of 29 patients treated with penicillin survived (Fig. 24). The survival rate continued to decline sharply, and a year after initiation of treatment only 27.5% of the patients were alive. After 2 years the percentage still was 27.5%. At the end of 4 years, survival was 24.1%, though this is not indicated in the figure. Only 1 of the patients who died received over 200,000,000 I.U. of penicillin; for the others the total dose was usually approximately 50,000,000 I.U., and it was the same for most of the surviving patients of this group.

The balance of 73 patients received penicillin combined with streptomycin or broad-spectrum antibiotics. The dosage followed no rigid scheme. The survival percentage in this group was 71.2% after 6 months, 60.3% after 1 year and 43.9% after 2 years. A few patients who died during the first 6 months had been given a total dose of 20,000,000-30,000,000 I.U. of penicillin; most received over 50,000,000 I.U., usually combined with 1-1.5 Gm. streptomycin/day. Of the patients in this group, 26 received broad-spectrum

(3) A.M.A. Arch. Int. Med. 100:419-422, September, 1957.

antibiotics at some stage of treatment. Of these patients, 65% were alive after 6 months, 34.7% after 1 year and 34.7% after 2 years. The slightly poorer therapeutic result for these patients weakens somewhat the over-all results for the combined treatment group, but the authors consider it necessary to retain them in the penicillin-streptomycin group, because broad-spectrum antibiotics were given

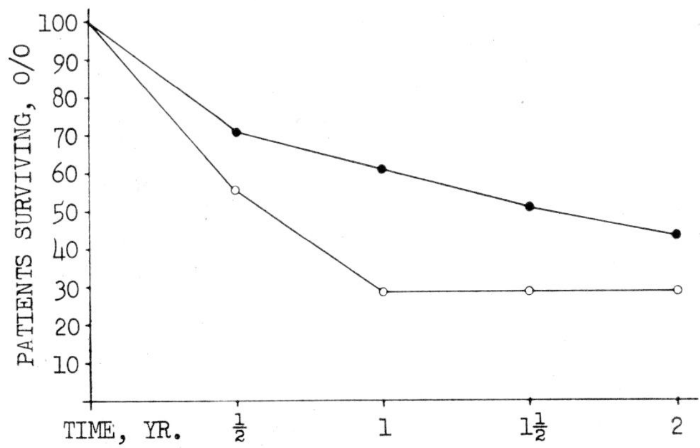

Fig. 24.—Therapeutic results in 102 patients with endocarditis lenta. Closed circles represent 73 patients treated with penicillin combined with other antibiotics. Open circles represent 29 patients treated with total over 20,000,000 I.U. of penicillin. (Courtesy of Kaipainen, W. J., and Seppälä, K.: A.M.A. Arch. Int. Med. 100: 419-422, September, 1957.)

mainly to patients who did not respond well to the combination of penicillin and streptomycin alone.

Of the total 102 patients, 40 (39.2%) were alive at the end of 2 years. To date, 3 of them have died before the follow-up period of 4 years. Twenty-four patients have been followed for over 4 years.

The cause of death was heart failure, embolism or uremia (1 patient) after clinical recovery from infection. The causes of death during treatment were identical; in some patients infection persisted. One who recovered clinically from the first infection was later reinfected and died 7 years after initiation of the first course of treatment.

Short-Term Penicillin and Dihydrostreptomycin Therapy of Streptococcic Endocarditis: Results of Treatment of 35 Patients are presented by Ralph Tompsett, William C. Robbins and Carl Berntsen, Jr.[4] (New York Hosp.-Cornell Med. Center). All patients had clinical evidence of valvular or congenital heart disease and all were febrile. Only cases were included in which bacteriologic confirmation of the diagnosis was obtained and in which the infecting organism was relatively sensitive to penicillin in vitro. In 33 cases, blood cultures showed viridans streptococci. A group H streptococcus was recovered in 2 cases and a "microaerophilic" streptococcus in another.

Treatment consisted in administering 500,000 units of potassium penicillin G intramuscularly every 2 hours (total daily dose 6,000,000 units) and 0.5 Gm. dihydrostreptomycin 4 times daily or 1 Gm. twice a day intramuscularly for 14 days. After completion of treatment, blood cultures were usually taken 3 times weekly for 2 weeks and at longer intervals thereafter for at least 3 months.

Of the 35 patients treated, bacteriologic cure was achieved beyond reasonable doubt in 24; i.e., the patient's response to therapy was entirely favorable, blood cultures were consistently sterile throughout treatment and for at least 3 months thereafter, and no additional antibiotic therapy was given for any reason.

Eight patients had a probable bacteriologic cure. In 4 of these persistent fever or other clinical signs of possible continued infection prompted further antibiotic therapy despite sterile blood cultures. In 3 patients further antibiotic therapy was necessary during the posttreatment period because of a new and unrelated infection. One patient died only 3 weeks after completion of therapy. Although there had been no clinical or laboratory evidence of continued or recurrent infection and none was found at autopsy, the result was classed as a probable cure because of the short follow-up period. Thus 32 patients (91%) had a certain or probable bacteriologic cure.

In the other 3 patients bacteriologically proved relapse occurred. One patient relapsed twice after short-term combined therapy. No significant change in the in vitro sensitivity to either penicillin or streptomycin was found in the strains isolated after unsuccessful treatment. This indicated that concurrent administration of the two antibiotics prevented emergence of streptomycin resistance.

(4) Am. J. Med. 24:57-67, January, 1958.

The results of this study afford additional clinical evidence for the decided effectiveness of combining penicillin and dihydrostreptomycin in the treatment of bacterial endocarditis caused by viridans streptococci and other streptococci which are reasonably sensitive to penicillin in vitro. The frequency of bacteriologic cure with the combined treatment for 14 days is comparable to that generally observed with penicillin alone for 28 days and probably is considerably higher than would be encountered with penicillin alone given for only 14 days. However, because of treatment failure in almost 10% of patients, and because it is not possible to predict in what patients short-term treatment will fail, it may be advisable to extend treatment for an additional 7-14 days, using either penicillin alone or combined therapy. By this regimen it may be possible to cure the remaining 10% of patients, and the risk of dihydrostreptomycin toxicity should not be significantly increased.

Antibiotic Therapy of Bacterial Endocarditis: VII. Vancomycin for Acute Micrococcic Endocarditis; Preliminary Report is presented by Joseph E. Geraci, Fordyce R. Heilman, Donald R. Nichols and William E. Wellman.[5] Vancomycin is bactericidal to micrococci and of low toxicity. Resistance to it develops slowly and to a small degree, if at all. It is effective against penicillin- and erythromycin-resistant micrococci and shows no cross-resistance with any other known antibiotic.

The authors gave vancomycin to 6 patients with acute endocarditis caused by coagulase-positive Micrococcus pyogenes (staphylococci). Therapy was guided by the results of serum bactericidal tests. In 5 patients a total killing effect was achieved in a serum dilution of 1:8 or greater, 3 and 6 hours, respectively, after the last doses when the medication was given intravenously in multiple doses of 0.5 Gm. every 6 hours; in 1 patient, the killing effect occurred in a serum dilution of 1:4.

Four of the 6 patients were considered cured on the basis of follow-up periods of 3-20 months. Two patients died, both of intractable congestive heart failure. In 1, the infection was severe and fulminating, with much toxemia and peripheral vascular collapse, and the infection was uncontrolled. The other patient died 2 weeks after therapy was terminated,

(5) Proc. Staff Meet. Mayo Clin. 33:172-181, Apr. 2, 1958.

with the infection under control, the blood cultures negative and the lesions healing.

There was a variable degree of phlebitis after intravenous injections. Use of a purified crystalline fraction of vancomycin eliminated chills. Occasionally, fever may be a manifestation of vancomycin toxicity.

Results suggest that short-term vancomycin therapy (2 weeks) may be practical and curative for micrococcic endocarditis.

► ↓ The number of hospital-acquired infections due to resistant staphylococci is rapidly mounting and already constitutes a major problem. J. W. Brown (J.A.M.A. 166:1185, Mar. 8, 1958), in an exhaustive consideration of the subject, well says that "the relatively successful measures for prevention by isolation are rusty from disuse, or were never learned in the first place."

In the several following articles there are offered measures for combating this menace to the modern therapy of infectious disease.—Ed.

Program for Prevention and Eradication of Staphylococcic Infections being carried out at Temple University Hospital is outlined by W. Emory Burnett, H. Taylor Caswell, Kenneth M. Schreck, Elsie R. Carrington, Norman Learner, Howard H. Steel, R. Robert Tyson and William C. Wright.[6] All infections are promptly reported to a central person. A committee meets weekly and investigates each case, recommending changes in procedures if necessary. Especially scrutinized are sterilization and laundry procedures, attending personnel, aseptic technics, indiscriminate use of antibiotics and routine use of antibiotics in surgery.

Contaminated linens are placed in specially marked containers and handled separately; workers wear gloves in handling this material. On the wards and private floors, patients with staphylococcic or other serious infections are placed under modified isolation technic. Blankets are sterilized between patients. Mattresses are encased in plastic covers that can be cleansed with antiseptic. Wet mopping of floors in the entire hospital was reinstituted to lessen dust. Doctors handling infected patients must use rubber gloves and avoid contact of their clothing with the bed or garments of these patients. Attendants of all types must use soap and water and alcohol freely on the hands. A special operating room is used only for patients who are infected, and these always are placed at the end of the operating lists. After use, the room is not used and is aired for 24 hours, if possible.

(6) J.A.M.A. 166:1183-1184, Mar. 8, 1958.

Medical personnel with infected lesions are encouraged to stay off duty. Local lesions are treated by compresses and drainage. Only when medical personnel are definitely ill are antibiotics used. Medicated soap (hexachlorophene) is prescribed for bathing. Surgical wounds are adequately drained early and topical antibiotics given. Nasal cultures in 640 members of the hospital personnel showed that 41% harbored a coagulase-positive staphylococcus, but that in only 4% were the organisms of the significant phage type 42B/52/81, which is the type responsible for 69% of the hospital infections. The nose was not an important source of infection, but these persons were warned to take special precautions; they were not treated with antibiotics.

In actual surgical procedures, all short-cut and easy-going procedures were abandoned and the strict aseptic technics of the preantibiotics era were reinstituted. Medicated liquid soap, although sterile in concentrated form, when diluted for use harbored a resistant Escherichia coli, as did the dispensers, and this source of liquid medicated soap was eliminated. A 10-minute scrub with white bar soap and sterile brush was reinstituted instead, followed by a hand bath in 70% alcohol for 1-2 minutes. Multiple layer gauze masks were replaced by thick filter types. Masks and caps are changed for each operation. Separate clean shoes for use only in the operating room are required of each staff member. All street clothing is exchanged for scrub suits. Visits outside the operating suite for rounds, to visit laboratories, etc., are discouraged. When necessary, street clothes are donned, then changed again on return.

Nurses carefully schooled in sterile technic again are in charge of dressing carts. Soiled dressings are placed in paper bags to be incinerated or autoclaved, and all instruments are placed in paper bags for sterilization before being handled.

With these measures, the previous alarming incidence of wound infections of 5% was reduced to a tolerable rate of 0.4-1%. This is a logical, practical although somewhat tedious program. There is no one source of error but many small facets that must be corrected and vigilantly policed.

Bacteriologic and Clinical Experiences and Methods of Control of Hospital Infections Due to Antibiotic-Resistant Staphylococci. H. Taylor Caswell, Kenneth M. Schreck, W. Emory Burnett, Elsie R. Carrington, Norman Learner,

Howard H. Steel, R. Robert Tyson and William C. Wright[7] found that the staphylococcus causing 69% of significant staphylococcic infections at Temple University Hospital was a strain lysed by three bacteriophages, i.e., 42B, 52 and 81. This bacteriophage type 42B/52/81 accounted for approximately 50% of all postoperative wound infections and pneumonias, 76% of cutaneous abscesses acquired by patients during hospitalization but not related to surgery and 80% of the typed organisms from cutaneous infections in hospital personnel. These figures compare with a 16% incidence of this bacteriophage type organism in patients admitted with staphylococcic infection. Only 4.1% of 265 nasal carriers of coagulase-positive staphylococci among hospital personnel were infested with organisms of this bacteriophage type. Thus nasal carriers of staphylococci among hospital personnel played an insignificant role in transmission of the organism.

It was found that bacteriophage type 42B/52/81 had an extremely high percentage of resistance to penicillin, streptomycin, tetracycline and erythromycin. It was sensitive to novobiocin, chloramphenicol, neomycin and bacitracin. The use of novobiocin, chloramphenicol and newly introduced antibiotics to which staphylococci are susceptible should be limited to patients with significant staphylococcic infection whose organisms are not susceptible to any other antibiotic or chemotherapeutic agent and whose infection cannot be controlled by other means, such as adequate surgical drainage. If this is not done, there will be a rapid increase in staphylococci resistant to these antibiotics also.

Infections with antibiotic-resistant organisms do not constitute a temporary epidemic but represent a problem which must be faced for an indefinite period in the modern antibiotic-saturated hospital society. Infected hospital personnel play a dominant role in transmitting these organisms. Successful control must be predicated on a return to strict sterile technics in addition to intelligent limitation of the use of antibiotics.

Trial of Penicillin V: Response of Penicillin-Resistant Staphylococcic Infections to Penicillin. Penicillin V is more stable in an acid medium than is penicillin G. Probably be-

(7) Surg., Gynec. & Obst. 106:1-10, January, 1958.

cause of this, blood levels reached after oral administration of penicillin V are higher and better sustained than those resulting from oral penicillin, G. J. I. Burn, M. P. Curwen, R. G. Huntsman and R. A. Shooter[8] (St. Bartholomew's Hosp., London) compared the efficacy of orally administered penicillin V with intramuscular penicillin in treatment of 346 patients with staphylococcic infections (furuncle on the face, abscess, carbuncle, infected wound, primary cellulitis, etc.). Patients treated by injection received a single daily dose of 600,000 units of procaine penicillin and 200,000 units of crystalline penicillin G. Those given penicillin V were instructed to take two 125-mg. capsules 3 times a day. On the basis of time required for healing of the lesions, results obtained with penicillin V were almost as satisfactory as those achieved with intramuscular penicillin. These results are not surprising in view of the reliable way in which penicillin V is absorbed.

Among the 346 patients were 66 infected with penicillin-resistant (penicillinase-producing) staphylococci. Infections due to these organisms responded as well to treatment with penicillin as infections due to sensitive staphylococci. Much has been made in recent years of the increase of penicillin-resistant staphylococci. If others confirm the present findings, it would appear that penicillin is still adequate for treatment of most staphylococcic sepsis. Other antibiotics are indicated only if the clinical condition warrants, and their use should not solely depend on a laboratory report of an in vitro penicillin-resistant organism.

Comparative in Vitro Studies of Hospital Strains of Staphylococcus Aureus with Oleandomycin, Tetracycline and Oleandomycin-Tetracycline Mixture. H. F. Hasenclever[9] (State Univ. of Iowa) studied the sensitivity to 1:2 oleandomycin-tetracycline mixture of 25 isolates of Staph. aureus that were resistant to 50 µg. or more tetracycline and of 12 isolates of Staph. aureus that were sensitive to less than 5 µg. tetracycline. Investigation was also conducted on the development of resistance to oleandomycin, to tetracycline and to the mixture of the two with the tetracycline-sensitive strains, and also to oleandomycin and to the olean-

(8) Brit. M. J. 2:193-196, July 27, 1957.
(9) Antibiotic Med. & Clin. Therap. 5:14-18, January, 1958.

domycin-tetracycline mixture with the resistant isolates. The tetracycline-resistant strains were generally more sensitive to oleandomycin than to the mixture. Observations on the emergence of resistance to these two agents showed little difference with these resistant strains. Tetracycline-sensitive strains of Staph. aureus were more sensitive to the mixture of oleandomycin and tetracycline than to either of the components. In vitro resistance developed most rapidly to oleandomycin, less rapidly to tetracycline and least rapidly to the oleandomycin-tetracycline mixture.

If in vitro studies are a reliable criterion for selection of a chemotherapeutic agent, oleandomycin generally would be more effective against tetracycline-resistant strains of Staph. aureus than the oleandomycin-tetracycline mixture. If judged on a similar basis, the mixture would be more effective against tetracycline-sensitive isolates than oleandomycin or tetracycline. These in vitro studies indicate that the problem of antibiotic-resistant staphylococci has not been solved by the combined action of oleandomycin and tetracycline.

Chemotherapy for Staphylococcus Aureus: Combined Use of Novobiocin and Erythromycin and Other Methods in Treatment of Burns led E. J. L. Lowbury[1] (Accident Hosp., Birmingham, England) to conclude that use of the combined antibiotics is undesirable if there is no particular indication for such therapy. Cultures of Staph. aureus originally sensitive to both erythromycin and novobiocin were serially subcultured in mediums containing the maximal tolerated concentration of the antibiotics alone and combined. Resistance promptly appeared with either agent alone, whereas a delay of about a week was observed when the two were used in combination. When the antibiotics were used separately, resistance developed only to the agent included in the medium; when both were used, greater resistance to novobiocin than to erythromycin developed. After subculture in the absence of antibiotic, there was some reversion to sensitivity among erythromycin-resistant but not among novobiocin-resistant strains.

The possibility of limiting the emergence of resistant strains during burn therapy was studied in all patients ad-

(1) Lancet 2:305-310, Aug. 17, 1957.

mitted during 1 month who had Streptococcus pyogenes or Staph. aureus sensitive to the two drugs. Adults were given 300 mg. erythromycin every 6 hours and 500 mg. novobiocin twice daily. Children under age 10 were given from one fourth to three fourths this dosage according to age. Comparison was made with records of former patients treated with tetracycline or erythromycin alone.

The burns were treated locally by one of three methods. In some, the closed method was used with penicillin cream on dressings changed every 5 days. In others, the exposure method was used with local insufflation of penicillin-lactose powder. The rest were exposed shortly before healing after treatment by the closed method.

In addition to these trials with combined antibiotics, two trials were made of the advantage of using chloramphenicol cream locally for staphylococcic infections of burns. This was found to be of value, particularly with out patients.

The combined therapy led to clearance of staphylococci from the burns in a significant number treated by the closed method, but not in those treated by the exposure method. Strains resistant to novobiocin began to appear after about 2 weeks and strains resistant to novobiocin in about 5 weeks.

Though the results of skin grafting were somewhat better in patients successfully treated to eliminate staphylococci, the organism does not constitute a sufficient threat to warrant routine use of novobiocin and erythromycin.

Ristocetin and Staphylococcus: Observations of Effects and Side Effects in 17 Cases of Staphylococcic Pneumonia are reported by George L. Calvy and L. Richard Schumacher[2] (US Naval Hosp., St. Albans, N. Y.). In nearly every case antibiotic-resistant staphylococci had been isolated. At the beginning, the dosage of ristocetin, a new antibiotic active against gram-positive pathogens, was 1-2 Gm. (15-30 mg./kg. body weight) daily. It produced prompt, measurable clinical improvement in 11 patients. No side effects were observed, except low-grade drug fever in 2 patients. Treatment averaged 15 days. In 6 patients, dosage averaged 2-4 Gm. daily for 15 days. At these levels, mild depression of the platelet count was noted in 2 patients and phlebitis in 3. No depression of granulocytes was found.

(2) J.A.M.A. 167:1584-1586, July 26, 1958.

The platelet counts returned to normal levels when dosage was reduced to about 25 mg./kg./day.

The drug was available in 500-mg. ampules, and the required amount was dissolved in 30-100 ml. of 5% glucose solution and administered over 10-30 minutes. The solution was injected into the tubing of an intravenous infusion system (5% glucose) ; 100-200 ml. glucose solution was usually flushed through the tubing at the end of the drug injection.

Blood cell counts, with particular attention to the white blood cells and platelets, should be determined on alternate days during therapy. Depression of the white cell count should call for a reduction in dosage or withdrawal of therapy in severe cases. With these precautions, ristocetin is a safe and potent agent against staphylococcic infections.

Intravenous Nitrofurantoin (Furadantin®) in Treatment of Systemic Infections Caused by Antibiotic-Resistant Bacteria can sometimes be lifesaving. Charles E. Friedgood[3] (Brooklyn) treated 26 patients with intravenous nitrofurantoin after other available antibacterial therapy had failed. The patients were aged 19-76 years. All were severely ill with infection, mostly superimposed on other pathologic conditions. Nine had malignant neoplasms and 13 various diseases of the genitourinary tract; disorders in the rest included peritonitis due to ruptured viscus, bacterial endocarditis, cholecystitis with cholangitis, empyema, phlebitis, pneumonia and mediastinitis. Positive bacterial cultures had been obtained from the blood of 9, urine of 12, bile of 3 and peritoneal fluid of 5. Most of the infections were due to Proteus sp. and were resistant, in vitro, to most or all the antibiotics but sensitive to nitrofurantoin. Other bacteria cultured were Escherichia coli, Pseudomonas sp., Aerobacter aerogenes, micrococci, enterococci, Streptococcus hemolyticus and Str. faecalis.

Nitrofurantoin is supplied as a sterile 0.6% solution in polyethylene glycol 300, each 10-cc. ampule containing 60 mg. nitrofurantoin. It is diluted, using sterile precautions, immediately before use and infused by slow drip. The recommended dose for the average adult is 3 ampules in at least 500 cc. diluent twice daily, making the daily dose 360 mg. The proportionate dose is 3.5 mg./kg. body weight.

(3) New York J. Med. 58:2044-2048, June 15, 1958.

Of the 26 patients, 18 were cured with nitrofurantoin alone and 2 with nitrofurantoin combined with chloramphenicol. Four were improved, but cultures remained positive, and treatment failed in 2. Of the 4 with persistent positive cultures, 1 had an alpha streptococcus, 1 Proteus sp. and the other 2 had pseudomonas associated with Proteus sp. or Str. faecalis. At the end of therapy, only the pseudomonas persisted in both.

Nitrofurantoin is one of the synthetic nitrofurans discovered during World War II. Generally, these are active against both gram-negative and gram-positive organisms, permitting comparatively little bacterial resistance and showing minimal toxicity to mammalian cells and organ systems. The highest reported blood level achieved by oral administration is 4 μg./cc., whereas by intravenous administration several patients achieved 10 μg./cc. This high concentration in the blood undoubtedly accounts for the success of the drug in systemic infection.

No toxic or allergic effects were noted in any of the 26 patients treated with intravenous nitrofurantoin. Oral therapy has induced nausea and vomiting in some patients, indicating a direct irritating effect on the gastrointestinal tract. Other adverse reactions previously reported have been malaise, headache, gastralgia and occasional drug rash. If saline is used as the diluent, close observation is necessary, since muscular irritability has occurred.

Intravenous nitrofurantoin appears to be valuable for the treatment of systemic bacterial infections caused by nitrofurantoin-sensitive organisms, especially if they are resistant to other antibacterial agents.

Clinical Trial of Tetracycline Phosphate Complex Combined with Nystatin in Treatment of Soft-Tissue Infections. The relation of fungi and yeastlike organisms to oral antibiotic therapy and the development of postmedication complications from the emergence of these microflora are still poorly defined. In the usual acute case of short duration, antimycotic agents may not be necessary. However, control of fungi and yeastlike organisms becomes more important in treatment of the young, the aged and the chronically debilitated. For this purpose, nystatin was combined with tetracycline phosphate complex in a single oral preparation.

Edwin A. Campbell, Aaron Prigot and Gladys M. Dorsey[4] (Harlem Hosp., New York) treated 123 patients with soft-tissue infections with the combined drugs. The capsules contained tetracycline phosphate complex equivalent to 250 mg. tetracycline hydrochloride activity and 250,000 units of nystatin. The dose schedule for adults was 2 capsules every 12 hours; children received proportionately less.

High serum concentrations were promptly achieved, inflammation and fever subsided rapidly and wounds healed quickly. In most patients, infections resolved without resort to operation. No evidence of toxicity appeared during courses of medication lasting 3-30 days. When the formulation was used in conjunction with operation, the magnitude of the procedures was lessened and morbidity decreased. No postoperative infections or other complications arose. For these reasons this combined therapy is recommended for acute soft-tissue infections in the young, the aged and the chronically ill.

Clinical Trial of Streptomycin Pantothenate in Treatment of Soft-Tissue Infections. Streptomycin, alone or with penicillin, is effective in soft-tissue infections, but damage to the 8th cranial nerve is a serious side effect. The pantothenic acid salt of streptomycin has been found to be considerably less toxic in acute experiments in mice and rats and in a clinical trial for 6 months in patients who had previously had severe side effects from both streptomycin and dihydrostreptomycin.

Rupert A. LaCaille and Aaron Prigot[5] (Harlem Hosp., New York) used streptomycin pantothenate, in conjunction with surgery, in treating 116 patients who had soft-tissue infections. Some were in the hospital but most were ambulatory. The dose schedule varied: all ambulatory patients received 1 Gm. intramuscularly daily, whereas hospital patients received 0.5 Gm. 3 or 4 times daily. The average duration was 7 days for ambulatory and 21 days for hospitalized patients. In all instances, the infection cleared rapidly, permitting definitive surgery when indicated.

Cultures of the infected areas grew Staphylococcus aureus, beta streptococcus, Escherichia coli, Staph. albus, paracolon

(4) Antibiotic Med. & Clin. Therap. 4:817-820, December, 1957.
(5) Am. J. Surg. 95:963-966, June, 1958.

bacilli, and Bacillus proteus. Four strains isolated were resistant to both streptomycin and streptomycin pantothenate. The rest were susceptible to both, but 6 were more sensitive to the pantothenate than to streptomycin. The antibacterial action of streptomycin is known to be enhanced by simultaneous administration of penicillin, and a similar synergism exists between Didrothenate and penicillin.

No allergy or toxicity could be demonstrated. None of the side actions usually associated with streptomycin or dihydrostreptomycin developed.

The inhibitory effect of pantothenate streptomycin on gram-positive and gram-negative organisms, the high level of patient tolerance and clinical response and the absence of toxicity make this new antibiotic a valuable adjunct in managing soft-tissue infections.

Treatment of Undulant Fever. J. Torres Gost[6] (Madrid) reports that all of 26 patients with undulant fever treated with Cathomycin were cured in about 5 days and none has had a recurrence. The adult dosage was 0.25 Gm. given every 4 hours until the day after the crisis (usually the 6th day) and then every 6 hours for 9 days to a total of 18 Gm.

The constant effect of Cathomycin was remarkable (Fig. 25). During the first 5 days of treatment no change was ap-

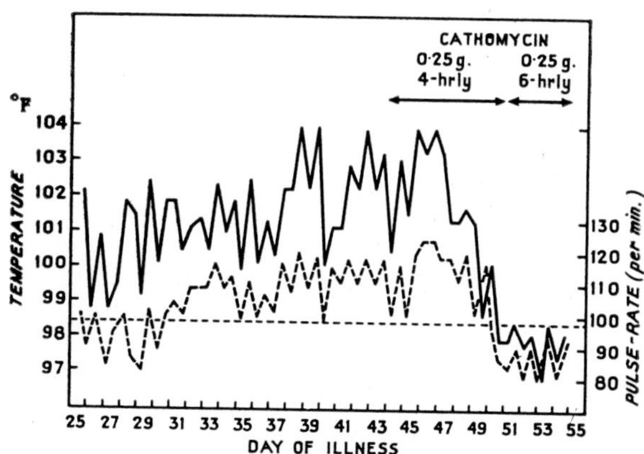

Fig. 25.—Typical chart of temperature and pulse rate in undulant fever before and during treatment with Cathomycin. (Courtesy of Torres Gost, J.: Lancet 1:191-192, Jan. 25, 1958.)

(6) Lancet 1:191-192, Jan. 25, 1958.

parent, pyrexia continued as before and the symptoms remained the same, but almost always on the 5th day the pyrexia resolved by crisis and all the symptoms (headache, insomnia, articular pain, anorexia, sweating, etc.) disappeared. Splenomegaly also disappeared, and by the end of treatment the spleen had returned to its normal size and shape, no matter how large it was. On the 3d day of treatment, liver function tests (Kunkel's, Maclagan's, Hanger's and Wührmann's), which were frequently made, were always normal. The leukopenia, which sometimes was extreme, rapidly disappeared. Anemia, which also is common in undulant fever, gradually returned to normal.

Many patients with chronic cases who had been pessimistic became cheerful and self-confident again after losing the fever and pain. So far urticarial eruption has been the only inconvenience caused by Cathomycin.

► [Remarkable as these results appear to be, it is nevertheless highly desirable that novobiocin (Cathomycin) be reserved for use only in infections of any sort that have been proved resistant to other antibiotics, for W. M. M. Kirby *et al.* found last year (1957-58 YEAR BOOK, p. 225) that when prompt healing did not occur in staphylococcic infections the organisms rapidly became resistant to the drug. It would be truly tragic if each of the new antibiotics that is effective against resistant strains of staphylococci were to be allowed to lose this advantage through widespread and thoughtless use. From this standpoint it seems difficult to justify such studies as those described in the 2 following articles.—Ed.]

Treatment of Pneumonia with Novobiocin. Joseph Van Der Meulen, Glenn Lubash and Ralph Tompsett[7] (Bellevue Hosp.) used novobiocin in treatment of 38 patients with pneumonia. In 24 with pneumococcic pneumonia who received adequate trial of therapy, results generally were satisfactory; in 2, results were difficult to assess and were considered indeterminate; in 1, apparent failure of therapy was associated with emergence of pneumococci resistant to novobiocin. In 3 patients in whom results were unsatisfactory, previous pulmonary disease may have contributed to the eventual outcome. In 7 of 8 patients with pneumonia of uncertain cause who were fully treated, results were good in 6 and fair in 1. The only untoward reaction was a skin eruption in 1 patient.

With the many drugs now available for treating pneumococcic pneumonia, it is apparent that for this purpose

(7) Antibiotic Med. & Clin. Therap. 5:26-35, January, 1958.

alone there is little need for new antimicrobial drugs. This study, however, provides information of value in two areas: (1) novobiocin may be useful in patients in whom pulmonary infection may be pneumococcic or staphylococcic. When it is difficult or impossible to establish the infective micro-organism, use of novobiocin may be lifesaving. Staphylococcic pneumonia is a dangerous infection, often caused by strains highly resistant to the older antimicrobial drugs. In this situation, novobiocin may have important use. (2) novobiocin is active in vivo on micro-organisms with in vitro sensitivities in the range of 1.5-3 μg./ml. These values are from 4 to 30 times higher than the sensitivities of most strains of staphylococci newly isolated from infections in man.

It seems reasonable to believe, therefore, that although novobiocin activity may be sharply reduced in vivo because of binding by serum protein, the degree of activity remaining must be great enough to provide potent antimicrobial activity against most strains of staphylococci.

Novobiocin in Common Pediatric Infections. Angella D. Ferguson, Gertrude C. Teixeira and Roland B. Scott[8] (Howard Univ.) treated 56 children under age 12 with novobiocin. The children had common pediatric infections including pneumonia, bronchitis, otitis media, tonsillitis and pharyngitis. The sodium salt of novobiocin was used in 47 cases and the calcium salt in 9. Dosage was 20 mg. novobiocin/kg./day in divided doses every 6 hours. Serial blood concentrations of novobiocin were obtained in 12 other patients given a single dose.

Satisfactory clinical and laboratory response was noted in all patients treated with novobiocin, except in 1 infant treated in the outpatient department for bronchopneumonia and acute gastroenteritis. In this patient, alpha streptococci and Escherichia coli were isolated from the nose and throat and E. coli was obtained from the stool.

Serum concentrations of novobiocin were all substantial, but higher levels were obtained with the calcium than with the sodium salt. The latter derivative, however, seemed to be more palatable and hence more acceptable to the children. The authors feel that this drug will probably find its great-

(8) J. Pediat. 51:655-663, December, 1957.

est usefulness in treatment of staphylococcic infections resistant to the older antibiotics.

Long-Acting Penicillin in Gonorrhea Control. Michael J. Takos, Lee W. Elgin and T. Elam Cato[9] (Miami, Fla.) report steady decline in the total incidence of gonorrhea in Dade County, Fla., after initiation of a program of using benzathine penicillin for treatment of gonorrhea in women. Benzathine penicillin G (Bicillin®), 2,400,000 units, was given in divided doses of 4 cc. (1,200,000 units) in each buttock. This allowed maintenance of effective therapeutic blood levels of penicillin for at least 6 weeks. The object of this therapy was to cure the patients of their neisserian infection and at the same time protect them from reinfection by the gonococcus for approximately 6 weeks. Only 6 treatment failures were noted. Men were given short-acting penicillin (600,000 units of 72-hour repository penicillin) in order that they be used for locating gonorrhea-infected women in the population.

Total Gonorrhea Cases, Population and Gonorrhea Morbidity Rates, Dade County, Fla., 1952-56

Year	Total reported cases	Estimated population [1]	Rate per thousand
1956	1, 554	734, 142	2. 1
1955	1, 663	703, 777	2. 4
1954	2, 030	658, 460	3. 1
1953	1, 994	617, 616	3. 1
1952	1, 808	576, 772	3. 1

[1] As calculated by vital statistics division, Dade County Health Department.

The best indication of the effectiveness of a control program was its effects on the community rates for the disease in question. The table presents data on total gonorrhea cases reported in Dade County at venereal disease clinics and by private practitioners and gives the estimated permanent population of the area and the gonorrhea morbidity rates. The morbidity rate was 2.1/1,000 in 1956 and averaged 3.1 during 1952, 1953 and 1954. If the average rate for 1956 had been 3.1/1,000, 2,276 cases of gonorrhea should have been reported, rather than the 1,554 actually reported.

(9) Pub. Health Rep. 72:976-980, November, 1957.

To be effective, the long-acting penicillin method requires that a fairly large proportion of infected women be brought to treatment. In Dade County nearly half the proved female gonorrhea cases were located by routine smear and culture examinations of women and girls in the local jails, of health card applicants and of persons coming to county maternity centers. Only about 35% of the laboratory-proved cases of gonorrhea in females were found through contact tracing. Female contacts of men with gonorrhea were treated with benzathine penicillin but were not counted as gonorrhea cases unless diagnosis was confirmed by laboratory studies.

The massive doses of benzathine penicillin used in the clinics apparently did not produce any more allergic reactions in patients than did the smaller doses of short-acting penicillins. Many complained of pain in the buttocks after injection, and an occasional patient had some difficulty in walking after Bicillin therapy. None of these effects lasted more than 24 hours, and those affected were usually highly excitable persons.

Streptomycin for Gonorrhea in London in 1956. R. R. Willcox[1] (St. Mary's Hosp.) treated 109 cases of acute gonorrhea with single injections of 0.5-1 Gm. streptomycin during 1956 and compared results with those in 62 cases reported in 1951. Follow-up (up to 3 months) was possible in 88 patients, in 53 of whom the condition at last visit was entirely satisfactory. Eighteen were later treated for nongonococcic infection and there were 11 gonococcus-positive failures (12.5% of those followed). Six patients were re-treated for reinfection. The failure rate was not significantly greater in 1956 than in 1951. There was thus no evidence of increasing resistance to streptomycin between the 1950 and the 1956 series.

When 0.5 Gm. streptomycin was used, the percentage of failures was 14.3 as compared with 10.2% when 1 Gm. was used. On the 1-Gm. schedule, the failure rates were not significantly greater in whites than in Negroes. With the 0.5-Gm. schedule, however, the failure rate in Negroes was significantly higher than that in white persons. The reason for this is obscure.

Sulfamethoxypyridazine in Urinary Tract Infections of-

(1) Acta dermat.-venereol. 37:332-337, 1957.

fers the advantage of maintaining a therapeutic level of the drug for a relatively long time, but it was not expected to produce a high urinary concentration, which has been considered desirable in such applications. A. Page Harris, Harris D. Riley Jr. and Vernon Knight[2] (Vanderbilt Univ.) verified the slow excretion of sulfamethoxypyridazine (Kynex®) as compared with sulfadiazine and sulfisoxazole (Gantrisin®). The average plasma level after a single oral dose of 2.5 Gm. Kynex in 6 subjects rose to 18 mg./100 ml. in 4 hours and remained at half that level at the end of 2 days, whereas a peak plasma level of less than 10 mg./100 ml. was achieved in groups of 5 subjects given 3 Gm. Gantrisin or sulfadiazine, either of which was completely excreted in about 48 hours. Conversely, the urinary level of Kynex rose relatively slowly and never reached the concentrations achieved with the other two drugs.

Chronic urinary tract infections from various causes in patients previously treated with antibiotics and other agents were treated with Kynex. The infections included those associated with indwelling catheters, chronic paralytic poliomyelitis, prostatic operations, pyelonephritis, chronic cystitis, urethritis and carcinoma of the bladder. Among 20 patients given 0.5 Gm. Kynex daily, the plasma concentrations varied considerably and were generally below the desirable therapeutic level of 10 mg./100 ml. or over. Only 4 patients showed clinical improvement, but 1 of these having negative bacterial cultures during treatment. With 5 patients given 1 Gm. daily, however, high plasma levels were maintained, associated with prompt clinical improvement and complete clearing of the urine in 3. No renal toxicity was noted; 1 patient acquired a morbilliform rash which improved promptly when the drug was withdrawn. No agranulocytosis or other hematologic difficulty was encountered.

Despite the low urinary concentration resulting from slow excretion of this drug, the authors believe that maintenance of a concentration of 10 mg./100 ml. or more in the plasma will prove effective in the treatment of urinary tract infections.

Prolonged Treatment of Urinary Tract Infections with Sulfamethoxypyridazine [Kynex®] was tried in 48 patients

(2) A.M.A. Arch. Int. Med. 100:701-708, November, 1957.

with urinary tract infections by Hans G. Grieble and George Gee Jackson[3] (Univ. of Illinois). This drug is readily absorbed from the gastrointestinal tract and slowly excreted in the urine, has a low degree of acetylation and is more soluble in acid mediums than are other sulfonamides. Its antibacterial activity in vitro, in human beings and in animals, is comparable to that of sulfadiazine.

Average duration of treatment was 35.5 days. Except for a few who were given daily doses of 1 Gm., all patients received an initial loading dose of 2.5 Gm. and then 0.5 Gm. daily. Children were given comparable doses calculated on a weight basis. Antibacterial concentrations of free sulfonamide (5-15 mg./100 ml.) were maintained in the serum in about 90% of patients with this dosage.

Eight of 10 patients with acute infections had a favorable symptomatic response. Prompt clearing of pyuria was observed in 5 and of bacteriuria in 7. Among patients with chronic infections, 9 of 38 showed a favorable response with respect to urinary symptoms and systemic manifestations. Ten of the 48 patients had bacteriologic cures as a result of treatment (freedom from infection for a minimum of 4-6 weeks). Only 1 patient of 24 with chronic pyelonephritis had a bacteriologic cure. None of the cured patients had a gross abnormality of the urinary tract, although 1 was pregnant. All 10 patients were infected with Escherichia coli, which was the only species recovered from the urine in 9. The antibacterial effect of sulfamethoxypyridazine was comparable to that of standard doses of other sulfonamides. In general, results with species other than E. coli were poor. Susceptible bacterial strains were eradicated after 1 or 2 weeks of treatment or not at all.

Adverse reactions were observed in 6.4% of patients during the first course of treatment. Headache and a diffuse erythematous maculopapular rash were the most common symptoms, but fever, abdominal pain and dizziness were also encountered. Sulfonamide crystalluria was observed in only 1 patient and without signs of renal toxicity. There was no leukopenia, and no signs of chronic toxicity were noted in patients who received full therapeutic doses for many weeks or months.

(3) New England J. Med. 258:1-7, Jan. 2, 1958.

Nongonococcal Urethritis in the Male Treated with Tetracycline. G. O. Mayne[4] (Royal Infirm., Edinburgh) reports results in 109 consecutive cases in which 250 mg. tetracycline hydrochloride was given every 6 hours for 5 days, a total dose of 5 Gm. The response was considered good if the discharge disappeared and the urine became clear in less than 7 days; and moderate if improvement was immediate and lasting but complete cure was delayed longer than 7 days. Failure was recorded if the urethritis did not respond to treatment or a relapse occurred immediately after a response.

No visible micro-organisms were present (including Trichomonas vaginalis) in 56 cases, and they were considered "abacterial." The other 53 were included in a heterogeneous group classed as "bacterial urethritis," in which bacteria other than gonococci were found.

Results of Treatment in 109 Cases

Type of Urethritis	Good		Moderate		Failure		Total	
	No. of Cases	Per cent.	No. of Cases	Per cent.	No. of Cases	Per cent.	No. of Cases	Per cent.
Abacterial	42	75	12	21·4	2	3·6	56	100
Bacterial . .	30	56·6	20	37·7	3	5·7	53	100
All Cases	72	66·1	32	29·3	5	4·6	109	100

The results (table) show that in cases in which a good response was obtained the difference between abacterial (75%) and bacterial (56.6%) urethritis was sufficiently large to be striking, almost 20%. The success rate of 75% in abacterial urethritis is considerably better than that obtained with any other treatment.

In only 1 case, in which vomiting and diarrhea developed on the 4th day, did treatment have to be suspended permanently. With this 5-day treatment, undesirable side effects were neither common nor troublesome.

Diagnosis of abacterial urethritis by microscopy should be regarded as an indication for tetracycline treatment. The use of previously unsuccessful therapy reduces the likelihood

(4) Brit. J. Ven. Dis. 33:244-245, December, 1957.

of satisfactory response. Therefore, tetracycline should be prescribed initially.

Trichomonas vaginalis infestation is high in female consorts of men with urethritis. However, it is unlikely that trichomoniasis plays a significant role in the cause of urethritis.

Place of Novobiocin in Genitourinary Tract Infections. Harry Seneca, John K. Lattimer and Anastasia Johnson[5] (Columbia Univ.) treated 60 patients with various urologic conditions, due to infections caused by a variety of pathogenic bacteria, with novobiocin. The dosage was 500 mg. 4 times daily after meals for a maximum of 10 days. This resulted in satisfactory serum levels, averaging 20-50 μg./ml. Ten patients received 250 mg. 4 times daily, but the results were not as good as with 500 mg. 4 times daily. Most patients had had previous antibiotic or chemotherapy but had failed to respond. Many were given other therapeutic agents after failure of novobiocin.

Novobiocin cleared the urine of 11 of 15 Micrococcus pyogenes aureus infections, 16 of 29 Streptococcus faecalis, 11 of 21 Bacillus proteus, 3 of 6 Gaffkya tetragena, 2 of 15 Escherichia coli, 1 of 7 diphtheroid and 1 of 6 Pseudomonas aeruginosa.

One patient had mild dermatitis medicamentosa and 2 had to discontinue medication because of vomiting or epigastric pain, but all others tolerated the drug well.

Bacteriuria and Diagnosis of Infections of Urinary Tract: Observations on Use of Methionine as Urinary Antiseptic. On the basis of observations on about 2,000 persons, Edward H. Kass[6] (Harvard Med. School) believes that true bacteriuria can be separated from contamination in most instances by bacterial counts of the urine. In general, patients with more than 100,000 bacteria/ml. urine have true bacteriuria. Bacteriuria is found in many asymptomatic persons, and its incidence is higher in persons known to have an increased incidence of clinically detectable pyelonephritis.

Pyuria is often absent when bacteriuria and pyelonephritis are present. Bacteriuria is often related to instrumenta-

(5) J. Urol. 79:882-891, May, 1958.
(6) A.M.A. Arch. Int. Med. 100:709-714, November, 1957.

tion and inlying catheterization of the urinary tract; single catheterizations are much less likely to induce infections. Voided specimens of urine are suitable for bacterial counts and yield valuable information which frequently may eliminate the need for catheterization.

When methionine in doses of 12-15 Gm./day is added to the normal diet, the urine pH may be lowered to 4.5-5 and kept at this level for months in patients with adequate renal function. The bacterial counts in the urine of patients with chronic urinary tract infections are reduced about 1,000-fold by administration of methionine alone, and occasionally complete eradication of bacteria may occur. This reduction in bacterial count appears to be due to the presence in the urine of an unidentified substance, probably a metabolite of methionine, that is bacteriostatic at pH 5.0.

If methenamine mandelate is given with methionine, the bacterial counts are usually lowered from about 10^8 bacteria/ml. urine to 10^3 to 10^4 bacteria/ml. The combination of drugs is generally well tolerated, although occasionally epigastric burning may occur. Lowering bacterial counts of the urine is usually accompanied by relief from dysuria. The sulfate ion is so active as a urinary acidifier that even alkaline urine of patients with proteus infections can usually be made acid and the infection brought under control.

► [Acidifying the urine in severe proteus infections is a very interesting achievement indeed. J. N. Hunt (Clin. Sc. 15:119, 1956) has shown that fed methionine has its sulfur oxidized to sulfate; the latter, excreted in the urine, apparently importantly affects urinary pH.—Ed.]

Furacin® Urethral Suppositories in Treatment of Non-Gonococcic Urethritis: Further Observations. R. R. Willcox[7] (St. Mary's Hosp., London) treated 23 patients who had acute, subacute or chronic nongonococcic urethritis with Furacin urethral suppositories containing nitrofurazone 0.2% and 2% diperodon hydrochloride, a local anesthetic dissolved in a water-dispersible base composed of glyceryl monolaurate and sorethytan monostearate. The pessaries, which are yellow, soft and slightly tapered, 2.5 in. long and 0.2 in. in diameter at the wider end, and 1.3 Gm. each, were used twice daily. Only 14 were used by 10 patients, whereas 11 used 28 and 2 used 42.

Immediate improvement was shown in 86.4% patients; 5

(7) Acta dermat.-venereol. 38:68-77, 1958.

had a relapse within 3 months of commencing treatment. The pessaries were well tolerated. It is felt that local Furacin therapy is capable of clearing residual discharge in a number of obstinate cases and provides a convenient substitute for urethral irrigations.

► [Furacin is not to be confused with Furadantin®, which is the subject of the 2 succeeding articles. Furadantin is given orally for its antiseptic action after excretion into the urinary tract; Furacin is used only locally in the urinary tract, the eyes and the ears. Both drugs are nitrofuran derivatives.—Ed.]

Proteus Infection of Urinary Tract, with Special Reference to Treatment with Nitrofurantoin. Nitrofurantoin is a relatively nontoxic drug, active in vitro against many gram-positive and gram-negative bacteria, including the proteus group, and is excreted in high concentration in the urine after oral administration. J. E. Middleton[8] (St. Thomas's Hosp., London) compared the effectiveness of nitrofurantoin with that of streptomycin or a sulfonamide in treating proteus infection of the urinary tract. Sensitivity tests were performed in vitro with nitrofurantoin and 12 antibiotics. All strains tested were sensitive to nitrofurantoin. Daily dosage of nitrofurantoin was 5-8 mg./kg., given in divided doses, most adults receiving 100 mg. every 6 hours.

Of 23 patients treated with nitrofurantoin, 12 had a laboratory and clinical cure. An additional 6 had clinical cure with relief from signs and symptoms, although the urine was not examined bacteriologically after treatment. Treatment failure occurred in 5 patients (22%). Of 23 patients treated with streptomycin, 13 failed to respond (57%). Of 22 treated with sulfonamides, 17 failed to respond (77%). Of the patients with urinary tract infection complicated by such factors as urethral stricture, prostatic hypertrophy, urolithiasis, hydronephrosis or automatic bladder, 8 of 12 were cured with nitrofurantoin, 3 of 13 with streptomycin and none of 13 with sulfonamides. The only toxic effect encountered with nitrofurantoin was vomiting in 2 patients, but in both it was severe enough to necessitate stopping treatment.

Effect of Therapeutic Dosages of Nitrofurantoin (Furadantin®) on Spermatogenesis in Man was shown by Warren O. Nelson and Raymond G. Bunge[9] (State-Univ. of

(8) Brit. M. J. 2:497-500, Aug. 31, 1957.
(9) J. Urol. 77:275-281, February, 1957.

Iowa) to be such that its use in urinary tract infections is unlikely to impair fertility. The drug, N-(5-nitro-2-furfurylidene)-1-aminohydantoin, produces temporary spermatogenic arrest at the stage of the primary spermatocyte in the rat testis.

In the present study, sperm counts were made before, during and after oral administration of 10 mg. Furadantin/kg. daily for 2 weeks to 36 healthy young men. Testicular biopsies were examined before and after treatment in all but 6. Half showed no significant variation in sperm count as a result of treatment. Of 12 subjects in this group submitting to biopsy, none showed histologic changes. A decrease in sperm count without appreciable change in the histologic picture was noted in 10 subjects; 5 of these counts were within the range of possible normal variation. Recovery was usually apparent within 3 months after initiation of treatment. In the rest, reduction of sperm production was apparent in decreased counts and, histologically, as a tendency toward arrest but not complete cessation of spermatogenesis.

About half the volunteers were from a prison population. The rest were medical students. Among the latter, the dosage used—a bit higher than the usual therapeutic dose—led to headache, nausea and some vomiting. The relative freedom from such effects among prisoners seemed to suggest a psychogenic factor in tolerance to the drug.

It may be said that Furadantin, in therapeutic doses, may produce moderate temporary spermatogenic arrest in unpredictable instances among healthy young Caucasians.

Results of Treatment in 1,086 General Paralytics, Majority of Whom Were Followed for More Than Five Years, have been compiled from 10 university hospitals by Richard D. Hahn, Bruce Webster, George Weickhardt, Evan Thomas, William Timberlake, Harry Solomon, John H. Stokes, Albert Heyman, George Gammon, Geraldine A. Gleeson, Arthur C. Curtis and John C. Cutler.[1]

Of 1,086 patients, 629 received penicillin alone, 457 penicillin plus fever therapy, usually induced tertian malaria. They were observed at 3, 6 and 12 months after treatment and yearly thereafter. Duration of syphilitic infection could not

(1) J. Chron. Dis. 7:209-227, March, 1958.

be determined in 50%, but in the others it was estimated to range from 2 to over 30 years, in most, from 10 to 24 years. Incidence ratio of men to women was 3:1, and over 2:1 of whites to Negroes. The cerebro spinal fluid complement fixation test was positive in all 327 who had been previously untreated. Almost all patients received 2,400,000 units and about half received over 6,000,000 units of penicillin. No untreated control group was available, but the end point in untreated general paralysis, with reference to the literature

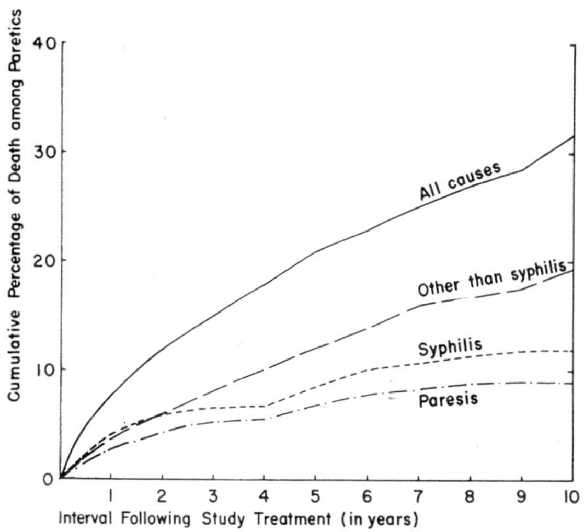

Fig. 26.—Probability of death among paretics after penicillin treatment, with or without fever. (Courtesy of Hahn, R. D., *et al.*: J. Chron. Dis. 7:209-227, March, 1958).

before malaria therapy was introduced in 1917, is death, usually within 4 years of detection.

Cumulative probability of death after treatment with penicillin (Fig. 26) was strikingly decreased. Probability of death 5 years after treatment was 10% for patients with severe psychosis when treated and zero for patients with moderate or mild psychosis. The effect of treatment on signs and symptoms of paresis (table) was strikingly beneficial. To avoid bias, improvement was not recorded, only complete disappearance of a sign or symptom. Impaired judgment, calculation, information, insight and speech were relatively resistant to therapy.

The trend in recent years in the United States has been toward treatment of paresis with penicillin alone. Possible additive effects of fever therapy are insufficient to justify its use in significant numbers of patients. Early diagnosis and prompt treatment with penicillin of incipient paresis result in clinical remission and ability to work in over 80% of patients and in practically eliminating death due to neurosyphilis. Even severely ill or institutionalized patients have one chance out of three of improvement and rehabilitation for work. In general, more than one course of penicillin is of no demonstrable additional value.

EFFECT OF TREATMENT ON SIGNS AND SYMPTOMS PRESENT

50%-60% Cleared up at 5 Yr.

Disorientation	Depression or euphoria
Convulsions	Untidy dress
Tremors	Incontinence
Inability to perform personal toilet	

40%-50% Cleared up at 5 Yr.

Impaired memory	Impaired retention
Impaired handwriting	Delusions, hallucinations
Illogical conversation	Psychotic on simple observation

30%-35% Cleared up at 5 Yr.

Impaired judgment	Impaired calculation
Impaired insight	Impaired information
Impaired speech	

Absence of clinical improvement, persistently abnormal cerebrospinal fluid protein level or persistently positive cerebrospinal fluid complement fixation reactions are not indications for retreatment. Retreatment with penicillin is indicated if initial therapy was less than 6,000,000 units, improvement was temporary after initial therapy but subsequently progressed or cerebrospinal fluid cell count of 5 or more persisted after the first posttreatment year. Routine repetition of treatment is not indicated.

Herxheimer's reactions, exacerbation of paretic psychosis or convulsions occur more often in the presence of cerebrospinal fluid pleocytosis than in its absence. Herxheimer's reaction does not appear to cause long-term damage.

A disease which was uniformly fatal within 4 years before 1917 has now become curable in some, and partially remediable in many, by brief treatment with penicillin.

► ↓ Since the methods of treating the various forms of syphilis are pretty well standardized and known to all in the United States, I have chosen for this YEAR BOOK 3 articles indicative of methods in use in France, Germany and Russia, respectively.—Ed.

Results of Treatment of Primary-Secondary Syphilis According to Personal Plan of Treatment Consisting of Preliminary Treatment by Three-Intravenous Injections of Cyanide of Mercury, Followed by 15 Million Units of Penicillin in Aqueous Solution: 10-Year Review is presented by M. Bolgert and G. Levy[2] (St. Louis Hosp., Paris). Each dose of mercuric cyanide was 10 mg. The first 1,000,000 units of penicillin was given in several daily injections within 3 days and 2 injections of 500,000 units each were given morning and evening daily for 14 days; thus the total dose was 15,000,000 units.

Since March 1947, 306 patients (62 with primary syphilis, seronegative 107 with primary seropositive syphilis and 137 with secondary syphilis) have been treated by this method. Of these, 63 (20.5%) are no longer being followed, but 43 of this group were negative over a long period. Of 243 patients still in follow-up, 213 are clinically and serologically cured. In 164, cure has persisted for 1,000-3,400 days. In 17, a definite reinfection occurred. There were 2 clinical failures, 4 doubtful cases and 7 serologic failures. Those who have not become serologically negative are free from clinical signs. All but 1 of the lumbar punctures performed gave normal results. None of the 37 children born to women treated by this method showed symptoms or signs of congenital syphilis.

Even when subjected to the strictest criteria of interpretation, this treatment was successful in 94.5% of the cases.

Results of Treatment of Neurosyphilis with Very High Doses of Penicillin Combined with Fever in Comparison with Usual Treatment with Penicillin Alone are better with the former method, according to Rudolf Degkwitz[3] (Univ. of Frankfort). During 1951-54, all patients in the author's series with neurosyphilis were given three courses of 10,000,000 units each of Aquacillin® (2 doses of 400,000 units) with intermissions of 2-4 weeks. In some cases, fever therapy was used concomitantly or afterward, when penicillin alone failed to arrest the infection in the central nervous system.

(2) Hautarzt 8:439-443, October, 1957.
(3) Nervenarzt 28:371-373, Aug. 20, 1957.

On the basis of experience with these methods, treatment was modified to consist of a single course of 30,000,000 units of Aquacillin (400,000 units regularly every 8 hours). Whenever a patient's condition permitted, Pyrifer was administered simultaneously. If this regimen did not arrest the process in the central nervous system, a supplementary course of malaria was given. Iodine was used to counteract inflammatory reactions of tissue defense.

Of 62 patients treated thus during 2 years, 56 had satisfactory follow-up; these included 30 with progressive paralysis, 9 with tabes dorsalis, 11 with cerebral syphilis and 6 with clinically symptomless neurosyphilis. In 33, predominantly those with progressive paralysis, Pyrifer was given in combination with penicillin, and in 9 a supplementary malaria cure was administered, with repetition in 1. In 18 further treatment was required to normalize the cerebrospinal fluid. In 14 a second course of 30,000,000 units of penicillin was given; in 4 of these it was with Pyrifer and in 4 with malaria.

The purpose of this intensive treatment was to arrest the syphilitic inflammation of the central nervous system as quickly as possible and thus to prevent further destruction of irreplaceable nerve tissue. Among cases studied, failures in progressive paralysis were 10% in patients who received combined penicillin-fever treatment and 20% in those who had penicillin alone. In ordinary types of neurosyphilis, inactivity of the cerebrospinal fluid can be achieved in 3-4 months. With intensive treatment, the cerebrospinal fluid cell count in progressive paralysis shows a more rapid decrease toward normal.

In Germany the incidence of neurosyphilis has not decreased markedly as it reportedly has in England and the United States where treatment of early syphilis with penicillin apparently has arrested progression and attack on the central nervous system. In this connection, the author notes that none of his patients with neurosyphilis had treatment with penicillin during the acute stage.

On Treatment of Early Forms of Syphilis. N. S. Smelov[4] (Central Dermato-venereological Scientific Res. Inst., Moscow) reports that among 184 patients with syphilis treated with 3,400,000 units of penicillin alone, follow-up 4 years

(4) Brit. J. Ven. Dis. 33:16-17, March, 1957.

later showed 3.7% relapses among primary seronegative cases, 5.5% among primary seropositive cases, 18.6% among cases of secondary fresh syphilis and 34.8% among cases of secondary recidive syphilis. Among 162 treated with 3,400,000 units of penicillin plus 1 or 2 courses of novarsenol and bismuth, follow-up 5 years later revealed no relapses among primary seronegative cases, 6% relapses among primary seropositive cases, 12% among secondary fresh syphilis and 30% in cases of secondary recidive syphilis.

Because of the higher relapse rate when syphilis is treated with penicillin alone, most Soviet syphilologists now insist on combined penicillin-novarsenol-bismuth therapy in patients without contraindications to use of Salvarsan®, bismuth or mercury. The main principles of this type of treatment are: (1) individual approach, (2) intermittent courses of treatment, (3) treatment beginning with penicillin, (4) penicillin followed by novarsenol-bismuth (or mercury), using 1-5 courses, depending on the stage of syphilis and the course of the disease during treatment, and (5) supplementary fever therapy, especially in cases of resistant syphilis.

Whatever method of specific treatment is used, much depends on the individual regimen of the patient. Sufficient sleep, fresh air, exercise, good nutrition and systemic polyvitamin therapy are of great importance.

Comparative Evaluation of Sustained Release Liquid Sulfonamide, Penicillin and Oral Tetracycline in Pediatric Practice is presented by Marvin McClellan[5] (Univ. of Cincinnati). Of 472 children (aged 4 months to 17 years) with moderately severe bacterial infections treated with 1 of 3 antibacterial medications, 233 were given a liquid, sustained release preparation containing sulfaethylthiadiazole, 207 were given penicillin, 25 were given penicillin (intramuscularly) and an oral pediatric suspension of tetracycline, 6 were given the sulfonamide preparation and penicillin simultaneously and 1 was given the sustained release sulfonamide prophylactically.

The maintenance dose of the sustained release sulfonamide preparation was based on ½ teaspoonful (0.32 Gm. or 5 gr.) for every 15 lb. body weight every 12 hours. Children over 75 lb. were given the adult dose of 1 tablespoonful every 12

(5) Ohio M. J. 54:41-44, January, 1958.

hours. Prophylactic doses were one-half the maintenance dose and also were given every 12 hours. All initial (priming) doses were twice the amount of the maintenance doses.

The initial dose of penicillin was given intramuscularly; subsequent doses were given orally. When patients showed a minimal response to therapy, a second and often a third dose was given intramuscularly even though the patient was taking penicillin orally. Intramuscular doses of penicillin varied with the size of the child and ranged between 300,000 and 500,000 units. Oral doses varied between 400,000 and 900,000 units/day.

In those treated with penicillin and tetracycline, penicillin was given only once, at start of treatment. This dose varied between 300,000 and 500,000 units and was given intramuscularly. Tetracycline was started immediately after penicillin. The doses varied betweeen 500 and 750 mg./day.

Of the patients treated with the sustained release liquid form of sulfaethylthiadiazole, 212 (90.9%) were cured; 188 (90.8%) treated with penicillin were cured; and 24 (96%) treated with penicillin and tetracycline were cured. The average number of treatment days required by each medication to bring about clinical remission of the infection was 6.9 days for the sustained release sulfaethylthiadiazole, 5.8 days for penicillin and 6.1 days for penicillin and tetracycline.

A statistical analysis (chi-square tests) of the number of patients cured with each medication failed to show any significant difference (chi-square=0.4579, P=0.75). Significant difference existed between the number of treatment days required for clinical remission of the infection for patients receiving the sulfonamide preparation and those receiving the other medications. The maximum difference between the number of treatment days for all of the medications was only 1.1 days and seemed to have little medical significance.

The reactions and number of reinfections observed with the sustained release form of sulfaethylthiadiazole and penicillin were about equal. The sustained form of sulfaethylthiadiazole thus offers a good alternative form of therapy in treating systemic bacterial infections in routine practice. Antibiotics then can be reserved to treat more serious infections.

ACTH and Adrenal Steroids in Treatment of Pneumococcic Meningitis in Adults. Failure of therapy in a large proportion of adults with this disease has continued, despite the use of antibacterial drugs which are known to sterilize the cerebrospinal fluid. Because pressure from the inflammatory exudate might be lethal and because clinical and experimental work indicate that ACTH and cortisone suppress the inflammatory reaction to pneumococci, John C. Ribble and Abraham I. Braude[6] (Southwestern Med. School) treated 12 consecutive cases of pneumococcic meningitis in adults with these drugs in combination with penicillin in an attempt to increase the percentage of cures. The usual dose of penicillin

Treatment

Day	Penicillin, Intravenously, (millions of units)	ACTH, Intravenously (units)	Hydrocortisone, Intravenously (mg.)
0	60	40	150
1	30	40	0
2	30	40	0
3	15	0	0
4	35	0	0
5	20	0	0
6	30	0	0
7	20	0	0

was 20,000,000-30,000,000 daily given as a slow intravenous drip. All patients received ACTH and 3 received hydrocortisone intravenously in the varying doses for varying periods.

The recovery rate of patients treated with the combined drugs was 92% ; 1 of the patients died 18 hours after admission. The results are offered as evidence, therefore, to support the concept that ACTH and adrenal steroids are beneficial in treatment of pneumococcic meningitis. This concept is based on the suppressive action exerted by these drugs in two potentially harmful features of pneumococcic infection: inflammatory exudation and bacterial hypersensitivity. No serious deleterious effects of ACTH were noted.

Woman, 34, was brought to the hospital in coma. Temperature was

(6) Am. J. Med. 24:68-79, January, 1958.

102.2 F., pulse 100 and respirations 32. Her neck was stiff. X-ray of the chest showed bronchopneumonia involving the right upper lobe. Hemoglobin was 6.3 Gm./100 ml., white blood cell count 20,000/cu. mm. with 6% lymphocytes, 81% segmented neutrophils and 13% nonsegmented neutrophils. Type 6 pneumococcus was demonstrated in the cerebrospinal fluid by capsular swelling with specific antiserum.

Therapy during the first 24 hours consisted of 60,000,000 units of penicillin, 40 units of ACTH and 150 mg. cortisone intravenously. The treatment is summarized in the table. Penicillin therapy was continued for 3 weeks. Because of low urine output, administration of potassium salts was not begun until 24 hours after admission.

Eight hours after admission the patient had two generalized convulsions which were controlled by barbiturates. Irregular, rapid respirations were corrected during the 1st day by lowering the cerebrospinal fluid pressure with repeated taps, and upper airway obstruction was treated with tracheostomy. Persistent tachypnea and episodes resembling carpopedal spasm were also present. For the first 2 weeks the course was complicated by a negative sodium balance, attributed to cerebral salt wasting. Improvement was gradual but marked. On discharge, 30 days after admission, the patient was well oriented, alert and co-operative. Her only symptom was moderate weakness. No residual lesions were noted when the patient was seen several months later.

Treatment of Mumps Orchitis with ACTH and Cortisone. To determine the efficacy of treatment by corticosteroids, Ian Maclean Smith and John W. Bishir[7] reviewed the charts of 85 patients who had mumps orchitis during 1954-55. This disabling complication develops in 15-40% of men with mumps. Apparently distention of the testis within the rigid tunica albuginea causes the pain, which can be relieved by incising the capsule. In 34 patients, only symptomatic treatment was given, consisting of bed rest, with support of the scrotum on an adhesive-tape bandage between the thighs, ice bags as indicated and acetylsalicylic acid in doses of 0.3-0.6 Gm. for temperatures greater than 101-102 F. A second group of 20 patients was given ACTH, 8 of whom received a single intravenous dose of 25 mg., 5 received this dose on each of 2 or 3 successive days and 7 received ACTH intramuscularly in divided doses totaling 50-500 mg. The other 31 patients received cortisone orally in doses of 50-100 mg.; 75 mg. 4 times daily was given to 22 of these patients for 4 days. Less than 900 mg. was taken by 12 patients and over 900 mg. by19.

Analysis of the three groups showed no significant difference in any characteristic. Those treated only symptomatical-

(7) New England J. Med. 258:120-124, Jan. 16, 1958.

ly had pain for a significantly longer period than those treated with cortisone. Treatment with ACTH had no significant effect on lessening any of the measurements compared with the control group. In none were signs or symptoms aggravated by ACTH or cortisone. Cortisone did not prevent onset of orchitis, neither in a second gonad nor in an unaffected gonad. Cortisone is analgesic for the pain of mumps orchitis, but it need not be used in most patients. In the natural course of a mild attack of mumps orchitis fever disappears in 4 days or less. The patient with mild mumps orchitis who has rectal temperature below 103 F. and a testis of less than twice its usual size need not be treated. An inadequate course of cortisone is worse than none because return of all the symptoms is most distressing to a patient who believes himself convalescent from the painful malady.

In this series, 9.8% of the hormone-treated patients had infections, but the controls had none. It is doubtful if treatment of a self-limiting, essentially benign disease is worth this risk. It is debatable whether the analgesia obtained is worth the infections incurred. In severe orchitis, a course of treatment is 300 mg. daily orally over 3 days.

Effects of Cortisone and ACTH in Mumps Meningoencephalitis in 5 patients were studied by John K. Spitznagel[8] (Fort Bragg, N. C.). Four patients received cortisone and 1 was treated with ACTH. Diagnoses were confirmed by lumbar puncture in all patients, and complement fixation titers were determined in 4. The dosage of cortisone was 200-300 mg./day and of ACTH, 60 mg./day. In all but 1 patient the drugs were discontinued by progressive decrements.

Cortisone and ACTH appeared to produce rapid remission of headache, nausea, anorexia, vomiting, photophobia, lethargy, delirium and nuchal rigidity. Fever, although it fell rapidly, tended to return to previous levels for short periods, accompanied by minor recurrence of other symptoms. Orchitis developed in 1 patient during cortisone therapy. This patient, and 1 other, also had salivary gland involvement during therapy. Abrupt termination of therapy in 1 patient after 3 doses of cortisone resulted in a dramatic recurrence of symptoms.

The duration of mumps in these patients did not differ

(8) Ann. Int. Med. 49:61-69, July, 1958.

from that in patients not receiving cortisone or ACTH. No evidence of residual disease of the nervous system could be detected in any patient.

The occurrence of remission 10-11 hours after institution of hormone therapy in 4 patients and after 18 hours in 1, regardless of duration of illness before therapy, appears to be convincing evidence of a definite palliative effect.

Management of Severe Tetanus: Use of Chlorpromazine in Two Patients. R. S. Packard, T. B. Cartmill and J. G. Henry[9] (Royal Prince Alfred Hosp., Sydney) treated 5 children with severe tetanus, using large doses of chlorpromazine. The drug was given by continuous intravenous infusion and supplemented by small quantities of amylobarbitone sodium. Further relaxant or sedative agents were unnecessary. All patients recovered.

Boy, 14, was hospitalized complaining of jaw stiffness and tightness in the chest for a day. Fifteen days previously he had had a splinter wound in the right ankle. Six days before being hospitalized he had been given tetanus antitoxin and penicillin; dosage of both was uncertain.

On physical examination, trismus was evident, with slight rigidity of upper abdominal muscles. He was confined to bed and given 50,000 units of antitoxin intramuscularly and 500,000 units of penicillin every 8 hours. There was no debridement of the wound. Sedation consisted of chlorpromazine, 50 mg. intramuscularly every 6 hours, combined with soluble phenobarbitone, 3 gr. intramuscularly, 3 or 4 times daily as required. Symptoms were at first well controlled, but within 48 hours several severe spasms occurred with marked opisthotonos, rigid abdomen and increase in extensor tone of lower limbs. Respiratory excursion was reduced, but laryngeal spasm and cyanosis did not occur.

By the 3d day as feeding by mouth was impossible, a polythene catheter was inserted in the right long saphenous vein and advanced into the inferior vena cava. For the next 2 weeks, all nutrition and drugs were given by this route and for 3 days soluble phenobarbital, 1½-3 gr., and chlorpromazine, 50 mg., were injected intermittently into the infusion set. Rigidity and spasm were controlled briefly, but the effect of the drugs in the doses given was transient and inadequate.

On the 6th day, tracheotomy was performed, followed by continuous intravenous infusion of chlorpromazine supplemented by amylobarbitone sodium. No subsequent major spasms occurred. Generally the patient lay with hypotonic limbs and ptosed eyelids, although varying degrees of rigidity of neck, spine and abdominal muscles persisted. Breathing was not depressed except when too much amylobarbitone was given; otherwise it was deep and effective, and his color remained good. No major pulmonary complications occurred. It was possible to

(9) Brit. M. J. 1:16-20, Jan. 4, 1958.

maintain good fluid and electrolyte balance. An intercurrent septicemia was controlled by antibiotics. During this period sedative requirements fell considerably. However, when septicemia was controlled, rigidity and minor spasms recurred and further intramuscular chlorpromazine was required. Tetanus gradually subsided, and by the 41st hospital day he was walking satisfactorily and eating well, with no trismus.

Chlorpromazine was effective in relieving major spasms, although modified minor spasms were often observed, especially if the trachea was aspirated roughly. The patient could be catheterized without provoking a spasm. Amylobarbitone was necessary, but the amounts required were small. When the amount administered was small, there was sign of respiratory depression, and the state of consciousness was never deep. When attempts were made to reduce the dose of chlorpromazine 3 days after it had been started, spasms recurred. Chlorpromazine diminished tracheobronchial secretions and caused no complications other than depression and irritability which persisted for 2 weeks after cessation. There was no jaundice, and liver function tests remained normal.

Effect of Chlorpromazine on Muscle Spasm in Human Tetanus proved to be more satisfactory than that of phenobarbitone for a child treated by Margaret N. Barr[1] (Univ. of St. Andrews).

Girl, 11, injured her foot on old wood and was hospitalized 2 weeks later with a suppurating wound, trismus and hunger. Muscle spasm held the foot in inversion and plantar flexion. The wound was cleansed, under general anesthesia, and she was given antitetanus serum, penicillin and intravenous infusion. Intramuscular phenobarbitone sodium, 5 gr. in divided dose, and oral phenobarbitone, 1 gr. 3 times that day, produced deep sedation, but trismus and spasm worsened.

Phenobarbitone was stopped and chlorpromazine substituted. Results were judged by the interdental distance (between the edges of incisors when mouth was opened, as widely as possible), the angle to which the injured foot could be dorsiflexed, compared with the angle achieved with the other foot and the degree of muscle spasm.

The interdental distance increased 150% immediately after slow intravenous injection of 20 mg. chlorpromazine and increased still farther in the next 6 minutes. Tendon reflex and spasm disappeared, and the patient became relaxed and sleepy but could be aroused easily. Respiration, pulse and blood pressure were not affected. After 15 hours, it was necessary to give further chlorpromazine (10 mg.), which reduced symptoms again, although less dramatically. The patient was then able to eat well. Chlorpromazine was given as needed, when, for

(1) Lancet 1:991-993, May 10, 1958.

various reasons, spasm and trismus returned. On the 6th day, 50 mg. thiopentone was given 2 hours after 20 mg. chlorpromazine. This resulted in reducing trismus and leg spasm further for a short time. This effect was demonstrated on two other occasions.

Chlorpromazine definitely modified the spasm and relieved trismus, thus permitting a normal diet, and left the patient conscious, results not obtained with phenobarbitone sedation. The effectiveness of the initial dose of chlorpromazine, given while the patient was under phenobarbitone sedation, and the observed effects of chlorpromazine and oral thiopentone indicate that combined therapy may be advantageous.

Comparative Value of Emetine and Chloroquine in Amebic Liver Abscess was studied by A. J. Wilmot, S. J. Powell and E. B. Adams[2] (Univ. of Natal). Alternate male African patients were given emetine or chloroquine. The series consisted of 19 patients treated with emetine, 5 of whom had amebic dysentery as well as liver abscess, and 16 treated with chloroquine, 3 of whom had associated dysentery.

Emetine, 1 gr./day, was given intramuscularly in two courses, the first lasting 10 days and the second 6 days, with 14 days intervening. Chloroquine was given as the diphosphate (250-mg. tablets equivalent to 150 mg. of the base) or the sulfate (200-mg. tablets equivalent to 150 mg. of the base) in a dose of 4 tablets immediately, followed by 2 tablets 6 hours later and 1 tablet twice daily for 29 days. In addition, all patients received 600 mg. diiodohydroxyquinoline 3 times daily for 20 days. When patients receiving chloroquine had active amebic dysentery in addition to liver abscess, tetracycline, 1 Gm./day for 10 days, was added.

Two patients who did not respond to chloroquine were given emetine. Both recovered satisfactorily. There was no apparent difference in initial response of the other patients to these two drugs. The relapse rate, however, was significantly different. In the emetine series there were no relapses, but in the chloroquine series 4 patients returned within 6 weeks with symptoms and signs of liver abscess. Pus was obtained at aspiration. The 4 patients were treated with emetine, with satisfactory results.

Aside from a moderate rise in pulse rate in some patients treated with emetine, no toxic reactions were noted with either drug.

(2) Am. J. Trop. Med. 7:197-198, March, 1958.

Treatment of Amebiasis with Camoform®. Laboratory evidence indicates that Camoform is effective against Endameba histolytica in vitro. Administered orally to animals infected with E. histolytica, the drug is effective against intestinal amebiasis in rats and dogs and amebic hepatitis in hamsters. Camoform is relatively nontoxic in animals after short-term administration, is rapidly absorbed, is stored in high concentration in the liver and lung and is slowly excreted largely by way of the bile (resulting in prolonged fecal levels).

J. María Bustamente y Rivero[3] (Arequipa, Peru) treated 40 patients with amebiasis, including 1 with pulmonary amebiasis. Camoform was given in a dosage of 250-500 mg. 3 times a day for 5 days. The drug was given with meals, since administration after meals may cause gastric intolerance.

All patients had a symptomatic cure and remained well over the subsequent several months of observation. All became free of E. histolytica after one course of treatment and there were no immediate relapses. It was found also that after the course of treatment the occurrence of E. coli, Chilomastix mesnili, Indolimax nana, Giardia lamblia and Trichomonas hominis was significantly reduced.

Camoform was well tolerated by most patients, although a few had occasional nausea, vomiting and abdominal distress. The symptoms were not sufficiently severe to warrant discontinuance of treatment.

Suppressive and Prophylactic Effects of Puromycin against Intestinal Protozoa were tested by Martin D. Young and Joe E. Freed[4] (Nat'l Inst. of Health) on patients in a mental hospital who were exposed to a high rate of infection. In an exposed group of patients receiving 100 mg. of the drug daily for 10 days, the amebic infection was cured in about half and suppressed in most of the rest. Weekly administration of as much as 500 mg. for 5 weeks effected few cures and failed to prevent new infections.

A group of patients in a heavily infected ward were then cleared of protozoa with 1 Gm. puromycin daily for 4 days; about half of these were continued on a prophylactic regimen of 250 mg. 3 times weekly for 6 weeks. The group in

(3) J.A.M.A. 165:829-830, Oct. 19, 1957.
(4) Am. J. Trop. Med. 6:808-812, September, 1957.

whom treatment had been stopped began to acquire infections during the 4th week after treatment cessation, but the treated group remained uninfected throughout the 6 weeks of prophylaxis, although constantly exposed. Two weeks after prophylaxis was discontinued, this group also began to acquire infections.

All who were receiving 1 Gm. daily had diarrhea on the 4th day and a few vomited, but these reactions disappeared when the drug was reduced or withdrawn. Lower dosages did not produce reactions.

Further Studies on Malaria Suppression by Monthly Drug Administration were undertaken by Max J. Miller[5] (Harbel, Liberia), since excellent results had been reported when antimalarials were administered weekly. It was hoped that the relatively rapid development of resistance to malaria in the native West African might make the more practicable monthly program successful.

Field studies were carried out in labor camps and native villages, assessing the value of pyrimethamine and chloroquine given at monthly intervals. In some cases, individual records were kept; in others a transient population was involved. Comparison was made with results in untreated control groups, with placebo administration and with the use of mosquito control measures without prophylactic drugs. For adults, the dose of pyrimethamine was 25 mg. and of chloroquine (base) 150 mg. Children under age 3 were given half these amounts. Results were observed in terms of malaria parasite rates obtained from thick blood film preparations, Giemsa stained. At least 150 oil-immersion fields were examined.

Control rates averaged somewhat over 20% (higher for children under age 15 years). Where pyrimethamine alone or with chloroquine was given to recorded populations, the rate dropped within 2 months to 3% and under and remained so during the period of the experiment, 16 months. In the shifting population study, 1 labor camp was subjected to house spraying with residual insecticide, in another pyrimethamine was given all subjects present at monthly intervals and 1 was left untreated.

The attempt at mosquito control had little if any effect on

(5) Am. J. Trop. Med. 6:625-637, July, 1957.

the parasite rate, whereas the rate dropped from an initial 40% to an average of 28% over 2 years of drug administration in the third camp. Similar evidence of the efficacy of the treatment was obtained from a thorough study of 20 young men during a year with no treatment and then during a year with pyrimethamine. Thirty-two attacks of malaria with 130 days of illness the 1st year contrasted with 1 attack which promptly cleared following administration of the usual dose of pyrimethamine the 2d year. The parasite rate was reduced from 21% to 0.1% of all blood films examined. The results showed that monthly administration of suppressive doses of antimalarial drugs could be relied on to reduce the rates of infection and clinical malaria and that drug-resistant strains of Plasmodium falciparum are less prevalent in West Africa than they have been reported to be in East Africa.

Ocular Complications of Chloroquine Therapy were investigated by H. E. Hobbs and C. D. Calnan[6] (Royal Free Hosp., London). Visual disturbances due to synthetic antimalarial drugs were first reported as corneal edema in airmen who took prophylactic mepacrine in suppressive doses. The disturbance was transient and disappeared as soon as the drug was withheld.

A more durable effect on vision was noted in workers engaged in the manufacture of mepacrine. Haloes were apparent from a deposit in the superficial layers of the cornea which was seen by slit-lamp microscopy to consist of fine yellowish dots. The deposits disappeared when the affected persons were withdrawn from this work.

In recent years the efficacy of such drugs, particularly chloroquine, in the treatment of some other diseases (notably lupus erythematosus and actinic dermatitis) led to their empiric use in higher dosage, with which visual symptoms tend to develop oftener. Bleil reported the transient appearance of opacification of the subepithelial layers and Bowman's zone of the cornea, producing partial blindness as one of a group of severe symptoms in a patient under treatment with amodiaquin (Camoquin®) for lupus erythematosus.

The authors observed a more insidious and less transient condition resulting from the administration of chloroquine. It develops after an interval and on a dosage which shows

(6) Lancet 1:1207-1209, June 7, 1958.

considerable individual variation; it consists of visual disturbance associated with haloes suggesting congestive glaucoma and characteristic deposits in the corneal epithelium. The details of the condition were determined after the examination of 30 patients to whom chloroquine was being given in various dosages and on different clinical indications. The commonest complaints were blurred or misty vision, blurred vision accompanied by colored rings around lights, and focusing difficulties.

Examination of 28 patients by slit-lamp microscopy showed corneal changes in 22. The changes, of several types, were confined to the epithelium of the cornea, with slight changes in the stroma immediately underlying Bowman's membrane in a few. The gradual evolution of these changes during chloroquine treatment and the more gradual recession seen in some when treatment was discontinued make it fairly certain that they arise as the result of treatment with chloroquine. The time needed for their evolution and relation to the dosage used are still uncertain.

► [It is unlikely that this description will be frightening to workers in the malaria field since the precise nature of the changes, their permanence and above all their relation to dosage and duration of treatment are, as admitted by the authors, still uncertain. None of the patients who were the subject of the study were being treated for malaria, and presumably the doses used, though not stated, were high since 23 of the 30 persons had lupus erythematosus, and 28 of the 30 had been under treatment for several weeks to 2 years. Furthermore, they were a selected group because at the beginning of the investigation they were those who complained of some disturbance.—Ed.]

Neostibosan® in Chronic Malaria. Mohd. Qudratullah[7] (Sylhet Med. School) treated 52 patients who had chronic tertian malaria with Neostibosan, an antimony compound, given intravenously in 5% solution. The patients had had relapses at varying intervals for 5-12 years. Patients of average build received 0.1 Gm. daily for 12 consecutive days. Heavier patients were given 0.1 Gm. daily for 6 days, followed by 0.2 Gm. daily for the next 6 days. Nitrite crises occurred in 3 patients after the 4th or 5th injection and were avoided or controlled by injection of epinephrine.

There has been no relapse of malarial fever in any patient following the course of Neostibosan, and no plasmodia have been detected in patients examined after treatment. Many who had been invalids have returned to active life.

(7) Medicus 14:176-179, August, 1957.

Neostibosan probably acts indirectly against plasmodia as it does against the Leishman-Donovan bodies in kala-azar. The drug either induces production of a substance in the reticuloendothelial cells that kills the parasite, or it goes into chemical combination, giving rise to a compound that kills the parasite or prevents further multiplication. In chronic malaria the exoerythrocytic form of the plasmodium is apparently destroyed or prevented from further growth.

Acquired Toxoplasmosis: Observations on Two Parasitologically Proved Cases Treated with Pyrimethamine and Triple Sulfonamides are presented by Donald E. Kayhoe, Leon Jacobs, Henry K. Beye and Norman B. McCullough[8] (Nat'l Inst. of Allergy and Infectious Diseases, Bethesda, Md.). One patient, a research worker in a toxoplasmosis laboratory, became ill 6 days after a laboratory accident. Myalgias, headache, a rash and fever developed. There was generalized lymphadenopathy with lymphocytosis, atypical lymphocytes and anemia. The serologic tests for toxoplasmosis became positive, and toxoplasma was recovered from the blood and later from an excised lymph node.

The second patient gave a history of thyrotoxicosis with removal of a thyroid adenoma and successful maintenance with 60 mg. desiccated thyroid daily for 5 months. Three weeks after thyroid treatment was discontinued peripheral neuropathy, ocular complaints, fever and lymphadenopathy developed. The patient was suspected of having acute lymphatic leukemia and during the study was found to have a high dye-test titer. Toxoplasma was isolated from lymph node and muscle tissue.

Both patients showed a prompt response to treatment with pyrimethamine and triple sulfonamides. The first patient had a rapid defervescence, with disappearance of skin lesions. Both had prompt diminution in size of lymph nodes and a fall in the dye-test titer, which later rose again. Anemia that developed in both before onset of treatment became worse during therapy and improved after the drugs were discontinued. In the second patient toxoplasma was present in the lymph nodes for 66 days after completion of treatment.

Treatment appears to be suppressive in the acute phase of the disease but may not prevent progression to the chronic

(8) New England J. Med. 257:1247-1254, Dec. 26, 1957.

form. The experimentally determined optimal dosage of pryimethamine is many times that safe for man. For this reason, dosage has been selected empirically at 25 mg. daily after a loading dose. Even at this level the drug is potentially dangerous, so that blood and platelet counts should be obtained often on patients under therapy.

Disseminated Coccidioidomycosis Apparently Cured with Amphotericin B. A case is reported by Margaret S. Klapper (Univ. of Alabama), David T. Smith and Norman F. Conant[9] (Duke Univ.).

Woman, 34, was exposed to dust while visiting in Arizona. Six months later she had left lumbar pain and was operated on for "acute osteomyelitis." Cultures were negative. She remained febrile, healing was incomplete and 3 draining sinuses persisted, despite intensive penicillin, sulfonamide and streptomycin therapy. New abscesses formed. Two years later a diagnosis of blastomycosis was made by skin test and complement fixation, and treatment with iodides and blastomycin vaccine produced slight clinical improvement, though low-grade fever persisted.

Four years after exposure, fever still persisted and the sinuses continued to drain. A pure culture of Coccidioides immitis was isolated from pus aspirated from a fluctuant, nondraining area. Complement fixation tests were slightly positive for blastomyces and strongly positive for C. immitis.

Over the next 5 years, the disease slowly progressed, despite various types of therapy. By the 10th year, the patient weighed only 86 lb., was able to get around only with crutches or a wheel chair, was in constant pain and required frequent transfusions. Treatment with nystatin, 10 Gm. daily, induced moderate improvement with weight gain of 10 lb., less pain and return of ambulation, but without evidence of healing.

Amphotericin B was then begun, 1 Gm. orally 4 times daily. At this time there were 30 draining sinuses over the left buttock and thigh, besides the incompletely healed operative site, and 8 over the right. Within 2 weeks of institution of amphotericin B, appetite and strength improved, the lesions drained less and fever disappeared. In 5 weeks the effects were dramatic. Some of the oldest lesions healed, the patient felt well and weight gain continued. In 7 weeks, the incision healed over for the first time in 10 years and all the left-side lesions were healed. In 3 months all lesions were healed and weight was 120 lb. Treatment was continued for 14 months. The drug was well tolerated with no evidence of untoward hepatic, renal or hemopoietic reactions.

Nitrofurazone Therapy of Trypanosoma Gambiense Sleeping Sickness in Man, used for the first time by F. Evens, K. Niemegeers and A. Packchanian,[1] gave encouraging results. The drug, 5-nitro-2-furaldehyde semicarbazone, known

(9) J.A.M.A. 167:463-466, May 24, 1958.
(1) Am. J. Trop. Med. 6:665-678, July, 1957.

to be an effective trypanocide in mice, was used alone or with other agents in 32 native Africans who had various stages of the disease. Daily doses in the form of 100-, 250- or 500-mg. tablets of nitrofurazone (Furacin®) were given with milk, bananas or water.

Three previously untreated adults without nerve involvement were successfully treated with Furacin alone in doses of 8.8-30 mg./kg. daily for 1-2 weeks. Two were free from parasites 4 and 10 weeks, respectively, after treatment; the 3d was not available to follow-up.

Three children, also untreated, with T. gambiense in the cerebrospinal fluid as well as in the blood and lymph nodes, were given 4 mg./kg. Lomidine intramuscularly daily or every other day for 6 days and 6.3-33.4 mg./kg. Furacin orally for 6-8 days. One did not respond to treatment and retained trypanosomes in the cerebrospinal fluid 2 months later. The other 2 were free from infection and showed normal cerebrospinal fluids and negative complement fixation tests 11 and 16 months after treatment.

Nine patients with chronic, relapsing cases refractory to previous treatment were given nitrofurazone alone. Marked improvement including normal cerebrospinal fluids resulted in each, but all but 2 showed parasitologic relapse. One died some weeks after treatment. The 2 without parasites were considered cured.

Three of those mentioned who had relapses and 17 other patients with hopeless relapsing cases of sleeping sickness were given a so-called cocktail treatment. Bayer 205 intravenously the 1st day was followed by intramuscular Lomidine for 3 days. The next 2 days, Furacin was given orally, and Arsobal was given intravenously on 1 of these days. Arsobal and Furacin were alternated with Furacin alone on days 7-9. Then Furacin alone was given for 4 more days. In some cases this course was repeated several times.

The 3 patients previously treated with Furacin alone again showed initial improvement followed by relapse some months after treatment. Of the others, 9 were considered probably cured. All showed a favorable immediate response with disappearance of trypanosomes from the cerebrospinal fluid and usually a return to normal cell counts. Two had relapses 3 and 6 months later; the other 6 did not return for follow-up.

Nausea and vomiting were encountered but were transient. In 2 of 3 patients so affected, these effects subsided before termination of therapy. Crippling muscular and arthritic pains occurred in some but were transitory; recovery was brought about sooner when vitamin B complex was used. Doses of 2.1-12.5 mg./kg. 3 times a day for 7-36 days were tolerated without permanent ill effects. The drugs combined seemed less toxic in some instances than when they were used alone. Most of these cases were originally considered hopeless. The cures effected recommend the use of nitrofurazon alone or with other trypanocides in treating African sleeping sickness.

Treatment of Leprosy with D-Cycloserine: First Results in 7 cases (1 tuberculoid and 6 lepromatous) are reported by M. Pestell and L. Chambon[2] (Saigon, South Vietnam). The first 4 patients were treated with three 250-mg. capsules of d-cycloserine/day for the 1st week and 2 capsules/day thereafter.

Man, 50, with symptoms of leprosy for 5 months, had lepromas over the entire body and large inflamed infiltrations below both breasts, on the left shoulder, in the right popliteal space and on the left ear lobe. There were no signs of peripheral nerve involvement. Hansen bacilli were found in nasal mucus and in the ear lesion.

After 2 months' treatment, the lepromas and infiltrations regressed but remained inflamed with desquamation. Nasal mucus and cutaneous biopsy specimens still showed Hansen bacilli. Histologic diagnosis was reactional tuberculoid leprosy. During the next 2 months, the patient's condition improved steadily. At the end of 3 months' treatment, the nasal mucus and a skin biopsy specimen showed no Hansen bacilli. After 4 months, the patient's appearance was completely transformed and bacteriologic examinations were normal except for a few isolated organisms in the popliteal region. After interruption for 1 month, treatment was resumed with 0.5 Gm., then 0.75 Gm. d-cycloserine/day.

After 8 months (96 Gm. d-cycloserine), the lepromas had completely disappeared on the face, back and arms and persisted only as small, brownish, nonanesthetic macules on the anterior trunk and legs. Infiltrations were reduced to large pigmented macules. Bacteriologic examinations were normal. Fernandez and Mitsuda tests were negative throughout.

The other patients also had prompt bacteriologic negativity and regression of skin lesions, as shown by histologic

(2) Presse méd. 65:1791-1793, Nov. 6, 1957.

serial examinations. Favorable effects were mitigated, however, by the occurrence of severe reactions in some patients which required postponement or cessation of treatment and presented the risk of aggravation of latent nerve lesions by sclerosis following reactional lesions affecting the nerve trunks. Hence the following dosage schedule was adopted: 0.25 Gm. for 15 days, 0.5 Gm. for 15 days and 0.75 Gm. thereafter. Even this dosage did not prevent the appearance of reactions, at first minimal and then more serious. In controlling such reactions, phenylbutazone seemed more effective than hydrocortisone. An attempt is being made to avoid such complications by simultaneous administration of anti-inflammatory substances with d-cycloserine. Preliminary results in several patients receiving this combined treatment appear promising.

Tuberculosis

Late Results of Prolonged Multiple-Drug Therapy for Pulmonary Tuberculosis. James W. Raleigh[3] (VA Hosp., Sunmount, N. Y.) reviews early and late results of initial chemotherapy in 550 patients with pulmonary tuberculosis who completed such therapy in 8 or more months without interruption. Chemotherapy consisted of streptomycin and PAS in 413 patients and regimens containing isoniazid in 137. Actual duration of therapy was 8-45 months and averaged 15.2 months. An initial observation point was established between the end of the 6th and 8th months of therapy. Follow-up information was obtained in 99% of patients 12 months after the observation point, in 90% at 18 months, in 78% at 24 months, in 70% at 30 months and in 55% at 36 months.

Though disappearance of tubercle bacilli as determined by culture and microscopy was observed in 86% of the patients, cavity closure at 8 months of therapy was obtained in less than half the entire group and in only 30% of the patients who had one or more cavities at the start. In patients in whom cavity closure was obtained at 8 months, the late prognosis was excellent with relapses few and benign and recovery of the inactive status in almost all cases. There were

(3) Am. Rev. Tuberc. 76:540-558, October, 1957.

no deaths from tuberculosis in this group, and the differences in relapse incidence and severity were only slightly in favor of the surgical group.

In the patients in whom cavity persisted, even though there was temporary bacteriologic remission lasting 3 months or longer, the relapse rate was high. The relapse rate in patients whose open lesions were resected was similar to that in the "closed-negative" group, but the relapse rate in patients whose cavities were not resected was much higher.

In patients with both persistent cavity and sputum positive for Mycobacterium tuberculosis after 6-8 months of initial chemotherapy, the prognosis was poor. Only about 50% achieved the inactive state, and in most of these inactivity of the disease was obtained only by addition of resection or thoracoplasty.

Of 27 patients who died of tuberculosis, all were in the "open-cavity" group at the observation point, and almost 80% of those with still active disease at the time of the last follow-up were in this category. The importance of cavity closure as a criterion of early therapeutic success in the treatment of pulmonary tuberculosis and the incidence of subsequent relapse is obvious. Appreciation of this fact may justify surgical risks to achieve the end which might heretofore have seemed excessive.

Artificial Pneumothorax as Aid to Chemotherapy in Treatment of Pulmonary Tuberculosis. Between 1937 and 1942, before the advent of antibiotics, 442 patients with unilateral artificial pneumothoraces were discharged from a sanatorium. A. F. Foster-Carter[4] (Frimley, England) reviewed the cases of 174 patients treated with chemotherapy and artificial pneumothorax and compared the results with those previously achieved with pneumothorax alone. In a 5-8 year follow-up artificial pneumothorax results were found to be good if cavities had been closed, with 90% of 230 patients surviving and with few complications. In contrast, if cavities failed to close, empyema, effusion and death were common. These results indicated that the unfortunate reputation attached to artificial pneumothorax by some physicians is undeserved, since it results from poor selection of cases. Cavity closure and not absence of adhesions is the

(4) Dis. Chest 33:382-397, April, 1958.

key to success. Adhesions which do not prevent cavity closure do not affect prognosis or complications. Yet the incidence of artificial pneumothorax has steadily decreased in patients discharged from the sanatorium (Fig. 27).

Of the 174 patients receiving both forms of treatment 17 (10%) relapsed, most of whom had been treated earlier when

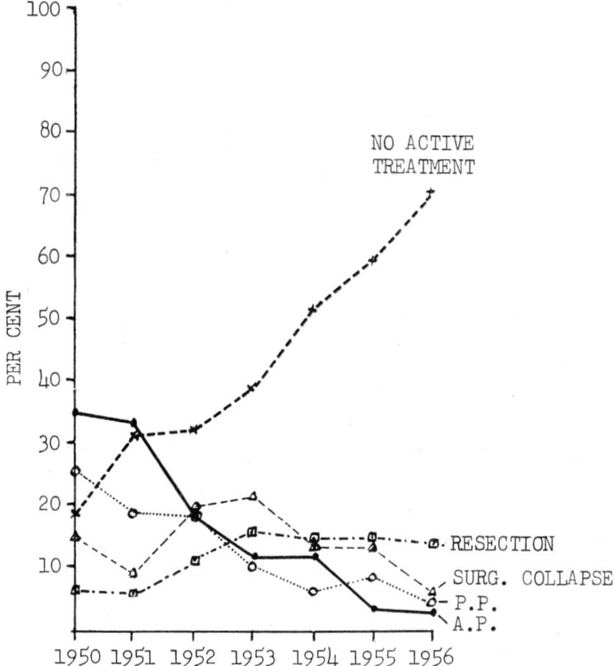

Fig. 27.—Various forms of treatment of pulmonary tuberculosis patients discharged from an English sanatorium in 6-year follow-up. (Courtesy of Foster-Carter, A. F.: Dis. Chest. 33:382-397, April, 1958.)

chemotherapy was of short duration. Only 8 had evidence of new activity in the treated lung. None had developed empyema. Pleural effusion occurred in 17%, contrasted with 25% without chemotherapy, but this lower percentage is still significant. A longer period of chemotherapy did not markedly decrease the incidence of effusions.

Most patients who would have been considered ideal for artificial pneumothorax 5 years before recovered with antibiotic treatment and rest alone, as shown by the increase in patients receiving no "active" treatment (Fig. 27).

Patients usually had 3 months' initial treatment with antibiotics. Those receiving artificial pneumothorax were selected from the relatively few who did not respond satisfactorily. Main indications were localized disease with cavities, localized cavities with widespread disease throughout the lung, localized cavities in one lung, with serious disease requiring surgical collapse in the other or the presence of local cavities in one lung, with the other virtually incapacitated by extensive surgery. Localized disease with cavitation was the most common indication.

Man, 29, had positive sputum, early tuberculous laryngitis, x-ray evidence of infiltration and cavity in the right upper lobe. After 3½ months' rest and daily treatment with streptomycin, isoniazid and PAS, the cavity was still present although smaller. Artificial pneumothorax was induced in the right lung. A few apical adhesions were present, but the cavity closed and sputum converted within a month. Four months later, with chemotherapy, he returned to full-time work. One year later, tomographs confirmed cavity closure and resolution of the lesions. Pneumothorax was no longer necessary.

Antibiotics have assumed paramount importance in tuberculosis therapy to the extent that all other treatment has become ancillary. Artificial pneumothorax still plays a small but important role in treating patients who do not respond satisfactorily to chemotherapy. Short-term pneumothorax may prove increasingly useful in promoting rapid closure of cavities.

Fate of Patient with Persistent Cavitation and Noninfectious Sputum ("Open-Negative") after Discharge from Hospital was studied by R. F. Corpe and F. A. Blalock[5] (Battey State Hosp., Rome, Ga.). It was found to be safe to discharge the patient with the "open-negative" syndrome to his home environment without creating a public health problem. The mortality rate among the 159 study patients was 3.8% and the reactivation rate 8.8%. No further bouts of suppuration or hemorrhage were reported.

To the present, there has been no discernible difference in the reactivation rate between the Negro and the white man. Men have not fared as well as women; 13 of the 14 reactivations were in men.

(5) Am. Rev. Tuberc. 77:764-777, May, 1958.

Only 2% of the patients were confined to their homes because of their physical disabilities; 45% had unlimited activity; over 25% were working full time. This serves as a counterbalance to the previous concepts that these cavities should be removed surgically or collapsed by thoracoplasty before the patients could return to their families and earn a living.

Of the group, 152 patients had received isoniazid while in the hospital. Only 3 had been advised to take streptomycin-PAS as postsanatorium drug regimen, whereas 153 had isoniazid-PAS and 3 isoniazid-streptomycin.

There are many unanswered questions, e.g., how long should a patient with the "open-negative" syndrome be continued on drug therapy? It is believed this must be highly individualized, but many patients should be continued on it indefinitely. However, among the 38 whose drug therapy has been stopped, there have been no reactivations to date.

Only 1 study patient has been considered a public health menace. If such people can be adequately cared for medically at home, they are much happier and it is cheaper to maintain them on drugs outside the hospital than to carry them as inpatients. Many of these, even those with cavitary disease, if given the opportunity, with public health clearance as to noninfectiousness, can become self-supporting and again take their place in society.

Place of Drug Therapy in Management of Unhospitalized Tuberculosis Patients is felt by Arthur B. Robins and Aaron D. Chaves[6] (Dept. of Health, New York) to be important. Antimicrobial therapy was given 1,631 patients who were awaiting admission, prematurely discharged or relapsing or who refused to be hospitalized. Of these, 831 were treated as clinic patients for 18 months and were available for study after 2 years. Most (75%) were instructed to take 5 mg. isoniazid/kg./day plus 12 Gm. PAS in divided doses. The rest were given isoniazid plus 1 Gm. streptomycin twice weekly, with or without PAS.

Of the group, 8% were under age 25, 48% over age 45, 66% male, 49% white, 36% Negro and 15% Puerto Rican. In 35%, the disease was far advanced, in 13% minimal. Most were active and a few were working.

(6) Ann. Int. Med. 47:774-781, October, 1957.

Of 537 showing positive serum cultures at the beginning, 62% had negative cultures at the end of 2 years. Improved x-ray status was achieved in 50%; deterioration in 11%. Among all cases 35% and among the most advanced 58% had active tuberculosis at 24 months. The same categories showed 55 and 28% of arrests, respectively.

There was no evidence that the program increased the incidence of drug-resistant infection in the community. No reduction in willingness to enter hospitals for treatment or to remain hospitalized as long as required was noted. Consequently, the authors feel such a program is an essential supplement to hospitalization among such patients.

Changing Concepts in Treatment of Pulmonary Tuberculosis are bringing us to the point at which good therapeutic results are consistently attained in patients excreting bacilli susceptible to the drugs used, according to Irving Kass, William F. Russell, Angeline Heaton, Terumasa Miyamoto, Gardner Middlebrook and Sidney H. Dressler[7] (Denver). Four factors contribute to the decrease in therapeutic failures: adequate combined drug therapy, assay to guide isoniazid dosage, physical activity as an adjunct to drug therapy and surgery of residual pulmonary lesions.

The authors report good, reproducible results from a program in which high doses of isoniazid combined with streptomycin were given to patients excreting bacilli sensitive to both and in whom physical activity was maintained. Streptomycin, 15-30 mg./kg./day for 90 days or more, was combined with a daily isoniazid dosage determined by bioassay which was continued for 18 months. Pyridoxine, 50-100 Gm./day, was given during isoniazid administration. In rapid inactivators, PAS or PABA, 10 Gm./day in divided doses, was added to this schedule.

The microbiologic assay method of Middlebrook which depends on the ability of known concentrations of isoniazid to render growing tubercle bacilli nonacid fast served to divide patients into four dosage groups. Six hours after a test dose of 4 mg. isoniazid/kg., a level of 1.6 μg./ml. calls for 4 mg. isoniazid/kg./day plus 25 mg. vitamin B_6; 0.8 μg. calls for twice this amount; 0.4 μg. for 4 times the dosage; and less than 0.4 μg. indicates the need for PAS or PABA as well.

(7) Ann. Int. Med. 47:744-761, October, 1957.

Since antimicrobial agents are most effective against multiplying organisms, physical activity is desirable during treatment when the infection is due to drug-sensitive strains of bacilli, but it is contraindicated otherwise. Activity is believed to promote cavity drainage as well and to improve the psychologic status of the patient.

In view of the inaccessibility to chemotherapeutic action of dormant bacilli in residual lesions, resection of such lesions is advocated to limit reactivation of infection after treatment is discontinued.

Seventeenth Veterans Administration-Armed Forces Conference on Chemotherapy of Tuberculosis was reported by Emil Rothstein[8] (Tufts College). This was the 12th year in which the Veterans Administration tuberculosis hospitals co-operated in a nationwide study group for tuberculosis. Interest in the last 2 years was in evaluating streptomycin administered daily combined with isoniazid and isoniazid plus PAS. Over 1,000 cases of pulmonary tuberculosis were randomly allocated to three treatment groups: streptomycin 1 Gm. daily, combined with isoniazid 300 mg. daily; isoniazid 300 mg. daily, combined with PAS 12 Gm. daily; and all three drugs in these dosages. Results were similar in all groups. Bacterial resistance was slight and identical in the three regimens. Toxicity was least with isoniazid; 7% had to stop PAS and 14% streptomycin because of toxicity. Toxicity was greatest when all three drugs were used. Triple drug therapy, even with daily streptomycin, had no special therapeutic value, did not decrease the chances of resistance, induced the greatest toxicity, was most difficult to administer and had the greatest danger of multiple-drug sensitization.

Previous evidence indicated that isoniazid alone might be effective in treating tuberculosis if tissue destruction was minimal and the chance of resistant bacilli emerging was slight. In 150 cases randomly distributed between treatment with isoniazid alone, 300 mg. daily, and combined with PAS, x-ray improvement, sputum conversion and "target point" occurred equally often in both groups. Isoniazid alone was better tolerated.

Cycloserine, 500 mg., combined with isoniazid, 300 mg.,

---

(8) New England J. Med. 258:1199-1204, June 12, 1958.

produced good results, comparable with those obtained with isoniazid combined with PAS, but a somewhat greater percentage of patients had x-ray evidence of worsening at the end of 8 months' treatment. By the criteria of cavity closure, sputum conversion and development of resistant bacilli, the isoniazid-PAS combination was superior.

Preliminary study showed the combination of 300 mg. isoniazid with 1.5 or 3 Gm. pyrazinamide to be therapeutically as effective as isoniazid-PAS. Hepatotoxicity occurred in about 10% of those receiving the 3-Gm. dose and in about 3% of those receiving 1.5 Gm. More extensive study of this drug is planned.

Streptovaricin, 3 Gm. orally in a single dose, with isoniazid, 100 mg. 3 times daily, was administered to 26 patients re-treated for cavitation whose tubercle bacilli were susceptible to isoniazid. Ten became isoniazid resistant at the end of 4 months and therapeutic results were no better than with isoniazid alone. Lethargy, anorexia and nausea caused difficulty and no further study of this drug is planned.

Thiocarbanidin and kanamycin are being studied further. Experience is still too slight to allow even tentative appraisal.

Infection with resistant tubercle bacilli is apparently not on the increase. About 2% of all patients with untreated tuberculosis continue to have organisms reported as resistant to isoniazid or streptomycin.

Corticosteroid therapy is beneficial when used in ample dosages for patients seriouly ill with tuberculosis, whether meningeal or otherwise. If effective antituberculosis drugs are used as well and steroids tapered off rather than stopped abruptly, this treatment is believed safe in all and perhaps lifesaving in many.

U.S. Veterans Administration-Armed Forces Co-operative Studies of Tuberculosis: VI. Survival among Patients with Miliary and Meningeal Tuberculosis (1948-55) has been significantly improved by the introduction of isoniazid, according to John H. Williams, Jr.[9] Records of 772 patients were divided in four groups based on the therapy used as new drugs became available. Patients in the earliest group were given streptomycin or dihydrostreptomycin alone; in the second, streptomycin and sulfone; in the third, streptomy-

(9) Am. Rev. Tuberc. 76:360-369, September, 1957.

cin and PAS; and in the fourth, isoniazid and streptomycin with or without PAS.

The influence of chemotherapy on the incidence of meningitis among patients with miliary tuberculosis was striking: on streptomycin and sulfone, 60% had meningitis; on streptomycin and PAS, 22%; and on isoniazid and streptomycin, none acquired meningitis, though it has been reported that the treatment will not completely prevent this development.

The 2-year survival rate for patients in the four groups was 56, 57, 81 and 95%, respectively, in the case of miliary tuberculosis. For meningitis without miliary tuberculosis the rates were 21, 15, 51 and 80%. Among patients with both, the rates were 10, 0, 33 and 77%. The 5-year survival data were essentially the same, though figures were not available for the most recent group. Besides the presence of meningitis, increasing age lowered survival. Race affected the incidence of tuberculosis but not the efficacy of treatment.

Superficial Glandular Tuberculosis: Treatment with Chemotherapy is reported by G. S. Kilpatrick and A. C. Douglas[1] (Univ. of Edinburgh) in 52 patients. Most patients received streptomycin and isoniazid daily, followed by PAS and isoniazid. All patients were followed for at least 1 year. In 31, retrogression of the adenitis was satisfactory. In 13, the end result was satisfactory, but the course of the disease was unsatisfactory because fluctuation or sinus formation occurred before an eventual satisfactory result was obtained. In 2, the end result was pending but treatment had so far failed. Six had a satisfactory end result but adenitis recurred after chemotherapy was discontinued. As these are not the results of a controlled trial, it is impossible to know with certainty whether chemotherapy hastened the healing process in these patients, but, on the basis of their experience, the authors believe that it did.

Patients with tuberculous adenitis should be hospitalized to insure adequate rest, supervision of chemotherapy and minor surgery at the optimal time if it is required. Patients under age 40 receive 1 Gm. streptomycin sulfate daily and 100 mg. isoniazid twice daily. To prevent onset of giddiness caused by streptomycin, older patients receive 1 Gm. streptomycin 3 times a week and 5 Gm. sodium PAS and 100 mg.

(1) Brit. M. J. 2:612-614, Sept. 14, 1957.

isoniazid twice daily. These regimens have been shown to prevent emergence of drug-resistant organisms in pulmonary tuberculosis. While streptomycin and isoniazid daily is the best and safest form of therapy, because of the risk of encountering primarily PAS-resistant organisms, it may be justifiable to use isoniazid with PAS when the patient is discharged from the hospital after a satisfactory initial course of treatment. In either instance, chemotherapy should be prolonged, at least 12-18 months' treatment being required.

When there is obvious fluctuation, the pus is aspirated or a small incision is made. Isolated large gland masses are removed surgically when they fail to respond to 4-6 weeks of chemotherapy.

Pyrazinamide Together with Oxytetracycline in Patients with Tubercle Bacilli Resistant to Streptomycin, PAS and Isoniazid. Sheila M. Stewart, J. McC. Murdoch, J. W. Crofton and David Hay[2] (Univ. of Edinburgh) treated 11 patients who had far-advanced, cavitated pulmonary tuberculosis with pyrazinamide plus oxytetracycline for at least 3 months. In all cases the sputum had been consistently positive for at least 15 months. Pyrazinamide was given in a dose of 40 mg./kg./day in 2 divided doses. Ten patients received 2 Gm. oxytetracycline twice daily and 1 received 1 Gm. twice daily (because of nausea and vomiting with the larger dose).

Except for 1 patient whose initial bacterial count was extremely high, all showed a marked drop in count in the first 14-40 days of treatment. Subsequently there was an equally steady rise with emergence of pyrazinamide-resistant organisms. No oxytetracycline resistance was encountered. Clinically there was some improvement in 8 patients, but there was an escape from the effect of the drug in each of these patients in the 2d month of therapy, after the emergence of drug-resistant organisms. No toxic effects attributable to pyrazinamide were noted.

Oxytetracycline apparently does not appreciably delay the onset of pyrazinamide resistance or prolong the short effectiveness of the drug. Until a drug can be found that will prevent pyrazinamide resistance, it is probably wise in patients whose bacilli are resistant to streptomycin, PAS and isoniazid to use the drug only for covering operations. It is un-

(2) Brit. J. Tuberc. 51:158-167, April, 1957.

likely to be effective for more than 4-6 weeks, but it may greatly improve the patient's condition during the early part of that time. The value of pyrazinamide combined with isoniazid in patients with streptomycin and PAS-resistant bacilli needs further assessment. It may be more effective than oxytetracycline in preventing emergence of isoniazid-resistant organisms.

Antibiotic Transosseous Perfusion in Severe Tuberculous Osteoarthritis is described, with 5 case reports, by A. Delahaye, A. Blanc and P. Treps[3] (Paris). Transepiphysial perfusion of antibiotics, with regular and repeated penetration of the drug through a shutter window covering the trephine orifice, is preferable to bone curettage followed by injection of the antibiotic through a small, fixed drainage tube. It constitutes minimal intervention without immediate risk and destruction which may be harmful in case the knee is later resected. The aim of treatment is to prevent amputation, to prepare the terrain for later conservative surgery if this is necessary or to obviate the need for operation. It should be regarded as conservative and expectant treatment, especially in cases of severe osteoarthritis with pulmonary foci.

Woman, 76, with bilateral recurrence of old pulmonary tuberculosis, had a white tibiotarsal tumor of the left foot, which had been immobilized for 6 months. Three months after streptomycin therapy was discontinued because of a facial eruption, the tuberculous osteoarthritis became worse and an abscess formed. The tibiotarsal lesion progressed, but amputation was postponed in view of the patient's poor general condition. When metaphysial trephine was done with institution of isoniazid dialysis, decalcification was extreme with tibial bulbar osteolysis and marked degeneration of the articular surfaces, extensive infiltration and cutaneous involvement. Local interosseous therapy included isoniazid, 10.8 Gm. during 54 days, streptomycin, 22 Gm. over 50 days, and PAS, 170 Gm. in 17 days. In addition, the patient received generally 20 Gm. streptomycin in 70 days (preceding development of the osseous lesion), 3,100 Gm. PAS intravenously and orally in 649 days and isoniazid, 100.6 Gm. over 554 days. Plaster immobilization was maintained for 725 days.

Within 2 months after the beginning of transosseous infusions, the patient's general condition was improved, with normal temperature and return of appetite. Three months later x-rays showed definite regeneration of bone and complete disappearance of the abscess. The condition of the joint and of the lungs steadily improved. Nine months after institution of local treatment, the patient began to walk and when discharged a year later was in good condition. Three years later the

(3) Presse méd. 65:1705-1707, Oct. 23, 1957.

patient, then aged 80, was well and active, caring for her own house. The tibiotarsal joint was completely ankylosed and painless.

In this case transosseous perfusion not only prevented amputation but also made conservative surgery unnecessary. In another case resection of the knee could be performed after improvement in the bone, and in 1, resection was done after synovial antibiotic therapy. In 1 case, however, of white tumor of the right knee which had been long neglected, transosseous and synovial perfusion for 3 weeks produced no improvement; amputation was followed by rapid general and pulmonary improvement.

Antituberculous Chemoprophylaxis with Isoniazid: Preliminary Note by A. Omodei Zorini[4] (Rome Univ.) indicates a preference for isoniazid prophylaxis over antituberculosis vaccination as a public health measure. Tolerance to high doses of isoniazid over a prolonged period was observed in the therapy of 20 teen-age patients. Even a mild liver disturbance was found not to contraindicate such treatment if careful watch was maintained permitting immediate interruption when necessary.

Tests in guinea pigs infected subcutaneously with virulent bacilli, some before and some after isoniazid treatment, and subsequently reinfected to determine immunity were not entirely conclusive, because of many nonspecific deaths and the use of too-large inocula. However, survival was 4 times as great among treated animals as among the controls, and animals infected while protected by isoniazid showed no more than a minimal lesion at the site of injection.

This background plus reports in the literature, led to a trial of isoniazid administered orally in several palatable forms to 600 children living with tuberculous relatives or in institutions. A daily dose of 20 mg./kg. was given for 6 months. The children, aged 4-11, were mostly skin positive but showed no signs of active tuberculosis. A similar group was untreated. The experiment was intended to show the degree of tolerance to such treatment, its eventual effect on the tuberculin reaction and the vaccinating effect of natural infection among those so protected. The report being preliminary, answers to these questions must depend on the results of follow-up studies. To date, the following may be reported.

(4) Dis. Chest 33:1-17, January, 1958.

Tolerance was excellent in nearly all cases; in 2 patients treatment had to be stopped because of relapsing dermatitis and in 2 because of gastroenteritis. Moderate eosinophilia in the peripheral blood of some patients was observed. Urinalyses were consistently normal. Vitamins, particularly of the B complex, were given with the drug. The method appears to be practical, and its success will be evaluated in the years to come.

Further Experience with Single-Drug (Isoniazid) Therapy in Chronic Pulmonary Tuberculosis: Initial Therapy with High-Dose Isoniazid. Clarence Jordahl, Roger Des Prez, Kurt Deuschle, Carl Muschenheim and Walsh McDermott[5] treated 32 unselected patients with moderately and far-advanced chronic pulmonary tuberculosis with isoniazid alone in daily doses of 10 mg./kg. for the initial 3 weeks and with 5 mg./kg. thereafter. During the year of treatment, 21 (65%) of the 32 patients completed the course with no other medical or surgical therapy. The roentgenographic extent of disease before therapy bore no significant relation to the success of treatment. In 11 the course was such that further therapy such as surgical excisions or changes in chemotherapy was used.

After 3 months of isoniazid therapy, two thirds of the total group had substantial x-ray improvement and three-fourths by the end of 6 months. Of the 29 patients who had demonstrable tubercle bacilli in the sputum, 23 (79%) became non-infectious, 19 during the first 3 months of therapy. Among 30 with cavities, they closed in 19. Of the 11 who required further therapy, 6 were not treatment failures in the strict sense. Four had considerable improvement before surgery was recommended and the results of surgery were excellent. Two patients did well on added chemotherapy. In only 3 was the final result unsatisfactory. These results are similar to those obtained with combined pyrazinamide-isoniazid. Drug toxicity was not observed in any patient treated with this isoniazid regimen.

Rising Incidence of Isoniazid Resistance: Its Clinical Significance. Among 322 patients, Jack Reiss and Sam M. Townsend[6] (VA Hosp., Coral Gables, Fla.) observed a 10%

(5) Am. Rev. Tuberc. 77:539-542, March, 1958.
(6) Dis. Chest 32:274-279, September, 1957.

incidence of primary resistance to isoniazid. None of the 33 patients with resistant tubercle bacilli had prior treatment with isoniazid as far as could be ascertained. Tuberculosis was far advanced in 25 and moderately advanced in 8.

Of 16 patients with newly discovered disease resistant to isoniazid, 15 became negative and the disease was arrested despite initial resistance to isoniazid. Ten of these patients received isoniazid plus streptomycin or isoniazid plus PAS, and 6 received streptomycin plus PAS. The rest of the 33 patients consisted of 17 with chronic cavitary disease. Only 8 became negative on chemotherapy, 5 showed arrested cases and 3 left the hospital against medical advice; 9 remained problems of therapy. Most patients with chronic cavitary disease require surgery at the proper time to arrest the disease.

Primary resistance to isoniazid in vitro does not necessarily indicate a poor clinical response.

Man, 30, had a history of productive cough for 1 year and fever and loss of weight for 30 days. He was acutely ill and was started on 300 mg. isoniazid daily and 1 Gm. streptomycin twice weekly. X-rays on admission revealed disease involving the entire right lung, with a 2.5 cm. cavity in the apex. The upper half of the left lung was also involved. Sputums were positive, and original culture was resistant to 5 μg. isoniazid. Sputums 1 and 2 months after start of therapy showed resistance to isoniazid and streptomycin. Sputums became negative by smear and culture 3 months after start of therapy and remained negative until 8 months later when the patient left. The final x-ray showed almost complete resolution of the pulmonary infiltrations and atelectasis of the right upper lobe. Follow-up film 3 years later showed atelectasis of the right upper lobe. He was working and had remained well.

Resistance to drugs in vitro does not necessarily indicate resistance in vivo. The period during which isoniazid remains effective in patients is still to be determined, but there seems to be a rising incidence of primary resistance to isoniazid in patients on admission to hospital. The problem of possible attenuation of isoniazid-resistant tubercle bacilli for human beings is a complex one, but this study indicates that isoniazid resistance may not have the fearful connotation connected with resistance to streptomycin and PAS.

Clinical Implications of Isoniazid Blood Levels in Pulmonary Tuberculosis are pointed out by Roger S. Mitchell and J. Carroll Bell[7] (Univ. of Colorado). The rate of metabolic alteration of isoniazid varies so in humans, the prod-

(7) New England J. Med. 257:1066-1070, Nov. 28, 1957.

ucts being without significant therapeutic value, that the free drug in the serum must be assayed after a test dose to gauge the quantity needed for treatment of a given case. Such substances as PAS compete with isoniazid for the acetylating mechanism and thus tend to increase the serum level of free drug.

Bioassay was performed at intervals after test doses of isoniazid alone or, if PAS was to be used in therapy, with the addition of a one-third the expected therapeutic dose. From a study of 226 persons, 209 of whom had active tuberculosis, the following criteria were proposed. With a test dose of 4 mg. isoniazid/kg. plus 4 Gm. PAS or 5.5 Gm. sodium PAS, a serum level of 3.2 μg. isoniazid/ml. 2 hours later and of 0.8 μg. at 6 hours indicates a slow inactivator. Patients showing 0.2 μg. or less at 6 hours are rapid inactivators. Those with levels between 0.2 and 0.8 μg. are intermediate.

When bioassay is not possible, it is suggested that at least 12 mg./kg. isoniazid daily, combined with PAS, be used. If clinical response is not satisfactory, this may be increased to 24 mg./kg. daily or more. With high dosage levels, pyridoxine must be given to avoid isoniazid neuritis.

Seven patients were observed to excrete isoniazid-susceptible tubercle bacilli after 6 months of therapy. Five of these were rapid inactivators.

Effects of Isoniazid Prophylaxis on Tuberculin Response and Local Lesion Following BCG Vaccination of Adults. Leo S. Palitz[8] (VA Hosp., Northport, N.Y.) reports that isoniazid prophylaxis in a continuous dosage of 10 mg./kg./day reduces the size of the local reaction, decreases the incidence of ulceration (with much of the effect coming between the 18th and 36th days) and significantly suppresses the level of tuberculous allergy following introduction in adult humans of an average immunizing dose of BCG vaccine. This suggests that the multiplication of living cells is altered by isoniazid prophylaxis under these conditions.

Nevertheless, 80% of the drug-treated subjects in the experiment acquired tuberculous hypersensitivity, as revealed by responses to 1 mg. tuberculin. Suppressive effects of the same order were noted when the drug was stopped at the time of BCG vaccine inoculation and restarted after 18 days.

(8) Am. Rev. Tuberc. 77:232-244, February, 1958.

In the drug-treated BCG vaccine-inoculated groups, allergy levels were maintained with relatively little loss (several actually gained allergy) following withdrawal of the drug, in contrast to the large loss of hypersensitivity in the nondrug-treated groups. It is possible that renewed multiplication of BCG cells was responsible for the individual gains in allergy. The remarkable ability of an attenuated organism such as BCG to "persist" under strong drug attack is noted.

Prolonged Blood Levels with Sustained-Action PAS. Harry L. Katz[9] (VA Hosp., Brooklyn) administered sustained-action PAS tablets to 38 patients in doses of 3 or 4 Gm. 3 times a day at 6 or 8-hour intervals. Patients who manifested symptoms of gastrointestinal irritation due to standard PAS preparations tolerated the sustained-action PAS tablets with minimal, if any, gastrointestinal side effects. Acceptance of the drug was excellent, since a 4-Gm. dose consists of only 4 tablets.

In dosage of 4 Gm. 3 times a day at 6-hour intervals, the tablets generally provided therapeutically effective blood concentrations for 24 hours. No other PAS preparation in equivalent dosage studied to date produced such sustained 24-hour PAS blood levels. It is emphasized that the sustained-action tablets should be administered every 6 hours rather than the customary 4 hours to gain the full benefit of this medication. These tablets are sodium and potassium free and therefore particularly suitable for treatment of tuberculous patients with associated cardiovascular-renal diseases.

The author lists the clinical implications and probable advantages inherent in the use of sustained-action PAS, administered concurrently with isoniazid or streptomycin. (1) Direct antimicrobial activity of PAS concentrations within tuberculous tissues is consistently maintained during the entire 24 hours each day. (2) The biologically active isoniazid blood and tissue concentrations are usually elevated, thereby enhancing the antituberculosis activity. (3) When administered concurrently with isoniazid, sustained concentrations of PAS and free isoniazid within the tuberculous lesions should potentiate their therapeutic efficacy and delay or inhibit the emergence of bacilli resistant to these drugs.

---

(9) Dis. Chest 32:626-635, December, 1957.

Hypersensitivity Reactions Associated with Sodium Para-Aminosalicylate Therapy: Four Case Reports and Review of Literature are presented by N. Matsaniotis, J. Jacobs and M. H. D. Smith[1] (New York Univ.). PAS can induce serious hypersensitivity reactions, with an incidence estimated at 2-3%. Occasionally drug fever may be the only symptoms. Most common is the appearance of both fever and rash, generally acute in onset. The height and duration of fever vary with the rate of elimination of the drug. The rash is most often maculopapular, starting from the face and extending to the neck, upper chest and extremities, but may be macular, papular, urticarial, vesicular, purpuric, frequently pruritic and of varying intensity, extent and distribution. Severe exfoliative dermatitis has occurred. Fever and rash are often accompanied by headache, chills, malaise, anorexia, conjunctivitis and generalized lymphadenopathy. Neutrophilic leukocytosis, neutropenia, eosinophilia and lymphocytosis have been reported. Jaundice is the most serious symptom associated with hypersensitivity to PAS, usually following the rash by 2-14 days. Characteristic of every hypersensitivity reaction is a certain incubation period. The earliest reaction attributed to PAS has been 8 days, the latest 73 days, but most occur between the 2d and 6th weeks.

The mechanism of hypersensitivity to PAS is poorly understood but probably is related to the aminophenol group in the para position. Desensitization, accomplished with ascending doses of PAS, has nearly always been successful. Only rarely need a patient be denied chemotherapy because of hypersensitivity, since this difficulty can generally be eliminated, usually within 3-4 weeks.

Patients or their parents should be warned to stop PAS at the onset of fever or any unusual symptom within 2 months of the start of treatment and to report immediately to their physician. Any fever during this period should be considered hypersensitivity until proved otherwise. The more severe reactions occur when PAS is continued in the presence of symptoms of hypersensitivity. Desensitization should be attempted unless specifically contraindicated.

Boy, 5, had pulmonary tuberculosis and scrofula. The neck lymph nodes were excised and treatment started with isoniazid, 20 mg./kg./

(1) Pediatrics 21:781-791, May, 1958.

24 hours, supplemented with PAS, 0.36 Gm./kg./24 hours. Within 10 days he acquired high fever, malaise, anorexia and an injected pharynx, which were treated with procaine penicillin and benzathine penicillin G. The fever seemed to decline but recurred next day with a rash which became progressively worse. The white blood cell count was 4,050 with 56% segmented neutrophils.

Within 8 hours after PAS was stopped, the rash disappeared. When PAS was reinstituted, the temperature again rose and the rash reappeared over the entire body. The white blood cell count rose to 17,200 with 92% neutrophils. Again the rash and fever subsided when PAS was discontinued. A test dose of 0.5 Gm. PAS 3 days later produced a macular rash on the legs and leukocytosis, but no fever. Desensitization was begun and successfully concluded in 16 days by starting with 5 mg. daily and gradually increasing to the full 8 Gm.

Two Cases of Methemoglobinemia and Acute Hemolytic Anemia with Death Following Ingestion of Solution of Para-Aminosalicylic Acid are reported by Francis X. Claps[2] (New York Univ.). Both patients had tuberculosis and had been receiving PAS. After ingestion of a stock solution of the drug that had been standing for some time and was black, the patients went into shock, became blue and died within 24 hours. One case is described here.

Girl, 17, had a palpable liver, enlarged axillary and inguinal nodes and multiple, small, deeply pigmented, cutaneous lesions, some crusted, scattered over the entire body. Biopsy of a skin lesion showed a granulomatous lesion, probably tuberculosis. X-ray examination of the chest was normal and cultures of gastric washings were repeatedly negative for acid-fast bacilli. Temperature was not elevated at any time. She was given isoniazid 100 mg. 3 times daily, streptomycin 1 Gm. twice a week and PAS 3 Gm. 3 times daily. One month later isoniazid was discontinued to evaluate the patient's mental status, and PAS was increased to 4 Gm. 3 times daily. Three days later PAS was given from a stock solution bottle that had been standing in the ward for an unknown period. Within 2 hours the patient was nauseated. She had vomiting and diarrhea. The temperature rose to 104.4 F. and the ventricular rate to 160. The skin became brownish, the serum chocolate colored and the urine black. The hematocrit fell to 25 mm. within 10 hours. Icterus appeared and the blood pressure slowly fell despite use of arterenol intravenously. A transfusion of 500 ml. whole blood was given, but the patient died 20 hours after receiving the PAS.

Just before death the blood nonprotein nitrogen was 43 mg. Carbon dioxide was 11 mEq./L. Chemical analysis of blood ante and post mortem revealed methemoglobin. The urine contained PAS, meta-aminophenol, salicyclic acid and a tarry black, phenolic type of material, otherwise unidentified. Autopsy showed disseminated tuberculosis regressing under chemotherapy. The single striking lesion was

(2) Am. Rev. Tuberc. 76:862-866, November, 1957.

pigment nephrosis with dark brown casts apparently representing the products of erythrocyte lysis and abnormal hemoglobin. Chemical analysis of the liver showed a tarry, phenolic substance which probably represented a degradation product of PAS or its breakdown products. A sample of the stock solution of PAS given to the patient contained 25% PAS and 75% degraded product consisting of meta-aminophenol (17%) and a tarry black, phenolic material (58%) which probably was the toxic substance.

Many reports of toxic reactions to PAS have appeared. Most have occurred in patients who received stock solutions of the drug. Solutions of PAS decompose rapidly at elevated temperatures and low pH. Light and high concentrations of carbon dioxide augment this breakdown. Solutions of PAS should be prepared at the time they are dispensed. The sodium salt would seem to be preferable, as it is much more soluble in water. If it is necessary to prepare stock solutions, they should be kept refrigerated in well-stoppered, dark bottles and not used after 5 days.

Fatal Hepatic Necrosis Associated with Aminosalicylic Acid: Review of Literature and Report of Case are made by David Paine[3] (Waltham, Mass.). The literature revealed 5 fatal PAS reactions, 3 of which were due to liver involvement. Four nonfatal cases of drug hypersensitivity hepatitis were seen; in 1 and possibly 2 of these, isoniazid was the offending drug.

Woman, 29, received chemotherapy for lung tuberculosis, including 300 mg. isoniazid and 10 Gm. sodium aminosalicylic acid daily. About 2 weeks later, she complained of headache and generalized pain in the extremities, and after another 5 days she had backache, was vomiting and had a temperature of 102 F. PAS therapy was discontinued. The eosinophil count was 8%. Two days later she became afebrile and that same day, through an error, she took 3.3 Gm. PAS after her noon meal. That afternoon the temperature rose to 103 F. and a morbilliform rash had appeared on the face, chest, abdomen and thighs. No further PAS therapy was given. The icterus index was 27 and cephalin flocculation 4+ in 48 hours. Clinical jaundice appeared a few days later and gradually deepened and she became stuporous and irrational. Despite therapy she died in about a week.

The postmortem diagnosis was acute toxic necrosis of the liver, bile necrosis, petechial hemorrhages of intestinal mucosa, gastromalacia, icterus, passive congestion of the spleen and moderately advanced active pulmonary tuberculosis.

Fever without eosinophilia or a rash may be the only symptom of a beginning PAS hypersensitivity reaction.

(3) J.A.M.A. 167:285-289, May 17, 1958

Arthralgia is another early symptom. By the time a rash has appeared and before the patient is jaundiced, irreversible and fatally progressive hepatitis may be under way. Unexplained fever in a patient taking PAS requires immediate withdrawal of the drug, which should be withheld until a hypersensitivity reaction can be ruled out. Test doses of PAS, unless minute, are dangerous.

Intoxication by Vitamin D_2 in Usual Therapeutic Doses in Case of Miliary Tuberculosis Treated by PAS is reported by R. Siegrist, W. Kaiser and K. H. Gedicke[4] (Univ. of Geneva).

Girl, 14½, received the following treatment for tuberculous meningitis: 2 Gm. dihydrostreptomycin/day intramuscularly; PAS, 10 Gm. orally and 12 Gm. intravenously; 2 infusions weekly of Bécozyme and Redoxon® intravenously, Arovit tablets (which patient said were difficult to swallow) and 2 doses of vitamin D_2 (each 600,000 units) orally 10 days apart. The meningitis was arrested, but about 5 days after the first dose of vitamin D_2, the patient had chills and later vomited after an infusion of PAS. The PAS was discontinued, but vomiting continued before and after meals and the patient lost 2-3 kg./week. It was then suspected that the symptoms were due to vitamin D, and this suspicion was confirmed by a high blood calcium level (172 and 168 mg./L.) with normal phosphorus (36 mg./L.) and slightly decreased phosphatase (2.2 Bodansky units). The urine calcium increased to 704 mg./24 hours, with phosphaturia of 530 mg. There was hyperazotemia of 0.60 Gm./L., traces of albumin and some granular casts in the urine. Polyuria was not marked and phenolsulfonphthalein tested 50%. Other biochemical blood tests showed chlorine 4 Gm./L., potassium 162 mg. and sodium 3.25 Gm., with alkalosis of 73.6 vol. %. Blood pressure increased to 140/80 and there were some changes in the ECG. The sedimentation rate increased to 40/76. Eosinophilia of 8% existed but later reached 29.5% when streptomycin was reinstated. Abdominal x-ray showed no renal calcification or bone changes. Pulmonary tubercles decreased in size. The cerebrospinal fluid 4 weeks after admission was normal, with negative cultures.

The patient received intramuscular injections of Arovit and intravenous glucose and physiologic saline. In the next 3 weeks, vomiting, thirst, constipation and signs of dehydration disappeared almost completely. The ECG, urea, chlorine and carbon dioxide values returned to normal. The urine still showed some casts and red cells. Urine calcium ranged around 300 mg./24 hours while hypercalcemia (120 mg./L.) persisted. Blood pressure was 135/80 and sedimentation rate still was rapid. The eyegrounds showed large "dysoric" foci bilaterally.

A week after the patient returned to her home, vomiting recurred. Lumbar puncture and clinical examination showed no change. Blood calcium of 138 mg./L. was accompanied by hyperazotemia of 0.52 Gm./L., hyperchloremia of 4.05 Gm. and hypokalemia of 94 mg., with

(4) Schweiz. med. Wchnschr. 88:9-13, Jan. 4, 1958.

a slight acidosis of 46.8 vol. %. Urine calcium was over 400 mg./24 hours; casts were constant, with occasional red cells. Chromatographic study showed pathologic cystinuria. Cessation of streptomycin and rehydration arrested vomiting immediately and the patient regained some weight. Then her condition began to deteriorate slowly. The urine showed red blood cells, leukocytes and colon bacilli, with occasional casts, but the culture was negative for tubercle bacilli. Two months later, an acute pyelitis with pain, chills, fever and oliguria was controlled with Terramycin®. Later the condition worsened steadily and the cerebrospinal fluid showed recurrence of tuberculous meningitis, which led to death. No autopsy was performed.

In supplementary experiments on mice, the authors showed that combined vitamin D_2 and PAS caused significant renal lesions in doses lower than toxic doses of either drug separately. With PAS alone, albuminuria of 0.7% was produced with 0.5-0.8 Gm./kg./day; with 2.5-4 Gm./kg., the albumin increased to about 2% and the urinary sediment contained leukocytes, red cells and casts. With vitamin D_2 alone, slight albuminuria was produced (0.7%) with a practically normal sediment, even when doses were increased to 5 mg.

The danger of intoxication in a tuberculous patient treated with vitamin D_2 and PAS should be kept in mind. This implies the necessity for strict observation and repeated examinations of renal function throughout treatment.

Treatment of Pulmonary Tuberculosis by Viomycin Combined with Oxytetracycline. Arnold Pines[5] (London Chest Hosp.) treated 20 patients with chronic, far-advanced, pulmonary tuberculosis. Previous treatment for a mean of 23 months with streptomycin, PAS and isoniazid had failed and in all cases high bacillary resistance had emerged. Viomycin was given as 1 Gm. twice daily 2 days a week. The dosage of oxytetracycline was 4 Gm. daily in 17 patients and 3 Gm. in 3. Because there are suggestions that isoniazid may retain some antituberculous activity despite decreased sensitivity of the bacilli, 2 patients were given 600 mg. isoniazid daily, and 12 were given 1.5-2 Gm. o-hydroxybenzal isonicotinyl hydrazone (Nupasal or Salizid®) daily. Treatment was continued at least 6 months in 16 patients.

Results were good, considering the apparently hopeless state of most of the patients. After treatment with viomycin and oxytetracycline there was striking x-ray and clinical

(5) Tubercle 38:189-193, June, 1957.

improvement in nearly half. In 4 there was cavity closure, and in 5 there was moderate to marked resolution, but "insurance operations" were performed afterward. In 5 there was little or no improvement, but operations were subsequently carried out without major incident. In 4 there was no x-ray change, in 1 there was deterioration and 1 patient died of amyloidosis.

These results are more favorable than those described by other authors, possibly because assessment has been after a much longer period of drug treatment. Whether addition of isoniazid or nupasal was helpful despite resistance is difficult to determine. In the patients whose sputum contained bacilli despite treatment, cultures continued to be fully sensitive to viomycin in all 9 tested.

In patients who have ceased to benefit from streptomycin, PAS and isoniazid, the combination of viomycin and oxytetracycline, perhaps with high doses of isoniazid or nupasal, may often be of great value. In those in whom operation may be indicated, these drugs provide good cover. Their effect is not as powerful as that of the standard drugs, and they are expensive, so they should not be given as initial treatment.

Viomycin as Operative Cover for Major Surgery for Pulmonary Tuberculosis is useful and reasonably safe, according to J. R. Edge, M. Kamiel, N. C. Scott and J. C. P. Weber[6] (Ulverston, England). Despite reports of toxic effects and of clinical response inferior to that obtained with streptomycin, patients infected with strains resistant to standard antituberculosis agents were protected by viomycin during resection (25 patients) and thoracoplasty (11 patients), as shown by absence of bronchopleural fistula in the former and of bronchogenic spread, Semb's space infection, wound infection or postoperative atelectasis in the latter. But 2 of the patients retained positive cultures in the sputum after resection and 4 after thoracoplasty.

Viomycin was given twice weekly, 1 Gm. in the morning and 1 Gm. in the evening, except in 3 patients whose dosage was reduced to 1 Gm. twice weekly because of side effects. Treatment lasted 5-61 weeks.

Some albuminuria with granular casts disappearing on

(6) Brit. J. Tuberc. 51:168-172, April, 1957.

cessation of therapy was noted, but no patient had to stop treatment because of renal disturbance. One patient had dizziness on 2 Gm. viomycin but not on 1 Gm., and no deafness was observed. There was no clinical evidence of electrolyte disturbance or liver damage. The most troublesome side effects were rash and bronchospasm with eosinophilia, which were controlled in 1 case with ACTH, permitting continuation of treatment.

The authors recommend that use of viomycin be reserved for operative cover in cases in which bacterial resistance indicates the need.

Pyrazinamide and Viomycin in Surgical Treatment of Pulmonary Tuberculosis. The proportion of patients who have tubercle bacilli resistant to streptomycin, PAS and/or isoniazid is increasing. Relatively few of these patients have had the benefit of continuous long-term antituberculous drug therapy from the time of initial chemotherapy.

When planning pulmonary resection in a patient in whom organisms were resistant to streptomycin, PAS and isoniazid, David V. Pecora[7] (Ray Brook, N.Y.) used pyrazinamide, 1 Gm. 3 times daily, and viomycin, 2 Gm. twice weekly. When the bacilli were susceptible to other drugs, these also were given. Occasionally cycloserine, oxytetracycline, thiosemicarbazone and/or a sulfone were used, but only when other drugs were not available. In 70 surgical procedures in 54 patients, best results were obtained in patients who received the multiple therapy in conjunction with effective pulmonary resection. Thoracoplasty was satisfactory for pulmonary disease and tuberculous empyema, provided surgery accomplished cavity closure or obliteration of empyema while effective drug therapy was being given. Multiple-drug therapy was beneficial postoperatively even in those in whom discharge of tubercle bacilli persisted, when there was no demonstrable operative complication or persistent pulmonary cavity.

Drug toxicity severe enough to necessitate cessation of therapy occurred in 3 patients whose bromsulfalein retention increased and in 2 in whom jaundice developed while taking pyrazinamide; 1 of these died. Viomycin was discontinued in 2 patients because of nausea and vomiting, diar-

(7) Am. Rev. Tuberc. 77:83-92, January, 1958.

rhea, erythema and dizziness. Several patients who had similar but milder symptoms tolerated the drug with little difficulty. In 1 patient, progressive hearing loss for the higher audible frequencies developed.

When pulmonary resection is planned, existing drug regimens should be replaced by 2 of the new drugs or 2 drugs to which the bacilli are known to be susceptible when (1) bacilli discharged in the sputum are known to be resistant to the existing regimen; (2) bacilli are present in the sputum and the patient has received treatment intermittently or for many months; (3) bacilli cannot be shown in the sputum, but previously organisms were shown to be resistant to the currently administered drugs; (4) discharge of bacilli in the sputum recently ceased, but the drugs had been used intermittently and the lung is greatly diseased; and (5) postoperatively, the resected specimen yields tubercle bacilli resistant to the current drug regimen, especially when much disease is present. Effective drug therapy must be combined with effective surgery.

Pyrazinamide and Cycloserine in Treatment of Pulmonary Tuberculosis. William S. Schwartz and R. E. Moyer[8] (VA Hosp., Oteen, N. C.) treated 44 patients with moderately or far advanced active pulmonary tuberculosis, previously treated unsuccessfully, with 3 Gm. pyrazinamide and 0.5 Gm. cycloserine daily for periods ranging from 12 days to 10 months or longer.

Hepatotoxicity associated with pyrazinamide occurred in 15%. There was no clear-cut instance of toxicity attributable to cycloserine. Unfortunately, it appeared that the combination of pyrazinamide and cycloserine was not superior to either cycloserine or pyrazinamide given as single drugs, when judged by roentgenographic change, reversal of infectiousness and delay in the emergence of cycloserine-resistant organisms.

Cycloserine-Isoniazid Combination Therapy in Virgin Cases of Pulmonary Tuberculosis. Cycloserine, an antibiotic produced by Streptomyces orchidaceous, is effective in vitro in higher concentrations than those obtained with isoniazid or streptomycin. It is easily absorbed into the blood and almost universally distributed in the tissues. It is effective in

(8) Am. Rev. Tuberc. 76:1097-1099, December, 1957.

previously untreated tuberculosis and is especially useful in chronic, resistant cases.

Israel G. Epstein, K. G. S. Nair, Linn J. Boyd and Paul Auspitz[9] (Metropolitan Hosp., New York) treated a series of patients with combined cycloserine 0.5 Gm. and isoniazid 0.3 Gm./day in 2 divided doses given morning and evening. In 84% fever was present, indicating the tuberculous process was severe and acute. All sputa were positive for tubercle bacilli on smear, confirmed by culture. Presumably, none of the patients had been treated with antimicrobial agents before admission.

About 40% of the x-ray films showed evidence of improvement within 6 weeks. This rose to 74% of 74 patients treated for 12 weeks and then rose to 93% of the other 48 patients within 6 months. Cough diminished and the amount as well as bacillary content of sputum decreased promptly and became less purulent. Within 3 months 80% of patients had bacteriologically negative sputa and by 6 months, 87%.

Toxic symptoms occur rarely with 0.5 Gm. cycloserine daily, whether given alone or combined with isoniazid. Doses of 1 Gm. or more daily induce central nervous system toxicity.

Results of this study, compared with previous studies of cycloserine alone and isoniazid alone, indicate an additive and possibly synergistic effect of cycloserine and isoniazid. Resistance to isoniazid when given with cycloserine developed at approximately the same rate as when isoniazid was given alone.

The combination of 0.25 Gm. cycloserine and 0.15 Gm. isoniazid twice daily was effective and safe in previously untreated pulmonary tuberculosis. Clinical results were superior to the usual isoniazid-PAS therapy in both speed and degree of response, as gauged by x-ray changes and sputum conversion.

Steroid-Treated Tuberculous Pleural Effusions. Acute tuberculous pleural effusions are treated with antibacterial drugs to reduce the risk of later tuberculous manifestations and to prevent loss of lung function and chest deformity. Attempts to hasten fluid absorption by repeated aspiration,

(9) Dis. Chest 33:371-381, April, 1958.

instillation of antibacterial drugs and physiotherapy have not always been successful.

Since pleural effusion is considered to be a by-product of the hypersensitive state, John Aspin and Helena O'Hara[1] attempted to control it by corticosteroid therapy. Of 30 patients, 16 received steroids. In each, pleural effusion had developed acutely and recently, and tuberculous etiology seemed to be beyond reasonable doubt. Peptic ulcer was excluded; weight, urine and chest films were checked weekly. Each patient was given streptomycin 1 Gm. and isoniazid 300 mg. daily, continued for at least 6 months after the steroids were stopped. Eight patients received corticotropin (ACTH), 2 cortisone, and 6 prednisone. Those treated with ACTH 40 units daily or prednisone 20 mg. daily showed dramatic clearing of even massive mediastinum-displacing effusions, without aspiration, down to the line of the 7th rib anteriorly or even farther into the costophrenic angle in 2-4 weeks. Only 1 minor loculation was left.

Of the 14 patients who had no steroids, 3 were treated by repeated aspiration, streptomycin and isoniazid and 11 were more conservatively treated. Fluid resolved to the line of the 7th rib anteriorly only after an average of 60 days, and 6 had residual loculations, 3 of considerable extent.

Steroid treatment of tuberculous pleural effusion is a real advance in management. In the year of follow-up, there was no evidence of extension of lung disease. Concomitant antibacterial therapy is indicated and should be continued after the steroids are stopped. Complications of steroid treatment can be avoided if proper precautions are taken.

Hinconstarch in Treatment of Pulmonary Tuberculosis. Hinconstarch is a polymer from periodate-oxidized potato starch by condensation with equimolar proportions of isoniazid and para-aminobenzalthiosemicarbazone. Vincent C. Barry, Noel C. Browne, Michael L. Conalty, Deirdre Waldron Edward, Brendan O'Brien and Arthur J. Walsh[2] treated 52 patients who had isoniazid-susceptible organisms and 10 who had isoniazid-resistant organisms with hinconstarch. The drug was administered orally, initially in gelatin capsules of 100 or 200 mg. or in tablets of 250 mg. Doses

(1) Brit. J. Tuberc. 52:81-84, January, 1958.
(2) Am. Rev. Tuberc. 77:952-967, June, 1958.

ranged from 0.5 to 4 Gm. daily if they were well tolerated.

Moderate or marked x-ray improvement was observed in 65% of patients at 3 months and 80% at 6 months, and the percentage increased with duration of therapy. In 55% cavities closed without resort to surgery. Tubercle bacilli disappeared from the sputum in 85% of the patients. In only 3 did hinconstarch have to be discontinued because of nausea and vomiting, though these symptoms appeared in 13 patients. Some found that by emptying the capsules onto food, discomfort was alleviated. Six patients had elevated serum bilirubin, 5 abnormal liver function tests and 3 disturbed renal function. Minor urticarial rashes appeared in 2 patients, which responded to an antihistamine cream or suspension of therapy.

Apparently a dose of 40-45 mg./kg. hinconstarch daily gives an adequate therapeutic effect without toxicity. Doses substantially larger than this may result in gastrointestinal or renal toxicity. If this agent were used first, it would leave other combinations of therapy such as streptomycin and PAS as effective alternatives should they be necessary.

Tuberculosis of Endometrium: Report on 250 Cases with Results of Drug Treatment. Genital tuberculosis is being recognized with increasing frequency, due partly to routine endometrial biopsy or diagnostic curettage in patients with infertility, irregular uterine bleeding and/or amenorrhea. The incidence among 5,521 curettages was 1.1% and among 864 uterine specimens examined histologically 1.4%. Among 65,943 patients admitted to a hospital for women, genital tuberculosis was proved in 0.56%, and in 3,804 admitted for investigation of primary infertility, the incidence was 5.6%. In 1,000 patients with functional endometrial bleeding, tuberculosis of the endometrium was found in 1%. In 200 women aged 20 years or less, endometrial tuberculosis was found in 4%. In 1,000 cases of abnormal uterine bleeding occurring in gross pelvic disease, the incidence was 0.9%, whereas in postmenopausal bleeding, the incidence was only 0.1%. Arthur M. Sutherland[3] (Glasgow) reviewed 250 cases of endometrial tuberculosis investigated during the last 7 years. Patients were aged 16-53 (average 28) years.

Infertility was the commonest symptom. Pain was fre-

(3) Obst. & Gynec. 11:527-536, May, 1958.

quent, varying in character and degree, but situated in the lower abdomen. The next symptoms in order of frequency were abnormal uterine bleeding and vaginal discharge. Pelvic examination revealed adnexal swelling in 120 patients, retroversion of the uterus in 32, erosion of the cervix in 27, cystic enlargement of one ovary in 7, uterine fibroids in 3, pyometra in 1 and no palpable abnormality in 85. Tubal insufflation was performed in 92 patients and the tubes were found to be blocked in 61.

Bacteriologic proof, sought in 229 patients, was found in 170. The endometrial system was injected into guinea pigs and inoculated into culture mediums. Routine vaginal swabs rarely established diagnosis and are not justifiable. Patients should be treated on the basis of the endometrial histology, without awaiting bacteriologic results.

Patients were treated almost always as outpatients, except for a few who had pelvic spread following initial curettage. These were admitted to hospital as emergency cases. Most were ambulant throughout treatment, and many continued their jobs. The recommended dosage schedule was streptomycin 1 Gm. daily and PAS 20 Gm. daily. Endometrial biopsies showed 102 patients were well at an average follow-up of 25 months and 32 had recurrence an average of 25 months after treatment was started. In 69 other patients, the medication was 1 Gm. streptomycin daily combined with isoniazid twice daily over the same period. After an average follow-up of 16 months, 59 were well. Nineteen patients received 12 Gm. PAS and 200 mg. isoniazid daily, but follow-up has not been long enough to allow evaluation.

Toxic drug reactions occurred in 35 patients (14%), most often streptomycin-induced vestibular disturbances or skin rashes. In 11 toxicity was due to PAS, usually manifested as gastrointestinal disturbance.

Pain, abnormal bleeding or amenorrhea were satisfactorily ameliorated in most patients. However, the most frequent symptom, infertility, was rarely benefited. Only 1 patient had a full-term pregnancy after treatment. Two had spontaneous abortions and 2 had ruptured tubal pregnancies.

It is not justifiable to withhold treatment from any patient with proved endometrial tuberculosis. If therapy is withheld, such patients will stay infected with active tubercle bacilli. A considerable number will show clinical deterioration within a year and require immediate treatment. Most patients treated will remain well and most are cured of principal symptoms.

Iproniazid as Adjunct in Treatment of Debilitated Patients with Tuberculosis is reported by Alfred S. Dooneief and George E. Crane[4] (Montefiore Hosp., New York). Twenty patients already on chemotherapy for tuberculosis received iproniazid [Marsilid®] in doses of 25-200 mg. daily. An average weight gain of almost 20 lb. was noted in 14 treated for 2 months to over 1 year; 6 treated under 2 months failed to gain weight. Significant relief from symptoms and improvement in general condition were noted in 13. A feeling of well-being, excessive appetite, marked increase in vitality and decrease in sleep requirements were the outstanding features of the typical reaction to iproniazid.

Although all patients received a psychiatric examination before administration of the drug to eliminate poor risks, there were severe psychotic reactions in 3. Some patients with emotional disturbances before treatment showed psychic improvement while taking iproniazid. Because of this, 13 patients with clear-cut psychiatric symptomatology were treated with this drug. In 5 there was intensification of the psychopathology. All others showed general improvement, which was especially marked in 3 with phobic neuroses.

Drug toxicity of a physical character was present to some degree in every patient. The commonest manifestations of toxicity were hypermotility (13), insomnia (9), dizziness (7), constipation (6), hypotension (4) and muscular rigidity and twitching (4). Tremor, paresthesia, urinary frequency, headache and anorexia were observed in 2 each and edema, palpitation, weakness, peripheral neuropathy, impotence and abdominal pain in 1 each. When side effects were severe, they tended to become progressively worse even when dosage was reduced, but all cleared in a few days when treatment was discontinued. All patients receiving 200 mg. iproniazid/day had serious side effects; 6 patients could not tolerate 100 mg./day and 1 had severe symptoms with only 25 mg./day. Eleven were able to take a maintenance dose

(4) New York J. Med. 57:3477-3480, Nov. 1, 1957.

of 100-150 mg./day, and this was continued for over 2 years in 2.

Iproniazid in carefully regulated dosage under close medical and psychiatric control is of value as adjunctive treatment in severely debilitated patients with advanced tuberculosis. It may also be useful in management of certain psychiatric conditions, notably severe anxiety states with acute phobic manifestations. This potent drug has many side effects, and its administration, except in hospitals or under supervision of a psychiatrist familiar with its use, is not recommended.

► [There are other articles dealing with this drug in the section on Neuropsychiatric Disorders.—Ed.]

KIDNEY DISORDERS

Survival in Group of Steroid-Treated Nephrotic Children: Preliminary Report of 79 children seen during 1953-57 is presented by Edmund C. Burke.[5] After diagnosis was made, treatment was started in the hospital, with 150 mg. corticotropin/sq. m./day for 8-10 days. Extra potassium chloride, 1 Gm./day, was given orally and penicillin or tetracycline was given in prophylactic or therapeutic doses. The diet was low in sodium. Treatment was then continued at home.

In nearly all instances proteinuria was absent at the end of treatment when diuresis occurred. Diuresis was obtained in approximately 85% of the children treated, 2-6 days after corticotropin was stopped. Occasionally, if diuresis had not occurred, paracentesis was performed and usually this was attended by increased urinary output. Hypertension, convulsions or azotemia did not occur to the degree that corticotropin had to be interrupted.

After patients were discharged from the hospital, they were given 100 mg. cortisone daily on 3 successive days/week for 6 weeks or longer if albuminuria persisted. Prednisone, 5 mg. 4 times daily, could be substituted for cortisone. When albuminuria returned, steroids were begun again until

(5) Proc. Staff Meet. Mayo Clin. 33:12-18, Jan. 8, 1958.

several urinalyses were normal in 4 or more weeks. Penicillin was given orally, 100,000-200,000 units daily by mouth, indefinitely.

Of 61 patients in whom adequate follow-up was available, 7 to 55 months after the initial treatment, 13 had died, 26 had neither albuminuria nor edema, 17 had no edema but some albuminuria and 5 had both edema and albuminuria. Thus 21% had died, 71% were in clinical remission and 8% in clinical exacerbation. A group of 47 patients were available for follow-up twice, 18 months apart, 19 to 55 months after the initial treatment. It was found that the mortality had risen from 15 to 31%, the percentage in remission remained about equal (64 and 62%), whereas the percentage in exacerbation had fallen from 23 to 5%. The rise in percentage mortality emphasizes the need for greater intervals if evaluation of survival is to be accurate. A statistically significant study of the efficacy of steroid treatment in the nephrotic syndrome must await a 20-year follow-up.

Children are not dying of infections but of progressive renal failure. Duration of life and reduced mortality suggest that steroids are improving the outlook for recovery. Despite intensive treatment with antibiotics and steroids and close medical supervision, some children progress to chronic renal failure and death. The specific factors which determine which children will progress and which will recover remain unknown. Intensive and prolonged intermittent treatment with steroids and antibiotics now seems to be the treatment of choice for the nephrotic syndrome.

► [In their study last year, K. Lange *et al.* (1957-58 Year Book, p. 284) found that when cortisone was given in 3 successive days of each week for 1 year after initial diuresis, the mortality in the 24 cases observed was reduced from the expected 5.6 deaths to 1 death.

Several points in prognosis under ACTH therapy are brought out in the following article.—Ed.]

Nephrotic Syndrome: Observations of Effects of ACTH in 40 Patients led Dorothy Charlton, A. L. Latner, J. W. Platt, G. A. Smart, R. B. Thompson and W. Walker[6] to consider ACTH valuable in patients free from proteinuria during treatment. Those studied, and followed for 7 months to 4 years, had generalized edema, proteinuria, low serum protein and high serum cholesterol but no chronic venous con-

(6) Acta med. scandinav. 161:33-56, 1958.

gestion, liver disease, severe hypertension or gross nitrogen retention. They were on a high protein diet, with less than 0.5 Gm. sodium/day for a control period, and some were given potassium chloride. Intramuscular injections of 25 I.U. of ACTH at 6-hour intervals or 40 I.U. of ACTH gel twice daily were given to adults, with smaller doses for children.

Response to ACTH was accompanied at first by water retention and increased edema, which was minimized by restricting salt intake. In some patients urinary protein output also rose. Later, diuresis and a reduction in urinary protein occurred. Body weight decreased to the point of emaciation, but increased appetite soon restored weight loss without edema. During therapy the eosinophil count fell to zero. Electrolyte changes and creatinine clearance corresponded to changes described by other investigators.

Diuresis occurred in 83% and proteinuria was relieved in 36.5% of patients. Two died, possibly as a result of therapy, 1 of whom definitely had symptoms of potassium intoxication. Six patients failed to respond to ACTH, and 2 of these died of uremia.

Relief of edema is appreciated by the patients and may permit some rehabilitation, although it may be minor in terms of cure. Prognosis is best for patients who respond to ACTH without subsequent residual proteinuria. Response to ACTH is accompanied by a rise in serum albumin and a fall in $alpha_2$ globulin. Most patients with the nephrotic syndrome display an elevated systolic pressure, and their response to ACTH seems to be inversely related to the degree of elevation.

Diuretics and Renal Disease. According to George E. Schreiner[7] (Georgetown Univ.), use of diuretics in renal disease involves many special considerations and requires a broad understanding of the physiologic mechanisms involved. Fluid retention in the nephrotic patient may defy any tubular blockade. Low filtration rates and hyponatremia may so reduce the filtered load of salt that blocking drugs become impotent. Fixed blood vessels may defy vasodilatation. Metabolic acidosis and hypoalbuminemia may completely negate otherwise effective drugs. The mildly uremic

(7) M. Ann. District of Columbia 26:623-632, December, 1957.

patient may present serious drug reactions or intolerance to regimens that are clinically successful in the cardiac or cirrhotic patient.

For purposes of diuresis, renal diseases may be divided into: (1) salt retention without gross impairment of glomerular filtration rate, as in nephrotic syndrome, membranous glomerulonephritis, mild pre-eclampsia and aldosteronism; (2) salt retention with moderate impairment of glomerular filtration, as in severe pre-eclampsia, nephrotic stage of subacute and chronic glomerulonephritis, amyloidosis, Kimmelstiel-Wilson disease, pyelonephritis, acute glomerulonephritis and lupus nephritis; (3) marked reduction of glomerular filtration, with or without clinical edema (often a function of diet), where increased urine flow may enhance the urea clearance and reduce azotemia, may aid in control of hypertension and may help in defense against secondary infection, as in chronic pyelonephritis, chronic glomerulonephritis and severe nephrosclerosis; and (4) special conditions such as polycystic disease and uric acid obstruction.

Schreiner presents 5 cases illustrating some problems of diuresis in renal disease, with particular emphasis on a new blocking agent, chlorothiazide (Diuril®), which may offer particular advantage in certain types of renal disease.

Case 1.—Girl, aged 15 months, had periorbital edema, oliguria, hematuria, reversal in albumin-globulin ratio, hypoalbuminemia, hypercholesteremia and urine and throat cultures positive for beta hemolytic streptococcus. There was no improvement after treatment with penicillin, chloramphenicol, diuretics and Meticorten®. Anasarca became massive. Blood pressure rose precipitously after administration of 2 units of albumin. She was placed on a salt-free glucose intake and given ACTH, 60 units daily. After treatment with chlorothiazide, 200 mg. daily for 4 days, potassium excretion rose, but there was no significant increase in sodium or urine volume. She was then given 2 units of albumin, which raised the serum concentration to 2 Gm., and a prompt diuresis ensued. Weight loss was equal to 45% of admission weight.

This case illustrates an instance of nephrotic syndrome in acute glomerulonephritis in which steroids alone, albumin alone, chlorothiazide alone and other measures failed to control progressive anasarca. However, with steroid preparation, elevation of serum albumin above 1.5 Gm. and chlorothiazide therapy, a prompt and massive diuresis ensued.

Case 2.—Man, 49, had progressive anasarca for 6 months. Examination showed 3+ edema of ankles, 1-2+ edema of the skin up to the midthoracic region, bilateral pleural effusion, ascites and a midline scar from a paracentesis 1 week before admission. Urinalysis showed albuminuria, hematuria, pyuria, cylindruria, oval fat bodies, fatty, waxy casts and renal tubular epithelial cells. Quantitative protein excretion ws 4.2 Gm./24 hours, and the Addis count was markedly abnormal in red blood cells, casts and white blood cells. Blood urea nitrogen was 16 mg. and total protein 3.2 Gm., with 1 Gm. albumin and 2.2 Gm. globulin. Diagnostic renal biopsy showed a membranous glomerulonephritis. The patient lost 8 lb. on bed rest and salt restriction alone. He then lost 20 lb. during 6 days on chlorothiazide. He received no steroids during diuresis but was placed on 80 mg. Meticorten daily as maintenance therapy after discharge. On high steroid dosage, the protein in the urine fell progressively.

This case is an excellent example of a marked diuretic response to chlorothiazide in a nephrotic patient with membranous glomerulonephritis and a good filtration rate who received no steroid therapy.

Case 3.—Woman, 45, had nephrotic syndrome due to amyloidosis. Onset was 2 years previously. Maintenance with a wide variety of diuretic regimens, including acidifying salts, plasma expanders and carbonic anhydrase inhibitors, had been unsuccessful. In the presence of a reduced filtration rate and a serum albumin concentration of 1 Gm., no significant diuresis could be achieved with chlorothiazide, although the chloride concentration in the urine was significantly elevated by the drug. However, with elevation of the glomerular filtration rate by adrenal steroids and expansion of plasma volume by injection of albumin, a massive diuresis was obtained and the patient could then be maintained satisfactorily on intermittent chlorothiazide therapy without signs of interim toxicity.

Case 4.—Man, 44, had recurrent abdominal pain, sudden sharp pains in the left kidney region, severe fatigue and recurrent chills. An intravenous pyelogram showed the infundibula of the right calyces to be elongated, and some of the calyces were dilated and deformed. There were multiple cystic deformities of the left kidney. Blood pressure was 170/120 and blood urea nitrogen 31 mg. Apresoline® reduced the blood pressure slightly. Chlorothiazide was then given, 0.5 Gm. every 12 hours 2 days a week. Average weight loss was 2-4 lb. on the diuretic day, with regain of weight in the interval. Headaches and abdominal pain disappeared. Two months later chlorothiazide was given 3 days a week. The patient remained asymptomatic and felt better than he had for years.

Case 5.—Man, 41, with a 7-year history of polycystic disease, had moderate hypertension, albuminuria, hyaline-granular casts, a urea nitrogen level of 34 mg. and phenolsulfonphthalein excretion of 6% in 15 minutes and 25% in 1 hour. He complained of abdominal pain and excessive fatigue. He was placed on an interrupted schedule of 1.5 Gm. chlorothiazide daily, at 2-day intervals. A weight loss of 1-3 lb., with reaccumulation, occurred regularly, but the patient had complete relief from symptoms. When the drug was stopped for 10 days there was an edema accumulation of 8 lb. and symptoms recurred. On reinstitution of chlorothiazide, the patient lost 7 lb. in 4 days and had complete relief from symptoms.

This case illustrates the effective control of symptoms by the intermittent use of chlorothiazide in a patient with proved polycystic disease.

Successful Treatment of Recurrent Uric Acid Renal Calculi with Probenecid (Benemid®) is reported by Arthur Bernstein, David Bronsky and Alvin Dubin[8] (Univ. of Illinois). Uric acid stones comprise 4-6% of all renal calculi. Treatment by surgical and dietary measures, by alkalinization of the urine and with salicylates has not been satisfactory. Such stones occur frequently in patients with gout. Probenecid, a potent uricosuric agent, may reverse the clinical course of gout. It may also be highly effective in treatment of recurrent uric acid stones in patients without symptomatic gout.

Man, 64, weighing 290 lb., had had recurrent kidney stones for 18 years. He had been well until age 46, when he had left lumbar pain with lancinating radiation to the groin. After 48 hours the pain subsided, and on micturition he passed a dark brown, pinhead-sized calculus. Six months later he observed another stone, and subsequently he continued to pass 1-3 similar stones/month. By age 61, the stones had become noticeably larger and more difficult to pass. Whereas previously they seldom exceeded pea size, they now were often ¼ in. in diameter and frequently star-shaped. Occasionally they would lodge in the urethra and have to be milked out or extracted through the meatus with a forceps. Hematuria sometimes accompanied passage of these large stones. At age 63, he had begun to pass gravel, i.e., 20 or more pinhead- to pea-sized stones during one micturition. These episodes occurred on the average of once or twice a month. Frequency of passage of large stones fell slightly. As at the onset, each passage of a stone or gravel was preceded by 48-72 hours of right or left lumbar pain with radiation to the groin. Episodes were unaccompanied by chills or fever. The patient denied ever having had joint pain, and there was no family history of renal calculi or gout. Throughout his illness he sought medical advice frequently. Therapeutic trials of low-purine diets, alkalinization of the urine, forced fluid intake and use of salicylates were consistently ineffective. In time he became inured to pain and seldom required analgesics.

The blood pressure was 154/120 mm. Hg. There were no tophi or joint deformities. The calculi consisted of pure uric acid crystals. Blood nonprotein nitrogen was normal and blood uric acid 8.3 mg./100 cc.

(8) Ann. Int. Med. 49:203-207, July, 1958.

An intravenous pyelogram revealed normal-appearing kidneys, ureters and bladder. Calculi were not visualized.

The patient was placed on 1.5 Gm. Benemid daily, and a low-calorie diet. An immediate effect was observed. Passage of large stones stopped at once. Gravel turned to sand, i.e., occasional passage of about ¼ teaspoonful of minute stones. The sand appeared intermittently at less frequent intervals for 29 months and then stopped. Small single stones were also passed less often and after 29 months stopped appearing. The patient has passed no stones of any type now for 5 months. The episodes of lumbar pain have been relieved. He has lost 30 lb. and blood pressure is normal.

Primary Chronic Interstitial Nephritis: Clinical, Experimental and Etiologic Investigation by O. Gsell, H. K. von Rechenberg and P. Miescher[9] (Univ. of Basel) suggests that phenacetin compounds play an important role in its pathogenesis. Of 28 patients (22 women) with chronic primary nonhypertensive, acidotic renal insufficiency observed during the past 2 years, 22 (80%) were habitual users of phenacetin analgesics, taking an average of 7.2 tablets daily, corresponding to 1.8 Gm. phenacetin, with an average total consumption to the time of clinical diagnosis of 37,000 tablets/patient or 1 kg. phenacetin.

Systematic questioning of all medical patients regarding use of phenacetin compounds revealed 33 who had consumed large quantities for years. These were divided into three groups after determination of erythrocyte survival: in 7, there was no evidence of clinical damage (average total consumption 21,000 tablets); in 9 with a shortened erythrocyte survival (20 days), the total average consumption was 35,500 tablets; in 17 with an erythrocyte survival of 18.5 days and signs of chronic acidotic renal insufficiency, phenacetin consumption had averaged 37,000 tablets.

In the 1st stage, represented by group 1, there were no clinical symptoms. In group 2, there was no basis for a diagnosis of renal insufficiency. Urinalyses and blood chemistry were normal. The erythrocyte count was 3,500,000-4,000,000 in 5 patients and over 4,000,000 in 4. In 4 of 7, the reticulocyte count was over 15%. In 1, there was a decreased alkaline reserve (43 vol.% CO_2). In 7 in whom renal function tests were performed, the phenolsulfonphthalein excretion was normal, but creatinine clearance was below normal in 3 and definitely pathologic (30 cc./minute in 1.) In group 3, the

(9) Deutsche med. Wchnschr. 82:1718-1726, Oct. 4, 1957.

clinical picture of renal tubular deficiency was well defined, with normochromic anemia, polyuria, hyposthenuria, azotemia and acidosis. Electrolyte imbalance was often observed but blood pressure increased only in terminal stages with total renal failure.

From clinical and experimental investigations, it appears likely that the toxicity of phenacetin is dependent on metabolic side products, e.g., paraphenetidin, which in animals had a much stronger effect on the erythrocytes than phenacetin. Two possible mechanisms of renal damage are (1) through a direct effect of substances like paraphenetidin on the kidney or (2) through the chronic precipitation of pathologic hemoglobin by the kidney. It seems highly probable that the toxic effect of phenacetin depends also on the presence of some other factors which potentiate the pathologic processes.

► [It seems to me that the evidence of a true causal relationship of phenacetin ingestion with the nephropathy in this series of cases is slim, but I have selected the article to emphasize the *possibility* that chronic use of familiar drugs is responsible for pathologic states in instances in which such an association is not frequently suspected.—Ed.]

LIVER DISORDERS

Effect of Cortisone and Hydrocortisone on Hepatic Coma. Leslie T. Webster, Jr., and Charles S. Davidson[1] (Harvard Med. School) gave large doses of cortisone or hydrocortisone to 7 alcoholics with hepatic cirrhosis and coma or impending coma. Four showed definite improvement within 12-48 hours, but relapsed within 4-10 days; 2 relapsed while still receiving steroid and 2 relapsed 3-6 days afterward. Subsequently, the last 2 patients received another course of steroid without improvement. Three showed no change or became worse. Of those who responded temporarily, 2 were in coma and 2 in impending coma when steroid was started. Of those who did not respond, including the 2 who received second courses of steroid, 3 were in coma and 2 in impending coma.

The temporary clinical improvement observed is presumed to have resulted from steroid administration, because ste-

(1) Gastroenterology 33:225-235, August, 1957.

roid was given when confusion or coma was stabilized or progressive, and clinical improvement, if it occurred, was always seen within 24 hours after initiation of treatment. Other medications lacked this time relation.

Response was observed in active and relatively inactive types of cirrhosis. Of those who improved, 2 patients had active liver disease characterized by a high serum bilirubin concentration and 2 others had relatively inactive disease with marked ascites and near-normal serum bilirubin concentrations. Depth of coma seemed to bear little relation to response. The initial dose was high (240 mg. hydrocortisone in 24 hours was the lowest) in all who improved, and seemed to be more important than the duration of steroid therapy. The mechanism of temporary favorable response to steroids is obscure.

All patients who improved had normal urine outputs before steroid initiation. Of those who did not improve, 2 of 5 were oliguric and 2 others were thought to be, though their urine volumes were not measured. Side effects of steroid treatment included changes in affect (usually euphoria) in 4 patients and appearance of moon facies in 1. The main complication, probably aggravated by steroids, which occurred in 3 patients during therapy, was infection.

The authors emphasize, as others have, that use of large quantities of steroids in hepatic coma, as in other conditions, is hazardous. Though these compounds did not reduce the mortality in the present group with hepatic coma, they might prove of permanent benefit if given early to patients who have sufficient hepatic reserve to survive after temporary improvement.

► [T. Pessar and J. W. Hessing (Ann. Int. Med. 48:1254, 1958) treated 6 comatose patients massively with cortisone; with the exception of 1 patient, inadequately treated, all came out of coma dramatically and quickly but all 6 died of various complications of cirrhosis, including coma.—Ed.]

Chlorothiazide in Control of Ascites in Hepatic Cirrhosis was studied by A. E. Read, R. M. Haslam, J. Laidlaw and Sheila Sherlock[2] (Postgrad. Med. School, London). Chlorothiazide was given orally, 2 Gm./day, in 15 courses to 13 patients with Laennec's cirrhosis complicated by ascites and peripheral edema (12 patients) or gross peripheral edema alone.

(2) Brit. M. J. 1:963-966, Apr. 26, 1958.

On 9 of the 15 occasions, the diuretic response to chlorothiazide was good. Patients lost at least 2 kg., and urinary sodium output increased by more than 39 mEq. In the other 6 instances, the response was poor; weight showed no change and, with 1 exception, the urinary sodium output little or no increase. In all patients, chlorothiazide resulted in a twofold to threefold increase in urinary potassium output, associated with a fall in serum potassium in every patient not receiving potassium supplements.

Anions excreted consisted mainly of chloride, but there was a considerable deficit between total urinary cations and chloride output. In 2 control and 2 cirrhotic patients, chlorothiazide caused a rise in urinary pH with a fivefold increase in bicarbonate excretion. These results suggest that chlorothiazide acted not only as a chloruretic (mercurial-like action) but also as a carbonic anhydrase inhibitor. The increase in bicarbonate and potassium loss resembled the action of the carbonic anhydrase inhibitor, acetazolamide. Potassium supplements (78-250 mEq./24 hours) were given 6 times. On 4 occasions, this proved insufficient to balance the urinary loss and serum potassium values fell. The other 2 patients showed a poor diuretic response to the drug.

Hepatic precoma and coma were noted in 7 of the 13 inpatients. It was usually associated with a good and rapid diuretic response to chlorothiazide. Deep coma after only 2 days' therapy developed in 2 patients.

Man, 47, an alcoholic with cirrhosis, was hospitalized for assessment of portacaval anastomosis following hemorrhage from esophageal varices. He had had previous hepatic precoma. Chlorothiazide resulted in a massive diuresis; 5 kg. was lost in 2 days. However, within 24 hours of start of the drug, fetor and tremor returned and the EEG showed slowing. The next day he passed into deep coma, regaining consciousness only after 36 hours.

Four outpatients were treated for longer periods with intermittent chlorothiazide and continuous potassium supplements. Neuropsychiatric changes were not seen, but 2 patients became refractory to the drug. Continuous chlorothiazide therapy should not be given to cirrhotic patients outside the hospital. Potassium chloride (3-6 Gm. daily) should be given to all patients with cirrhosis receiving the drug. Particular care should be taken in patients with a previous history of neuropsychiatric complications of liver disease.

► [There are, of course, more articles dealing with this drug in the sections on congestive heart failure and hypertension.—Ed.]

Antibiotic Therapy in Management of Hepatic Coma. Development of hepatic stupor with increased protein intake and its response to several antibiotics were studied in 2 patients during repeated episodes of stupor and recovery. Bernard B. Fast, Stanley J. Wolfe, James M. Stormont and Charles S. Davidson[3] (Boston) found that arterial blood ammonia concentrations tended to parallel the clinical state, but the relationship was inconstant. Of 9 patients with hepatic coma associated with hepatic failure and/or massive gastrointestinal hemorrhage treated with a regimen designed to reduce absorption of toxic nitrogenous metabolites, including oral antibiotics, protein restriction, enemas and purges, 7 improved but only 3 recovered.

The oral antibiotics used, especially neomycin and paromomycin, were effective therapy for hepatic coma, unless some liver failure or massive uncontrolled gastrointestinal bleeding was underlying, when outcome often was fatal. In hepatic coma associated with hepatic failure, antibiotics are recommended; they allow administration of protein, which may be essential to liver cell recovery.

► [The matter involved here is that a major source of ammonia—which is highly toxic as a blood constituent but quickly detoxified by the normal liver—is the intestinal tract in which it appears as a byproduct of bacterial enzymatic action on nitrogenous compounds. Antibiotics which act on these intestinal organisms reduce the production and hence the absorption of intestinal ammonia; the subfunctioning cirrhotic liver is thus spared a part of its work load.—Ed.]

Treatment of Ascitic Atrophic Cirrhosis of Liver with High Dosages of Testosterone Propionate results in clinical cure in a large percentage of cases, according to Mario Girolami[4] (Univ. of Rome), who treated 50 patients (28 men), aged 33-75, each of whom had ascites. Some had advanced disease and were in poor condition. Most had atrophic (Laennec's) cirrhosis, 2 had Banti's disease, a few Wilson's disease and some had pigmentary cirrhosis.

Testosterone propionate was given intramuscularly, 100 mg. daily for 12 days, then reduced to every other day for another 12 days. The courses were repeated if required. Oth-

(3) A.M.A. Arch. Int. Med. 101:467-475, February, 1958.
(4) J. Am. Geriatrics Soc. 6:306-323, April, 1958.

er therapy was given or continued as indicated, such as diuretics, paracenteses, vitamins, insulin and glucose. Any intercurrent infection was treated promptly. If liver insufficiency supervened, glutamic acid or nicotinic acid amide was given intravenously in isotonic or hypertonic glucose solution.

Despite severity of the disease in these patients, symptoms completely disappeared in 30. Best results were obtained in those whose symptoms had recently appeared and who had paracenteses only a few times. Patients who improved and remained well have been followed for up to 6 years. Those who did not benefit from testosterone had far-advanced and severe cirrhosis or concomitant unfavorable conditions, such as heart disease and syphilis.

Man, 62, with cirrhosis of the liver and syphilitic aortitis was in poor condition with dyspnea, edema, hydrothorax, tense ascites and venous collateral circulation. He received 100 mg. testosterone propionate daily for 40 days, amino acids, penicillin, glucose solution, vitamins and cardiotonic and diuretic substances. At first he had weekly paracenteses, but later the interval could be lengthened. Pleural fluid was spontaneously reabsorbed during the first 10 days. Six months later he was discharged in fair condition without edema, ascites or visible superficial venous circulation.

He was well for the next 2 years, then he died of carcinoma of the lung. At autopsy the liver showed no gross signs of cirrhosis. Histologically, changes of Laennec's cirrhosis were found, but in modified form with the connective tissue relaxed and rich in fibroblasts, indicating that it had been converted from a fibrocytic to a fibroblastic connective tissue.

Testosterone therapy must be started early to get best results, preferably before ascites develops. The dose must be at least 100 mg. daily. Small doses and intermittent therapy are ineffective. Treatment must be continuous and prolonged, because improvement may occur only after several months of testosterone administration. It should be continued for several months after clinical cure. After signs of cirrhosis have disappeared, 1-2 injections/week should be continued. Appropriate concomitant treatment should be given for cardiovascular disease.

► [In all instances in which testosterone has, or is alleged to have, some efficacy in therapy on any basis other than that of true replacement of the missing hormone, it is probable that the action is purely anabolic, i.e., the protein store is recruited. The Italian group around the present author have been reporting their use of the agent in treating hepatic cirrhosis since 1953, but to my knowledge this is the first of the articles to appear in an American Journal. I saw the article in *Minerva medica* (47:411, Feb. 11, 1956), and am now wondering whether I should have been more impressed. At any rate, a thorough trial with adequate controls could easily be made and it would seem that this should be done.—Ed.]

NEOPLASTIC DISEASES

Triethylene Thiophosphoramide (Thio-TEPA) in Treatment of Neoplastic Disease involves toxicity hazards outweighing therapeutic value except for ovarian cancer, in the experience of John E. Ultmann, George A. Hyman, Charles Crandall, Horst Naujoks and Alfred Gellhorn[5] (Columbia Univ.). N-N′-N″-triethylene thiophosphoramide, variously referred to as TSPA, S-TEPA or thio-TEPA, was administered in 109 courses to 100 patients with biopsy-proved neoplasms, including Hodgkin's disease, lymphosarcoma, carcinoma and malignant melanoma.

A 1% solution, sterilized by filtration, was used full strength for intramuscular injections or diluted with saline to provide 5 or 10 mg. in about 5 ml. for the intravenous route. Dosage varied widely according to diagnosis, previous therapy and hemopoietic function, ranging from 3.5 to 20 mg./day intravenously (91 patients) or larger single doses in a few intracavitary injections. The authors favor systemic administration with a view to controlling malignant cells wherever they may be.

Measurable improvement was observed in only 32 patients and striking improvement in only 7. Hodgkin's disease, reticulum cell sarcoma and ovarian carcinoma were the only conditions that showed any response to the drug. Of 27 patients with advanced ovarian carcinoma, 13 had observable regression, as demonstrated by decrease of abdominal masses and resolution of ascites and pleural effusions. The duration of remission was 6 weeks to 10 months at the time of writing.

Thio-TEPA caused no local reaction intramuscularly, nor were local or general toxic effects observed when it was injected intravenously or into a serous cavity. In the 109 courses of injection, hematologic depression occurred in 47 patients, the platelets dropping below 75,000/cu. mm. in 14,

(5) Cancer 10:902-911, Sept., Oct., 1957.

white blood cell counts below 2,000 in 5 and both being decreased in 28. Thrombocytopenia was more frequent, appeared later and persisted longer than leukopenia. Clinical manifestations, including purpura, ecchymoses, gastrointestinal bleeding, genitourinary bleeding, pneumonia, infection and liver abscess, were observed in 17 of the 47. Toxicity was a major factor in the death of 2 patients in whom initially high uric acid levels rose higher during treatment. Judgment of safe dosage was difficult, because the hemopoietic depression was often delayed. In general, the least tolerant were patients with prior radio- or chemotherapy or with a poor initial hematologic status.

► [Despite the feeling of these authors that toxicity outweighs therapeutic achievement in all types of malignancy except ovarian cancer, there is record in the two following articles of apparently five results in both disseminated melanoma and metastatic cerebral malignancy.—Ed.]

Triethylene Phosphoramide in Treatment of Disseminated Melanoma. The effects of administering triethylene phosphoramide (TEPA) and a related sulfur compound (thio-TEPA) were studied in 13 of 15 patients treated for malignant melanomas by James L. Tullis[6] (Harvard Med. School). The distinguishing clinical features were diversity of presenting symptoms, including central nervous system disease, rapidity of death after metastasis to abdominal and thoracic organs and a high incidence of reddish complexion among the patients or their immediate relatives. The drugs were given intravenously or orally in doses sufficient to decrease the leukocyte or platelet count.

Of the 13 patients, 9 were unimproved and 4 improved (table). All 9 unimproved patients died 6 days to 5 months after institution of therapy. Of the 4 improved patients, 2 died. One died after 13 months of complete resolution of metastases and outwardly normal health. The average duration of life of the 4 improved patients (at the time of writing) has been 16 months, the intervals ranging from 5 to 30 months after treatment was begun.

The interval between removal of the primary lesion and later occurrence of metastases in remote organs averaged 4.3 years. Duration of life after evidence of metastasis was observed, however, averaged only 140 days in those patients who did not benefit from therapy. This was in contrast to an

(6) J.A.M.A. 166:37-41, Jan. 4, 1958.

average 16 months' survival of patients after metastasis was observed in the organs of those who showed a favorable response to TEPA and thio-TEPA. Once malignant melanoma has disseminated to the thoracic and abdominal organs, the duration of life, even in patients who outwardly appear healthy, is less than for patients with acute leukemia. However, this is not true of patients showing only skin metastases or local recurrence in the area of the original disease.

DATA ON PATIENTS WITH DISSEMINATED MALIGNANT MELANOMA

Case	Age	Sex	Interval Between Appearance of Primary and Organ Metastases, Mo.	Drug	Interval Between Appearance of Organ Metastases and Death, Mo.	Results
1	56	F	27	TEPA	13	Successful remission
2	49	M	48	TEPA	3	Died 7 days after starting therapy
3	54	F	108	TEPA	5	Died 6 days after starting therapy
4	55	F	...	TEPA	Living	Successful
5	50	F	36	TEPA	4	Unsuccessful
6	34	F	24	TEPA	3	Unsuccessful
7	33	M	25	TEPA & ThioTEPA	2	Unsuccessful
8	36	M	15	ThioTEPA	3	Unsuccessful
9	60	F	96	ThioTEPA	2	Unsuccessful
10	60	M	18	ThioTEPA	6	Temporary remission
11	67	M	13	ThioTEPA	1	Unsuccessful
12	31	M	100	ThioTEPA	5	Unsuccessful
13	28	M	12	ThioTEPA	Living	Successful

One case implied that an advanced stage of the disease would not preclude successful treatment.

Woman, 56, had undergone surgery for removal of a melanotic mole of the right foot 27 months before admission. She was admitted with a diagnosis of virus pneumonia, which was followed by recurrent pleural effusion. Melanoma cells were demonstrated in the pleural fluid. The patient also had nausea and vomiting, presumably due to gastrointestinal involvement, and generalized convulsive seizures from central nervous system metastases. Treatment with TEPA was instituted, despite the poor condition of the patient. Twelve days later, concurrent with pancytopenia and depigmentation, the metastases began to decrease. This was followed shortly by cessation of convulsive seizures, dyspnea and vomiting and improvement in general strength. All evidence of the disease disappeared during the next 3 weeks. The pleural fluid cleared and the lung masses and subcutaneous nodules could no longer be found. The patient returned home and received intermittent maintenance treatment with TEPA. There was sudden generalized recurrence of the disease 13 months later with no further response to treatment.

Triethylene Thiophosphoramide in Treatment of Metastatic Cerebral Malignancy. Perk Lee Davis, Margaret H. Shumway and Barbara Siu[7] (Paoli, Pa., Med. Center) injected triethylene thiophosphoramide (thio-TEPA) into the carotid arteries of 8 patients with cerebral metastases from cancer of the breast, of 3 with such metastases from cancer of the lung (all 11 were unconscious at the time of initial treatment) and in 1 patient with diabetes insipidus from metastatic cancer of the pancreas. All patients responded dramatically; the 11 regained full consciousness 4-6 hours after injection and returned to full activity within 6 days. Only 1 patient died, 6 months after the first treatment; the others remained well. Remissions were maintained by repeated intracarotid injections of the drug every 7-9 weeks. Local skin metastases responded to local injections into the tumor.

Woman, 68, had diabetes insipidus for 6 months and lost 42 lb. For several months before and continuously after onset of symptoms she had vague and occasionally severe pain in the left upper part of the abdomen. Complete physical and laboratory studies were normal, except for persistently low specific gravity. Intravenous injection of hypertonic saline confirmed the absence of antidiuretic hormone. The diabetes insipidus did not respond to inhalations of posterior pituitary powder, injections of vasopressin in oil or administration of 600 mg. aminopyrine 4 times daily. Presumptive diagnosis was metastatic carcinoma to the supraoptic region from a cancer in the tail of the pancreas.

Thio-TEPA, 40 mg., was injected into the right common carotid artery in the manner used in angiography. Improvement was noted in 3 days, and in 9 days, the patient was apparently normal. She stayed well for 5 months 21 days, gaining 21 lb.; then symptoms of diabetes insipidus returned. Injection of 40 mg. thio-TEPA into the left common carotid artery again induced clinical remission lasting 3 months 19 days. Thereafter, the patient was kept comfortable by vasopressin injections 1-3 times weekly for the next 2 months, after which she became totally refractory. Another 50 mg. thio-TEPA given in the right common carotid artery again induced remission, but this time lasting only 28 days. She received 3,600 r which induced a partial remission lasting 3 weeks, but she became progressively weaker and died. Autopsy revealed a 1-cm. carcinoma of the tail of the pancreas densely adherent posteriorly and with a 4-mm. metastasis in the pituitary stalk in the region of the hypothalamic supraoptic nuclei.

Relative Frequency of Several Types of Chronic Leukemia and Their Management. Frank H. Bethell[8] reviewed 1,179 cases of leukemia in persons over age 13 seen at the Univer-

(7) J.A.M.A. 167:726-727, June 7, 1958.
(8) J. Chron. Dis. 6:403-420, October, 1957.

sity of Michigan during 1927-56. The leukemia was chronic in 734 cases and acute in 455. The ratio of acute to chronic cases showed a steady rise during the period studied, so the incidence of acute leukemia seems to be definitely increasing. No inference concerning over-all increase in chronic leukemia is justified, since, although in terms of total hospital registrations the number of chronic cases has increased, it is not possible to weigh accurately factors which affect the referral of patients with a particular disease to a medical center. This review has afforded no evidence that the relative frequency of chronic granulocytic and lymphocytic leukemia is changing, or that there has been any change in sex distribution or age incidence in the chronic leukemias.

Ionizing radiation continues to be the standard of reference when new forms of treatment for chronic leukemia are proposed, and it has not been conclusively demonstrated that survival times are increased or even equaled by use of drugs when compared with x-radiation or radioactive phosphorus. Nevertheless, chemotherapy has largely supplanted radiation in the treatment of chronic granulocytic and lymphocytic leukemias in recent years. With passage of time and increased experience, use of these agents has received increasing justification.

The alkylating agents, Myleran®, triethylene melamine and chlorambucil, are the preferred compounds. There is no evidence of qualitative difference in biologic actions of these drugs, but there are quantitative variations which affect dosages, absorption rates, duration of effects and likelihood of severe myeloid depression. At present, because of advantages of administration, dosage control and relative safety, Myleran is generally preferred in chronic granulocytic and chlorambucil in chronic lymphocytic leukemia. Continuous drug administration on individually determined maintenance dosage is superior to intermittent therapy.

Colcemid® may be useful in some cases of advanced proliferative granulocytic leukemia and the antimetabolite 6-mercaptopurine (Purinethol®) may be used in these situations. The adrenal cortical steroids are mainly of value in controlling secondary hemolysis and thrombocytopenia which occur in some patients with chronic lymphocytic leukemia and malignant reticuloendotheliosis. When these agents do not prove effective, splenectomy may be beneficial.

Hyperuricemia Associated with Treatment of Acute Leukemia was observed by G. Lennard Gold and Richard D. Fritz[9] (Nat'l Inst. of Health) in 2 patients. In the first, hyperuricemia was related to administration of 6-mercaptopurine and methotrexate on one occasion and of hydrocortisone during a second episode. In the second, hyperuricemia was concomitant with administration of 6-mercaptopurine, cortisone and ACTH.

The marked rise in serum uric acid and excretion of uric acid following antileukemic treatment may be explained by the following hypotheses. (1) The drugs may actually cause lysis of the leukemic cells in the blood, bone marrow and other tissues and release large amounts of nitrogenous products and uric acid, causing an acute uremic picture. (2) Large amounts of uric acid and other purines and pyrimidines may of themselves interfere with normal renal function. (3) Chemotherapeutic agents may interfere with the re-use of nucleic acid breakdown products derived from white blood cells. Pre-existing renal disease or leukemic infiltration of the kidney may aggravate the magnitude of the metabolic changes.

In every case of acute leukemia the possibility of an acute uremic episode concomitant with antileukemic therapy should be considered. The risk is apparently greatest in patients with acute lymphocytic leukemia with high white blood cell counts. The following plan is suggested to ameliorate or prevent such an occurrence: (1) obtain urinalysis, blood urea nitrogen and uric acid determinations before therapy; if these are abnormal, undertake further evaluation of the renal status; (2) force fluids during treatment if marked uricosuria is present, and administer alkali by mouth to prevent precipitation of uric acid crystals; and (3) observe closely the levels of serum uric acid during treatment.

Cortisone in Treatment of Hypercalcemia in Neoplastic Disease. W. P. Laird Myers[1] (Cornell Univ.) administered cortisone, prednisone or hydrocortisone to 11 patients with hypercalcemia and hypercalciuria secondary to widespread cancer. The neoplasms treated included carcinomas of the

(9) Ann. Int. Med. 47:428-434, September, 1957.
(1) Cancer 11:83-88, Jan.-Feb., 1958.

kidney and breast, lymphosarcoma, multiple myeloma, metastatic adenocarcinoma of unknown primary origin and rhabdomyosarcoma. There was complete reversal of the calcium changes in 5 patients, partial reversal in 2 and no response in 4.

Initial doses of cortisone ranged between 200 and 400 mg. daily, and doses were then tapered, depending on the responses observed. The 5 patients who responded to treatment all did so within the first 2 weeks, and in general, longer periods of treatment (in 1 instance as long as 54 days) did not increase the chances of obtaining a positive effect. Route of administration of steroid had no consistent effect on response observed, and prednisone, used in 1 instance proved to be as effective as cortisone. Of 5 patients who died while still under treatment, 4 had received cortisone for 14 days or longer and therefore had adequate trials of therapy. Of these, 1 showed a positive calcium response, 2 a negative and 1 a partial.

Inhibition of the rate of growth of tumor appears to be responsible for the observed changes in some patient, but other possible mechanisms, although not clearly defined, cannot be excluded. It is felt that cortisone is useful in the management of hypercalcemia of neoplastic origin.

Treatment of Acute Leukemia in Adults with Massive Doses of Prednisone and Prednisolone. Norma B. Granville, Fernando Rubio, Jr., Asuman Unugur, Edward Schulman and William Dameshek[2] treated 20 adults with acute leukemia in the following schedule:

Method.—Prednisone and prednisolone, used interchangeably, were given orally in doses of either 250 mg. every 6 hours or 125 mg. every 12 hours. This schedule was maintained for 2 weeks, after which the dose was gradually reduced to a maintenance dosage of 5-50 mg./day. Two patients given 1,000 mg. daily had received small doses of steroids earlier in the course. Five of the 10 patients in the 1,000-mg. group and 3 of the 10 in the 250-mg. group received 6-mercaptopurine, 100-200 mg./day, at various times after completing the initial course of massive prednisone therapy. Unless there was evidence of salt retention, no effort was made to restrict salt intake, and potassium chloride was not administered routinely. All patients received supportive care.

Only 3 of the 10 patients treated with 1,000 mg. prednisone/day were able to tolerate the medication for the entire

(2) New England J. Med. 259:207-213, July 31, 1958.

2-week period. In 5, the drug was decreased or discontinued at the end of 8 days because of undesirable side effects; 2 patients died less than a week after starting therapy. The 250-mg. dosage was better tolerated, 9 of the 10 patients receiving the full 2 weeks' course. The tenth patient died during the 1st week of therapy. Remarkable symptomatic improvement was evident within the first 24-48 hours of treatment in most patients. Outstanding changes were the development of a striking sense of well-being, marked increase in appetite and, objectively, defervescence and decreased bleeding. Three complete remissions occurred in the 1,000-mg. group. Since corticosteroids or ACTH had been used before massive prednisone therapy in 2 patients, and a short course of 6-mercaptopurine had been given in the third, it cannot be stated unequivocally that remissions were due to the use of prednisone alone. An additional patient had a partial remission and might have continued to complete remission, but he died of acute myocardial infarction 4 months after therapy began. In the 250-mg. group, no patients with remissions received previous therapy; however, in 1 patient, clear-cut remission appeared only after a brief course of 6-mercaptopurine therapy. These patients continued normal activities, such as farming, practicing medicine, housekeeping, etc., during remissions.

In 5 patients receiving 1,000 mg. prednisone daily, agitated depression bordering on frank psychosis developed. This did not occur in the 250-mg. group.

The earliest hematologic response to therapy was initiated by a fall in the high white cell count and a reduction in the number of blast forms in the peripheral blood except in patients showing initial leukopenia, in whom there was usually a rise in the white cell count. Reticulocytosis (counts of 8-10%) was then noted in most patients, usually followed by an increase in hemoglobin and in the red cell count. The return of platelets to normal values in patients in whom remissions developed took 3-6 weeks. Bone marrow, which had been hypercellular, usually showed a striking decrease in cellularity shortly after treatment; in several instances no marrow material could be obtained. As remission progressed, and after reduction in the prednisone dose, the marrow returned to normal cellularity. With relapse, the marrow again became intensely hyperplastic.

The over-all figure of complete remissions was 25%, which is not considered striking. Nevertheless, it compares favorably with that obtained by other therapeutic methods (folic acid antagonists, 6-mercaptopurine, x-rays, etc.) used in acute leukemia of adults.

Use of 6-Mercaptopurine in Treatment of Acute Leukemia in Late Pregnancy. Over 115 cases of leukemia associated with pregnancy have been reported in the literature. Harold R. Schumacher[3] (US Naval Hosp., Portsmouth, Va.) presents a case in which 6-mercaptopurine was used in the management of this disease in late pregnancy. Results suggest that the drug can be used for acute leukemia complicating late pregnancy without apparent ill effects on the fetus.

Woman, 23, gravida II, para II, whose last menstrual period was Apr. 17, 1955, was hospitalized on August 8 with severe anemia (hemoglobin 4 Gm. hematocrit 15 vol.%) and a chief complaint of "dizziness and giddy feeling for 1½ months." On bone marrow biopsy, a diagnosis of acute myelocytic leukemia was made. During a month's stay, she received 8 pt. of fresh whole blood, 25 mg. cortisone 4 times daily, low-sodium diet, potassium supplement, vitamins and iron medication. On discharge in late August, hemoglobin was 10 Gm., hematocrit 29 vol.% and a white cell count 10,500. In the next 3 months she received 8 pt. of fresh whole blood.

In October, at 26 weeks' gestation, while cortisone was continued, 6-mercaptopurine (25 mg. orally 4 times daily) was started in an attempt to obtain a temporary remission. A month later she was readmitted and given a transfusion of 4 pt. of fresh whole blood. On November 28, a low platelet count of 36,000/cu. mm. (Fonio method) was discovered, and 6-mercaptopurine was discontinued. Cortisone was continued, 25 mg. 4 times daily, along with a low-sodium diet, potassium supplement, vitamins and blood transfusions. On December 10, after 5 more transfusions of fresh whole blood, the platelet count rose to 90,000/cu. mm.

The patient did well until 2 weeks before delivery, when hydronephrosis, paresthesias in both legs and paraplegia developed in 72 hours. Because of rapid deterioration, labor was medically induced and she was delivered, at 39 weeks' gestation, of a living infant, weight 7 lb. 14 oz., whose hemoglobin was 18 Gm. and hematocrit 63 vol.%. The infant's blood count and differential were normal. The mother's condition continued to deteriorate rapidly, and she died a week after delivery. Autopsy revealed the classic findings of acute myelocytic leukemia.

---

(3) Am. J. Obst. & Gynec. 74:1361-1362, December, 1957.

Intrathecal Amethopterin in Neurologic Manifestations of Leukemia. Failure to control the central nervous system involvement of acute leukemia with conventional chemotherapy and hesitancy by some radiotherapists to use irradiation for this purpose stimulated search for a different approach to the problem. It was postulated on the basis of preliminary data that the therapeutic agent given orally or parenterally might not gain access to the cerebrospinal fluid or brain parenchyma in the same relative concentrations as in the serum and somatic organs. Therefore, James A. Whiteside, Fred S. Philips, Harold W. Dargeon and Joseph H. Burchenal[4] (Mem'l Center for Cancer, New York) experimented on dogs and humans using intrathecal instillations of the antimetabolite amethopterin.

Dogs tolerated up to 0.5 mg./kg. amethopterin (methotrexate) intrathecally, yet exhibited megaloblastosis and depression in the nucleated cell count in the bone marrow. One dose of 1.8 mg./kg. intrathecally caused death from marrow depression and damage to gastrointestinal epithelium.

Five patients with neurologic symptoms due to leukemia and lymphosarcoma improved markedly on 0.1-0.5 mg./kg. intrathecally. The neurologic remissions began about 1 week after instillation and lasted about 6 weeks. Repeated neurologic remissions were obtained in all patients. The EEG tracings improved in 2 patients after amethopterin intrathecally. Intrathecal amethopterin produced neurologic remission in 2 patients who were considered refractory to the drug given orally. Intrathecal instillation yielded extremely high cerebrospinal fluid levels (30-100 times those obtained after even a massive single oral dose) and prolonged serum levels of amethopterin. Intrathecal therapy produced no change in the peripheral blood picture and did not significantly alter the differential count in the bone marrow except for producing megaloblastosis. Amethopterin was given to patients in repeated doses with no ill effects.

Treatment of Leukemia Cutis with Demecolcin. Demecolcin is an alkaloid of Colchicum autumnale. Experimental evidence demonstrates that it inhibits mitosis in metaphase, but

(4) A.M.A. Arch. Int. Med. 101:279-285, February, 1958.

its toxicity appears to be 30 times less than that of colchicine. Unlike other cytotoxic agents used in treatment of leukemia, its action on hemopoiesis is a unique selective inhibition of granulocyte production. Demecolcin has been used with some success in acute granulocytic leukemia, and some suggestive benefit has been observed in Hodgkin's disease and other tumors. Most authors, however, agree that it may be harmful in lymphocytic leukemia. The best therapeutic results are seen in chronic granulocytic leukemia and are characterized by a striking improvement in general clinical condition, rapid decrease in splenomegaly and diminution in the total number of granulocytes. Remissions are short lived if the drug is stopped, but prolonged remission may be obtained by continued maintenance therapy. The dosage of demecolcin is not well established but has averaged about 5 mg. daily. To date, toxic effects have been minor and usually subside after discontinuance of the drug.

Edward Shanbrom and Daniel Kahn[5] (VA Hosp., West Haven, Conn.) report resolution of skin lesions in 2 patients with leukemia cutis treated with demecolcin. One had chronic granulocytic leukemia and was moribund when demecolcin therapy was instituted. After 3 days of therapy the total leukocyte count dropped from 250,000 to 30,000. The differential count was essentially the same, and there was no decrease in the number of blast forms seen. The general condition of the patient improved temporarily and there was a dramatic regression of the nodular skin and mucous membrane lesions. However, hemorrhagic manifestations of epistaxis, purpura and melena increased; the patient became confused, had persistent tonic seizures and died.

The other patient had acute monocytic leukemia of the Naegeli type with extensive leukemia cutis. Demecolcin was given in doses of 5 mg. daily for 5 days and resulted in a rapid decrease in the total leukocyte count from 67,000 to 5,-900, but no change in the systemic condition of the patient. The skin nodules showed a rapid resolution. Severe aphthous stomatitis developed but subsided rapidly. The patient became progressively worse, fulminant uremia developed and he died 20 days after hospitalization.

(5) Ann. Int. Med. 47:565-576, September, 1957.

Treatment of Polycythemia Vera with Radioactive Phosphorus. Irving I. Cowan[6] (Marquette Univ.) reports results with P^{32} in 38 patients. Thirty-four were successfully treated, but hematologic complications developed in 6 of these and in 1 of the 4 who were not benefited. The doses used were computed on the basis of 50 μc./kg. body weight and given in 2 or 4 mc. every 2-3 weeks until clinical and hematologic responses were satisfactory. Most patients had a good remission with 3-7 injections and within 6-10 weeks.

With symptomatic relief and reduction of the hematocrit, redness of the skin disappeared or diminished and the spleen decreased in size. The remission induced with the 1st course of treatment may last 6 months or as long as 2 or more years; the average is about 18 months. Recurrence of symptoms and increase in the hematocrit are indications for a 2d course of therapy.

Radioactive phosphorus is easily administered and can be given orally or intravenously. The patient does not require hospitalization during treatment. Because P^{32} becomes concentrated in the bone marrow, liver, spleen and lymph nodes, it provides a method for irradiating the overactive hemopoietic tissues more selectively than can be done with external irradiations.

There is no local or systemic reaction when P^{32} is given intravenously if the solution is isotonic. Symptoms such as are noted in radiation sickness do not occur. The chief complication from P^{32} administration is severe depression of the hemopoietic tissue, which may occur when the dose is too high or when the patient is unusually sensitive to this substance. Other complications include thrombocytopenia with petechiae and anemia. None of these occurred in the 38 patients. A late complication of polycythemia vera may be leukemia, which also occurs in patients not treated with P^{32}. The etiologic relationship between P^{32} therapy and leukemia is not established but remains a possibility.

Therapy of Polycythemia Vera with Myleran®. Niel Wald, Takashi Hoshino and Mary E. Sears[7] used Myleran in the treatment of 9 relapses of polycythemia vera in 5 patients. The average dosage that produced full remission was 29.4

(6) Wisconsin M. J. 56:501-505, December, 1957.
(7) Blood 13:757-762, August, 1958.

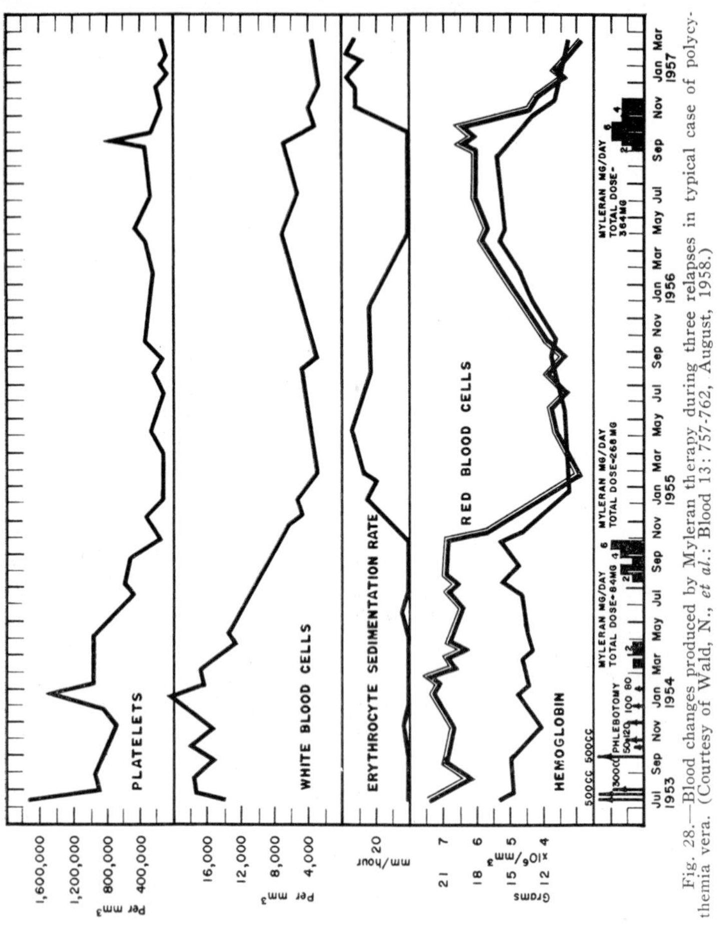

Fig. 28.—Blood changes produced by Myleran therapy during three relapses in typical case of polycythemia vera. (Courtesy of Wald, N., *et al.*: Blood 13: 757-762, August, 1958.)

mg./week (range 22-40 mg./week). Only partial remissions resulted in 2 instances in which 14 and 17 mg./week were used. When more than one fully effective course of Myleran was given, subsequent remissions were produced without significant dosage increase.

The 7 complete remissions were characterized by disappearance of clinical symptoms and abnormal physical findings, including hypertension and splenomegaly when these were present. Results of hematologic tests were also improved. In the 2 instances of incomplete remission, clinical improvement occurred, but hematologic tests showed a fall in leukocytes and platelets without much change in red cell values. Individual variation in the response to a given dose level was evident, but no significant difficulty in control was found, nor did any complications of therapy occur.

Figure 28 shows a typical clinical course. Occasional phlebotomy was ineffective in this patient, resulting in microcytosis but producing no significant fall in erythrocyte count or hemoglobin level. The initial dose of Myleran produced only incomplete remission, reducing the leukocyte and platelet counts alone. The second trial of Myleran, in a higher dosage, gave a complete remission, as did the third after a second remission ended.

Myleran effectively reduced the red cell volume in all 3 patients studied by tracer methods, though other findings were not as consistently affected. However, the plasma iron turnover was reduced in 2 and the plasma volume increased in 2 after therapy. The possible contributing role of moderate overtreatment in the production of these results must be considered but cannot be assessed accurately.

Evaluation of Some Factors Affecting Estrogen Response in Treatment of Advanced Cancer of Breast is presented by J. L. Hayward.[8] The study material consisted of 92 patients, aged 42-84, treated with estrogens during the past 10 years. Assessment was by means of the mean clinical value method, which consists of an initial objective survey of each individual lesion before treatment starts and the selection of some of these for accurate monthly assessment. Most of the patients received 100 mg. stilbestrol daily by mouth. Ethinyl estradiol in doses of 1 mg. daily was given to a few patients who could not tolerate stilbestrol. Estrogen therapy was applied only to patients who were unsuitable for any other form of treatment or in whom other treatment had failed. Observations were made only during the first 2 years after start of treatment.

Resolution of the mean clinical value records according to

(8) Guy's Hosp. Rep. 106:254-263, 1957.

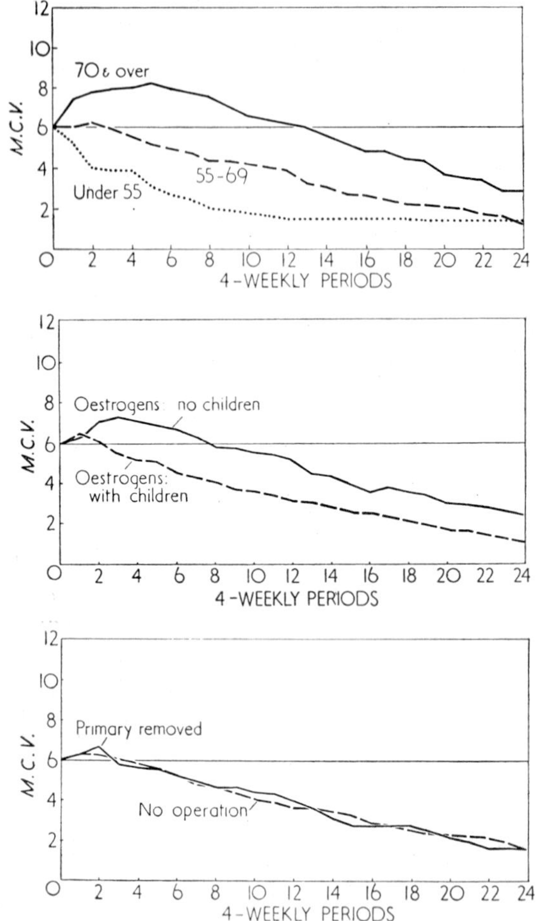

Fig. 29 (top).—Resolution of mean clinical value records according to age.
Fig. 30 (center).—Resolution of mean clinical value records according to presence or absence of children.
Fig. 31 (bottom).—Resolution of mean clinical value records according to presence or absence of primary.
(Courtesy of Hayward, J. L.: Guy's Hosp. Rep. 106:254-263, 1957.)

age (Fig. 29) showed that reponse to estrogen therapy increased with age. The increased benefit derived by older patients may reflect an increased dependence of their tumors on prolactin, for by taking estrogens the prolactin levels would fall. A greater response was obtained in patients who had no children (Fig. 30). It would be reasonable to expect that the reason why nulliparous women show greater response than parous might also be reflected in the prolactin output. Previous removal of the primary lesion had no effect on the response to estrogen therapy (Fig. 31). The main value in this part of the investigation is that the method will definitely show that an aspect of the disease has no bearing on response to treatment. No significant difference was noted in response to treatment by secondary lesions at different sites.

Use of Prednisolone in Treatment of Disseminated Breast Carcinoma in 45 patients is discussed by Sydney Kofman, Devanaboyina Nagamani, Richard E. Buenger and Samuel G. Taylor III[9] (Chicago). Eleven patients with symptoms of cerebral metastases received orally 100 mg. prednisolone daily, 50 mg. on awakening and 50 mg. at bedtime. The other 34 patients received 50 mg. daily in 2 doses. Treatment was continued for 3 months unless side effects or rapid progression of the disease necessitated a change. Sodium was not restricted, and potassium was not given except when specifically indicated. Because of the high incidence of gastric and duodenal ulcers noted in the early part of the study, a modified ulcer diet and antacids were used later.

Significant healing of some lesions without simultaneous progression of others or development of new lesions was considered the main criterion of regression. Three patients had a generalized regression of metastases for 3 or more months; 2 are still in remission after 1 year of therapy. Regressions for less than 2 months occurred in 5 other patients. Previous surgical or radiation castration did not increase the number of regressions.

Patients treated with prednisolone showed marked subjective improvement. There were decreased pain and increased ambulation, strength and appetite. In some patients subjective improvement lasted for months, even though the malignant disease was definitely progressing. Lymphedema of the arm decreased in a number of patients.

Clinical improvement was most often seen in patients with cerebral metastases (6 of 11). Although tumor regression probably occurred in at least 1 patient, reduction in inflam-

(9) Cancer 11:226-232, Jan.-Feb., 1958.

matory reaction and cerebral edema were probably the mechanisms that resulted in clinical improvement in most patients.

Six patients with hypercalcemia, with serum calcium values ranging from 14 to 25 mg./100 cc., were treated with 200 mg. prednisolone daily for 1-2 weeks. In 4 patients the serum calcium returned to normal. It is questionable whether this change necessarily indicated tumor regression, since there was no evidence of regression.

Almost all patients treated more than several weeks had weight gain, moon facies, hirsutism and abnormal fat deposition. Two patients discontinued therapy because of sleeplessness and nervousness. Psychotic symptoms occurred in 2 patients with cerebral metastases. Prednisolone-induced or -aggravated diabetes was not uncommon but usually could be controlled easily with diet and insulin. Gastric or duodenal ulcers developed in 5 patients. Quadriceps weakness was seen in several. Frequency of edema was low, and neither hypertension nor aggravation of pre-existing hypertension was seen.

The percentage of patients with disseminated breast carcinoma reported to have tumor regression from bilateral adrenalectomy varies from 15 to 45%. However, the endocrine changes produced by prednisolone and other corticosteroids are not similar to those produced by adrenalectomy, and the term "medical adrenalectomy" may be misleading. For example, corticotropin secretion is depressed by corticosteroids, whereas in adrenalectomy the secretion is increased. Regression has been observed after adrenalectomy in patients unsuccessfully treated with corticosteroids.

Subjective improvement seen with prednisolone is important not only from the standpoint of comfort but also because it may allow bedridden patients and those in the terminal stages to obtain other forms of therapy such as adrenalectomy or oophorectomy.

Prednisolone causes relatively little salt retention. It is inferior to cortisone in the maintenance of patients who have undergone adrenalectomy. Those on relatively large doses (200 mg./day) may experience adrenal insufficiency under a stressful situation. The greatest danger of this is in a patient with poor adrenal function or none at all. Therefore, in patients under stressful situations, prednisolone should not be used to control adrenal insufficiency.

Nonspecific Cortisone Effects from ACTH Administration in Advanced Prostatic Carcinoma. Frank Hinman, Jr., and Gilbert I. Smith[1] (Univ. of California) treated 8 patients who were in relapse after orchiectomy plus stilbestrol administration (and in some instances after cortisone therapy) with 80 units of ACTH/day. This amount of ACTH causes adrenal secretion of urinary 17-hydroxycorticoid titers comparable to those occurring after administration of 100 mg. cortisone acetate daily, which was the standard dose of cortisone used in a previous series.

Administration of ACTH produced clinical improvement comparable in quality but not in duration to that with cortisone therapy in 3 of the 8 patients. Of the 3 patients with proof of the greatest adrenal stimulation, 2 had remission despite the concomitant rise in 17-ketosteroid excretion (and presumably similar rise in biologic androgens, which would be expected to exacerbate the disease. It is felt, therefore, that this clinical improvement is due to the effect of the adrenal corticoids which are perforce released along with the androgens. This, in turn, indicates that it is not adrenal suppression but the direct action of cortisone which produces the clinical changes with cortisone therapy of advanced prostatic carcinoma.

The authors believe that the effectiveness of cortisone and, to a less degree, of ACTH therapy is exerted through a shift in the hormone environment of the tumor. This hormonal shift by ACTH would be anticipated to be less great than that of cortisone, because of the concomitant secretion of androgens, in contrast to their suppression by cortisone. Cortisone therapy, in turn, would be less effective than adrenalectomy. Clinical observations have shown a similar gradation.

Preliminary Evaluation of Radioactive Colloidal Gold in Treatment of Carcinoma of Prostate is presented by Willis H. Carter and Robert G. Bogen[2] (Brooks Army Hosp.) on the basis of results in 20 patients. All had carcinoma extending beyond the prostatic capsule but showed no evidence of

(1) J. Urol. 77:305-311, February, 1957.
(2) Ibid. 78:483-486, October, 1957.

distant metastasis. If obstructive symptoms were present (as they were in 4) transurethral resection was done 3-4 weeks before injection of radioactive gold.

Colloidal Au^{198}, with particle sizes of 0.003-0.004 μ., was used. The isotope has a half-life of 2.7 days and possesses suitable radiation characteristics. Epinephrine hydrochloride, 1 ml., and 150 units of hyaluronidase were added to the isotope and isotonic saline was used to dilute the material to a concentration of 5 mc./ml. solution. An intravesical approach through a lower abdominal midline incision was used. Through a lead-walled syringe, the gold was injected in 12 areas around the bladder neck into the prostate and in 1 area in each seminal vesicle. From 2.5 to 3 mc./Gm. prostatic tissue was injected, with a maximum of 150/mc. Follow-up injections, as indicated, were done transperineally.

Of the 20 patients treated, 16 are alive. Of the 4 who died, 3 died of widespread carcinoma arising from the prostate and 1 of carcinoma of the pancreas. These patients died 6, 21, 34 and 35 months after the initial injection. Five patients have positive Silverman needle prostatic biopsies and have been re-treated by the perineal route 1-4 times. The average survival period of the 20 patients is 22 months. Of 7 patients living more than 2 years after operation, 4 have positive Silverman needle biopsies and 2 have demonstrable bony metastasis.

Though no definite conclusions are possible, the authors believe that this treatment has merit if the proper criteria for selection of cases are followed. They have been impressed by the immediate improvement of the prostate on digital examination and postoperative negative Silverman needle biopsies. Subjectively, the patients have shown improvement and are more comfortable. Though most patients are not cured, the disease may be controlled for varying periods.

Intra-arterial Nitrogen Mustard in Treatment of Pelvic Cancer. Nearly all agents capable of slowing growth or producing temporary regression of tumor tissue also have toxic effects on the bone marrow, liver or other organs when given systemically. Host toxicity is the limiting factor in dosage. Klopp *et al.* reported that in inoperable cancer largely localized to a single area nitrogen mustard could be given in a larger total amount by repeated small doses into the arteries which supply the area than could be safely administered intravenously.

Irwin H. Krakoff and Robert D. Sullivan[3] (New York) report their experiences with intra-arterial nitrogen mustard in 29 cases of metastatic or nonresectable cancer in which the principal manifestations were in the pelvis. The aorta was catheterized by percutaneous puncture of the femoral artery. Each patient received a single dose of 0.4 mg./kg. The catheter was then withdrawn.

In 15 patients the tumor caused discomfort and 3 had intestinal obstruction due to extrinsic pressure. Four had uremia due to ureteral obstruction by tumor mass. Three had severe pelvic pain, usually due to osseous metastases, and 3 had compression of the spinal cord, cauda equina or sacral roots.

Of the 29 patients, 18 (62%) obtained some benefit. The therapeutic response lasted 3 weeks to 6 months. A measurable decrease in tumor size, an increase in urine flow or some other objective measure of improvement was found in 21 patients. The best results were in lymphomas and carcinomas of the ovary and uterus. Carcinoma of the cervix responded less well and that of the rectum not at all. These are the same malignancies which respond to intravenous nitrogen mustard.

In about one third of the cases leukopenia occurred 7-14 days after treatment, but in none did the count fall below 1,000/cu. mm. Transient thrombocytopenia occurred in only 7 cases. There were no instances of femoral artery bleeding. In 1 case the distal end of the catheter was sheared off when it was removed before the needle was withdrawn. The safest practice is to remove the needle first, then withdraw the catheter, then apply firm pressure for 2-3 minutes. Nausea and vomiting occurred in nearly all patients and was of the same severity and duration as is commonly encountered when the drug is given intravenously. It was easily controlled by sedation with barbiturates and chlorpromazine.

Intra-arterial administration of nitrogen mustard is a useful procedure in palliation of pelvic neoplasms of ovarian, uterine or lymphomatous origin. The technic is simple, easily mastered and safe.

---

(3) Ann. Int. Med. 48:839-850, April, 1958.

Girl, 20, had right lower monoplegia and a large osteolytic lesion of the sacrum previously proved to be reticulum cell sarcoma. She had severe sacral pain. Nitrogen mustard, 0.4 mg./kg., was administered intra-arterially. Within 14 hours some function returned to the extremity. Therapy was then started with Co^{60} and within 24 hours she could move her leg freely. Seven days later she could walk. After 3,000 r tumor dose to the osteolytic lesion she was discharged. X-rays showed bone healing. The only residual neurologic sign was slight persistent right footdrop. Three months later she died of widely disseminated disease, but without evidence of recurrence of the sacral lesion.

Nitrogen Mustard in Treatment of Pleural and Peritoneal Effusions was used by Charles W. Fullerton and Peter I. Reed[4] (Montreal Gen'l Hosp.) in 8 patients.

TECHNIC.—Half an hour before the injection give 0.2 Gm. secobarbital and 25 mg. chlorpromazine orally. Mix the HN2 at the bedside: one 10 mg.-vial with 10 cc. sterile water. Give 0.4 mg./kg. Insert the needle or trocar into the pleural or peritoneal cavity. Be sure of a free flow of fluid. Inject HN2. Change the position of the patient every 5 minutes for 1 hour. If there is any further nausea, repeat the secobarbital and chlorpromazine. Tap and remove all fluid possible 24 hours later.

Of 8 patients, 4 responded well. The only ill effect noted was nausea in those patients receiving HN2 intraperitoneally. No depression of the blood cell count was observed.

The HN2 may be adsorbed by protein in the cavity and only a little be absorbed into the blood stream. This would explain the lack of harmful effect on the bone marrow. Patients most likely to respond are those in whom ascites or peritoneal effusion is the only evidence of metastatic carcinoma, especially if the breast or ovary is the site of the primary tumor.

Therapy of Choriocarcinoma and Related Trophoblastic Tumors with Folic Acid and Purine Antagonists is discussed by Min Chiu Li, Roy Hertz and Delbert M. Bergenstal[5] (Nat'l Inst. of Health). Tumors of trophoblastic origin may arise in the uterus or in the gonads. They are characteristically highly malignant and spread rapidly by direct extension and by metastasis to the lungs and brain and less commonly to many other sites.

Intensive, intermittent therapy with the folic acid antagonist methotrexate or with 6-mercaptopurine was studied in 6 women with far-advanced choriocarcinoma or chorioadeno-

(4) Canad. M. A. J. 79:190-191, Aug. 1, 1958.
(5) New England J. Med. 259:66-74, July 10, 1958.

ma destruens and in 5 men with embryonal carcinoma of the testis. Methotrexate was administered orally or intramuscularly in daily doses of 15-25 mg. for 5 consecutive days; 6-mercaptopurine was administered orally in daily doses of 600-800 mg. for 5 days. No further therapy was given until all signs of induced toxicity, such as stomatitis, leukopenia, thrombocytopenia, enteritis and drug rash had in most instances completely subsided. Subsequent 5-day courses were repeatedly administered with similar precautions. The necessary interval between courses was 7-12 days. Supportive medical and nursing management was provided throughout treatment. This included frequent oral lavage, parenteral infusion of fluids, extra nourishment and semiliquid diets when required.

Criteria for therapeutic response included regressive changes in the x-ray appearance of metastases, regression of visible and palpable tumor masses, reduction of urinary gonadotropin titer and general clinical rehabilitation of the patient. All 6 women showed a marked drop in gonadotropin titer associated with other evidence of tumor regression. Five have been in clinical remission for 3-23 months. Two of these present no residual evidence of disease, and 3 manifest some residual disease by a sustained but low titer of gonadotropin excretion, despite absence of any other symptomatic, x-ray or physical manifestations of recurrence. One patient died of methotrexate toxicity during the final phases of therapy and after having given unequivocal evidence of marked tumor regression. No male patient exhibited a significant response to identical forms of therapy.

Of 79 courses of methotrexate and 14 of 6-mercaptopurine, only 1 of the former was accompanied by irreversible toxic effects. Stomatitis was the most regularly produced toxic effect. Its intensity was highly variable from patient to patient and from course to course in the same patient. With sustained fluid and caloric intake and frequent oral lavage this problem and its sequelae were readily managed in all. Bone marrow depression was variable; though many courses were unaccompanied by appreciable bone marrow effects, in others, marrow depression was extreme. Erythematous drug rash and a characteristic acneiform eruption occurred irregularly and with varying severity. Gastrointestinal manifestations included anorexia, nausea and occasional vomiting.

Prophylactic Treatment of Cancer at Time of Operation. Francisco Morales, Millar Bell, Gerald O. McDonald and Warren H. Cole[6] (Univ. of Illinois) reported previously that nitrogen mustard and triethylene thiophosphoramide (thio-TEPA) will prevent or diminish the percentage of "takes" in rats inoculated with a suspension of Walker 256 cells, when the drugs are given within an hour after inoculation. In the present experiments, they found that when nitrogen mustard was given to three groups of animals 48, 24 and 6 hours after inoculation of cells, the difference in "takes" between the control and treated animals was only 5, 8 and 11%, respectively. This indicates that unless the drug is given to rats at the time of inoculation of cancer cells, the effect will be greatly diminished and perhaps not significantly different from the percentage of "takes" in the control animals.

Studies were made on the effect of nitrogen mustard when the dosage of cells was varied. Nitrogen mustard was given in 4 daily doses of 0.25 mg./kg. intraperitoneally after intraportal inoculation of 110,000 cells in one group of animals and 220,000 cells in another group. The percentage of "takes" in the former group was 62% compared with 31% in the latter, indicating that the effect of the anticancer agent is influenced sharply by the number of cells injected.

Prophylactic or adjuvant therapy with nitrogen mustard given at the time of operation has been used in 65 patients with cancer of the gastrointestinal tract or breast. Only 1 death has occurred. This patient received only 1 dose (6.5 mg.) in the peritoneal cavity at the time of completion of the abdominal portion of a combined Miles resection. The cause of death 11 days later was fulminating enterocolitis due to a staphylococcus with no apparent relation to the nitrogen mustard. Four patients exhibited slightly increased bleeding tendencies and 4 had transient leukopenia, with leukocyte counts below 3,000. Two patients receiving intraperitoneal mustard had increased postoperative ileus.

Although complications are greater in treated patients than in controls, the authors are convinced that adjuvant therapy at the time of operation is safe, provided certain precautions in the use of nitrogen mustard are taken. Patients

(6) Ann. Surg. 146:588-595, October, 1957.

past age 70 are eliminated. The total dose used is 0.4 mg./kg., but not more than 30 mg. Half the total dose (0.2 mg./kg., but not more than 15 mg.) is given at the time of surgery. The other half is given intravenously in divided doses on the 1st and 2d postoperative days. The hematocrit is watched closely, and blood is given postoperatively if necessary.

Blood studies have revealed cancer cells in the peripheral venous blood of surprisingly many patients, including some in whom a 5-year survival is expected. Nitrogen mustard appears to destroy these circulating cells temporarily, but more data are needed before conclusive statements can be made.

Use of l-Triiodothyronine as Pituitary Depressant in Management of Thyroid Cancer, according to Colin G. Thomas, Jr.[7] (Univ. of North Carolina), offers advantages over other methods. Adequate suppression may be deduced from measurements of the serum protein-bound iodine, since endogenous thyroxin is firmly associated with alpha globulin, whereas the binding of l-triiodothyronine is not firm.

After study of the type, extent and functional activity of the neoplasm in 10 patients, serum protein-bound iodine levels and I^{131} uptake were determined. l-Triiodothyronine was then given by mouth, beginning with 25 μg. twice daily and increasing the dose every 1-2 weeks until the tolerated maximum (200-300 μg. daily) was reached. This dosage was continued for 6 weeks to a year or more. Periodic determinations of protein-bound iodine showed that endogenous hormone was reduced to the hypothyroid range within 6 weeks, leveling off at an irreducible minimum beyond which increased dosage and prolonged administration produced no effect. This probably represented complete suppression of the pituitary effect. The dosage required was variable: as little as 50 μg. daily in some.

In 1 patient, whose metastases exhibited autonomy of growth, a level below 2 could not be reached. In 2 patients with total thyroidectomy, functioning pulmonary metastases showed a decreased output of iodinated protein after therapy was begun, and 1 showed decrease in size of the metastases.

Tolerance varied; some patients had symptoms of hyperthyroidism at 100-150 μg. daily and others tolerated 300-350 μg. without sign of symptoms. The action of the drug per-

(7) Surg., Gynec. & Obst. 106:137-144, February, 1958.

sisted for several days after it had been discontinued.

Suppression of I^{131} uptake was accomplished in all patients with functioning carcinoma. There was no autonomy of iodine uptake as in Graves' disease.

When thyroidectomy was possible, the morphology of normal and neoplastic gland tissue was studied. After 1 year, involution and atrophy were apparent in the normal thyroid and to a lesser degree in the neoplastic gland. The cells of the latter were more columnar and showed no colloid production.

The uptake of P^{32} in normal, hyperplastic, carcinomatous and treated glands was studied. The increased uptake in cancerous tissue approximated that of the hyperplastic gland. When normal and cancerous thyroid tissue coexist, the uptake is more readily suppressed in the normal than in the neoplastic tissue.

Abnormal Responses to Muscle Relaxants in Carcinomatous Neuropathy in 5 patients are reported by P. B. Croft[8] (London Hosp.).

Case 1.—Woman, 65, had carcinomatous neuromyopathy of the mixed type (motor and cerebellar). Clinically, the muscular wasting and weakness preceded and was always more prominent than the cerebellar disorder. After the use of gallamine during bronchoscopy, the patient had prolonged respiratory difficulty with only partial response to neostigmine. She did not regain normal consciousness for 2 days. Autopsy confirmed the presence of a bronchial carcinoma. In the nervous system, cerebellar degeneration appeared to be the most important pathologic feature. The myopathy was unspecific. Changes in the myocardium were reminiscent of myasthenia gravis, but the complete absence of lymphorrhages in the voluntary muscles and of any germ centers in the thymus was against this diagnosis. Examination of the heart did not disclose any evidence of myocardial infarction, despite the ECG changes seen shortly after bronchoscopy.

Case 2.—Man, 54, with long-standing quiescent pulmonary tuberculosis, acquired a neuromyopathy in association with an oat cell carcinoma of the left lung. During pneumonectomy d-tubocurarine was used; afterward, the patient was apneic for 3 hours despite the use of neostigmine. Though spontaneous respiration returned, it was never normal, and he died 5 days after operation. The neurologic disturbances could not be attributed to the secondary carcinoma of the brain, since the foci observed were small and remote from one another. The cerebellum was not affected. Changes in the posterior root ganglions were too slight to be significant. Those in the voluntary muscles

(8) Brit. M. J. 1:181-187, Jan. 25, 1958.

examined appeared trivial in relation to the degree of clinical disturbance observed.

CASE 3.—Man, 65, showed a clinical picture of carcinomatous neuropathy. During the search for the underlying carcinoma, muscular weakness increased greatly after the use of suxamethonium during bronchoscopy, and this increased weakness did not disappear for 2 weeks. The neurologic condition later improved further, but he died after operation for carcinoma of the sigmoid, 21 months after the first neurologic symptoms had been noted.

CASE 4.—Man, 68, was admitted for surgical treatment of carcinoma of the prostate. He had general weakness for 1 month before admission, but there were no striking neurologic abnormalities. After the use of gallamine during endoscopic resection he became extremely weak, with signs of widespread impairment of function of the spinal cord, peripheral nerves and muscles. The condition persisted and was ultimately fatal, though the muscular weakness showed a partial clinical and electromyographic response to neostigmine. Histologic proof of prostatic carcinoma was not obtained, but the clinical diagnosis was not in doubt.

CASE 5.—Woman, 46, was admitted for investigation of a hilar mass seen on chest x-ray examination. Three weeks before admission she had complained of general weakness, but no obvious neurologic abnormality was noted on admission. After the use of d-tubocurarine during exploratory thoracotomy she had generalized muscular paralysis with apnea. She showed a partial response to neostigmine but died 2 days later. An oat cell carcinoma of the bronchus was found at autopsy, but no significant abnormalities were present in the central nervous system or muscles.

The author emphasizes that anesthetists and surgeons should be aware of the possible risk of using muscle relaxants on patients in whom carcinomatous neuropathy is suspected.

NEUROPSYCHIATRIC DISORDERS

TRANQUILIZERS AND STIMULANTS

► One recent writer said that at his state hospital 39 new drugs in these categories had been investigated during the past 2 years, but he nevertheless recommended that practitioners concentrate on but one drug in each of the two classes. This seems to indicate that his "investigations" were really only trials and that his personal confidence did not extend beyond the one tranquilizer and one stimulant with which he had had the most experience. I find it difficult to plumb the real meanings in the current literature because too few comparative studies of the older drugs with the new are being made. We already know rather well what is to be expected of chlorpromazine and reserpine in certain of the psychoses and schizophrenias, and of meprobamate in certain neuroses and tension states;

could not this knowledge be used as a backdrop against which to compare the more recent competitive drugs? Instead of pursuing such a course, the published studies reveal clinical investigators quickly dropping each drug they "investigate" in order to hurry into print a report on the newest one urged on them by its manufacturer. This is all very well in the sense that these drugs must have their trials, but why not perform those trials in a considered, unhurried and scientific manner? Whole wards in large institutions are being placed on a single drug, and then there quickly follows a breathless report transparently betraying its author's desire to get into print before the other fellow does. It would really be so much better if a third of the patients received one of the established drugs, a third the new drug and a third a placebo, the study being protracted and "double-blind" throughout. My friends assure me that this is difficult to accomplish, and I am sure they are correct. But why should it be easy, why just this, when truth is ground out so tediously in all other departments of life? Never has mankind verged so closely on disaster as now when the advances of science have placed in its hands all sorts of potent agents with which to disturb the internal and external economies. Such of these things as come within the medical province *must* be studied according to the rules—rules which require (a) the employment of an unprejudiced (because uninformed) personnel to make the objective determination, (b) adequate control and (c) a certain leisurely ease in the procedures. Some of the studies described in the following articles have been performed in this manner, but too few, and the situation is therefore a disquieting one.—Ed.

Effects of Analeptic and Depressant Drugs on Psychologic Behavior. G. T. Hauty and Robert B. Payne[9] (Randolph Air Force Base) investigated the effect on fatigue and proficiency of d-amphetamine, mephentermine, pipradol [Meratran®] and methyl-caffeine in normal, healthy young men. They were required to monitor several simulated aircraft indicators and to correct for random driftings by appropriate manipulation of simulated aircraft controls. Sustained alertness and continuous exercise of judgment were required.

In placebo and drug-free groups, deterioration of proficiency began during the 1st hour of this exacting work and was strikingly progressive. All analeptic preparations significantly postponed onset of deterioration, but the two most effective were mephentermine and d-amphetamine.

When the air breathed contained only 12% oxygen, the deterioration was even more marked, yet the deleterious effect of the hypoxia was completely counteracted by Dexedrine®. There was no demonstrable difference in performance of subjects taking Dexedrine between those breathing air containing 21% oxygen and those breathing 12% oxygen. This finding, plus reported electrophysiologic studies, suggests

(9) Am. J. Pub. Health 48:571-577, May, 1958.

that the characteristic ability of Dexedrine to sustain proficiency is almost wholly derived from enhancement of subcortical arousal activity and consequent maintenance of alertness.

d-Amphetamine clearly restored proficiency once it had deteriorated due to fatigue. Extent of restoration depended on dosage. A given dose increased proficiency by the same amount regardless of the level of decrement prevailing at the time the gain was induced.

A standard dose of Dexedrine intelligently administered to a normal, healthy person engaged at a task requiring vigilance and judgment will mitigate the degradation of proficiency resulting from prolonged work, with little likelihood of inducing extremes in emotional and attitudinal behavior.

Several of the most commonly used motion sickness preventives were given to a large population of Air Force personnel who were then subjected to various standardized tests, carefully controlled. The most profound adverse effects involved the higher intellectual processes. Adverse effects were least pronounced on processes requiring the least intellect, such as the perceptual motor type of task. Addition of 5 mg. d-amphetamine to a preparation of Benadryl®-hyoscine attenuated practically all the deleterious effect which Benadryl-hyoscine normally exerts on proficiency. Barring frank idiosyncrasy, the adverse drug effects could also be overcome by using technics or policies which increased and maintained worker motivation or by appropriate job-training programs.

Neuropharmacologic Agents in Rehabilitation of Patients with Chronic Mental Illness: Three-Year Clinical Evaluation is reported by John T. Ferguson[1] (Traverse City, Mich., State Hosp.). The biochemical processes by which these new compounds exert their peculiar effect on human behavior are as obscure as are the biochemical abnormalities at the root of the disease or group of diseases under treatment. This makes the evaluation of these drugs, on a strict comparison of percentages of mentally ill patients helped, almost analogous to what might have happened had the antibiotics been evaluated similarly in a group of febrile diseases of unknown etiology many years before the development of the science of bacteriology.

(1) J.A.M.A. 165:1677-1682, Nov. 30, 1957

Ferguson treated 1,003 psychiatric patients, aged 14-96, who had spent an average of 9 years in the hospital. Previously, their psychiatric treatment was custodial, supplemented by shock, sedation and seclusion. During the first 3 years of the program, 28 tranquilizers, 14 central stimulants or analeptics, 2 hallucinogens and 2 antihallucinogens were evaluated.

Six drugs were found sufficient to control, ameliorate or resolve the abnormal behavior manifestations of those chronic mentally ill patients who respond to chemotherapy. These drugs produced what may be called a "deep change" It is a change within the patient that enables him to respond to other therapeutic measures and participate in a rehabilitative program. Of the 6 drugs, reserpine (Serpasil®) and chlorpromazine (Thorazine®) hydrochloride, are psychosedatives, or true tranquilizers. They are of greatest value in treating overactivity and/or aggressiveness. Ectylurea (Nostyn®) and doxylamine succinate (in 100-mg. capsules and to be distinguished from the same compound, known as Decapryn®, available in tablets of 12.5 and 25 mg. for the treatment of allergic diseases) are neurosedatives or mild tranquilizers. These are of greatest value in treating tension and anxiety if minimal overactivity and/or aggressiveness are present. Ectylurea is the drug of choice for mildly disturbed ambulatory patients because of its low-sedative and high-hypnotic dosage range and its absence of untoward side effects. Doxylamine succinate is the best single drug for the confused, disoriented and mildly overactive elderly patient.

Since the behavior of patients is mixed, or more specifically, because their behavior is a combination of overactivity and underactivity, a central stimulant or analeptic is needed to not only handle the underactive behavior but also balance the psychosedatives and neurosedatives to produce an "active tranquility." Methylphenidylacetate (Ritalin®) hydrochloride is the author's drug of choice.

Azacyclonol (Frenquel®) proved to be the best antihallucinogen. In about 50% of the patients, clinical improvement in the delusional and/or hallucinatory pattern occurred within 5-45 days on oral therapy. Injectable solution may produce the same improvement within hours, after which the patient can be maintained by oral administration of azacyclonol tablets. Azacyclonol therapy, in most cases, requires the addition of a tranquilizer and/or an analeptic to control the patient's behavior.

By controlling the overactivity and aggressiveness of some patients and inducing a new interest in life in others, these drugs made it possible practically to eliminate the use of shock, sedation and seclusion. It thus became possible to channel the time of the hospital personnel into a more effective program of rehabilitation. Accidents to patients and personnel were reduced, the life span of the patients was extended and their well-being enhanced, and the destruction of furniture, fixtures, and clothing in certain wards was reduced to a tenth of what it was before.

Use of Sustained-Release Chlorpromazine in Management of Hospitalized Chronic Psychotic Patients. Recently a sustained release form of medication was introduced under the name Spansule®. The preparation consists of capsules containing hundreds of tiny pellets, about two thirds of which are coated with different thicknesses of a digestible material. From the uncoated pellets, the medication is readily assimilated to produce the initial therapeutic effect, whereas the coated ones disintegrate gradually in the process of digestion to release the medication continuously during 8-10 hours. The advantages are many: greater convenience in administration; avoidance of peak concentrations by providing a blood level plateau with better continuity of drug action; elimination and reduction of undesirable side effects resulting from peak concentrations after administration of drugs 3 or 4 times daily; avoidance of what is known as the "missing pill" and consequent exacerbation of symptoms; avoidance of rousing sleeping patients for medication; and alleviation, to some extent, of anxiety in tense pill-conscious patients.

John Vasconcellos and Albert A. Kurland[2] (Spring grove State Hosp., Baltimore) tried Thorazine® Spansule capsules on 36 chronic psychotic patients who had been on various dosages of Thorazine for several months or longer. In switching over to Spansule capsules, the Thorazine dosage was not changed. The initial dose ranged from 200 to 1,200 mg. administered in 1-6 of the 200 mg. Thorazine Spansule cap-

(2) Dis. Nerv. System 19:173-177, April, 1958.

sules given in 1 dose in the morning. If a patient's status appeared to have reached a plateau on regular medication, dosage was increased to determine whether further improvement could be obtained. In no case was the 1,200 mg.-exceeded. It was subsequently observed that after several weeks' treatment the dosage could be lowered in many patients who had started with 800-1,200 mg. At the end of 12 weeks, patients were again evaluated.

Of the 31 completing the course of Spansule medication, 5 were kept on the dosage level maintained for the multidosage medication. There were 11 patients whose dosages were decreased from the original level and 15 whose dosage requirements fluctuated due to changes in clinical course. In general, patients who had been reasonably well stabilized on regular medication could be maintained as well on Spansule capsules with about half the original dosage.

Skin rash developed in 2 patients but responded to Pyribenzamine®. In 1 whose normal blood pressure usually averaged 100/65, a marked hypotensive reaction developed after several weeks of relatively high dosage of Thorazine Spansule capsules (1,200 mg. daily) and treatment was discontinued. If a patient has a reaction that cannot be controlled within a comparatively short time, it may be necessary to wait until the medication has cleared the gastrointestinal tract. Some patients complained of drowsiness in the afternoon after taking a 600-1,000-mg. Thorazine Spansule capsule in 1 dose. This gradually disappeared, however, and no particular benefits were noted in dividing the number of capsules into 2 doses given morning and evening. In 4 patients, medication was discontinued when the white blood cell count fell below 5,000.

A survey of subjective impressions with respect to decreased number of drug administrations showed that most patients preferred receiving the Spansule form.

Treatment of Drug and Alcohol Withdrawal Effects with Thorazine® (Chlorpromazine) is discussed by Anthony A. Sainz[3] (Marcy, N. Y., State Hosp.) In acute alcohol intoxication, 100-200 mg., according to the patient's state, is administered by mouth and the dose is repeated once or twice at 3-hour intervals until confusion and agitation disappear or

(3) Psychiat. Quart. 31:275-284, 1957.

the patient goes to sleep. Un-co-operative patients and those with gastritis are given 50 mg. intramuscularly.

The acute intoxication stage is followed by true withdrawal symptoms, including irritability, tremulousness, mild depression, anxiety and insomnia. During this period chlorpromazine is most valuable and far superior to the usual sedatives. The optimum dose is usually about 50-100 mg. orally with meals and 100-300 mg. at bedtime. Chlorpromazine is used as an ego stabilizer and "psychic modifier" but is not used to the exclusion of needed ancillary measures such as maintenance of hydrostatic and electrolyte balances, and adequate diets and vitamin supplements.

Treatment of delirium tremens is similar to that of acute intoxication, but greater effort is required to maintain electrolyte, protein and vitamin balances and to prevent intercurrent infections, exhaustion and injuries from hyperkinesis. Of 56 patients treated with paraldehyde, Tolserol®, ACTH, Amytal® sodium and/or ether, several died and many failed to respond to a particular drug or combination of drugs. However, of 38 treated with chlorpromazine, all recovered, treatment averaging 3 days. The only side effect was benign, transient hypotension, which could be controlled by placing the patient in bed with the legs slightly elevated. The maximum oral doses required in delirium tremens were 200 mg. with meals and 600 mg. at bedtime, but many patients were controlled with smaller dosage. Un-co-operative patients with mild to moderate overactivity were given 50 mg. intramuscularly every 3-4 hours; those with severe excitement or impending exhaustion were given injections of 50 mg. hourly until they fell asleep.

Chlorpromazine is the drug of choice in cases of opiate withdrawal. In 16 patients who received a combination of chlorpromazine and "weaning" treatment, the dosage was started at 100 mg. orally every 4 hours round the clock. Opiates could be discontinued in 4 days without discomfort. Of 10 patients treated with chlorpromazine alone, 4 did not require further medication after the 1st week. Five patients required increases up to 250 mg. at 4-hour intervals but were able to discontinue all medication after 7 days. One patient required 400 mg. every 4 hours but for only 3 days. The only problem was constipation which required strong cathartics.

Definite conclusions concerning treatment of barbiturate withdrawal with chlorpromazine cannot be reached because of the few patients treated, but it seems that chlorpromazine is as effective as, or more effective than, any other method and much preferable to barbiturate "weaning."

Study of Photosensitivity Occurring with Chlorpromazine Therapy. John H. Epstein, Louis A. Brunsting, Magnus C. Petersen and Bert E. Schwarz[4] (Mayo Clinic and Found.) studied the effect of chlorpromazine therapy on the skin-erythema response to a "B" carbon arc exposure in 72 patients, mostly schizophrenics. Group A consisted of 58 patients with no history of previous chlorpromazine intake or no known reaction to the drug if they had taken it. Group B was made up of 14 patients with histories of possible previous cutaneous reactions to chlorpromazine. The eruption in 2 appeared to have been induced by exposure to sun. Each patient was given an average minimal erythema dose to an area on the back from a "B" carbon arc source. A comparable site also was exposed for 5 minutes, from the same distance, through a "7740" Corning glass filter which absorbs almost all the effective erythemogenic ultraviolet rays shorter than 3,100 A.

Abnormal reactions to the "B" carbon exposures while taking chlorpromazine were observed in 8 patients in group A; 1 patient in group B showed an increased response to the carbon arc exposure only while not taking the medication. These reactions appeared to be exaggerations of the normal sunburn response. No reactions other than those attributed to heat occurred in any patient when the erythemogenic ultraviolet rays were absorbed by the "7740" Corning glass filter.

A 1% solution of chlorpromazine hydrochloride, examined spectrophotometrically, showed complete absorption of the wave-lengths between 2,000 and 3,700 A. Thus the absorption pattern of the drug included the ultraviolet rays shorter than 3,100 A.

Examinations of the urine of 19 patients revealed no abnormal porphyrins. No subject showed clinical evidence of hepatic dysfunction or porphyria. Dermatitis medicamentosa of a maculopapular, urticarial type occurred in about 10% of

(4) J. Invest. Dermat. 28:329-338, May, 1957.

the subjects. In 2, these reactions were apparently precipitated by exposure to natural sunlight.

Effects of Oral Sex Hormones and Reserpine in Elderly Men were assessed in a double-blind experiment reported by Raymond Harris[5] (Ann Lee Home, Albany, N. Y.). Examinations were made before the study, during the initial period of placebo administration, during and after therapy with placebo, placebo plus reserpine, Femandren® plus reserpine, and Femandren plus placebo. Oral treatment consisted of two apparently identical tablets a day. Patients included 40 men, aged 59-87, with chronic geriatric conditions.

Improvement was noted in 75% of 12 patients receiving the combined androgen-estrogen (Femandren) and reserpine therapy and in 72% of 8 on hormones alone, judged by strength and well-being. Weight gain was experienced by more patients on the combined therapy.

No adverse effects on cardiovascular conditions, even when pre-existing, were observed with the combined treatment, and only 1 patient on Femandren alone became worse in this respect during the experiment.

Of 7 patients in the combined therapy group who had osteoporosis before treatment, 3 improved, judged by comparison of x-ray pictures. One of 14 in the Femandren group showed similar decreased osteoporosis.

Judging by the appearance of slight gynecomastia in a few patients and of an enlarged prostate in a few others, the dosage, adequate for most, may have been excessive in some and insufficient in others. It should be adjusted to the individual patient. Hormone replacement therapy by the oral route proved satisfactory in a significant number of the older men.

Allergic Reactions to Tranquilizing Drugs are discussed by Leo E. Hollister[6] (VA Hosp., Palo Alto, Calif.). Tranquilizing drugs which may act as allergens are classified as: (1) phenothiazine derivatives (Thorazine®, Sparine®, Vesprin®, Pacatal®, Compazine® and Trilafon®); (2) rauwolfia alkaloids, notably reserpine and (3) substituted propanediols or butanediols, notably meprobamate. In the first and third classes, the major complications encountered are due to allergic reactions.

(5) J. Am. Geriatrics Soc. 6:297-305, April, 1958.
(6) Ann. Int. Med. 49:17-29, July, 1958.

Sensitivity to chlorpromazine may be manifested by agranulocytosis, jaundice, dermatitis and other minor reactions. Strong circumstantial evidence suggests that agranulocytosis from chlorpromazine is of immunologic origin, though this has not been proved. Chlorpromazine jaundice has been reproduced often enough by the challenge test to implicate drug allergy as the mechanism.

In evaluating claims that new phenothiazine derivatives may produce less jaundice or agranulocytosis than does chlorpromazine, the time relation of these complications to treatment should be considered. Statements as to prevalence of jaundice can be made with certainty only in patients treated for at least 5 weeks. In agranulocytosis, at least 3 months' treatment is necessary before it can be assumed that this complication would not otherwise have appeared. At present, introduction of the piperazine ring into the structure of these drugs (Compazine, Trilafon) appears to increase their therapeutic potency and decrease their allergenic potential.

Reserpine barely qualifies as an allergen on the basis of the comparatively few reports of reactions. It does appear to have the potential of producing immunologic thrombocytopenia, like quinidine, Sedormid® and some sulfonamides. Aggravation of such allergic disorders as chronic urticaria, bronchial asthma or atopic rhinitis may be expected from the parasympathomimetic action of the drug.

Meprobamate sensitivity is manifested by fever, skin rashes and constitutional signs, including vascular collapse. This sensitivity is peculiar in that it commonly is produced by the initial dose of drug, implying that the carbamate groups of the meprobamate molecule determine this type of sensitivity.

Unexpected Asphyxial Death and Tranquilizing Drugs. Leo E. Hollister[7] (VA Hosp., Palo Alto, Calif.) reviewed all unexpected asphyxial deaths at a 1,325-bed neuropsychiatric hospital in the past 6½ years. Only those cases were included in which the mode of death or its time was not expected. The midpoint of the series, 1954, was the year in which tranquilizing drugs were started in many patients.

This type of death was no more common during the period of tranquilizing drug therapy than before. There was a high

(7) Am. J. Psychiat. 114:366-367, October, 1957.

incidence of asphyxial death in patients with brain damage, particularly those with convulsive disorders. Such an association of brain damage and unexpected asphyxial death was clearly present before tranquilizing drugs were used.

Of the 3 patients who died while on tranquilizing drugs, only 2 deaths raised the possibility of these drugs being contributory. One man, 66, a syphilitic, had had many near-fatal aspirations before taking proclorperazine. A man, 43, appeared to have drowned during a convulsion while swimming. He had been receiving chlorpromazine without any previously noted increase in seizure frequency. A woman, 34, had been on intensive chlorpromazine therapy. The day before death she had a seizure (though she had others recorded before receiving chlorpromazine) and was placed on anticonvulsants. Next day she was found dead less than 1 hour after the evening meal. Though food particles were present in the trachea, the amount was insufficient to have caused major obstruction. Death was attributed to glottal spasm from a seizure and irritation from aspirated food.

The risk of using tranquilizing drugs may be increased in brain-damaged patients or in those with known seizures. This increased risk should be measured against the potential benefit from the drug.

Convulsions Complicating Ataractic Therapy: Their Incidence and Theoretical Implications are discussed by Leon D. Hankoff, Harvey E. Kaye, David M. Engelhardt and Norbert Freedman[8] (State Univ. of New York, New York City). Clinical observations and experimental findings suggest that the initiation or increase of convulsive activity is a significant complication of therapy with the current ataractic drugs. The neurophysiologic and clinical action of ataractic drugs suggests both sedating and activating qualities. Though clinically these drugs produce a tranquilizing and an attenuated hypnotic effect, they lack anticonvulsant properties; in fact, they facilitate or produce seizures. Promazine induces an appreciable incidence of convulsions, suggesting epileptogenic properties inherent in the drug. Convulsions with ataraxics seem to be directly related to the drugs' action on the central nervous system and not to be secondary to orthostatic hypotension.

(8) New York J. Med. 57:2967-2972, Sept. 15, 1957.

The possibility of convulsions must be considered, especially in patients with a history of brain damage or previous convulsions. It is probably advisable to use small doses of barbiturates or anticonvulsants in the early days of treatment, which seems to be the danger period with chlorpromazine and promazine. If large doses are used, the dosage should probably be built up gradually. Reserpine, chlorpromazine and promazine do not have primary anticonvulsant properties. When used for epileptics, the existing regimen of anticonvulsants should not be radically changed. However, some reduction of barbiturates may be necessary, because of the sedative potentiation of the ataraxics. During ataractic therapy central nervous system stimulants should be avoided when treating the syncope due to orthostatic hypotension. Chemical activation of the EEG in the presence of ataraxics should be done with caution.

The seizure activity observed both in ataractic and shock therapies may be related to a common physiologic process leading to clinical improvement.

Psychomotility and Parkinsonism in Treatment with Neuroleptic Drugs were studied by F. A. Freyhan[9] (Univ. of Pennsylvania). Chlorpromazine and reserpine are most effective in treating psychiatric disorders which have in common hypermotility, hypernormal initiative and increased affective tension. Both drugs inhibit psychomotor activity in a manner which involves changes in the functional balance of the extrapyramidal motor system. If pronounced, these changes are associated with a clinical picture of parkinsonism.

A 2-year study of 653 psychiatric patients under treatment with chlorpromazine and reserpine revealed the incidence of parkinsonism to be 10.7 and 16.9%, respectively. Diagnosis, age, duration of treatment and total dosage showed no correlation with parkinsonism. The incidence of parkinsonism was twice as high in women, regardless of which drug was used. No explanation can be offered at present.

Parkinsonism recurs in certain patients during each course of therapy with chlorpromazine and reserpine, given singly or interchangeably. Such recurrence devaluates further the assumption of a toxic reaction, since it eliminates desensiti-

(9) A.M.A. Arch. Neurol. & Psychiat. 78:465-472, November, 1957.

zation, which plays a significant part in jaundice and skin reactions. Moreover, antiparkinsonian drugs, of which procyclidine hydrochloride is especially effective, ameliorate tremors and rigidity successfully. Therefore, a polarity of pharmacologic action between the neuroleptic and antiparkinsonian agents is postulated.

Several patients had multiple evidences of familial mental and nervous diseases. In at least 2 and probably 3 instances, the patient had a parent with paralysis agitans. Several patients had previously had traumatic, toxic or infectious encephalopathies. Personal psychomotor patterns, in the sense of a consitutional extrapyramidal endowment, may exert a predisposing influence. It is conceivable that there are individual differences in the manner in which cortical and subcortical motor systems are functionally integrated. The qualitative or quantitative representation of component systems would then account for the continuum of normal to abnormal psychomotor patterns. Such elements of individuality must be considered in the experimental search for neurophysiologic causes of drug parkinsonism.

Breast Changes in Male and Female with Chlorpromazine or Reserpine Therapy. Bruce Robinson[1] (Univ. of Melbourne) observed breast enlargement in both sexes and secretion of a milklike fluid in women during chlorpromazine or reserpine therapy. Among 66 women receiving chlorpromazine, a milklike fluid could be expressed from the breasts of 7. Of 26 on reserpine, 2 had such fluid. All patients who lactated were below age 42, and all were receiving large doses of chlorpromazine or reserpine. The complication is, therefore, most likely to be seen in severely disturbed, young, psychotic women. The changes are not related to parity. The secretion had features of both milk and colostrum; the urine did not contain lactose. Gynecomastia was seen in a man, 56, after 9 months of reserpine treatment.

The mode of action of chlorpromazine or reserpine is not clearly known, but certain effects of both are presumed to be mediated through the hypothalamus. Thus both indirectly could affect the adenohypophysis, which could initiate the breast changes. Possibly, chlorpromazine and reserpine can themselves act as hormones and directly affect the breast.

(1) M. J. Australia 2:239-241, Aug. 17, 1957.

Promazine Treatment of Chronic Psychoses in 100 Hospitalized Patients, aged 20-76, is reported by Marie Kershaw Frain[2] (Bryce Hosp., Tuscaloosa, Ala.). Patients were not selected or grouped in any way. The sole criterion for medication need was the presence of abnormal attitudes or conduct, such as hostility, resistiveness and un-co-operativeness; untidy habits and neglect of personal appearance; overactiveness, noisiness and overtalkativeness; negativistic, combative, destructive or denudative behavior; idleness and inertia; or severe delusions or hallucinations. Previously, 71 had received electric shock therapy and 67 had been treated with reserpine. Among the latter patients, the behavior of 66% had been favorably altered. Promazine (Sparine®) was begun with 25-50 mg., 2-3 times/day, and was increased or adjusted as necessary. In about 90%, medication was given for 6 months.

Promazine was directly responsible for improvement in 83%, of whom 9 were furloughed; 17% were not benefited. Of those who had been treated with reserpine, 96% responded as well or, in most cases, better to promazine. Of the entire series, 63% gained weight. Side effects were remarkably few, consisting mainly of drowsiness. A mild blush or rash appeared over the face, neck, arms and upper trunk in 2 patients. This cleared in 48 hours and ataractic medication was not interrupted. A maximum daily dose of 800 mg. is recommended.

Treatment of Chronic Schizophrenia with Promazine Hydrochloride. John Paul Sibilio, Gwen Andrew, Dorothy Dart, Kenneth B. Moore and Vernon A. Stehman,[3] divided 93 women with chronic schizophrenia into three matched groups and assigned them to different treatment schedules —promazine, placebo and no treatment (basic design)—for 28 days. The basic design was extended to form six matched groups and each was given a different treatment schedule using promazine hydrochloride (Sparine®). The experiment lasted 4 months. Nine measures of adjustment were obtained, using the Gardner Behavior Chart. Besides a prestudy measure, ratings were made on the 7th and 28th days of the 4 consecutive months.

(2) J. Nerv. & Ment. Dis. 125:529-533, Oct.-Dec., 1957.
(3) A.M.A. Arch. Neurol. & Psychiat. 78:419-424, October, 1957.

During the 1st month, in carrying out the basic design, promazine was given orally, in capsule form, 4 times daily. All patients were started on a daily dose of 150 mg. On the 3d day, this was increased to 300 mg. and on the 6th, to 600 mg. On the 15th day, the dose was increased or decreased, depending on the requirements and tolerance level of each patient, as determined by the clinical impression. Most patients were maintained on 900 mg., which was increased to 1,200 mg. on the 3d day. The maintenance dose was 400-1,400 mg.

In general, there were no behavioral changes which could be associated with administration of promazine or a placebo or with no treatment. No difference as to amount and frequency of dosage was noted between regular and irregular patterns of administering medication.

Delirium Tremens: Reduction of Mortality and Morbidity with Promazine. Francesco A. Figurelli[4] (Med. Center, Jersey City) treated 180 patients for fully developed delirium tremens. All were actively drinking until hospitalization; 96% were hospitalized while in delirium; 4% went to delirium 1-48 hours later. The first 434 were treated by conventional methods. Their delirium averaged about 7 days and hospitalization 2-4 weeks.

Subsequent patients without complications were treated by complete withdrawal of alcohol and the administration of promazine hydrochloride. Experience led to a program consisting of an initial intramuscular injection of 200 or 300 mg., a second injection of 100 mg. within 4 hours or less and oral administration of 100 mg. 4 times daily for maintenance.

The death rate with conventional treatment was 10%. The over-all mortality with promazine treatment, both oral and parenteral in all dosages, was 4.5%. After the practice was started of giving larger parenteral doses initially and larger oral maintenance doses, the mortality fell to 0.6%. Among the last 87 patients there were no deaths.

Many patients recovered from delirium tremens in the first 24 hours, most of them in 48 hours. Seven in whom delirium had cleared in the first 24 hours relapsed on the 2d to 4th day.

No precipitous drop in blood pressure nor orthostatic hy-

(4) J.A.M.A. 166:747-750, Feb. 15, 1958.

potension, which had been a problem with chlorpromazine, were encountered. Nausea and vomiting were eliminated; thus pulmonary complications were reduced. Hepatic coma did not develop during the course of medication, despite the severe cirrhosis present in many patients. Gastrointestinal disturbances did not recur after initial control of vomiting, which was acute in several on admission. All were able to start eating as soon as their confusion cleared.

Promazine and Azacyclonol in Treatment of Chronic Psychotics: Clinical Note. A. J. Graffeo[5] (State Hosp., Rochester, N. Y.) treated 22 patients, aged 25-61 (average age 44), for 9 months. Each was unpredictable in behavior, often upset, irritable, agitated, restive, resentful, antagonistic and each had hallucinations and/or delusions. Duration of illness was 2-27 (average 16) years.

The study was divided into five phases. (1) Azacyclonol, 20 mg. 3 times daily, was given for 7 weeks. Response was minimal. (2) Azacyclonol was abruptly withdrawn and promazine hydrochloride, 100 mg. 3 times daily, was substituted. Behavior began to improve. After 5½ weeks of daily promazine, the dose was increased to 200 mg. 3 times daily. Psychic tension and stress were largely relieved without evidence of central nervous system depression. (3) For 46 days no drug was administered and 15 of the 22 patients lapsed into their original state, whereas 6 remained quiet and improved. (4) During the final 16 days of the control period, lactose tablets were given 3 times daily as a placebo. No improvement was noted. (5) Promazine therapy, 200 mg. 3 times daily, was resumed in the 16 who had regressed when the drug was stopped. Behavior began to improve within 48 hours. Improvement has persisted and several patients have continued to show progress at this dose level.

Promazine substantially improved the behavior in 19 of 22 patients treated. They became more co-operative, less restless and less destructive. They remained alert and responded to questions. Psychotic trends were less pronounced. Patients showed more interest in individual and group psychotherapy. No blood dyscrasia was observed in any patient. No complications or side effects were noted after more than 9 months of therapy.

(5) New York J. Med. 58:2056-2057, June 15, 1958.

Comparative Study of Promazine and Chlorpromazine for Hospital Management of overactive, disturbed psychotic patients was made by Ralph H. Archer[6] (Mayview, Pa., State Hosp.). The investigation, extending over 10 weeks, included 40 patients (average age 40), who previously had benefited from chlorpromazine.

The series was divided into two groups: 20 patients (controls) were continued on chlorpromazine in the dosage previously given and 20 were transferred to promazine (Sparine®). The total daily dose of either drug, averaging 300-400 mg., was increased or reduced according to the response of the patient; it never exceeded 800 mg.

Observations were made by lay attendants working under the supervision of scientifically trained personnel. The patients were evaluated, in three periods of 4, 4, and 2 weeks, respectively, for activity range, ward relationships and side effects. There was no measurement of psychiatric improvement.

Results showed no important differences in the usefulness of the two drugs. Although variations in performance tended to occur, these seemed to offset each other. The chief difference between the drugs was in the incidence of adverse side effects. In patients receiving chlorpromazine, these effects occurred first in 20%; later when the dosage was reduced, the incidence decreased to 10%, but management difficulties recurred. The promazine-treated patients experienced no side effects.

Agranulocytosis Associated with Promazine Administration: Report of Three Cases. According to Gerald L. Glaser and Donald A. Adams[7] (Univ. of Rochester), the incidence of agranulocytosis following chlorpromazine administration is estimated at less than 0.3%. Promazine differs structurally from chlorpromazine only in the absence of a chloride radical in the 2-position of the phenothiazine ring. Reports of complications associated with promazine began to appear only recently.

The authors studied 2 women and 1 man with these complications.

Case 1.—Woman, aged 73, received 6.5 Gm. promazine in 42 days.

(6) Pennsylvania M. J. 60:1343-1345, October, 1957.
(7) Ann. Int. Med. 48:372-379, February, 1958.

No other medication described as associated with agranulocytosis was taken and the leukocyte response was prompt on withdrawal of the promazine. The marked eosinophilia which developed during the recovery phase may be evidence to support a hypersensitivity mechanism or may possibly be an unusual recovery response of this patient's marrow to insult. Mild jaundice was also present.

Case 2.—Woman, 74, who had known allergies, took promazine intermittently for 7 months. Besides she took a small daily dose of glutethimide (Doriden®) for a month. The bone marrow lacked all myeloid elements. The immediate cause of her death was a sudden generalized monilial infection occurring after several days' therapy with penicillin, broad-spectrum antibiotics and prednisone.

Case 3.—Man, 58, received 2.75 Gm. promazine for 31 days and 0.2 Gm. chlorpromazine was given just before onset of symptoms leading to his second hospitalization. Promazine was thought to be the principal offender though chlorpromazine might have contributed.

Possible etiologic mechanisms may be of the immunoallergic variety, or may encompass a direct toxic effect on the marrow.

Comparative Study of Four Tranquilizing Agents, Phenobarbital and Inert Placebo was made by John H. Moyer, Keith Pevey, Charles H. Heider and Vernon Kinross-Wright[8] (Baylor Univ.) on 63 patients with nervousness, tension, anxiety, insomnia and various somatic disorders indicative of psychoneuroses. No psychotic patients were included. For comparison, 40 similar patients received placebo.

Regardless of diagnosis or symptoms, the patients received a course of meprobamate (Equanil®), phenaglycodol (Ultran), benactyzine (Suavitil®), a benactyzine-related compound (CT-840) or phenobarbital in random manner. Some received an experimental drug initially, whereas others received the phenobarbital placebo initially. The "active" placebo (30 mg. phenobarbital in an identical capsule) was given 4 times daily in an attempt to standardize the placebo response. One fifth of the patients received two or more active drugs to determine the relative efficacy of different drugs in the same patient. Minimal psychotherapy was extended.

Therapy lasted from 2 to 16 weeks with total daily dosages of 800-2,400 mg. meprobamate, 600-1,600 mg. phenaglycodol and 3-8 mg. benactyzine and its related compound.

All the tranquilizers used are clinically comparable, with each eliciting improvement in about two-thirds the patients treated. Incidence of side effects is less with meprobamate

(8) Geriatrics 13:153-170, March, 1958.

than with the other agents, although benactyzine in low doses also produces a low incidence of side effects at the expense of reduced therapeutic value (Fig. 32, *A* and *B*).

Phenobarbital was equally effective in one-half the patients who responded to meprobamate and in about one third of all patients treated. This is of particular importance, since it has been used for many years, and it is not likely that any

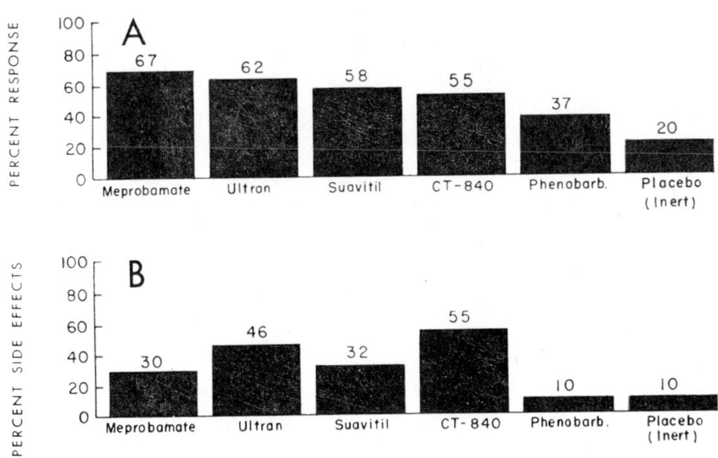

Fig. 32.—*A*, comparison of various ataraxic agents with phenobarbital and inert placebo, using objective criteria for estimating beneficial effects. *B*, incidence of side effects as compared to phenobarbital and inert placebo. (Courtesy of Moyer, J. H., *et al.*: Geriatrics 13:153-170, March, 1958.)

new serious, untoward effects of this drug will be forthcoming. In contrast, the newer and experimental neurosedatives have been tried for fairly short periods. It must also be kept in mind that relatively small doses of phenobarbital were used.

Results of Treatment of Psychotic States with Newer Phenothiazine Compounds Effective in Small Doses. Douglas Goldman[9] (Longview State Hosp., Cincinnati) investigated four phenothiazine compounds, related to chlorpromazine, in the treatment of a group of patients with chronic psychosis who were confined to a mental hospital. Compazine® (proclorperazine) was given to 667 patients, Trilafon® to 206, Vesprin® to 176 and Winthrop 13,645-5 to 94. Most patients

(9) Am. J. M. Sc. 235-67-77, January, 1958.

received less than the following amounts per day: Compazine, 150 mg.; Trilafon, 65 mg.; Vesprin, 300 mg.; and Winthrop 13,645-5, 150 mg.

The chief differences between these compounds and phenothiazine derivatives, such as chlorpromazine, promazine and mepazine are (1) more intense pharmacologic and therapeutic activity and thus smaller dosage level and (2) fewer side effects and toxic complications. Jaundice and agranulocytosis were not seen. There was little or no sedation. Side effects were allergy-like manifestations, "trophic" and endocrine effects, and neurologic disorders. The chief neurologic effect, parkinsonism, is often (but not always) an accompaniment of psychotherapy and should be managed by regulating dosage and using Cogentin® along with the active drug.

The drugs used were particularly effective in treating schizophrenia, manic-depressive psychoses in the manic group, and synergistically with electric shock in the depressed group, also organic delirium.

Compazine and Trilafon are in many respects similar in their general clinical effect, except that Compazine tends to be somewhat more stimulating. Trilafon when first used occasionally produces somnolence of minor degree that is rare with Compazine. Both produce "turbulence" at times, but this is more often clinically important with Compazine. Parkinsonism can be produced by smaller doses and apparently more quickly with Trilafon than with Compazine. The effectiveness of the two drugs in treating psychotic symptoms is at present not clearly distinguishable.

Vesprin seems to be much milder in producing side effects than either Compazine or Trilafon. Winthrop 13,645-5 is extremely effective and has a marked tendency to allay psychotic manifestations without actually influencing the level of consciousness. It is the only drug which produces hypotension similar to that produced by chlorpromazine.

Proclorperazine in Hospitalized and Private Psychiatric Patients. Frank Wilcox[1] (Oregon State Hosp.) tried proclorperazine (Compazine®) in 109 patients, including acute and chronic psychotics, psychoneurotics, patients with tension states and children with behavior problems. The psychotics were assaultive, denudative, overactive, deluded, con-

(1) Dis. Nerv. System 19:118-121, March, 1958.

fused, and generally speaking, difficult management problems. The psychoneurotics manifested a mounting uneasiness of mind, heightened tension and many somatic complaints, including headache, insomnia, vertigo, gastrointestinal disorders, eczema, asthma and various allergies. The group was about evenly divided between men and women, aged 12-100; most were between 30 and 50. Duration of illness ranged from several months to 15 years or more in the psychotics and from 1 month to 5 years in the psychoneurotics and children. About half the group, chiefly the chronic psychotics, had been treated previously with sedatives, other neuroleptic agents and electroconvulsive therapy, but failed to show or maintain any appreciable improvement.

Most patients were started on oral medication, 10 mg., at meals and at bedtime. Dosage was increased gradually in increments of 10-20 mg. every other day until clinical improvement resulted or bothersome side effects supervened. When rapid control of agitation and excitement was necessary, proclorperazine was given intramuscularly, 10-20 mg., repeated every 3-4 hours, as necessary. Although dosages as high as 300 mg. were given, the usual oral maintenance dosage was 75-150 mg. for psychotics and 30-75 mg. for psychoneurotics. As a matter of convenience, patients once stabilized on proclorperazine were given the drug in sustained release capsule form.

During an 8-month study period, proclorperazine controlled psychotic manifestations of severely disturbed patients and reduced mounting tension and anxiety of psychoneurotic patients. No untoward reactions of jaundice, agranulocytosis or hypotension attributable to the drug were observed. Combined use with electroconvulsive therapy appeared safe as well as beneficial to relieve agitation and excitement. Extrapyramidal symptoms, such as tremulousness, drooling and masked facies, occurred in excited psychotics on high dosages (100-300 mg.); anti-parkinsonian agents given concomitantly or reducing dosage usually provided relief. In lower dosages, given ambulatory patients, drowsy side effects were absent; in fact, a few patients appeared stimulated on taking proclorperazine. Use of the drug in sustained release Spansule® form provided, with 1 capsule, a therapeutic effect lasting about 12 hours.

Treatment of Anxiety and Agitation with Proclorperazine in Geriatric Patients. Edward Settel[2] (Forest Hills, N. Y., Nursing and Rehabilitation Center) administered proclorperazine (Compazine®) to 70 agitated geriatric patients, 47 of whom were under custodial care in a nursing home and 23 of whom were in their homes. The over-all effectiveness was 77%. The optimum dosage was 5-10 mg., 3-4 times daily.

Results were most outstanding in mild to moderately severe senile agitation; 91.6% of the patients in the institutional group and 83% in the home group were benefited. Among the 23 nursing home patients classified as having severe agitation bordering on psychosis, only 56.5% showed improvement.

Mild side effects appeared in 7 patients. There was transient drowsiness in 4, in 3 of whom it disappeared after the 4th day of treatment. The 4th patient was receiving 10 mg. 3 times daily and his tendency to sleep was overcome by reducing the dosage to 5 mg. 3 times daily. Two patients had vertigo; 1 was relieved by reducing each dose from 10 to 5 mg.; the other case was mild and transient. There was no evidence of mouth dryness, blurred vision, hypotension or bradycardia on either the 5- or 10-mg. dosage schedule. Transient pruritus, subsiding after the 4th day, was reported by 1 patient. In 1 case of accidental overdosage, there was evidence of a mild extrapyramidal effect, notably muscular disco-ordination, which promptly disappeared on reduction of the dosage to the usual level.

Proclorperazine appears to be a safe and effective therapeutic agent for the relief of geriatric agitation, whether from a primary emotional source or secondary to somatic disease.

Clinical Trial with Hydroxyzine (Atarax®) on Group of Maladjusted Educationally Subnormal Children was conducted by Leslie J. Segal and A. E. Tansley[3] (St. Francis Residential Special School, Birmingham, England). Rats receiving Atarax became quiet but retain their usual agility and alertness and respond to the threat of danger by flight. It has been suggested that the drug acts by depressing the reticular formation of the brain stem.

A clinical trial was carried out on 16 matched pairs of edu-

(2) J. Am. Geriatrics Soc. 5:827-831, October, 1957.
(3) J. Ment. Sc. 103:677-681, July, 1957.

cationally subnormal children who were maladjusted and under-functioning. One of each pair was given 10 mg. Atarax after breakfast and 10 mg. after luncheon. The other of each pair was given a dummy tablet in appearance similar to the drug. This was continued for 3 weeks. At the end all the children were given dummy tablets for 2 weeks, after which Atarax and dummy tablets were given as in the first period for another 3 weeks.

All children in both experimental and control groups were rated by the class teachers on 5-point rating scales for activity, application and progress in the basic subjects. In deciding whether or not a child had improved, both his behavior in class and performance in basic subjects were considered. The teachers were asked to say which of the 32 children were receiving treatment. They were aware that 16 matched pairs had been selected, but did not know which children had been matched or were receiving treatment. The results are shown in table.

TEACHERS' CLASSIFICATION OF CHILDREN IN STUDY GROUP

	ON TREATMENT	CONTROLS
Absolutely sure receiving treatment	4	—
Reasonably sure receiving treatment	10	2
Unable to decide	—	2
Reasonably sure *not* receiving treatment	2	8
Absolutely sure *not* receiving treatment	—	4

At the end of the trial, before the identity of the matched pairs was disclosed, all 32 children were case-conferenced to ascertain changes in behavior and school progress. Of those on treatment, 14 showed improvement in both behavior and school progress and in 2 there was no change. Among the controls, 2 showed improvement and 14 no change.

Periodic white cell and differential counts did not reveal a degree of leukopenia or granulopenia warranting interference with treatment. A transient eosinophilia and monocytosis cleared quickly.

Clinical Investigation of Pacatal® in Open Psychiatric Settings is reported by G. J. Sarwer-Foner and E. K. Koranyi[4] (Montreal). Pacatal is a substituted phenothiazine compound and has both parasympatholytic and sympatholytic actions, with the former predominating, thus producing

(4) Canad. M. A. J. 77:450-459, Sept. 1, 1957.

a marked atropine-like effect. The drug was given to 42 patients. It was the only variable introduced into an otherwise formalized psychotherapy technic. The patients were selected because of marked disorders of affect irrespective of diagnosis. Administration was oral or intramuscular. Dosage range was 100-800 mg. 4 times daily. Treatment lasted 3-164 days.

A good result on affect was shown by 34 patients, a poor result by 8. Subjectively, 33 patients felt they were helped by the drug. The main changes produced on the target symptoms were reduction in energy output and motor activity (27 patients), reduction in anxiety (26), improvement in sleep (27) and better appetite (15). Fifteen patients stated they felt more relaxed and calmed. Agitation was controlled in 7, and 4 showed alleviation of depressive symptoms. Seven lost their tremor and shakes. Two patients' asthma attacks were markedly reduced.

The commonest side effects were dry mouth (21 patients), dry throat (16), sore throat (7), blurred vision (12), constipation (8), stomach upset—heartburn, burning, dyspepsia—(10), vomiting (2) and nausea (1). No significant changes in pulse, blood pressure, respiration or laboratory screening tests were found.

Fatal Agranulocytosis during Treatment with Pacatal® is rare, but should be considered a possibility in view of a case reported by Paul E. Feldman, James Bertone and Hildegart Panthel[5] (Topeka State Hosp.).

Woman, 73, was admitted as a catatonic schizophrenic and was hospitalized for 12 years. After this period, stasis edema and dermatitis of the lower extremities developed and was relieved by digitoxin, an elastic bandage and lanolin ointment. Digitoxin was discontinued 4 months before Pacatal, 100 mg. twice daily, was prescribed for hyperactivity and combativeness. The patient improved and blood studies after a month were normal.

Three weeks later, the patient had fever and appeared acutely ill. The skin and mouth were dry, the mucous membranes and nail beds pale and the pharynx swollen and covered with a thick yellow exudate. Pulse was 110, blood pressure 120/70, respirations 24, rales were absent and breath sounds diminished. The abdomen was distended, tympanic and tender on deep palpation. There was no adenopathy or neurologic abnormality. Blood study showed 3,760,000 red

(5) Am. J. Psychiat. 113:842-843, March, 1957.

cells and 350 white cells with 96% lymphocytes and 4% basophils. Hematocrit was 36, sedimentation rate 42 mm., nonprotein nitrogen 37 mg./100 ml. and blood sugar 107 mg./100 ml. Three days later, the white cell count had risen to 550 with 97% lymphocytes, 2% basophils and 1% monocytes. After 2 more days the count was 180 with 98% lymphocytes and 2% monocytes. The patient died the next day. Autopsy revealed bilateral bronchopneumonia, pleural effusion, fibrous pleurisy, gastric and colon ulceration and agranulocytosis.

The findings resemble those noted in 0.067% of patients treated with chlorpromazine, as reported by Pollack. If biweekly blood studies are not feasible, fever, sore throat or lesions of mucous membrane in patients receiving such drugs should be treated as agranulocytosis until such diagnosis can be excluded.

Therapeutic Trial of Azacyclonol (Frenquel®) was carried out by S. Gray and A. D. Forrest[6] (Royal Edinburgh Hosp. for Mental and Nervous Disorders) on 56 patients with schizophrenia and 2 with alcoholic hallucinatory states.

A controlled trial was conducted on 40 patients (four groups of 10 each) with schizophrenia who appeared to have hallucinations. Azacyclonol (20 mg.) and placebo tablets

CONTROLLED TRIAL (40 PATIENTS)

Treatment	No. of Patients	No Change	Improved	Worse	Total
Azacyclonol ..	30	19 (63·4%)	10 (33·3%)	1 (3·3%)	30
Placebo	30	15 (50%)	14 (47·7%)	1 (3·3%)	30
Total ..	60	34 (56·7%)	24 (40%)	2 (3·3%)	60

$\chi^2 = 0{\cdot}556$. $P < 0{\cdot}5 > 0{\cdot}2$.

were put into bottles labeled A and B. Group 1 had 5 weeks on A, then 5 weeks on B. Group 2 went through the reverse sequence. Group 3 had tablet A and group 4 had tablet B for the whole 10 weeks. The dose was 1 tablet 3 times a day. The results (table) suggest that azacyclonol is not of great value in treating this type of patient.

Four patients were studied outside the controlled trial. They were kept in bed and given azacyclonol, 60 mg. daily. Temperature, pulse, blood pressure, liver function, blood urea nitrogen, white blood cell count, fluid intake and output and possible skin rash were investigated.

(6) Brit. M. J. 1:374-377, Feb. 15, 1958.

Subsequently, in a clinical trial, 18 more patients were treated with azacyclonol for 4-12 weeks. The dosage varied from 60 to 180 mg. daily. The diagnoses were schizophrenia (16 patients) and alcoholic hallucinatory states (2 patients). In these patients, the illness was of more recent onset than in those involved in the controlled trial. Results showed that 13 patients improved, 6 sufficiently to leave the hospital.

It is felt that azacyclonol has a central stimulant action and that part of the poor result of the drug in the controlled trial was due to the masking effects of excitement and overactivity. The only toxic effect observed was a rise of blood urea nitrogen in 2 of the 4 patients. In 1, the elevation was insignificant; in the other, evidence of chronic nephritis was later established.

Treatment of Acute Complications of Chronic Alcoholism: Use of Azacyclonol (Frenquel®) Hydrochloride in 100 Consecutive Cases is reported by Julius C. Travis[7] (San Francisco). Of the 100 patients treated with this antihallucinatory drug, 57 were considered recovered and 27 improved, a total of 84. At the time of assay, 51 were again employed. However, it is assumed that more would be employed if a later assay had been done. Only 6 patients were sent to the hospital. Six discontinued treatment and 4 were unimproved. Most patients in the latter three groups continued to drink and were thus unchanged or worse after initiation of treatment. No patient was considered to have been made worse by treatment. Of the 75 who had hallucinations, 60 (80%) recovered quickly and 8 (11%) were improved (total 91%).

The drug was given primarily by mouth in a dose of one 100-mg. tablet 4 times daily, besides the medication usually given patients who are psychologically and biologically in extremis. Duration of administration as determined by recovery from symptoms was generally less than 4 days.

Azacyclonol is of considerable help in treatment of such chronic alcoholics in any situation, primarily through shortening the recovery period and making it tolerable. Azacyclonol injected intravenously reduces fear and anxiety immediately by halting the hallucinatory images or sensations; orally it achieves the same result in a similar but slower fashion.

(7) J.A.M.A. 167:156-159, May 10, 1958.

Clinical Report on Benactyzine Hydrochloride. Frank J. Ayd, Jr.[8] (Franklin Square Hosp., Baltimore) evaluated benactyzine hydrochloride (Suavitil®) in 29 women and 11 men, aged 20-50, who had one of the following: anxiety neurosis, phobic reactions, obsessional neurosis, obsessive-compulsive neurosis, agitated depressions with obsessive thinking and schizophrenia with obsessive-compulsive symptoms. Anxiety and obsessive thinking were the predominant symptoms of their illnesses. Clinically, each case was in an acute stage. All patients, regardless of the severity of illness, were started on an oral dose of 1 mg. 2-3 times a day. Dosage was increased as needed until improvement occurred or toxic side effects appeared. The daily dose range was 3-50 mg., average 6-9 mg. Except for those who were intolerant of the drug or refused to take it because of annoying side effects, all patients received it for 2 months, after which it was discontinued and the cases evaluated.

Therapeutic results were inconsistent, variable and difficult to evaluate. In some patients anxiety was relieved, in others enhanced. Even when anxiety was diminished, obsessive thinking, phobias and compulsive behavior persisted. After initial improvement in some patients, anxiety recurred as treatment continued and was resistant to larger doses. Patients who obtained the most symptomatic relief were those with an acute illness of recent onset or those anxious to recover.

The medication caused various side effects due to its anticholinergic action. These were not serious but sufficiently annoying so that 30% of the patients refused to take the drug, which often caused some blocking of thought, unpleasant psychologic reactions such as depersonalization and enhanced anxiety, impairment of concentration, dizziness, lassitude and a subjective sensation of muscular weakness.

Perphenazine (Trilafon®) Treatment of Psychoses. P. O. O'Reilly, H. M. Wojcicki, W. Hrychuk and R. P. Keogh[9] (Saskatchewan Hosp.) carried out a double-blind study on 20 men. Group I, including 9 chronic schizophrenics and 1 epileptic, received a placebo and chlorpromazine. Group II, including 9 chronic schizophrenics and 1 epileptic, received

(8) New England J. Med. 257:669-670, Oct. 3, 1957.
(9) Canad. M. A. J. 77:952-955, Nov. 15, 1957.

perphenazine. Dosage of all drugs was 8-20 mg. twice daily for 12 weeks.

Patients in group I showed no significant changes and those in group II fairly marked changes. Among the latter, 1 was markedly improved, 4 moderately or mildly improved and 1 unchanged. The most striking feature of perphenazine medication appeared to be its relative freedom from side effects. The only side effect encountered was mild parkinsonian features in 2 patients, which developed shortly after their dosage was increased to 40 mg./day. After a small dose of trihexyphenidyl hydrochloride (Artane®) was added and/or the dose of perphenazine decreased, the extrapyramidal syndrome quickly disappeared.

After the project was completed, all group II patients were left without perphenazine or any other tranquilizer for 2 weeks. During that time 4 of the 9 patients who had responded favorably to treatment showed slight but definite trends toward regression to the previous mental condition. Administration of 16 mg. perphenazine caused return to the previous degree of improvement in a few days. Thus the optimal length of administration of perphenazine may be greater for proper therapy. This may warrant consideration of perphenazine for so-called maintenance therapy in the chronic mentally ill, particularly because of the freedom from side effects.

Use of Perphenazine (Trilafon®) to Control Anxiety and Agitation in Aged Patients is discussed by Edward Settel[1] (Forest Hills, N. Y., Nursing and Rehabilitation Center). Tranquilizers are valuable for short-term amelioration of acute emotional crises and enhancement of a patient's receptivity to other psychotherapeutic modalities. They should not be used in place of definitive psychotherapy. A new and most promising tranquilizer is perphenazine, a phenothiazine compound which is 5 or 6 times as potent as chlorpromazine and much less toxic. According to early clinical reports, perphenazine is an effective and comparatively safe tranquilizer suitable for the full range of psychiatric indications, from mild tension and anxiety states through frank psychoses.

Perphenazine was given to 60 patients, aged 60-93, who

(1) J. Am. Geriatrics Soc. 5:1003-1008, December, 1957.

had anxiety and agitation. Ambulatory patients received 12 or 16 mg. daily and hospitalized patients 24-48 mg. daily. Average duration of therapy was 16 weeks.

Good or excellent results were achieved in 51 patients (85%). Results were generally good in moderate or severe senile agitation and in anxiety with tension or with depression. Results in 4 patients with agitation and terminal carcinoma were disappointing; however, the antiemetic properties of the drug were useful in this group.

Side effects occurred in 5 patients. Three patients who received 24 mg. perphenazine had extreme lassitude, fatigue and drowsiness. In 2 of these, the side effects were reversed by reducing the dosage to 12 mg. daily; in the 3d, vertigo supervened and necessitated discontinuance of therapy. The vertigo disappeared 48 hours later, but reappeared when the drug was resumed. Two patients receiving 24 mg. perphenazine daily had gross trembling of the hands and feet, extreme salivation and unstable gait. These symptoms, which probably indicated extrapyramidal involvement, were sufficiently disturbing to necessitate withdrawal of the drug. When therapy was resumed 5 days later, antiparkinsonian drugs were administered concomitantly and largely controlled the side effects.

Repeated laboratory tests (hemograms, urinalyses and renal and hepatic function tests) revealed no instance of toxicity. There was no evidence of accentuation of the primary symptoms, even in the 9 patients in whom anxiety was associated with depression.

Unusual Complication Following Use of Trilafon® in Children is reported by Reginald V. Berry, Sheldon H. Kamin and Alan Kline[2] (US Naval Hosp., Jacksonville, Fla.). Trilafon, like other phenothiazine derivatives, is used in anxiety and tension states, in agitated psychoses and in schizophrenics. It also is considered a potent antiemetic. The authors observed a boy, 10, and a girl, 6, who reacted in a bizarre manner requiring hospitalization, to three 4-mg. doses of Trilafon. The outstanding symptoms were a peculiar cataleptoid state with the phenomenon of waxy flexibility in each case. Both patients recovered spontaneously about 12 hours after hospitalization.

(2) U. S. Armed Forces M. J. 9:745-749, May, 1958.

Boy, 10, was seen because, though active and apparently healthy, he continually complained of physical discomforts. Several years before, after a blow on the head, he was unconscious for several hours. Neurologic and EEG examination findings were reported as normal, and physical examination and laboratory findings were within normal limits.

The child was started on Trilafon, 4 mg. 3 times a day. About 24 hours later, he was carried into the clinic, rigid, unresponsive and apparently dissociated from his surroundings. He had taken the third dose of Trilafon that morning before going to school and at school complained to his teacher of headache and stiff neck. Soon thereafter he was seen to stare fixedly, holding himself stiffly in his chair, immobile.

Shortly after he was hospitalized, he was seen in neuropsychiatric consultation. He was lying rigidly on his side, with one leg elevated in extension and without motion. The face was expressionless and he looked fixedly into space. There was no meningismus. His head could be bent forward and backward with the type of resistance designated as waxy flexibility. Moving his extremities produced the same bizarre mobility. Releasing the extremities resulted in fixational positions at levels in which they were released. There was no response to questioning and no outward show of pain. The patient could be moved into a sitting position, head flexed back and arms outstretched. Occasionally there was a parkinsonian-like twitching of the thumb. Neurologic examination, including cerebrospinal fluid examination, was otherwise normal. The appearance of the patient was best described as cataleptoid, not unlike the picture of catatonia.

About 3 hours after hospitalization, the child began to respond by moving the extremities on command but otherwise continued to be uncommunicative. During the night, brief episodes of torsion spasm were observed, which gradually subsided and 16 hours later he was entirely symptom free. His only remark in referring to his illness was, "I was awfully afraid."

Chemotherapy of Depression: Use of Meprobamate Combined with Benactyzine (2-Diethylaminoethyl Benzilate) Hydrochloride was evaluated by Leo Alexander[3] (Boston State Hosp.). Depression, defined as a state of sadness with self reproaches, psychomotor inhibition, sleep disturbance and impaired appetite, was treated in 35 patients by simultaneous use of meprobamate and benactyzine hydrochloride (Deprol). Meprobamate was given initially in doses of 400 mg. 4 times daily and, when necessary, gradually increased to 1,200 mg. 4 times daily; its purpose was to relax and reduce excitability without exerting a significant inhibitory effect. Benactyzine was given initially in dose of 1 mg. 4 times daily and, when necessary, gradually increased to

(3) J.A.M.A. 166:1019-1023, Mar. 1, 1958.

3 mg. 4 times daily. It is a mild antidepressant particularly effective in relieving the ruminative, obsessive aspects of depression. Close daily supervision extending over the entire 24 hours was required to offset the risk of suicide. The usual supportive psychotherapy was given concurrently. Average duration of treatment was 8 weeks. Twenty patients (57%) made a complete and/or social recovery. This is higher than the rate of spontaneous recovery under comparable conditions, but not so high as the recovery rate obtained by electric shock therapy.

In patients responding favorably, the early effect of the drug combination was a marked reduction of tension and depressive rumination as well as a striking reduction in hostility toward self and in suicidal trends. Resumption of normal sleep rhythm was also one of the striking early effects. Before eventual recovery supervened, it was possible to discontinue the nocturnal use of hypnotics in patients who had started using them before treatment began. No patients had to be hospitalized and none attempted suicide.

The meprobamate-benactyzine treatment for depression is recommended as a step which allows those patients to recover for whom this treatment is sufficient, thus screening out and reducing the number requiring electric shock therapy.

Effect of Meprobamate (Equanil®) on Brain-Damaged Patients was studied by C. H. Carter[4] (Gainesville, Fla.). Meprobamate, a mephenesin derivative, possesses both skeletal muscle-relaxant and ataractic properties. By virtue of its dual activity, it was tried on 105 brain-damaged patients of three types: (1) those with neuromuscular disorders, including athetosis, spasticity, ataxia and paralysis agitans; (2) those with behavior problems ranging from mild anxiety and tension because of a handicap to frank psychoses; and (3) those combining the more severe features of the other two groups. The only criterion was brain damage demonstrable by abnormal EEG.

Dosage of meprobamate was adjusted to individual needs, based on clinical appraisal of severity of symptoms. The goal was optimum improvement without drowsiness. Twelve patients were given meprobamate 4 times daily, the others, 3

(4) Am. J. M. Sc. 235:632-638, June, 1958.

times daily. The predominant daily dose was 1,200 mg., ranging from 400 to 3,600 mg. Neither age nor body weight determined dosage. No other drug was given during the study. More than 80% of spastic and 97% of athetoid patients responded with at least moderate remission of neuromuscular symptoms. Behavior problems almost vanished in 57% and were moderately relieved in 94%. Improvement was maintained over a 2-year period while medication continued at dosages up to 3,600 mg. daily. Many patients improved sufficiently to benefit from physiotherapy or psychotherapy for the first time. The only side effect, occurring in 11 patients, was drowsiness.

Meprobamate in Treatment of Stuttering was tried by Roy D. H. Maxwell and James W. Paterson[5] (Western Infirm., Glasgow) in 18 patients. All, severely affected by stuttering, had defects in social adjustment and had been treated by speech therapy previously, with little improvement. All had secondary tonic or tonoclonic stuttering. Meprobamate was given in tablets of 400 mg.; 1 tablet 3 times a day was used initially, with increased dosage where needed. The study covered 8 months.

Results were very good in 6 patients (33%), good in 8 (44%) and poor in 4 (22%). For most patients, 1 tablet 3 times daily was adequate. After active drug therapy, placebo tablets could be substituted with continued benefit to a variable extent. Meprobamate had no effect without speech therapy.

Meprobamate is useful in relaxing tension which provokes and perpetuates the condition. It is of value in restoring speech confidence, facilitating treatment and shortening the period of speech therapy.

Use of Double-Blind Study Investigating Clinical Merits of New Tranquilizing Agent. Herbert Koteen[6] (Cornell Univ.) investigated the effects of Miltown®, a member of the propanediol group and chemically identical with Equanil®, on emotional tension and muscle discomfort. Miltown and a matching placebo were dispensed in capsules to 25 patients by the double-blind method. About 3,600 capsules were distributed for a total of 1,000 patient days. All patients took

(5) Brit. M. J. 1:873-874, Apr. 12, 1958.
(6) Ann. Int. Med. 47:978-989, November, 1957.

between 1,200 and 1,600 mg. daily, the currently recommended dose.

Results revealed that Miltown in this dosage had no greater effect in relieving symptoms than did the placebo in this group of unselected patients. The effects of larger dosages on the central nervous system were not explored.

It has been stated that tranquilizing agents significantly alter the quantitative expression of anxiety and panic but do not modify learned behavior patterns. Whether there actually are tranquilizing agents remains to be determined, but it appears that the tranquilizing agent that has been used longest, oftenest and most effectively is still the placebo.

Possible Habituating Properties of Meprobamate: Clinical Study in Institutionalized, Highly Susceptible Population. Austin R. Stough[7] (State Prison, McAlester, Okla.) carried out two programs using meprobamate in 60 prison inmates. Most were highly unstable with a history of injury, illness or other physical or psychologic abnormality, including previous addiction to alcohol or narcotics. Meprobamate was given first in dosages far in excess of clinical need, then abruptly withdrawn, then given in the more common dosages and, finally, gradually withdrawn. The discomforts that occurred in a few subjects in the first 24-36 hours after the larger dosages were stopped reflected a resurgence of previous psychosomatic symptoms. All subjects returned to pretreatment clinical status in 48 hours. No true habituation developed. No permanent effects resulted from the medication in any dosage or from abrupt withdrawal A few patients, especially those with serious nervous or other abnormalities, may react undesirably to abrupt cessation of ataractic therapy, for the ataraxics are not curative and improvement under medication is no guarantee against subsequent relapse.

There is no way to predict who will react with an increase of tension to termination of ataractic therapy and who will be unaffected. The EEG alone cannot be used as an index. However, in these subjects, history of physical or emotional abnormalities or both, resurgence of discomfort in the placebo period and instability of the EEG seemed definitely related. The development of any type of dependence on a

(7) J.A.M.A. 166:882-888, Feb. 22, 1958.

drug apparently is determined largely by the character structure of the person.

Gradual withdrawal of any ataraxic is recommended. If the total dosage of meprobamate required to control emotional disturbances exceeds 1.6 or even 1.2 Gm./day, withdrawal at the rate of 400 mg./day may be desirable. Thus, return to pretreatment subjective symptoms, if it occurs, will be gradual and the patient will adjust with less difficulty.

Clinical and Cerebral Action of Promethazine and Methylphenidate Hydrochloride. Promethazine (Phenergan®), an isomer of promazine, is used therapeutically as an antihistamine and as a premedicant for anesthesia. James G. Shea, John D. Schultz, Edward Lewis, Jr., and Joseph F. Fazekas[8] (District of Columbia Gen'l Hosp.) administered promethazine intravenously in doses of 200-400 mg. to 27 patients with delirium tremens and 18 acutely disturbed patients with various psychoses. The total dose was given in 5-10 minutes.

A state of deep sedation from which patients could not be aroused was induced in 5-10 minutes after administration. Immediately after the injection, all patients had a transient excitatory phase which lasted 1-2 minutes and was characterized by myoclonic-like involuntary motor activity. Sedation lasted 4-6 hours and was usually followed by a return of increased psychomotor activity. Administration of promethazine was associated with a decrease in total cerebral blood flow and oxygen consumption and an increase in cerebral vascular resistance and mean arterial pressure. With continued administration of the drug, patients with delirium tremens could be kept under sedation until their delirium subsided spontaneously. Repeated injection was often followed by venous thrombosis, but this complication could be obviated by diluting the drug (200 mg. in 5 ml.) or by injecting it slowly.

Seven patients were given 400 mg. methylphenidate hydrochloride (a new analeptic) intravenously 30-45 minutes after promethazine administration. This drug did not change appreciably either the clinical or experimental effects induced by promethazine.

If promazine is used in dosages adequate to induce a qui-

(8) Am. J. M. Sc. 235:201-205, February, 1958.

escent state in patients with increased psychomotor activity, they can be aroused by external stimuli, whereas after promethazine they cannot be aroused. Further, patients with delirium tremens resistant to promazine can be made unconscious by administration of equivalent concentrations of promethazine. Methylphenidate hydrochloride (which was not effective in arousing patients made quiescent by promethazine) is effective in arousing patients quieted by promazine.

These observations suggest that promethazine, unlike other phenothiazine derivatives, may depress both cortical and subcortical centers if given intravenously in fairly large doses. In view of this action, the drug appears to have considerable therapeutic value in managing patients with increased psychomotor activity not clinically controlled by promazine or chlorpromazine.

Practical Mood Stimulant is needed to counteract depression, particularly in elderly patients, according to Milton E. Landman, Rudolph Preisig and Maximilian Perlman[9] (Bloomfield). Functional depression not severe enough to warrant shock therapy has, in the past, been treated largely with amphetamine or caffeine. The former is less than satisfactory because of side actions, including anorexia and sympathomimetic effects. The latter is variable in efficacy and may also have undesirable side effects.

Methyl-a-phenyl-2-piperidineacetate hydrochloride (Ritalin®) has a psychic stimulatory effect in animals and increases co-ordinated activity. It has an analeptic and respiratory stimulant effect against certain narcotics. In double-blind tests, placebos or 10 mg. Ritalin 3 times a day for 4-day periods were given to 23 normal subjects, to 28 patients with mild depression secondary to short-term illness and to 61 elderly, chronically ill, institutionalized patients.

Marked mood improvement appeared in 83% of the normal subjects. Lethargy, fatigue, crying spells, chronic complaints and resistance to rehabilitation were used to judge efficacy in the other two groups. Among those with mild depression, 64% obtained obvious benefit, whereas 11% showed improvement that could not be clearly differentiated from that with placebos. In the geriatric groups, 61% showed marked benefit, but again 11% were questionable. Even

(9) J. M. Soc. New Jersey 55:55-58, February, 1958.

treating the latter as negative, results were statistically favorable to the drug in all three groups. No serious side effects or influence on blood pressure or pulse was observed.

Combined Ritalin® and Serpasil® Therapy in Chronic Psychoses was studied by Tibor W. Wodraska, John C. Saunders and Nathan S. Kline[1] (Rockland State Hosp., Orangeburg, N.Y.). A comparative evaluation of reserpine, methylphenidate and a combination of reserpine and methylphenidate was made in 220 chronic psychotic patients. The 100 patients selected for combined therapy with reserpine and methylphenidate included 84 chronic schizophrenic patients with a history of hospitalization for many years; of these, 51 previously had other forms of chemotherapy without favorable results. In this group, 17% failed, 70% improved moderately and 13% markedly. In the group of 40 patients on methylphenidate alone, 45% failed, 47.5% improved moderately and 7.5% markedly. In the group of 80 who received reserpine only, 18.75% failed, 71.25% improved moderately and 10% improved markedly. Thus the best therapeutic results were obtained with the combined chemotherapy.

The effect of methylphenidate follows not a linear but rather an exponential curve. The optimal therapeutic dosage of methylphenidate with minimum side effects is between 40 and 60 mg. daily, given orally or parenterally. Apparently in certain depressive states, except in agitated depression, methylphenidate is beneficial.

Another advantage of the combined therapy is due to the pharmacodynamic properties of methylphenidate and reserpine in combination. The undesirable and disturbing side effects of either drug can be eliminated or markedly reduced. Even in prolonged treatment, no adverse side effects were observed (table). It appears also that this form of combined chemotherapy has a somewhat wider range of effectiveness in the treatment of chronic psychoses, inasmuch as some favorable therapeutic results were obtained in patients with psychoses associated with mental deficiency and in those with epileptic deterioration. The combination of reserpine and methylphenidate was well tolerated, even in prolonged use, by patients in the older age group with psychoses due

(1) Dis. Nerv. System 19:122-136, March, 1958.

COMPARISON OF COMMON SIDE EFFECTS WITH RESERPINE, METHYLPHENIDATE AND COMBINATION OF RESERPINE AND METHYLPHENIDATE*

RESPONSE	RESERPINE (80 PATIENTS)			METHYLPHENIDATE (40 PATIENTS)			RESERPINE & METHYLPHENIDATE (100 PATIENTS)		
	None	Mild to Moderate	Marked	None	Mild to Moderate	Marked	None	Mild to Moderate	Marked
"Turbulent phase"	22.5	62.5	15	100	0	0	59	41	0
Increased motoricity	62.5	37.5	0	15	55	30	45	55	0
Allergic phenomena	10	77.5	12.5	100	0	0	81	19	0
Parkinsonism	3.75	75.25	21	100	0	0	72	28	0
Bulimia	22.5	58.75	18.75	100	0	0	100	0	0
Anorexia	97.5	2.5	0	12.5	67.5	20	89	11	0
Drop of blood pressure	21	75.25	3.75	80	20	0	65	31	4
Tachycardia	2.5	95	2.5	25	75	0	42	54	4
Depressive states	46.25	50	3.75	100	0	0	97	3	0
Hyporeflexia	75	25	0	100	0	0	94	6	0
Hyperreflexia	100	0	0	37.5	62.5	0	88	12	0

*Expressed in relative percentage.

to cerebral arteriosclerosis with hypertension, with the advantage that methylphenidate does not essentially inhibit the hypotensive action of reserpine.

Ritalin® and Chlorpromazine in Chronic Schizophrenia: Controlled Clinical Trial is reported by Barbara J. Salisbury and E. H. Hare.[2] Ritalin (methylphenidate) resembles amphetamine in its central stimulant and sympathomimetic action but has a different chemical structure. It was used in a 5-month study of 48 schizophrenic patients, 13 of whom were mainly overactive and aggressive and 23, mainly apathetic. Fourteen had undergone leukotomy. During the trial patients received no other drugs or special therapy except that 4 who previously had epileptic seizures continued to receive anticonvulsant drugs.

The drugs tested were: Ritalin, 10 mg. 3 times daily; Ritalin, 20 mg. 3 times daily, and chlorpromazine, 50 mg. 3 times daily. These were administered in a syrup which, when given without the addition of a drug, served as the inert control. For the 1st month, all patients received only the control sirup. For the succeeding 4 months, every patient received these drugs, including the inert control, for a month at a time.

Compared with the control period, patients on Ritalin (both dosages) showed no significant difference in behavior or in severity of symptoms. On chlorpromazine, however, a significant number improved, compared with their state during the control period, in 8 of the 18 symptoms rated. Behavior also tended to improve, although singly none of the 7 aspects of behavior examined showed a significant degree of improvement. The symptoms showing most marked improvement with chlorpromazine were those related to sociability and social use of language.

At different stages in the trial 16 patients were markedly confused or drowsy; in 13 instances this occurred while the patient was on chlorpromazine, in 1 instance while a patient was on 10 mg. Ritalin 3 times daily and in another on 20 mg. Ritalin 3 times daily and on the control sirup. Of the 13 patients who became markedly drowsy on chlorpromazine, only 3 showed general improvement compared with that shown in the control month; this should discount any

(2) J. Ment. Sc. 103:830-834, October, 1957.

marked bias toward favorable rating of patients thought to be on chlorpromazine.

At different stages 14 patients were described as unduly restless or agitated, 10 while they were on Ritalin, 3 while on chlorpromazine and 1 while on the control. In 5 instances the dosage was halved for a few days because of a patient's untoward behavior; in 3 of these instances the patient was on chlorpromazine, in 1, Ritalin (20 mg. 3 times daily) and in 1, the control. No other noteworthy complications occurred during the trial.

Indications for Use of Iproniazid in Psychiatric Practice are discussed by P. J. Dally[3] (St. Thomas' Hosp., London). Iproniazid (Marsilid®; 1-isonicotinyl-2-isopropylhydrazine phosphate) is a derivative of isoniazid and was originally introduced because of its similar activity on tubercle bacilli. In the early clinical trials of iproniazid in pulmonary tuberculosis, using doses of 300 mg. daily, increased appetite associated with large weight gains was noticed, accompanied in some patients by mood changes which sometimes developed into frank psychosis. These changes were reversible on stopping the drug. Iproniazid is thought to inhibit monoamine oxidase.

Dally used the drug on 131 patients with depressive and allied psychiatric disorders. Each patient was started on 150 mg. (3 tablets) daily, in 3 divided doses, but was warned to reduce the dose to 100 mg. daily if side effects developed and to stop altogether if these continued. This daily dosage was continued for 4 weeks and then reduced by 50 mg. at intervals of a month, until either the patient was off the drug completely or symptoms of depression reappeared. If the latter happened, the daily dosage was increased by 50 mg. weekly until the patient was symptom free and maintained for another month before again being reduced.

Iproniazid was of value in treating certain patients showing symptoms of mild depression associated with weight loss. There was a time lag of 7-10 days after the treatment was started before improvement was noticed. The advantage of iproniazid over amphetamine or electroconvulsive therapy in this type of depression is that improvement appears to be maintained as long as the drug is given in ade-

(3) Brit. M. J. 1:1338-1339, **June 7, 1958.**

quate dosage. Severe depressions, however, were not helped and depressive states associated with agitation were often made worse.

Side effects depended largely on dosage and occurred increasingly when 150 mg. or more of iproniazid a day was given. Constipation, impotence, decreased need of sleep, dryness of mouth and blurring of vision were all reported. Postural hypotension was seen in 6 patients. The side effects disappeared when the drug was stopped.

Therapeutic Trial of Iproniazid (Marsilid®) in Depressed and Apathetic Patients was conducted by R. L. DeVerteuil and H. E. Lehmann[4] (Verdun Protestant Hosp., Montreal). The study included 31 patients, aged 32-83, who were depressed, with or without anxiety, or apathetic. All but 4 received 150 mg. daily in tablet form (50 mg. 3 times daily) for most or all of the treatment period. These 4 received 100 mg. daily (50 mg. twice daily). In 11, dosage was reduced or treatment discontinued as a result of toxic reactions. Eventually all patients were taken off iproniazid because of the high incidence of toxic reactions and one fatality. Treatment thus varied from 14 to 112 days.

Significant improvement was seen in 11 patients (35%); this was sustained in 7. The incidence of side effects was 35%. Dizziness, loss of muscular tonus and ataxia, with or without hypotension, occurred in 7. Ataxia resulted in frequent falls in a young woman, whereas cerebral thrombosis was suspected in 1 man. Because of these symptoms, which persisted as long as iproniazid was given, another man was investigated for an expanding intracranial lesion. Syncope was observed in 2 patients and asymptomatic hypotension in 1. A fatal necrosis of the liver occurred in 1 of the 4 patients receiving the smaller dosage of 100 mg. daily. Because of improvement, the dosage in this patient had been reduced to 50 mg. daily 14 days before the onset of jaundice, and the drug had been immediately discontinued when jaundice appeared. Nevertheless, the hepatitis progressed to fatal liver necrosis in 12 days. At autopsy, this necrosis was found to be the type sometimes seen in response to toxic agents.

(4) Canad. M. A. J. 78:131-133, Jan. 15, 1958.

Liver Damage Concurrent with Iproniazid Administration is discussed by Louis Zetzel and Herman Kaplan[5] (Harvard Med. School). Iproniazid (1-isonicotinyl-2-isopropyl hydrazine) was originally introduced for treatment of tuberculosis. Because of its toxicity in the dosage used, it has been replaced by its chemical relative, isoniazid. However, its observed effect as a central nervous system stimulant has led to renewed interest and use. As a psychic energizer it has been used in treatment of depressive and debilitating states and, more recently, in the management of hypertension, ulcerative colitis, rheumatoid arthritis and angina pectoris.

The authors observed 5 women in whom jaundice developed while they were receiving iproniazid. The amount of drug taken by each patient varied between 1,350 mg. over 11 days and 2,500 mg. over 50 days. Liver function tests were consistent with hepatocellular disease. At autopsy of the patient who died, the liver had an appearance consistent with that described in the fulminant form of hepatitis or in severe toxic damage.

Woman, 32, had progressive anorexia and discomfort in the upper abdomen 12 days, and dark urine, light stools and scleral icterus 7 days before hospitalization. During the preceding 2½ months, she had been taking the following drugs daily for treatment of a schizophrenic reaction: iproniazid, 150 mg.; meprobamate, 800 mg.; and pyridoxine, 50 mg. About 2 days before beginning this course of drug therapy, she received an injection of methacholine and epinephrine as part of the Funkenstein test. There was no known exposure to patients with hepatitis or obvious hepatotoxins.

On physical examination she was deeply jaundiced but afebrile and in no distress. The liver edge was felt 8 cm. below the right costal margin and was smooth, firm and nontender. The spleen was palpable 6 cm. below the left costal margin. Physical findings were otherwise normal. A scout film of the abdomen revealed no abnormalities. The abnormal liver function studies suggested hepatocellular damage. Reticulocyte counts were consistently elevated, and the red blood cells showed increased osmotic fragility to hypotonic saline solution, but there was no anemia. Throughout the hospital course she was afebrile, maintained a good appetite and, aside from intermittent depressive moods, felt well. Treatment consisted, at first, of bed rest and a normal house diet, supplemented by daily intramuscular injections of 75 mg. menadiol until the blood prothrombin concentration was normal. Seven weeks after hospitalization, the liver was barely

(5) New England J. Med. 258:1209-1211, June 12, 1958.

palpable, the spleen was no longer felt, and the scleras were still mildly icteric, corresponding to a serum bilirubin of 2 mg./100 ml.

Comparative Effects of Relaxant Drugs on Human Skeletal Muscle Hyperactivity. Francis A. Vazuka[6] (Temple Univ.) performed clinical observations, motion picture recordings and electromyographic and myometric studies on 11 patients with neuromuscular disorders before, during and after oral administration of 1,250 mg. Robaxin® 4 times a day, 500 mg. Equanil® 3 or 4 times a day and 500 mg. Flexin® 3 or 4 times a day. Alterations were noted in spasticity, ankle clonus, clonic extensor spasms, flexor spasms and functional capacity as manifested by self-care and ambulation abilities. Variations were recorded when each subject received the three drugs in series.

VARIATIONS IN CLONUS, SPASMS AND SPASTICITY INDUCED BY MEDICATION

	Control	*Robaxin*	*Equanil*	*Flexin*
Mean weight producing ankle clonus (LBS)	10.9	5.7	3.3	4.5
Mean amplitude of ankle clonus (M.V.)	267	180	148	172
Clonus on resting legs on balls of feet (number of patients)	9	5	4	8
Spasms on stroking feet				
Severity	25.1	9.6	14.0	17.9
Duration (seconds)	3.2	1.8	2.4	2.6
Spasticity on passive stretch				
Severity	33	20	16	22
Duration (seconds)	2.5	2.0	1.5	2.2
Clinical clonus (with daily routines)	28	17	10	24
Clinical spasms (with daily routines)	24	9	14	23
Clinical spasticity (with daily routines)	34	23	20	28

As shown in the table, each modality of muscle hyperactivity was not depressed to parallel levels. Equanil was more effective than Flexin and Robaxin as a muscle relaxant. In the dosage used, Robaxin was more effective in relieving muscle spasticity than Flexin. The major benefit derived by the 11 patients was partial alleviation of muscle hyperreactivity which allowed greater self-care and easier ambulatory capabilities. Urinary frequency was lessened. Wheelchair patients could sit more comfortably and manipulate the chair without aid. Movements no longer threw the extremities into severe clonic extensor spasms.

Reflex spasms and clonus showed considerable fluctua-

(6) Neurology 8:446-454 June, 1958.

tions in severity on different days, depending on the variations in the state of central excitability. This was especially prominent with Robaxin and Flexin. Tranquilizing properties of Equanil tended to produce more stable conditions of emotional tension during the formal testing procedures, resulting in more uniform results.

Robaxin in dosages of 5 Gm./day produced subjective tiredness, fatigability, exhaustion and weakness in 6 patients. The degree of weakness was not proportional to the amount of muscle relaxation attained. Nervousness, anxiety, inward tension, shakiness and jittery nerves were symptoms described by 8 of the 11 patients at varying intervals while on Robaxin. Patients taking Equanil did not note anxiety, but 3 had drowsiness and 1 persistent weakness. Nausea and vomiting occurred in 4 patients taking Flexin, nervousness in 4, tiredness and weakness in 3 and a cutaneous eruption in 2.

Drugs in Other Neuropsychiatric Entities

General Principles for Drug Therapy in Childhood Epilepsy, based on follow-up studies of about 9,000 children with epileptic seizures of all types, are outlined by Samuel Livingston[7] (Johns Hopkins Univ.). Treatment should be instituted as soon as diagnosis has been established. In most instances, the degree of success in controlling seizures bears a direct relation to duration of epilepsy.

Seizures in a patient in whom a specific cause, such as hypoglycemia, hypocalcemia or fever, cannot be determined should be considered epileptic unless repeated examinations and time prove them to be a manifestation of another disorder. This is true whether the EEG is normal or abnormal.

Even for patients who have had only one epileptic seizure, immediate, prolonged therapy is indicated. If treatment is started immediately after the initial convulsion, and parents are told that seizures are less likely to recur if regular medication continues for a long period, parents and patient soon return to normal living.

Selection of the drug of first choice depends on the type of seizure. Some anticonvulsants are more effective than oth-

(7) Journal-Lancet 78:182-184, May, 1958.

ers in controlling certain types of seizures, whereas some drugs increase the frequency of certain types of convulsions. The drug of choice should be selected on the basis of relative effectiveness, toxicity and cost (table).

Treatment should begin with one drug. Others should be prescribed only after it has been determined that the maximum tolerated dosage of the initial drug failed to produce satisfactory clinical response. In patients who suffer relatively infrequent seizures, the conventional starting dosage should be prescribed and increased, if necessary, until satisfactory control of seizures is attained or limit of tolerance is reached. For those who experience relatively frequent and severe seizures, the average maximum dosage should be prescribed initially, decreased or increased, if necessary, depending on the patient's tolerance and frequency of seizures. The therapeutic dosage of anticonvulsant medication varies. The proper dosage for any given patient is that which controls seizures without producing untoward reactions. The same dosage which controlled seizures should be taken daily for at least 4 years after the last convulsion. If the 4-year period of freedom from seizures should coincide with the onset of puberty, the medication should be continued through

DRUGS IN CURRENT USE FOR CONTROL OF DIFFERENT TYPES OF EPILEPTIC SEIZURES, IN ORDER OF PREFERENCE AS TO RELATIVE EFFECTIVENESS, TOXICITY AND COST

MAJOR MOTOR	PETIT MAL	MINOR MOTOR	PSYCHOMOTOR
Phenobarbital* (or Mebaral®)	Benzedrine® (or Dexedrine®) sulfate	Phenobarbital* (or Mebaral)	Dilantin
Dilantin®	Paradione®	Miltown (Equanil)	Phenobarbital (or Mebaral)
Mysoline®	Tridione®	Bromides	Benzedrine (or Dexedrine) sulfate
Bromides	Dimedione	Benzedrine (or Dexedrine) sulfate	Mysoline
Peganone®	Celontin®	Celontin	Peganone
Gemonil®	Diamox®	Milontin	Celontin
Mesantoin	Milontin®	Gemonil	Phenurone®
	Miltown® (Equanil®)		Tridione
	Atabrine®		Mesantoin
	Prenderol®		

*Mebaral is given to patients who show untoward reactions to phenobarbital.

adolescence. This is particularly important in girls. Medication should be discontinued gradually. Following the 4-year period of freedom from seizures, dosage should be reduced gradually over a period of 1-2 years.

Periodic physical and laboratory examination should be made on all patients receiving certain drugs, including complete blood counts on those taking Mesantoin, Tridione® and Paradione®, which are known to have an adverse effect on the hemopoietic system. Periodic urinalysis should be done on patients receiving drugs known to impair the genitourinary system, such as Tridione and Paradione, and liver function tests made before and at regular intervals during Phenurone® therapy. A drug should be discontinued immediately if any type of cutaneous reaction appears. When the drug is stopped, another should be started immediately, as sudden withdrawal may precipitate recurrence of seizures or produce status epilepticus.

New Method of Phenobarbitone Administration in Treatment of Epilepsy is described by Desmond C. J. O'Connor.[8] Barbiturates are the least toxic of all the anticonvulsant drugs and are still the first choice in treating major, temporal lobe and other focal seizures. The hydantoins and primidone, alone or in combination, may succeed where

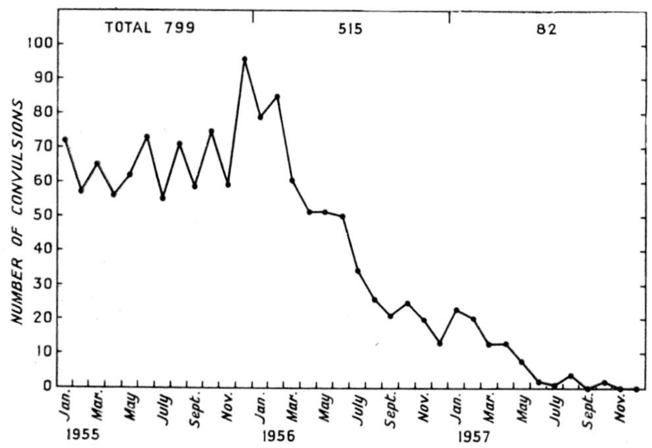

Fig. 33.—Number of convulsions in entire group of patients throughout trial. (Courtesy of O'Connor, D. C. J.: Lancet 1:609-611, Mar. 22, 1958.)

(8) Lancet 1:609-611, Mar. 22, 1958.

DATA ON 18 CASES OF EPILEPSY

Case no.	Age (yr.)	Diagnosis	Results of treatment					
			No. of convulsions				Personality	
			1955	1957			1955	1957: Improvement
				Total	Jan.–June	July–Dec.		
1	33	Traumatic jacksonian; unsuccessful operation	82	0	0	0	Violent	Striking
2	39	Idiopathic grand mal	48	12	11	1	Violent	Moderate
3	37	Idiopathic grand mal	66	4	4	0	Retarded	Striking
4	47	General paralysis with major and minor convulsions	25	4	4	0	Retarded	Slight
5	32	Idiopathic grand mal	32	3	3	0	Violent	Striking
6	37	Idiopathic grand mal	91	7	7	0	Retarded	Striking
7	48	Idiopathic grand mal	48	4	4	0	Violent	Moderate
8	43	Idiopathic grand mal	28	3	3	0	Retarded	None
9	54	Idiopathic grand mal	17	1	1	0	Retarded	Striking
10	48	Idiopathic grand mal	15	9	6	3	Violent and retarded	Striking
11	36	Idiopathic grand mal with hysterical overlay	30	10	8	2	Retarded	Striking
12	48	Post-traumatic grand mal	67	0	0	0	Violent	Striking
13	52	Idiopathic petit mal	53	2	2	0	Retarded	Moderate
14	24	Idiopathic grand mal; episodes of status epilepticus	57	1	0	1	Violent	Striking
15	55	Idiopathic petit mal	49	6	6	0	Retarded	Striking
16	64	Idiopathic grand mal	3	0	0	0	Retarded	Slight
17	55	Idiopathic grand mal	10	2	2	0	Retarded	Striking
18	45	Idiopathic grand mal	78	14	14	0	Retarded	Striking

barbiturates have failed, but they produce toxic reactions. Major effects of barbiturates, and particularly phenobarbitone, are increased recovery time and, in general, increased threshold for cerebral neurons. Phenobarbitone has, in addition, a selective anticonvulsant effect unrelated to its depressive and sedative qualities.

Available phenobarbitone preparations, however, have not been universally successful in abolishing seizures and often are toxic. Because toxicity may be related to changes in blood levels of the drug, a preparation was used that releases phenobarbitone slowly over long periods. This was done with Spansules® containing 1½ gr. phenobarbitone in coated granules which release the drug at a uniform rate, ensuring slow, steady absorption over a long period.

Eighteen hospitalized psychotic men with epilepsy who had persistent convulsions, despite daily phenobarbitone in total dose of 1-4½ gr. or primidone, 0.25-1.25 Gm./day were gradually given Spansule phenobarbitone. Before changing, the mean daily dose of phenobarbitone was 2.8 gr.; with Spansules it was 5.8 gr.

The use of Spansules was accompanied by slight, immediate reduction in the number of convulsions, mental improvement and a striking reduction in toxicity. In most cases the only new effect was slight drowsiness, which was overcome in a few days. The number of convulsions, major and minor, gradually and progressively decreased (Fig. 33) and by the 3d year of treatment no patient had convulsions. Blood levels of barbiturate during treatment with Spansules were found to be much higher than could be tolerated without either unconsciousness, ataxia or both, in nonepileptic persons. Personality and mental state improved in most cases (table).

Use of Parenteral Diphenylhydantoin (Dilantin®) Sodium in Control of Status Epilepticus. Parenteral phenobarbital sodium to suppress convulsions is dangerous, because of its severe depressant effect on respiration. Diphenylhydantoin, however, neither depresses respiration nor is an anesthetic. C. H. Carter[9] (Gainesville, Fla.) treated 121 episodes of status epilepticus in 85 patients with parenteral diphenylhydantoin.

(9) A.M.A. Arch. Neurol. & Psychiat. 79:136-137, February, 1958.

The 5 cc. of solvent was added to the diphenylhydantoin sodium in the Steri-Vial® and shaken. The resultant solution contained 50 mg./cc. diphenylhydantoin sodium or 250 mg. in the ampules. It must be used within a few hours of preparation. It was injected intravenously, 1 cc. of solution/minute. After consciousness returned, diphenylhydantoin or other therapy was continued orally. Occasionally, 250 mg. had to be given intramuscularly for 2 or 3 days every 4-6 hours to maintain control.

Of the 121 episodes, 97 were controlled by a single injection. Of the other 24, 17 were controlled by a second dose, and 7 episodes in 5 patients also required a barbiturate or other medication for control. These 5 were controlled on 250 mg. intramuscularly every 6 hours for 2 or 3 days. No sedative or other side effects were noted. Even with multiple doses, the patients did not show staggering gait or other disturbance of balance. Respiration was not depressed.

Lupus Erythematosus Disseminatus after Administration of Mesantoin: Report of Two Cases. Mesantoin has been of considerable advantage in treating epilepsy. Side effects are absent or slight, even if the drug is given in comparatively large doses. The most dreaded complication is granulocytopenia, occasionally resulting in agranulocytosis. Lupus erythematosus has not previously been reported associated with Mesantoin treatment. Two patients described by Torsten Lindqvist[1] (Univ. of Göteborg) acquired typical lupus. In 1, symptoms began about 1 year after the start of Mesantoin and severe pathology developed rapidly about 6 months later. In the other, symptoms appeared within a few weeks after Mesantoin was started and were fully developed in a year.

Epilepsy is a well-known symptom of lupus erythematosus, but usually the convulsions are terminal, and such seizures are a late symptom of lupus. In a few patients, however, the epilepsy has antedated the lupus. No information is available in these cases as to the type of treatment used. In the author's 2 cases, there was little doubt of the causal connection between administration of Mesantoin and the appearance of clinical lupus erythematosus.

Many cases have been reported in which skin eruptions

(1) Acta med. scandinav. 158:131-138, 1957.

and mucous membrane lesions combined with fever, adenopathy and eosinophilia have developed acutely after Mesantoin was given the patients. These alarming symptoms have caused the drug to be stopped. In the 2 patients described by the author, initial symptoms were mild, and therapy was continued until the more severe disorder became apparent. Dilantin® is known to cause pathology similar to periarteritis nodosa if continued in patients who acquire skin symptoms. An obviously benign skin reaction may indicate a more dangerous disseminated vascular response to hypersensitivity. Serious complications are rare, partly because the drug is discontinued as soon as symptoms appear and partly because the symptoms of the more serious cases are not always recognized.

When epilepsy is being treated with Mesantoin, slight symptoms of intolerance should be considered as possible initial signs of serious lupus erythematosus. Treatment should be interrupted. If more serious symptoms occur, it is necessary to be aware of them and to begin ACTH or cortisone early.

Symptoms of lupus erythematosus disseminatus may appear after Apresoline®, Mesantoin or other substances through a mechanism similar to that known for polyarteritis nodosa. The cryptogenetic cases probably have a similar mechanism. Lupus erythematosus disseminatus probably is not an etiologic entity but a specific reaction to various noxious substances.

Macrocytosis and Macrocytic Anemia Caused by Anticonvulsant Drugs. Megaloblastic anemia in epileptic patients taking anticonvulsant drugs has been increasingly recognized during the past 2 years. Diagnosis is based on exclusion of known causes. C. F. Hawkins and M. J. Meynell[2] (Birmingham, England) made a hematologic survey of 72 institutionalized epileptics. Controls consisted of nonepileptics—30 healthy persons and 30 other inmates of the same institutions. The epileptics showed a significant tendency toward macrocytosis; one-third had a mean corpuscular volume of 94 cu. μ. and over. The mean among all epileptics was 92.2 cu. μ., whereas the mean among controls was 86.6 cu. μ.

(2) Quart. J. Med. 27:45-63, January, 1958.

Macrocytosis was confirmed by diameter measurements of blood films photographed at a magnification of 2,000. All epileptics were taking phenytoin or phenobarbitone. As no other cause for macrocytosis could be found, it was believed that the change in red cells resulted from a metabolic disturbance due to these drugs. In 3 patients who were able to discontinue the anticonvulsant drugs, macrocytosis concurrently disappeared. Since most epileptics take anticonvulsant drugs, it was impossible to find an untreated group to compare with that being studied.

Both macrocytosis and megaloblastic anemia are corrected by folic acid, and either may be present without any known toxic effects of anticonvulsant drugs such as skin lesions, central nervous system signs, bone marrow aplasia or liver disturbance. Macrocytosis itself does not appear to be of practical significance, but megaloblastic anemia is often fatal. It is not known why some patients taking anticonvulsant drugs have macrocytosis alone, others have anemia and the rest maintain a normal blood picture.

A number of patients with epilepsy who were treated with folic acid and vitamin B_{12} because of macrocytic anemia showed marked improvement. It is probable that the reduction in the number of seizures in treated patients is significant and that vitamin B_{12} and folic acid are important in lowering the threshold for the cerebral discharge producing epileptic attacks.

Effects of Nydrane on Epilepsy in Mental Defectives were studied by D. S. Sharpe, G. Dutton and J. R. Mirrey.[3] Nydrane is the English name for N-benzyl-β-chloropropionamide, known as Posedrine in Europe and as Hibicon® in the United States. A 6-month study was made of 18 male patients with idiopathic epilepsy, 6 having the traumatic type and 1 epiloia, all of whom had chronic grand mal seizures before treatment with barbiturates and/or hydantoins. A 0.5 gr. tablet of Nydrane was added to daily therapy for 7 days, then Nydrane was gradually increased and other drugs reduced. Maximum dosage was 4 gr./day. No hemopoietic or liver function disturbance could be detected, although kidney disturbance was noted in 6 patients by transient albuminuria. Blood urea showed a slight increase in 4.

(3) Brit. M. J. 1:1044-1046, May 3, 1958.

A 25% decrease in the number of attacks over that observed in a similar pretreatment period was considered evidence of improvement. On this basis, 68% showed improvement, 20% no change and 12% deteriorated. This was considered significant evidence of the value of Nydrane as an anticonvulsant in epilepsy. In only 3 patients, however, was it possible to dispense with barbiturates entirely. Eight showed improvement in general behavior. In some patients, better conduct and emotional stability were obtained on dosages not affording maximal anticonvulsant protection. It is suggested that such dosages may represent a truer optimal level of medication.

Methsuximide in Psychomotor and Petit Mal Seizures. Elizabeth G. French, Jean Rey-Bellet and William G. Lennox[4] (Harvard Med. School) administered methsuximide (Celontin®) to 106 well-studied patients, aged 6 months to 60 years, whose seizures had defied full control by other medications. All but 3 had had seizures for at least 2 years. Previous drugs used included trimethadione, paramethadione, acetazolamide, phensuximide, quinacrine, phenacemide, phenobarbital, mephobarbital, metharbital, benzchlorpropamide, diphenylhydantoin, primidone and methylphenylethylhydantoin. Drugs that gave partial control were retained, and methsuximide was added in slowly increasing doses, starting with 0.15 or 0.3 Gm. Final amounts ranged from 0.15 to 2.4 Gm. daily. Most patients received 0.9-1.2 Gm./day for 5-24 months.

Among the 76 patients who were able to continue medication and were available for follow-up, seizures in 12 were completely controlled, in 18 markedly and in 19 somewhat improved and 27 were not benefited. Thus, 40% had less than half the previous number of seizures and 35% were not improved. Marked benefit was obtained by 55% of patients with petit mal and by 33% of those with psychomotor seizures. This last group is of special interest, since it is unusually resistant to drug therapy.

Side effects were noted in 40 of the 106 patients; in 14 they were severe enough to demand discontinuance of the drug. Drowsiness was noted by 19; anorexia, nausea, vomiting or constipation by 9; ataxia and dizziness, 7; irritability, 6;

(4) New England J. Med. 258:892-894, May 1, 1958.

confusion, 4; and headaches, diplopia, hiccups and sweating, 1 each. Most of the side effects were transient and disappeared spontaneously when the drug was reduced and usually did not reappear when full dosage was resumed. In general, the frequency of side effects increased sharply with increase of daily dosage, especially if over 1.2 Gm./day. Methsuximide warrants further clinical evaluation in early epilepsy and in cases not easily controlled by standard drugs.

Spirodon (Tetrantoin): New Anticonvulsant of Hydantoin Group. Tracy J. Putnam and John Jacobs[5] (Los Angeles) review the experimental data on Spirodon and present results of a clinical trial in patients with epilepsy. Hidalgo and co-workers found that no fatalities resulted in mice and rats after oral doses of this drug as large as 12 Gm./kg. Dogs tolerated a single dose of 0.8 Gm./kg. with only an occasional slight ataxia. No changes in liver or kidney function were found in rabbits receiving 0.5 Gm./kg. 5 times weekly for 2 weeks. No inhibition of growth and no significant changes in hematology or in organ weights were observed in young rats given varying doses. The drug was found to have significant anticonvulsant potency by the maximal electric shock seizure pattern test and Metrazol® seizure threshold test in mice, rats, rabbits and cats. The minimal electric shock seizure threshold was also elevated.

Untreated patients whose seizures are of recent origin respond as a group more satisfactorily to any new drug than patients who have had seizures over many years, despite treatment with a variety of medications. Therefore, 40 patients who had not responded to the "standard" treatment with the commonly used medicines were selected for study. All had been under treatment for 6 months to 15 years and had had repeated neurologic examinations and EEG studies. Spirodon was administered in single daily doses of 0.5 Gm. in addition to the medicines the patient was already taking with incomplete success. The dose was then increased by 0.5 Gm. weekly until tolerance was reached. In all cases toxic symptoms were deliberately provoked by systematically increasing the dosage until they occurred, usually 5-6 Gm. daily. They consisted of drowsiness, dizziness, ataxia, nystagmus and nausea. The patient was usually comfortable

(5) Neurology 7:784-788, November, 1957.

when the dosage was reduced by 0.5 Gm. Most patients were comfortable on 2-3 Gm. daily. In 13 patients, however, toxic symptoms occurred with 0.5-2 Gm. A rash developed in 8 patients, nausea and vomiting in 4, confusion in 4 and fever in 3. In only 1 was there any significant change in the blood count, and in this patient the outcome was fatal. Of 17 patients who remained on Spirodon, 15 were seizure free.

The largest proportion of good results were seen in patients in whom grand mal was the presenting symptom, but the petit mal and psychomotor attacks were not sufficiently numerous to justify more than an impression. In patients with focal attacks, results appeared excellent. Five patients with fairly clear histories of encephalitis or mental deterioration did poorly.

The effect of Spirodon on the EEG was tested in 10 cases and proved the best available drug in 4. This is comparable to the results with phenytoin, which was best in 14 of 47 cases and second best in 7. Phenobarbital was best in 9 of 40 cases and second best in 6.

► [This drug was tried by G. Frank and F. Morrell (Neurology 8:529, 1958) in 29 patients who had been otherwise inadequately controlled. Significant improvement occurred in 15 instances, the most striking effects being in psychomotor cases. Toxic reactions, insufficient to cause cessation of therapy, occurred in 17 patients. In 9 of 16 cases in which the drug was suddenly withdrawn there was an exacerbation of symptoms within 72 hours.—Ed.]

Celontin® in Treatment of Convulsive Disorders. Experimentally, Celontin protects rats against Metrazol® convulsions, and clinically it has been found effective in controlling petit mal seizures. Haddow M. Keith and Joseph G. Rushton[6] treated 21 children and 20 adults who had petit mal, minor motor seizures, psychomotor seizures and a few cases of grand mal. The youngest patient was age 3½, the oldest 61 years. The smallest amount of Celontin administered was 0.3 Gm. daily, the largest 1.8 Gm. and the usual dose was 0.3 Gm. 3 or 4 times daily.

Five cases (12%) were completely controlled when Celontin was given alone or added to existing treatment. About half the patients were definitely improved, but 3 had to stop the drug because of rash, nausea or drowsiness. Thus about 66% of the cases were benefited or completely controlled.

All patients had previously taken one or more anticonvul-

(6) Proc. Staff Meet. Mayo Clin. 33:105-108, Mar. 5, 1958.

sants including phenobarbital, mephobarbital, Dilantin®, Tridione®, Paradione®, Mesantoin, Diamox®, Milontin®, Mysoline®, Phenurone®, Hibicon®, Desoxyn®, Peganone® and Dramamine®.

Of a total of 48 patients receiving Celontin, 33 had no side effects. Dizziness, drowsiness and rash each occurred 4 times. Ataxia occurred in 2 children. Irritability and tiredness occurred in 2 patients and each of the following in 1: headache, abdominal pain, dyspnea, nausea, restlessness and poor memory. All patients had EEGs, but no relation was seen between EEG findings and therapeutic results.

Ethotoin (Peganone®): New Anticonvulsant. No anticonvulsant is completely effective in all cases of epilepsy or even in all cases of one specific type, and each has objectionable side effects. Therefore, new anticonvulsants are constantly being introduced. Frederic T. Zimmerman and Bessie B. Burgemeister[7] (Columbia Univ.) used ethotoin for almost 2 years in 60 children and adolescents, all resistant to various standard and experimental drugs.

Most were subject to both petit and grand mal attacks. All were aged 4-18 (average 11) years at the start of treatment. Ethotoin was given initially as 0.5 Gm. daily and gradually increased over several weeks until the maximum effect in reducing seizures was obtained or toxicity appeared. In most cases an average daily dose of 1 Gm. gave optimal results, though individual doses reached as much as 4.5 Gm. daily.

On an average daily dose of 1 Gm. for an average of 21 weeks, grand mal seizures were reduced an average of 71%. Some patients have now received the drug for 1½ years. Complete control (absence of seizures for at least 8 consecutive weeks) was achieved in 20% and practical control in another 10%. Some benefit was seen in a further 12%. Thus some improvement was noted in 42% of the patients.

Only 5 patients reported any side actions. Toxicity was unrelated to dosage and apparently was due to personal idiosyncrasy to the drug. Side effects were vomiting, anorexia and abdominal distress and rash. No blood dyscrasias appeared and urines were normal.

Combined with other hydantoins, ethotoin provided com-

(7) New York J. Med. 58:2054-2056, June 15, 1958.

plete control in 29% of the cases and some control in another 29%. Ethotoin has anticonvulsant activity of its own, gives good synergistic anticonvulsant action when combined with other drugs and permits reduction of the more serious side effects of other medication. It seems to hold promise as a grand mal anticonvulsant.

► [But S. J. Saltzstein *et al.* (J.A.M.A. 167:1618, July 26, 1958) have reported an instance in which Peganone induced a lymphadenopathy that clinically and pathologically mimicked malignant lymphoma. All the findings disappeared when the drug was stopped.—Ed.]

Clinical Evaluation of Acetazolamide (Diamox®) in Treatment of Epilepsy in Children is presented by Jean Holowach and Don L. Thurston[8] (Washington Univ.). The anticonvulsant action of Diamox (2-acetylamino-1,3,4-thiadiazole-5-sulfonamide) is probably due to its inhibition of carbonic anhydrase in the central nervous system and not exclusively by way of renal acidosis. The mechanism of anticonvulsant action by inhibition of carbonic anhydrase at the neuron level is not certain. It may be related to the demonstrated effects of carbon dioxide on nerve sensitivity and propagation of nerve impulses. The superiority of carbonic anhydrase inhibitors in control of seizures peculiarly sensitive to changes in carbon dioxide tension or associated wth marked hyperventilation buildup is not unanimously agreed on.

Diamox was given to 56 epileptic children refractory to standard anticonvulsive therapy. Ages ranged from 3 months to 16 years and duration of attacks from 2½ months to 13 years. Only 6 had more than one type of seizure at the start of Diamox therapy. Dosage was empiric, 250-1,000 mg./day.

Seizures were completely controlled in 62.5%; 16% were improved and 21.4% were unchanged. Undesirable reactions occurred in 7 patients; 2 had lethargy or drowsiness and a third great excitability, all necessitating dosage reduction. Two patients had numbness and tingling of the extremities. In 1, these symptoms were transitory; in the other, the drug had to be stopped because numbness of the face affected speech. Increased seizures developed in 1 patient, so Diamox was stopped after 10 days. One patient had had nocturnal enuresis before Diamox therapy, and the impression was that this increased while the drug was being taken.

(8) J. Pediat. 53:160-171, August, 1958.

Eight patients had striking improvement in disposition, motor co-ordination and mental capability. Considering pre-existing status epilepticus and/or repeated, often prolonged postictal mental and physical exhaustion, one cannot determine whether this particular effect of Diamox therapy is primary or secondary to seizure control.

► [In their study of acetazolamide in epilepsy, Lombroso *et al.* (1956-57 YEAR BOOK, p. 357) found some suggestion that the agent directly interfered with cerebral neuron metabolism, the beneficial effects being correlated with neither dosage of the drug nor level of carbonic anhydrase activity in the blood.—Ed.]

Control of Petit Mal by Acetazolamide. With the advent of electroencephalography, respiratory alkalinization made clear the influence of pH on the occurrence of epileptic concomitants. Carbon dioxide has a demonstrable inhibiting effect on some continuous epileptic discharges, and there is some evidence of sympathetic conditioned cerebral vasoconstriction. Attention was therefore directed toward the effects of reduction of pH therapeutically by any practicable biochemical procedure. Acetazolamide (Diamox®) proved to be the most potent and least toxic substance available to effect the maximum inhibition of carbonic anhydrase. Its effect on body pH had been studied in the treatment of glaucoma. Its inhibiting power is several times greater than that of more toxic sulfonamides which had yielded inconclusive results when used previously by the authors to treat epilepsy.

F. L. Golla and R. Sessions Hodge[9] (Stapleton, England) selected 78 patients, aged 6-35, with symptoms of centrencephalic epilepsy with a seizure pattern generally described as petit mal lapse and with a primary bilateral electroencephalographic synchrony exhibiting a wave and spike rhythm of about 3/second. Seizures in these patients ranged from 2 to 100 daily. All 78 patients were refractory to every form of treatment, but only 2 failed to respond to a 250 mg. daily tablet of acetazolamide supplementing previous treatment. During observation periods of 3-10 months, 34 patients had completely overcome minor attacks and the others had a decrease in attacks from 5 or more daily to 1 or 2 a month. Increasing the dosage from 250 mg. to 500-750 mg. did not noticeably decrease the number of attacks. In 5 patients with a low incidence, reinforcement of the acetazola-

(9) J. Ment. Sc. 103:214-217, January, 1957.

mide with ammonium chloride in 0.5 Gm. doses 3 times daily stopped attacks altogether. The abnormalities of the EEG response to stroboscope stimulation did not indicate noticeable improvement for a long period, often weeks, after clinical cessation of the petit mal attacks. From experiments in rats it was concluded that acetazolamide is probably of little value in the treatment of cortically conditioned epilepsy. No toxic side effects were noted. Paresthesias, somnolence and diuresis were infrequent complaints, all of which disappeared after the first few days of treatment.

Meprobamate in Treatment of Epilepsy of Children. Samuel Livingston and Lydia Pauli[1] (Johns Hopkins Univ.) treated 128 epileptic children, 59% of whom also had hyperactive behavior disorders, with meprobamate for 9 months to 2 years. Maximum dosage of one or more other anticonvulsants, administered for 6 months or longer, had previously proved ineffective in controlling seizures in 86 (67%) of these patients. The daily dose of meprobamate varied from 400 mg. to 2,400 mg., administered in 2-4 divided doses. The amount was increased every 2 weeks, at the rate of 200 mg. daily, as necessary, to the maximum dose used. Routine blood cell counts and urinalyses were done monthly on all patients.

Meprobamate controlled or reduced minor motor seizures in 4 of 14 patients not previously treated with anticonvulsant drugs, in 6 of 18 whose condition was partially controlled by other drugs and in 3 of 9 in whom the disease was completely refractory to maximum dosage of other anticonvulsants. Behavior difficulties were alleviated in 42% of 76 patients. Patients with major motor disturbances, petit mal or psychomotor seizures were not significantly relieved. Except for drowsiness in a few patients, no significant side actions occurred. No abnormalities developed in the blood picture, and urinalyses remained within normal limits.

Comparison of Hypnotics—Doriden® and Nembutal®. Doriden is 1-phenyl-1-ethyl-glutarimide, not a barbiturate, and the manufacturer claims a hypnotic effect of medium duration, the patient awakening at his normal hour, refreshed and without hangover. F. N. Fastier[2] (Otago Univ.) com-

(1) A.M.A. J. Dis. Child. 94:277-280, September, 1957.
(2) New Zealand M. J. 57:171-175, April, 1958.

pared Doriden and Nembutal with placebos issued to healthy student volunteers on different nights. One third of the capsules contained only lactose, the rest either Doriden or Nembutal. The subjects were told that the trial was to compare the hypnotics but were not informed which drugs they had been given or that a placebo had also been issued. The results were tabulated by a questionnaire which was issued to the volunteer with the drugs.

In one trial, 500 mg. Doriden was not more effective than the placebo, whereas 200 mg. Nembutal had a powerful hypnotic effect on almost all the students who took it. In another trial on other volunteers, increasing Doriden to 700 mg. and reducing Nembutal to 150 mg. resulted in almost identical results in the test. About half the subjects who took them stated they felt drowsy within an hour of swallowing the capsule and slept more soundly than usual. The incidence of hangover drowsiness was no less with Doriden in this dose than with Nembutal. About 80% indicated that the placebos had no effect, compared to only 30% who said this of Doriden or Nembutal. The only side effect of note was dry mouth after 700 mg. Doriden.

These results indicate that Doriden is about one-fifth as potent as Nembutal by weight. When they were given in comparable doses, there was no significant difference in speed of action, duration of effect or incidence of hangover sensation. With both Doriden and Nembutal, a dose large enough to produce sleep reliably in a healthy young adult is likely to cause hangover drowsiness.

► [Controlled studies, as discussed last year by L. Lasagna (1957-58 YEAR BOOK, p. 363) suggest that the newer hypnotics do not differ qualitatively from barbiturates in their desirable or undesirable attributes. The barbiturates are still the drugs on which most practitioners place greatest reliance, but I think that old fashioned chloral hydrate has much to recommend it: efficacy; bad taste and gastric disturbance to discourage too frequent use; lack of addicting properties.—Ed.]

Acute Glutethimide (Doriden®) Poisoning: Use of Bemegride (Megimide®) and Hemodialysis is discussed by George E. Schreiner, Leonard B. Berman, Renato Kovach and H. Allan Bloomer[3] (Georgetown Univ.). Glutethimide (Doriden®), a hypnotic and sedative, is poorly soluble in water but highly soluble in alcohol and acetone. In large doses, the gastric absorption may be irregular. This makes it difficult

(3) A.M.A. Arch. Int. Med. 101:899-911, May, 1958.

to establish dose-toxicity relationships in human glutethimide poisoning. Once absorbed, glutethimide is eventually excreted in the bile and up to 85% can be recovered from a biliary fistula. It is presumably available for reabsorption from the intestine and then excreted in the urine as a conjugate or metabolite.

The authors observed 5 women and 1 man, aged 24-47, with severe acute glutethimide poisoning who were managed with varying combinations of supportive measures, bemegride (Megimide®) and external hemodialysis. Among these, deep coma, areflexia, severe hypotension and hypoventilation occurred after ingestion of 7-12 Gm. glutethimide. Death occurred in 1 patient, to whom it is reasonably certain only 10 Gm. was available, but potentiation by alcohol was likely. In 3, there was a complicating synergism of other tranquilizing drugs taken in small amounts. Two others had secondary infections.

Glutethimide was identified and measured in the serum of all patients by the method of Goldbaum and associates.

METHOD.—The stimulant β,β-methylethylglutarimide (Megimide®) in a dilute solution of 5 mg./ml., was injected into the tubing of a running intravenous infusion of 5% dextrose in distilled water. Over a 3- to 5-minute period, with 10-15 minutes between doses, 10-ml. increments were injected. The injection was stopped when anesthesia was satisfactorily lightened, as evidenced by good respiratory excursions and return of reflexes. Plantar withdrawal was considered to be the single most valuable sign. Injection was also stopped when excessive grimacing, muscle twitching or clonus heralded the danger of convulsions. Reflex changes were graded on a scale of 0-5 and, when presented in serial fashion, represent the judgment of a single observer.

There were cyclic variations in the clinical level of anesthesia in these patients. Such cycles are much more prominent than in comparable degrees of barbiturate poisoning and can lead to difficulties in evaluating the patient and effect of treatment. A talking patient may become completely unresponsive in a matter of minutes. Glutethimide is largely excreted in the bile, but it is not certain whether the intestinal resorbate represents inert metabolite or active drug. It is possible that intestinal anesthesia may slow initial absorption, a mechanism which has been observed in severe phenobarbital poisoning.

The authors observed violently pruritic petechial rash in

a patient who had never before received the drug or had a clinical allergy. Two patients were successfully treated with external hemodialysis, which proved that glutethimide is dialyzable.

Patients with mild glutethimide poisoning have normal blood pressure and deep tendon reflexes and can be aroused by painful stimuli. The blood level will probably be around 0.5-1 mg./100 ml. Such patients can be treated with symptomatic therapy, but patience is required. They will waken after a period of prolonged sleep.

Patients with moderate poisoning may manifest hypotension, shallow or abdominal breathing, absent or variable deep reflexes and some plantar withdrawal. Pain response and corneal reflex should be present. The blood level will probably be 1-3 mg./100 ml. Treatment should include early lavage of the stomach, but the physician should desist immediately if apnea or respiratory irregularity occurs. The use of endotracheal suction and oxygen and pressor drugs for hypotension are valuable—care is necessary to avoid overhydration. Cerebral edema represents a major threat. The patient may be titrated with bemegride, using 50-mg. increments every 10-15 minutes and maintenance doses as needed to keep a "safe" state of anesthesia. It is well to be suspicious if more than 1,500 mg. bemegride is required to lighten anesthesia. The bemegride should be stopped immediately if clonus or convulsions are produced.

Patients with severe poisoning show hypotension, areflexia, deep coma, absence of plantar withdrawal and pain response. The blood level will probably be above 3 mg./100 ml. Such patients should be titrated with bemegride immediately after a sample is taken for glutethimide blood level before bemegride is given. Other measures should be instituted, if possible. In event of failure to elicit light reflex or plantar withdrawal, a bemegride requirement greater than 1,500 mg. on titration, convulsions from bemegride, or later deterioration of clinical state, plans should be made for external hemodialysis on an emergency basis.

Clinical Aspects of Susceptibility to Methylpentynol. Methylpentynol (Oblivon) is a vinylethynl carbinol, described as an important sedative, producing mental relaxation and diminished anxiety. Early reports unanimously emphasized the paucity of toxic complications. Recently, however, a number of publications have drawn attention to toxicity. Edward Marley and Allen A. Bartholomew[4] (London) prescribed 0.5 Gm. methylpentynol 4 times daily for 5 days to 54 subjects who had received inert capsules for the 5 days immediately preceding the test period.

Toxic effects appeared between the 3d and 5th day of the regimen in 32 subjects, all of whom recovered completely within 4 days of withdrawal of the drug. Toxicity was manifest as pupillary abnormalities, nystagmus, suffusion of the conjunctivas, ptosis, loss of facial muscle tone, dysarthria, tremor of the protruded tongue and cerebellar ataxia in the limbs and/or posterior column ataxia. Muscle tone and tendon reflexes were diminished. Abnormalities appeared in the EEG's. Mood change, particularly depression with irritability, dominated the mental status. The subjects were oriented, but concentration and attention were impaired. Dysphasia, paraphasia and distorted time experience and body image were noted. Illusions or possibly hallucinations occurred. Retrospective memory for the toxic episode was impaired. One patient had prominent withdrawal features. The drug probably accumulates in the body, and doses of 2 Gm. daily are too high for long-term sedation.

Medical Control of Tic Douloureux: Preliminary Report on Effect of Mephenesin on Facial Pain is presented by Robert B. King[5] (Washington Univ.). Experiments with cats prompted the administration of mephenesin (Tolserol®) or the carbamic acid ester of mephenesin (Tolseram®) and Dilantin® to patients with trigeminal neuralgia. A dosage schedule was developed gradually as experience was gained. Recently, patients were started on mephenesin carbamate suspension, 1 Gm. 5 times a day, increasing the dosage if necessary to 3 Gm. Occasionally, another 1-3 Gm. was taken during the night if the patient awoke with pain. Intravenous mephenesin was given 3 times a day before meals if a patient was having too much pain to eat during the 1st week on oral medication. Dilantin®, 0.09 Gm., was given to those having unusually severe or frequent pains or unpleasant side effects from the larger doses of mephenesin.

(4) J. Neurol., Neurosurg. & Psychiat. 21:129-140, May, 1958.
(5) J. Neurosurg. 15:290-298, May, 1958.

Unpleasant side effects were reported by 18 patients. Usually mild transient dizziness or unsteadiness occurred only after the early morning dose taken on arising. These complaints were minimized by drinking a glass of milk or orange juice on arising and tended to subside after the first few days of treatment. Four patients complained of nausea; 1 vom-

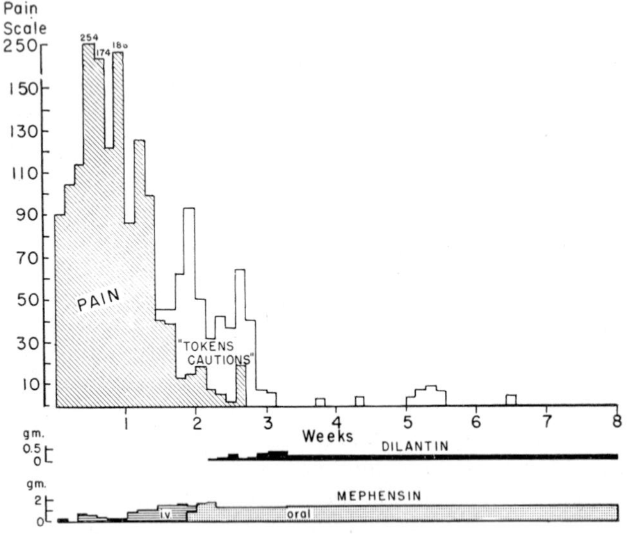

Fig. 34.—Pattern of response in man, 72, with severe tic douloureux. (Courtesy of King, R. B.: J. Neurosurg. 15:290-298, May, 1958.)

ited; 3 noted a mild generalized macular erythematous rash after 1-3 months of medication, which cleared in 1 despite continued treatment but persisted to a mild degree in the other 2.

Of the patients with typical trigeminal neuralgia, 86% gained satisfactory relief from pain. In 1, moderate pain persisted but was sufficiently controlled to prompt him to refuse surgical intervention. Two gained moderate relief but required section of the posterior root. Eight with trigeminal neuralgia and marked anxiety or depression did not improve on medication to the same degree as those not requiring psychiatric care. Half of those with tic douloureux and psychiatric overlay gained major relief. Three patients with paroxysmal facial pain and organic disease of the central nervous system were improved. Two required section of the posterior root despite moderate improvement. Six of 7 patients with atypical facial pain were not improved after taking large amounts of these drugs. The seventh was not greatly relieved.

The pattern of symptomatic relief after the use of these drugs was reasonably consistent.

In man, 72, with frequent severe tic douloureux, the pattern of response (Fig. 34) was recorded by asking him to mark on an hourly check sheet each pain during each 24 hours. He had eaten little solid food for over a week and was completely free from pain for 40 minutes to 1½ hours after each intravenous dose of mephenesin. Pain gradually subsided in intensity and later in frequency. Thirteen days after treatment was begun he resumed chewing tobacco and eating soft foods without requiring intravenous mephenesin before mealtime. "Tokens" occurred at first on the 10th day and persisted periodically throughout the 12 months of observation. Dilantin® was given to try to control the paroxysmal paresthesia, but without success, and was discontinued after 3 months. Occasionally, he has mild pain, frequently associated with periods of stress, which he reports on his weekly check-up. With minor adjustments in dosage of Tolseram®, these attacks have been readily controlled.

Dilantin® in Treatment of Trigeminal Neuralgia. Dilantin was given to 4 patients with trigeminal neuralgia and to 1 with glossopharyngeal neuralgia. Anthony Iannone, A. B. Baker and Frank Morrell[6] (Univ. of Minnesota) report that in all who received adequate dosage definite relief from pain was obtained and the paroxysms of pain controlled.

Man, 62, had lancinating pain above the right eye and in the right cheek in 1954. The pain was intermittent and appeared in attacks several times daily. Injections of vitamin B_{12} were given and the pain subsided after 2 weeks. In September 1956, the pains recurred, became more intense, occurring 3 or 4 times daily, and lasted about 1 hour. The attacks could be triggered from the forehead, eyelid or roof of the mouth. No relief was obtained from intramuscular vitamin B_{12} or intravenous procaine. In October 1957, he was hospitalized. Neurologic examination was normal except for areas of hyperesthesia in the forehead, eyelid and roof of the mouth. An attack of pain could be reproduced by stimulating these areas. The patient was placed on 0.1 Gm. Dilantin 3 times daily. The clinical picture at different stages of treatment appeared to depend on drug level. On doses of 0.3 Gm./day the pain in areas of radiation tended to disappear, though it could be reproduced by stimulation of the trigger area. Pain in the region of the trigger point tended to persist and still caused distress. At 0.4 Gm./day, the patient noticed localization of paresthesia in the region of the trigger point. This was not par-

(6) Neurology 8:126-128, February, 1958.

ticularly painful. Raising the dosage above this level produced complete relief from symptoms, but with corresponding signs of Dilantin toxicity. Attacks were reproduced on 3 separate occasions by withdrawal of the drug, and relief was obtained by administration of Dilantin. The patient was discharged on 0.4 Gm./day and by February 1957, dosage gradually was cut without initiating a paroxysm. He remained pain free without medication until April 1957. At that time he again felt some twinges of pain in the right face and immediately resumed Dilantin, 0.3 Gm./day. He had relief within 24 hours. He remained on this drug for 1 month and then was able to discontinue it without recurrence of pain. He has been pain free since.

The pain-relieving properties of Dilantin are not due to a placebo effect because relief from the drug is reversible and does not occur until 24 hours after administration and the pattern of response depends on the dosage given.

Treatment of Myasthenia Gravis: Prolonged Action with Multiple-Dose Tablets of Neostigmine Bromide and Mestinon® Bromide. Neostigmine, by injection or in 15-mg. tablets, is effective for only 1-3 hours in myasthenia gravis. The frequent dosage necessary in severe cases leads to inconvenience during the day and interruption of sleep at night. Prolonging the parenteral effect of neostigmine by the use of oil was not successful because of the uncertain absorption which resulted in serious over- or underdosage. Enteric-coated tablets, which lose the protective coating in the small intestine, are absorbed as rapidly as is an ordinary compressed tablet. Mestinon bromide has fewer gastrointestinal side effects than does neostigmine bromide, and in some patients it has a longer action. However, many patients must take frequent doses of Mestinon during the day, and some must be awakened for medication at night.

At the suggestion of Robert S. Schwab, Kermit E. Osserman and J. Edward Tether,[7] prolonged-action tablets were manufactured. Neostigmine bromide was supplied in tablets containing the equivalent of 3 doses of 15 mg. each and 3 doses of 7.5 mg. each. Mestinon bromide was supplied in tablets containing 3 doses of 60 mg. each and 3 doses of 30 mg. each. Neostigmine bromide in the prolonged-action tablets was administered to 85 patients with myasthenia gravis, 54 of whom found the tablets superior to their regular medication and continued to take them. Mestinon bromide in the prolonged-action tablets was administered to 109 patients,

(7) J.A.M.A. 165:671-674, Oct. 12, 1957.

82 of whom found these tablets superior to their regular medication and continued to take them. The greatest value of this type of medication is that it eliminates the need for doses during sleeping hours. Severe toxic or accumulative effects were not encountered, and variability in absorption, once the satisfactory dosage was established, did not occur.

Treatment of Anticholinesterase Intoxication with Oximes: Use in Normal Subjects and in Patients with Myasthenia Gravis is discussed by David Grob and Richard J. Johns[8] (Johns Hopkins Univ.). Intoxication by anticholinesterase compounds may occur in normal subjects after accidental exposure to organophosphorus insecticides (e.g., parathion and tetraethylpyrophosphate [TEPP]) and chemical warfare agents (e.g., sarin, one of the "nerve gases," isopropyl methyl phosphonofluoridate). Similar intoxication may occur as a result of overtreatment of patients with myasthenia gravis with anticholinesterase medication, whether organophosphorus (TEPP or octamethyl pyrophosphoramide [OMPA]) or quaternary ammonium (neostigmine [Prostigmin®], bis-neostigmine [BC-40], pyridostigmine [Mestinon®], bis-pyridostigmine [hexamarium, BC-51] or ambenomium [Mytelase®]). These compounds inhibit cholinesterase enzymes throughout the body, resulting in local accumulation of acetylcholine, which produces increased activity of smooth muscle and secretory glands (manifested by nausea, vomiting, diarrhea, sweating and increased salivary and bronchial secretion), bradycardia, central nervous system symptoms, muscular weakness and fasciculations in normal subjects and increased strength which may be followed by weakness in patients with myasthenia gravis. In the management of the latter disease, graded doses of anticholinesterase compound are administered until a maximal level of strength is attained in the affected muscles. Unfortunately, in patients with severe myasthenia, the maximal strength attained may be far below normal. Increasing doses may result in no further increase in strength, and excessive use may produce generalized weakness which is accompanied by less muscular fasciculation and gastrointestinal symptoms than in normal subjects.

The authors found that intravenous administration of

(8) J.A.M.A. 166:1855-1858, Apr. 12, 1958.

1,000-2,000 mg. pyridine-2-aldoxime (2-PAM) or diacetyl monoxime (DAM) ameliorated generalized weakness produced by quaternary ammonium or organophosphorus anticholinesterase compounds in normal subjects and in patients with myasthenia gravis. These oximes are valuable adjuncts to atropine in the management of anticholinesterase intoxication and should diminish the necessity for, or duration of, artificial respiration and endotracheal intubation. More cautious administration is necessary in myasthenic patients in whom overtreatment with oxime returns strength to the basal level present before administration of anticholinesterase compound.

Use of Citrated Calcium Carbimide (Temposil®) in Treatment of Chronic Alcoholism. Jackson A. Smith, Jack A. Wolford, Marilyn Weber and Dougald McLean[9] observed reactions to 154 alcohol tests in 73 male alcoholics taking citrated calcium carbimide. Reactions began 5-10 minutes after the alcohol was given, reached a maximum in about 30 minutes and lasted 60-90 minutes. Conjunctival injection, flushing of the face, headache and dyspnea were routinely seen. The patient usually became somewhat apprehensive, although less so than with disulfiram. A few patients experienced palpitation, tremor, vertigo and drowsiness. After the reaction patients felt lethargic, but less so than after a disulfiram-alcohol reaction. Only 4 reactions were accompanied by nausea and vomiting.

In only 6 patients were the objective findings such as to cause concern; 4 became cyanotic, 1 had generalized tremor with "chilling" and marked apprehension and the sixth, a known asthmatic, became dyspneic. The marked fall in blood pressure frequently seen in disulfiram-alcohol reactions was not observed. There was no evidence of bone marrow depression after prolonged administration, but leukocytosis occurred in several patients. Abdominal discomfort and impotence were not observed.

An average daily dose of 50 mg. seems adequate, but a few patients may require 100 mg. There is no evidence that citrated calcium carbimide is habituating or addicting.

The tests were carried out to determine the toxicity of this medicament when alcohol is taken. There is little cause to

(9) J.A.M.A. 165:2181-2183, Dec. 23, 1957.

believe that the discomfort of reaction from citrated calcium carbimide or disulfiram and alcohol is of its therapeutic, since alcoholics often have more unpleasant reactions after a bout of drinking without the discomfort influencing in the least their drinking pattern.

Galactose Treatment of Multiple Sclerosis: Preliminary Report. Prominent among the component substances of myelin are the cerebrosides, some of which are fairly well characterized as galactolipids. Their formation depends on an adequate supply of galactose. In multiple sclerosis there is a decreased cerebroside content in and around the demyelinated areas of the cerebral cortex. It has been suggested that demyelinating diseases of adults may be related to defective myelin structure laid down in infancy. Infants fed cow's milk may have less galactose available during rapid growth, and myelin formation and the myelin sheath may be synthesized from glucose. Another suggestion is that there may be a primary disorder of metabolism that has only a secondary effect on the central nervous system. An increase in thyroxin level makes difficult the assimilation of galactose. The role of pregnancy, often considered a precipitating cause of exacerbation, gains support from this hypothesis in terms of depleting body galactose stores through the secretion of milk by lactation.

On the supposition that there is an abnormality of galactose metabolism in multiple sclerosis, Jack Hartstein and George A. Ulett[1] (Washington Univ.) gave galactose to 11 patients. All were hospitalized and given 1,000 cc. of 5% galactose (50 Gm. in water to which was added 2 cc. Betolake®, 1 ampule of Ascorbin-B and 1,000 mg. vitamin B_{12}) intravenously/day for 30 days at a rate not exceeding 10 cc../10 lb. body weight/hour, and 25 units of regular insulin daily. Ten patients also received 50 Gm. galactose orally in orange juice. Two additional patients were given the intravenous galactose at a faster rate but did not receive the oral galactose or insulin. Ten patients showed a significant reversal of symptoms with intravenous therapy. After the initial treatment phase, 9 patients were continued on 50-100 Gm. galactose/day orally with insulin for 70-90 days, but this treatment regimen was discarded because of extreme nausea and

(1) Dis. Nerv. System 18:255-258, July, 1957.

weakness. The 6 patients who remained in the hospital showed a steady decline in function and a reversal of symptomatology, although all were still somewhat better than when admitted. One patient had further intravenous treatment on 3 occasions for 5-7 days, with improvement after each. Because of lack of suitable veins for repeated injections, treatment was continued with 50 cc. of 5% galactose solution by clysis with 150 units of hyaluronidase daily, and the patient continued to improve. Although the initial observations were inconclusive, this treatment warrants further investigation. It is possible that multiple sclerosis patients have a defect in galactose metabolism related to absorption of galactose from the alimentary tract.

Treatment of Myotonia with Procainamide was evaluated by D. Stuart MacRobbie and Walter J. Friedlander[2] in 6 patients with myotonia dystrophica and 1 with myotonia congenita. All had definite myotonic reactions after voluntary contraction of the hand ("voluntary contraction myotonia"). In addition to a neurologic work-up, pertinent endocrine and ECG studies were made. After a base line of behavior and activity was recorded, the patient was usually started on 2 Gm. procainamide hydrochloride USP daily by mouth in 4 divided doses, and the dose was then increased by 0.5-1 Gm. increments until the effective maintenance dose was reached. The patients were observed daily in the hospital for several weeks and followed after discharge. Opinions of the nursing staff, other patients and at least three physicians were recorded. Frequent blood counts were obtained.

Oral procainamide produced significant diminution of the voluntary contraction myotonia in all except the patient with myotonia congenita, who had only a minimal degree of myotonia at the outset. Although voluntary contraction myotonia was virtually abolished, the myotonia after percussion ("percussion myotonia") was not appreciably altered. The 5 patients with well-advanced myotonia dystrophica were helped enough to warrant definite continuation of this rather expensive drug. Improvement started within 1 hour after oral administration of a single dose and continued noticeably for about 4 hours. Some patients claimed additional benefits such as relief from chronic muscle stiffness and aching, and

(2) A.M.A. Arch. Neurol. & Psychiat. 78:473-475, November, 1957.

increase in strength, stamina and alertness. Follow-up studies for a year revealed no significant changes in the effectiveness of the drug, though the feeling of well-being decreased. There were no side effects unfavorable enough to necessitate stopping the drug. Epigastric distress and nausea, the most common, were eliminated by slight reduction of dosage. No change in the hemogram was noted, although agranulocytosis was reported.

Hexafluorodiethyl Ether (Indoklon)—an Inhalant Convulsant: Its Use in Psychiatric Treatment. Pharmacologic agents formerly used have had many disadvantages compared with electroconvulsive therapy. However, the convulsant action of a recently synthesized compound, Indoklon, led John C. Krantz Jr., Augusto Esquibel, Edward B. Truitt Jr., Alfred S. C. Ling and Albert A. Kurland[3] (Univ. of Maryland) to its clinical evaluation in 75 patients receiving convulsive therapy. The compound is a colorless, mobile liquid, readily volatile, which emits a pleasant ethereal odor and is soluble in alcohol. The vapor is noninflammable. A standard course of 12 treatments, 3 a week, was given to all 75 patients.

TECHNIC.—After fasting, the patient is given 0.6 mg. atropine sulfate parenterally. A close-fitting Stephenson mask is used, modified with an activated charcoal exhalant adsorber. The drug is dispersed in a measured amount over absorbent gauze in a plastic reservoir with air inlets. The patient breathes oxygen for about 30 seconds, a rubber mouth gag is then inserted, the mask strapped on and the hexafluorodiethyl ether reservoir shunted into the respired air. The reservoir is initially loaded with 1.5 cc. hexafluorodiethyl ether saturating the gauze. Subsequent convulsions may be induced by resaturating with 0.5 cc. of the solution.

The onset of convulsion is preceded by unconsciousness, then a series of myoclonic movements lasting 2-5 seconds, opisthotonic arching of back lasting 15-30 seconds and clonic movements lasting 15-35 seconds. The patient responds to his name 2-15 minutes later.

Every time hexafluorodiethyl ether was used, it produced a convulsive seizure. The same therapeutic results were achieved as in electroconvulsive therapy, with apparently less apprehension and less postconvulsive confusion. The onset of convulsion was slower but the gradual onset obviated the "jackknifing" frequently seen with electroconvulsions and thought to produce many compression fractures. Also, the period of apnea appeared shorter and cyanosis less

(3) J.A.M.A. 166:1555-1562, Mar. 29, 1958.

marked. Subjectively, patients appeared less fearful of this treatment, despite anxiety occasioned by delayed onset, and requested the treatment in preference to electroconvulsions.

There was no evidence of toxicity in blood, urine, liver function tests or electrocardiograms. Previous intensive studies in experimental animals had shown no drug-induced toxicity in lungs, liver, spleen, brain, heart, kidneys, adrenals or bone marrow. The mechanism of action of hexafluorodiethyl ether is unknown.

OBESITY

Phenmetrazine Hydrochloride: Clinical Evaluation of New Anorectic Agent is presented by Robert Feldman, Edmond C. Alberton and Leela Craig[4] (Univ. of California). Phenmetrazine (Preludin®) was given in doses of 25 mg. 3 times a day 30 minutes before meals to 49 patients attending the Obesity Clinic. No specific dietary restrictions were made, except that patients who were already following dietary regimens were advised to make no changes. No other anorectic agents were used during the study, but previous therapy such as administration of diuretics, desiccated thyroid and sedatives was not discontinued. All patients had been observed for long periods, during which their weight had fluctuated little.

Thirty-nine patients (80%) lost weight while taking phenmetrazine. Ten failed to lose weight, and some of these gained weight while taking the drug. Average weight loss/week in the total group was 0.82 lb. A placebo was given 33 patients for a total of 145 patient-weeks, and these patients showed an average weight gain of 0.44 lb./week during this period.

An average weight loss of 1.1 lb./week occurred in 25 patients under age 45 during a mean study period of 9.7 weeks of treatment with phenmetrazine. An average weight loss of 0.42 lb./week occurred in 24 patients over age 45. The smaller weight loss in the older age group was in keeping with general experience that it is harder to obtain weight reduction in older subjects.

(4) California Med. 87:408-410, December, 1957.

No serious side effects or allergic or toxic reactions were noted. Occasional subjective complaints were noted in 10 patients. They consisted of nausea, gaseousness, nervousness, insomnia or metallic taste and were not serious enough to warrant discontinuation of the drug except in 1 patient, for nervousness. In the others, the side effects could be controlled by decreasing the dose and/or altering the time of administration.

It has been noted by others that most regimens that include anorectic agents are effective for 1-2 months, then the efficacy of the regimens drops sharply. No such loss of efficacy of phenmetrazine was observed in the present study. The mean weight loss/week in 33 patients studied 10 weeks or less was 0.77 lb.; in 16 studied 11-18 weeks, it was 0.88 lb./week.

► [Side effects were noted by M. E. Rossman *et al.* (New York J. Med. 58:2394, 1958) in 29 of 91 patients who co-operated to the end of the study, but among 13 additional patients who discontinued treatment early there were some for whom "intolerable" side effects provided the excuse. Most frequent complaints were nervousness and insomnia.—Ed.]

Treatment of Obesity with Phenmetrazine Hydrochloride, a New Anorexiant. Phenmetrazine hydrochloride (Preludin®) is an oxazine derivative with sympathomimetic properties, and its reported action is suppression of appetite with minimal cardiovascular and central nervous system stimulation. In animal experiments the lethal dose was about five times that of amphetamine, whereas the stimulative effect was about one-sixth.

Charles Ressler[5] (Cornell Univ.) reports results of a clinical study in which phenmetrazine, 25 mg. 3 times a day before meals, or a similar-appearing placebo tablet was given to 30 obese patients in a double-blind procedure for an average of about 12 weeks. During the first interview the elements of a balanced, 1,100-calorie regimen were explained orally, and from then on no special stress was placed on diet. With phenmetrazine, every patient lost weight. This was accomplished smoothly and consistently with an average weekly loss of 1.34 lb. The average total weight loss for all patients receiving the drug was 15.25 lb. (table). With the placebo, some patients lost and others gained, so that the average weight loss was 0.24 lb./week. The average total

(5) J.A.M.A. 165:135-138, Sept. 14, 1957.

weight loss for all patients receiving the placebo was 3.02 lb. for the duration of the study (table).

The incidence of side effects and subjective symptoms in patients taking phenmetrazine was negligible, and examination, including pulse, blood pressure, blood cell count and

ANALYSIS OF FINDINGS IN 2 GROUPS OF PATIENTS TREATED FOR OBESITY

	Tablet A (Phenmetrazine)	Tablet B (Placebo)
No. of patients	14	16
Distribution by sex	2 male; 12 female	1 male; 15 female
Av. age, yr.	50.6	48.6
Total no. of wk. of dieting	159	206
Av. no. of wk. of dieting	11.4	12.6
Total weight loss, lb.	216.25	50.25
Av. weight loss, lb.	15.25	3.02
Av. weight loss per wk.,* lb.	1.34	0.24
(Standard error of av.)	(0.343)	(0.113)
Incidence of side-effects	4	2

*Average weekly weight loss for phenmetrazine group was statistically significant at 1% level. For placebo group, it was of borderline significance at 5% level. Difference was also statistically significant at 1% level.

urinalysis, showed no signs of toxicity. Phenmetrazine was found to be an effective and seemingly harmless anorexiant for routine therapy in obese patients.

► [G. Brandan reported (Nervenarzt 29:83, 1958) the interesting case of a patient who became addicted to Preludin, having previously been addicted to opiates.—Ed.]

Study of 1-Phenyl-2-Aminopropane Alginate (Levonor), New Anorectic. Raymond J. Gadek, Harold S. Feldman and Ralph J. Lucariello[6] (New York Med. College) gave one 5-mg. tablet of Levonor 3 times a day ½ hour before meals to 80 overweight patients who were on a diet designed to reduce weight. Many received an added dose at 8 or 9 p.m. to curb nighttime eating. There were no signs of restlessness from this late dosage schedule. Many patients had previously been on therapy with amphetamines or amphetamine-like drugs with diet and had little success.

This drug has been found to delay the feeding reflex in animals without significant stimulation of motor activity. In the human subjects studied, the combined treatment was accompanied by a mean weight loss of 0.9 kg. (2 lb.)/week. Side effects were noticeably absent.

The drug is of no value for the depressed obese patients or for patients for whom psychic stimulation is indicated.

(6) J.A.M.A. 167:433-437, May 24, 1958.

Use of Derivatives of Rauwolfia serpentina in Treatment of Malnutrition. Leon G. Dinkin[7] (Mount Sinai Hosp., New York) treated 42 patients in whom the primary diagnoses were diverse. All had been given high-calorie diets and intermittently multivitamin formulas, liver and vitamin injections, sedatives and in some instances, antibiotics and testosterone for long periods without weight gain. Two varieties of rauwolfia were administered, the whole root of R. serpentina and the alkaloid reserpine. After treatment for 4-24 weeks, the drug was discontinued and usually a placebo was substituted for 8-10 weeks. Administration of rauwolfia or reserpine was then resumed. The dose used was 100 mg. rauwolfia twice daily or 0.25 mg. reserpine 3 times daily.

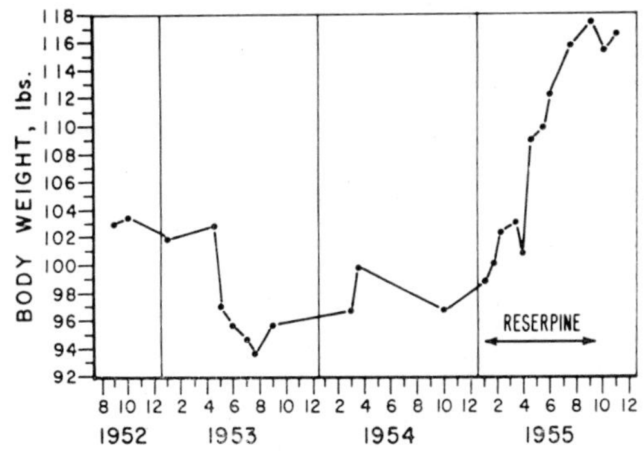

Fig. 35.—Effects of reserpine on body weight of 1 patient. (Courtesy of Dinkin, L. G.: New York J. Med. 58:505-510, Feb. 15, 1958.)

Of the 42 patients treated, 35 gained weight. The total weight gain ranged from 2.5 to 20 lb. (average 6.6 lb.). An especially rapid and marked increase in weight was observed in 13 patients (Fig. 35). Under 26 courses of rauwolfia, the average weekly gain was 0.38 lb., and under 16 courses of reserpine, 0.46 lb. Parallel with increased body weight was improvement in the patients' general condition. They felt stronger, ate more and showed decided improvement in mental attitude. After rauwolfia therapy was stopped, there was usually an arrest in weight gain or a weight loss. Many patients maintained an appreciable weight increase for many months after discontinuing rauwolfia.

(7) New York J. Med. 58:505-510, Feb. 15, 1958.

Few side effects were observed during rauwolfia therapy. In some patients bowel function was stimulated, but this was considered desirable by many. Stuffiness of the nose, often observed in patients treated for hypertension, was not noted in this group. No changes occurred in the skin or in the blood count.

OBSTETRIC AND GYNECOLOGIC DISORDERS

Fertility Control with Oral Medication. Published studies by Pincus and co-workers indicated that norethynodrel suppresses ovulation. When given cyclically in low dosages, combined with a subeffective estrogen, it regulates menstrual cycles. In the present investigation, Gregory Pincus, John Rock, Celso-Ramon Garcia, Edris Rice-Wray, Manuel Paniagua and Iris Rodriguez[8] studied 1,857 cycles of 265 Puerto Rican married women. In 1,467 cycles, tablets were given containing 10 mg. norethynodrel and 0.22 mg. ethinyl estradiol 3-methyl ether or, in a very few instances, 0.23 mg. of the latter. In the other 390 cycles, the estrogen supplement was somewhat lower, i.e., 0.08 mg. in 157 cycles, 0.15 mg. in 61 cycles and 0.18 mg. in 172 cycles. (Tablets containing 10 mg. norethynodrel and 0.15 mg. 3-methyl ether of ethinyl estradiol are marketed under the name Enovid.)

Every woman was given 1 or 2 vials, each containing twenty 10 mg. tablets, with instructions to take 1 tablet daily beginning on day 5 of the menstrual cycle, until 1 vial of 20 tablets was consumed, i.e., through day 24 of the cycle. If a tablet was skipped on any given day, the subject was instructed to continue with the 1-a-day regimen until all 20 tablets were taken.

A schedule of visits by a trained social worker was arranged, so that in every medication cycle every woman was seen shortly after the last tablet should have been taken.

It was found that ingestion of 10 mg. norethynodrel supplemented by varying amounts of estrogen on a prescribed day 5 through day 24 regimen resulted in a normal distribution of menstrual cycle lengths. Observations also indicated that if the regimen is altered by omission of medication, the

(8) Am. J. Obst. & Gynec. 75:1333-1346, June, 1958.

menstrual cycles may be shortened, presumably due to withdrawal bleeding, or lengthened, due to adequate maintenance of the endometrium despite intermittent lack of medication or to extension of treatment by use, after the 24th day, of the tablets missed earlier.

Presumption of suppression of ovulation is strengthened by the fact that conception did not occur in any woman in whom the medication schedule of day 5 through day 24 was followed faithfully. Among those who omitted medication

REASONS GIVEN BY 123 PUERTO RICAN WOMEN FOR DISCONTINUING TREATMENT

	NO.	% OF TOTAL DISCONTINUING	% OF TOTAL SUBJECTS
(a) Reactions	37	30.1	14.0
(b) Moved or too distant	19	15.4	7.0
(c) Pregnant with disuse	14*	11.4	5.5
(d) Pregnant during use	5	4.1	2.0
(e) Sterilized	11	8.9	4.0
(f) Separated from husband	10	8.1	4.0
(g) Husband sterilized	7	5.7	2.5
(h) Unrelated illness	7	5.7	2.5
(i) Husband against practice	4	3.3	1.5
(j) No interest	3	2.4	1.0
(k) Religion	1	0.8	0.5
(l) Miscellaneous causes	5	4.1	2.0
Total	123	100.0	46.5

*Four of these stopped medication because of reactions.

for 3 days or longer, the low incidence of pregnancy was roughly proportional to the number of unused tablets.

No pathologic endometrial changes were observed in specimens taken at different times in the cycle and after varying periods of medication up to 10 months. The sequence of endometrial response to medication, as well as of regression after medication, was generally regular, and no distinction could be made between endometrium from short-term and that from long-term treated subjects.

During or after medication, no significant differences in hemoglobin level were noted in comparison with those of untreated women. The average bleeding time, however, both during and after medication was found to be significantly shorter than in the controls.

Reactions which may be attributable to the drug were breast tenderness, nausea, dizziness, vomiting and pelvic pain. About 18% of the women studied stopped medication because of side effects. Other reasons for discontinuing medication are listed in the table.

In practice, several difficulties were encountered in maintaining complete fertility control. As a result, 19 pregnancies occurred, 5 of them in women who had omitted 3-17 tablets from the regimen and 14 in those who had stopped medication because of "reactions" or carelessness.

Fourteen women who discontinued medication after 1-17 cycles became pregnant within 1-3 months. This suggests that the drug, as used, does not interfere with subsequent fertility.

Male Subfertility: Treatment with Liothyronine (Cytomel®). Liothyronine, 3,5,3'l-triiodothyronine, was isolated from the plasma of normal persons and hyperthyroid patients. It is considered to be the ultimate thyroid hormone, with l-thyroxin becoming effective at the cellular level through deiodination to the liothyronine form. Liothyronine has been successfully used in treating hypothyroidism and simple goiter and has reportedly increased the number and speed of spermatozoa in subfertile men.

D. Cramer Reed, William H. Browning and Harold F. O'Donnell[9] (Wichita, Kans.) evaluated liothyronine treatment in 45 men with oligospermia. Living, active cells with good forward motility were counted in the ejaculate. Fewer than 80,000,000 in the entire ejaculate was arbitrarily considered as indicating subfertility, 80,000,000-185,000,000 as relative fertility and above 185,000,000 as high fertility. Thirty-two patients had deficiencies in both number and speed of spermatozoa and 13 in speed or number. Treatment was begun with one 5 μg. tablet daily and, depending on individual response, the dose was gradually increased to a maximum of 15 μg. daily. Treatment lasted 3-26 weeks.

Of the 32 men who had spermatozoa deficient in number and speed, 24 improved with therapy, 14 in both factors and 10 in one factor without significant change in the other. Of the other 13, therapy increased the number of spermatozoa in 4 and motility in 3, whereas 6 showed no improvement or slight decrease.

Although all 45 patients were classed as subfertile before therapy, 12 improved sufficiently to be reclassed, as relatively fertile and 6 as highly fertile. Conceptions were reported among the wives of 8 of these 18 men.

(9) J. Urol. 79:868-872, May, 1958.

There was no detectable correlation between duration of therapy and response. Only 1 patient reported undesirable side effects—increased pulse rate and nervousness. Both subsided when the drug was discontinued.

Progesterone-Induced Withdrawal Bleeding as Simple Physiologic Test for Pregnancy. According to Glen E. Hayden[1] (Univ. of Chicago), the use of progesterone in the diagnosis of early pregnancy is predicated on its ability to induce withdrawal bleeding in patients with proliferative or estrogen-prepared endometrium. Application of this method to the differentiation of pregnancy from other causes of amenorrhea is necessarily based on the premise that one of the three principal structures, namely, uterus, ovaries or pituitary, may be responsible for the amenorrhea. Menstruation after progesterone therapy in a patient with amenorrhea indicates that the pituitary must be in a more or less normal functional status, since it is producing sufficient follicle-stimulating hormone to cause the ovary to secrete sufficient estrogenic hormone. Finally, the endometrium must be capable of responding and developing to the point of proliferative endometrium. Hence, the patient has a comparatively normal genitoendocrine system. In the absence of proliferative endometrium, as with decidua or the undeveloped endometrium of premenarche or the atrophy of the menopause, no withdrawal bleeding will occur.

Hayden selected 120 patients, aged 18-35, on the basis of previously regular menstrual periods and the distinct possibility that a conception had occurred. They were instructed to report any unusual bleeding and to bring in any clots or tissue passed. All the patients were amenorrheic for 35-70 days from the 1st day of the last menstrual period. The medication was given to 102 patients according to one of the following modes of administration: (1) anhydrohydroxyprogesterone orally, 200-400 mg./day for 4-5 days; (2) progesterone USP vaginally, 75-250 mg./day, for 4-5 days; (3) 17α-hydroxyprogesterone caproate intramuscularly, 125-500 mg./day for 2-5 days.

After this procedure, withdrawal bleeding did or did not ensue within 14 days. The accuracy of progesterone-induced withdrawal bleeding as a simple physiologic but nonspecific

(1) Am. J. Obst. & Gynec. 76:271-278, August, 1958.

test for pregnancy or secondary amenorrhea was 100%. The oral or vaginal mode of administration is preferred to the intramuscular route, since with the former onset of bleeding occurred between the 3d and 7th day in 85% of the patients.

No alteration in the course of a gestation was noted with either standard or excessively large dosage. No abortion can be attributed to use of the progesterone. In secondary amenorrhea, the progesterone test was not only accurate diagnostically but therapeutically, since in 72% of the nonpregnant patients the menstrual cycles were restored to normal regularity.

Antihistaminics in Management of Abortion. During pregnancy the histaminolytic power of the serum increases over a thousand times; histaminase increases sharply from the end of the 2d month to the end of the 5th and continues in a rising level up to term. The purpose of this increased histaminase production might be to counterbalance an increased production of histamine during pregnancy. Such increased production might exceed the physiologic limits, leading to a high level of histamine in the blood, which might excite uterine contractions.

Abdel Hamid Badawy and Beatrice Gabrawy[2] (Cairo), determined the plasma histamine level and histaminolytic index of 50 patients with threatened abortion, 15 of whom were habitual aborters. All were given 50 mg. Pyribenzamine® tablets, 3/day, until bleeding stopped completely; thereafter only 1 tablet was given daily.

In the 15 patients who habitually aborted, plasma histamine was raised to many times its normal level. This high level was brought down by Pyribenzamine, and all but 1 pregnancy continued to term. Thus the fetal salvage rate was 93.3%. In similar patients treated by rest, sedatives and progesterone, pregnancy continued in 17 of 52, a fetal salvage rate of 30.68% (table).

Of 35 patients with threatened abortion who either had no abortion before or had only one, 22 had successful pregnancies. In 5, bleeding stopped as long as the antihistamine was administered. When it was discontinued, bleeding started again and abortion quickly occurred.

The absence of detectable histaminase in the serum after

(2) J. Obst. & Gynaec. Brit. Emp. 65:260-265, April, 1958.

RESULTS OF TREATMENT WITH ANTIHISTAMINES IN 15 CASES OF HABITUAL ABORTION

Case Number	Week of Gestation	Number of Previous Abortions	Number of Days of Medication	Duration of Bleeding After Start of Treatment	Histaminolytic Index Before Treatment Per cent	Histaminolytic Inde After Treatment Per cent	Plasma Histamine Before Treatment Micro-gramme/ ml.	Plasma Histamine After Treatment Micro-gramme/ ml.	Result
1	16	10	12	1	30	40	0·06	0·028	Pregnancy continued
2	24	3	10	5	30	75	0·13	0·035	Pregnancy continued
3	12	3	17	1	20	30	0·125	0·03	Pregnancy continued
4	20	4	2	2	30	50	0·06	0·04	Abortion after two days
5	12	5	18	2	10	—	0·09	—	Pregnancy continued
6	8	8	13	3	Not detected	10	0·075	0·032	Pregnancy continued
7	14	3	13	1	10	30	0·19	0·1	Pregnancy continued
8	8	4	18	2	Not detected	12	0·115	0·06	Pregnancy continued
9	12	3	13	1	12	30	0·15	0·05	Pregnancy continued
10	12	3	14	1	10	28	0·1	0·04	Pregnancy continued
11	12	3	5	2	8	25	0·125	0·06	Pregnancy continued
12	8	3	11	11	Not detected	12	0·1	0·04	Pregnancy continued
13	20	3	13	1	20	50	0·2	0·07	Pregnancy continued
14	22	8	13	5	20	54	0·05	0·032	Pregnancy continued
15	8	3	11	2	Not detected	10	0·4	0·15	Pregnancy continued

the 10th week is a poor prognosis for pregnancy. This can be explained by a high level of histamine in the blood, unopposed by histaminase, leading to irritation of the uterus and abortion.

Intravenous Pitocin® in Late Abortion and Immature Delivery, when the product of conception is too far developed for convenient removal by curet or ovum forceps, is advocated by H. E. Atherton, Albert Alexander and Phil C. Schreier[3] (Univ. of Tennessee). The recommendation is based on experience with 33 patients with little or no dilatation or effacement of the cervix, considered "inoperable from below," 1 of whom had a hydatid mole of 40 weeks' duration, 3 immature labor at 22-28 weeks and the remainder inevitable or incomplete abortion at 16-22 weeks.

Distilled water containing 5% glucose and 0.5-2 cc. Pitocin/L. was administered in an antecubital vein at approximately 15-30 drops/minute, under continuous observation, for not more than 4 hours a day. Each was delivered spontaneously, requiring the assistance of artificial rupture of the membranes in 4, sponge forceps removal of placenta or placental fragments in 9 and a prophylactic dilatation and curettage in the patient with the mole. With no dilatation or ef-

(3) Obst. & Gynec. 10:576-578, November, 1957.

facement, the average time required was 6½ hours, 13 hours being the maximum. Those with some dilatation and effacement averaged 2 hours 15 minutes.

CASE 1.—Multigravida, aged 36, 18 weeks' gestation, had malignant hypertension. She showed no dilatation and effacement of the cervix and no uterine action. Pitocin drip, 4 hours on each of 2 successive days, led to sufficient dilatation and effacement of the cervix to permit artificial rupture of the membranes on the 3d day, followed in 40 minutes by spontaneous delivery.

CASE 2.—Primigravida, aged 23, had spontaneous rupture of the membranes with prolapse of umbilical cord at 18 weeks. There was no effacement and minimal dilatation of the cervix. Pitocin drip for 3 hours produced some ripening of the cervix, and the next day, after a 4-hour drip, spontaneous abortion of a breech presentation was accomplished.

Intravenous Use of Demerol®, Scopolamine and Nalline® in Labor was studied in 265 cases by Herbert Harris, Carl H. Tafeen, Henry L. Freedman and Edward Fogarty[4] (Long Island, N. Y., College Hosp.). When labor was established, 5% glucose in water was started intravenously. A mixture containing 100 mg. Demerol, 0.3 mg. scopolamine and 10 mg. Nalline was drawn into a 10-cc syringe. When the patient asked for sedation, one-third to one-half of this solution was slowly injected through the intravenous tubing. The injection was repeated every 10 minutes or more until the desired effect was obtained, regardless of the imminence of delivery.

PAIN RELIEF IN 265 PATIENTS

	No. Cases	%
Subjective relief		
Excellent	206	77.7
Good	55	20.7
Fair	4	1.6
Objective relief		
Excellent	221	83.4
Good	37	13.9
Fair	7	2.7

In 190 patients (72%), the 1st stage of labor lasted less than 10 hours. Pain relief was evaluated as noted in the table.

In this series 254 infants (96.8%) uttered a sustained cry within 1 minute of delivery. Eleven (4.2%) infants required resuscitation and responded in 2-4 minutes. None of these babies was markedly depressed (only 3 below Apgar 7) and there were no deaths.

(4) Am. J. Obst. & Gynec. 75:39-42, January, 1958.

The minimum total dosage of Demerol was 33 mg. and the maximum 200 mg. Within 1 hour before delivery 102 patients received 66 mg. of Demerol or more. In this series there were 3 slightly depressed infants (Apgar 8). The patients were further evaluated according to the interval between the last dose of the mixture and delivery. There were only 2 depressed babies (Apgar 7 and 8). An irritative excessive cry was noted in 14 cases. The cause and significance of this are not known.

Use of Intravenous Dramamine® to Shorten Time of Labor and Potentiate Analgesia was studied by Carl W. Rotter, Jack L. Whitaker and Joseph Yared[5] (Euclid-Glenville Hosp., Cleveland.) Dramamine was given intravenously to all patients with vertex presentations delivered vaginally

EFFECT OF DRAMAMINE ON LABOR

	NUMBER CASES	TOTAL AVERAGE LENGTH OF LABOR	RATE OF DILATATION
Group 1	47	540 minutes	77.0 min./cm. dil.
Group 2	135	352 minutes	43.0 min./cm. dil.
Group 3	198	386 minutes	55.1 min./cm. dil.
Group 4	125	224 minutes	27.8 min./cm. dil.

who had cervical dilatation of about 2 cm. and intact membranes and whose contractions were becoming established, entering the active phase of the 1st stage of labor. Four groups were compared: primigravidas and multigravidas not receiving Dramamine and primigravidas and multigravidas receiving Dramamine. The duration of the 1st stage of labor was recorded for each patient and the rate of cervical dilatation calculated. Results are listed in the table.

The average length of labor of the treated patients compared with that of the controls was decreased by 3.13 hours in the primiparas and 2.7 hours in the multiparas. This decrease was attributed to the relaxation afforded by the drug. The use of Dramamine also decreased the amount of sedative and analgesic drugs needed, probably due to its tranquilizing effect, by diminishing pain perception and by substantially potentiating the effect of analgesics.

Clinical Evaluation of Phenergan® in Management of Labor was made by William J. Fitzgerald, Rogelio R. Garcia and James J. Cassidy[6] (A. N. Brady Hosp., Albany, N. Y.)

(5) Am. J. Obst. & Gynec. 75:1101-1104, May, 1958.
(6) New York J. Med. 58:1514-1515, May 1, 1958.

in 150 unselected patients given 75 mg. Demerol® and 25 mg. Phenergan as premedication in active labor. Phenergan is known to have the most potent antihistaminic and sedative effects. One hundred controls were given Demerol and scopolamine.

The following results were observed: (1) relief from emotional stress and apprehension, (2) satisfactory analgesic effect, (3) absence of uterine inertia, (4) lowered incidence of nausea and vomiting, (5) shortened labor (the average median length being shortened by 4 hours and 30 minutes compared with that in the 100 controls, in whom it was decreased by 2 hours and 10 minutes), (6) no untoward blood pressure variation, either systolic or diastolic, (7) no tachycardia, (8) absence of postpartum mental depression effects, (9) no postpartum hemorrhage, (10) no allergic reaction and (11) no localized pain, tenderness, swelling or infection at the injection site.

Analgesic-Potentiating Effect of Chlorpromazine during Labor. A study of 1,881 charity patients given chlorpromazine, meperidine and scopolamine in varying proportions every 2 or 3 hours was carried out by John E. Lindley, Stanley F. Rogers and John H. Moyer[7] (Baylor Univ.). Five dosage programs were used: (1) 25 mg. chlorpromazine; (2) 25 mg. chlorpromazine plus 25 mg. meperidine; (3) 25 mg. each of chlorpromazine and meperidine plus 0.4 mg. scopolamine; (4) 12.5 mg. chlorpromazine, 50 mg. meperidine and 0.4 mg. scopolamine; and (5) 25 mg., 50 mg. and 0.4 mg., respectively, of the three drugs. Scopolamine was given only with the initial injection. Evaluation was based on the opinion of the physician at the end of labor and on that of the patient on the 1st postpartum day.

Results with the last program (1,049 patients) were the most satisfactory. Satisfactory sedation and pain relief were reported by 84% of the patients; the physicians reported good results in 89%. Apprehension, nausea and vomiting were reduced and patient co-operation was improved.

Of the 1,887 infants delivered, active resuscitation was required in 2.6%, and 1.6% were stillborn. Moderate respiratory depression was noted in 11.9%; 83.8% were born in good condition.

(7) Obst. & Gynec. 10:582-586, November, 1957.

Side effects attributed to chlorpromazine were seen in less than 3% of the 1,881 patients. Secondary uterine inertia, responding well to Pitocin®, was noted in 0.85%. Unduly profound sedation occurred in 9 patients, transient nuchal rigidity ascribed to involvement of the extrapyramidal nervous system in 2 and transient urticaria in 1. Un-co-operative, disoriented, hyperactive behavior of the type usually ascribed to scopolamine was noted in 19 women. However, in view of the fact that only 1 initial dose of scopolamine had been given, it was felt that chlorpromazine was a definite contributory factor. The incidence of hypertension was only 0.32%. This low incidence was probably due to the fact that all patients remained supine during therapy. No jaundice or blood dyscrasia was encountered.

A series of 212 private patients were also treated, with good results.

On the basis of their results, the authors believe that use of barbiturates for patients in labor is unnecessary.

Preliminary Clinical Evaluation of Dihydrocodeine Bitartrate in Normal Parturition. James D. Myers[8] (Univ. of Tennessee) studied the effect of dihydrocodeine in 50 patients in whom normal labor with no complication was anticipated. No patient was included if a secondary medical or obstetric diagnosis were known. There were 22 primiparas and 28 multiparas whose previous parity ranged up to 8.

On hospitalization, the patients were given 100 or 200 mg. Seconal® orally. Dihydrocodeine, 30 mg., was given subcutaneously to all regardless of weight when labor had progressed to about 5 cm. of cervical dilatation and the presenting part was at zero station. Of these, 34 received a single injection, 11 received 2-4 injections on the basis of individual duration of action, and 5 had injections every 2½ hours to study the effect of a continuous level of analgesia and accumulated dosage.

Dihydrocodeine was found to be an effective, safe and potent analgesic agent in labor, essentially free from side effects. Cardiovascular and pulmonary depression in the mother and a depressing effect on the fetus in utero were absent.

Dihydrocodeine was associated with 55% less over-all fetal depression than was 100 mg. meperidine, given to a similar

(8) Am. J. Obst. & Gynec. 75:1096-1100, May, 1958.

group of patients. The degree of depression, as indicated by the time required to establish normal cry and respiration, was notably less in the dihydrocodeine group. For the level of analgesia obtained, dihydrocodeine is indicated as the safer drug.

Preliminary Report on Dihydrocodeine-Scopolamine in Obstetrics, based on clinical impressions drawn from use in 115 patients in 1st and 2d stage labor, is made by Walter A. Ruch and Robert M. Ruch[9] (Baptist Mem'l Hosp., Memphis, Tenn). Saturation of the ring carrying the hydroxyl radical changes codeine to dihydrocodeine, the bitartrate salt of which is a very soluble white crystalline powder. Solutions of this are stable and may be autoclaved.

With pain as an indication for beginning medication, an initial dose of 30 mg. dihydrocodeine and 0.4 mg. scopolamine was followed in 45 minutes by another 0.4 mg. scopolamine. Larger doses of dihydrocodeine cause some respiratory depression without much increase in analgesia. Scopolamine, 0.2 mg. every 1 or 2 hours, was then continued until delivery. The dihydrocodeine was repeated at about 4-hour intervals, depending on the patient's condition. Eight patients were also given 0.3 Gm. vinbarbital. The only babies showing delay in respiration were those of 3 women in this group.

Ability of dihydrocodeine to limit the wildness which, in part, results from the use of scopolamine to produce amnesia serves as a criterion of analgesic effectiveness. Complete quiet and rest between contractions with almost no activity during a contraction was achieved in 64% of the patients, while 16% showed a high level of excitement. Amnesia was poor in only 7 patients, 2 of whom were given medication only a short time before delivery.

Labor varied from 3 hours or less (30%) to 13-18 hours (5%). Most of the deliveries (78%) were effected under cyclopropane; pudendal anesthesia with Xylocaine was used in the remainder.

The analgesic properties of dihydrocodeine administered as described were found comparable to those of meperidine, with fewer side effects and with little respiratory depression in the baby.

(9) Am. J. Obst. & Gynec. 74:1125-1127, November, 1957.

Tranquilizers in Obstetrics and Gynecology: Studies with Trilafon®. W. Benson Harer[1] (Fitzgerald-Mercy Hosp., Darby, Pa.) used Trilafon, a new tranquilizer, which experiments have shown to be about 5-10 times as potent and only half as toxic as chlorpromazine, in 250 patients in labor at term and an additional 250 obstetric and gynecologic patients.

Trilafon was first used in 50 unselected patients in labor. When labor was well established and analgesia seemed indicated, each patient received 3 gr. Tuinal® orally and 10 mg. Trilafon, 50 mg. Demerol® and 1/100 gr. scopolamine hydrobromide intramuscularly. This provided adequate analgesia and amnesia in all patients. Hypotension occurred in 2, but neither required treatment. Analysis of results in 50 patients and comparison with those obtained with 50 mg. chlorpromazine, together with the same doses of Tuinal, Demerol and scopolamine, showed remarkably similar results. It also established the safety of the drug.

In a double-blind study on 400 women, the 200 who took an 8-mg. Trilafon tablet at onset of labor before leaving for the hospital were calmer, quieter and more co-operative than were the 200 controls who took a placebo. Hypotension was not encountered. Few of the patients in the Trilafon group asked for or needed sedation until late in the 1st stage of labor, when they required 30% less Demerol than did the controls. Labor proceeded normally, and no evidence of harmful effects on mother or child was found. The length of labor was shorter, and its mechanism and the type of delivery were not altered. Adequate analgesia and amnesia were obtained in most instances with a single injection of 50-100 mg. Demerol and 1/100 gr. scopolamine after oral ingestion of 8 mg. Trilafon. Additional smaller amounts of Demerol and scopolamine were required in 12%. No after-effects were encountered.

Trilafon, 4 mg. 3 times a day, for 2-14 days was administered to 56 patients for nausea and vomiting in early pregnancy. Good to excellent results were obtained in about 60%.

Twenty women with premenstrual tension and dysmenorrhea were treated for 2-10 months with 4 mg. Trilafon and 500 mg. ammonium chloride 3 times a day for 7 days preced-

(1) Obst. & Gynec. 11:273-279, March, 1958.

ing the expected onset of the menses. Results were better than with any other method.

Trilafon, 4 mg. 3 times a day, was given orally to 101 menopausal women. Some took the drug for as long as 10 months with no toxic effects. Good or excellent results were obtained in 92 patients. There were 3 failures among patients under age 40 with surgical menopause. Two patients had severe numbness, tingling and pain in hands, arms and shoulders, which cleared up within a week after stopping Trilafon.

► [I suggest that the reader turn to the articles dealing with Trilafon in the section on Neuropsychiatric Disorders; the drug occasionally manifests disturbing side actions.—Ed.]

Synthetic Oxytocin: Critical Evaluation in Labor and Post Partum of a preparation synthesized by the method of Boissonnas was undertaken by Emanuel A. Friedman[2] (Columbia Univ.). The oxytocin, 10 units intramuscularly, was first given to 100 consecutive patients post partum. Of these, only 11% showed uterine atony, as compared with 22% in a similar untreated group. Blood loss estimated at less than 250 cc. was observed in 79.3% of all cases in which the drug was used, as contrasted with 58.8% among the controls, approximately 2% of the patients in both groups losing over 500 cc. Nausea and vomiting were equally frequent in the two groups. Elevation of blood pressure in the oxytocin group was similar to that in the control group and to that observed when natural oxytocin is used.

Intravenous infusion of the drug in a concentration of 7 I.U./500 cc. of 5% aqueous glucose, with flow adjusted to uterine response, was used to induce labor in 126 cases. In 102 of these induction was elective, and in the remainder it was indicated by diabetes mellitus, severe pre-eclampsia, essential hypertension, Rh incompatibility, myasthenia gravis or gouty nephritis. Induction was successful in 109 cases. The same treatment when used in 110 cases to stimulate progress in desultory labor, primary inertia or secondary arrest of cervical dilatation was successful in 107. Statistical analysis based on phases of cervical dilatation versus time, presented graphically, shows a significant reduction of the duration of each part of the curve: the latent phase, acceleration, linear phase and deceleration in the first stage of labor.

(2) Am. J. Obst. & Gynec. 74:1118-1124, November, 1957.

The second stage appears to be shortened but not to a significant degree. These conclusions apply to primiparas or multiparas, except that in the latter group the deceleration phase is not shortened.

The drug was administered with great caution, excessive and possibly harmful stimulation being avoided. No obvious fetal damage was sustained, and cervical laceration in labor and postpartum hemorrhage were not excessive.

Intravenous Pitocin® Infusion: Attempt to Use Pitocin in Semiphysiologic Manner in Induction of Labor and in Treatment of Uterine Inertia. A method of administration of intravenous Pitocin infusion in extremely dilute solutions based on the physiologic responses of the myometrium and the fetus is presented by Brooks Ranney[3] (Univ. of South Dakota).

METHOD.—Each patient is evaluated by obstetric examination. If it is judged the myometrium will respond to a dilute solution of Pitocin, an initial dose of 2 minims (0.123 ml.) is placed in 1 L. of 5% glucose in water, making a concentration of 1:8097. If examination indicates that the initial dose should be more concentrated, 3 minims (0.185 ml.) is placed in 1 L. of 5% glucose in water, making a concentration of 1:5405.

Intravenous infusion is started slowly, while the attendant places his finger tips on the patient's abdomen over the fundus. Even with these dilute solutions there is usually an initial hyperreaction. The uterus contracts strongly and relaxes poorly. The fetus may become somewhat more active, but fetal heart tones are rarely affected. This initial sensitivity usually lasts for 5-15 minutes, during which the fluids are administered slowly or stopped temporarily. When this initial phase has passed, the uterus is more relaxed between contractions, and the contractions are more efficient and rhythmic.

Now the speed of the infusion is titrated against the patient's myometrial response. The infusion is dripped fast enough to produce a firm uterine contraction every 3-5 minutes, each lasting 30-45 seconds, yet slow enough to allow myometrial relaxation between contractions and to avoid any signs of fetal distress. In 93% of patients this semiphysiologic level of myometrial function was achieved and maintained with the original liter of fluids or less.

Within 15-30 minutes after analgesic agents are given, there is often a small modification of the Pitocin requirement; usually the speed of drip must be increased slightly. If fetal membranes rupture spontaneously or are ruptured artificially, Pitocin infusion should be diminished, as labor is thus stimulated. In toxic and some nontoxic patients, Pitocin infusion is followed by a rise in blood pressure. In some cases the speed of the infusion must be slowed.

---

(3) Obst. & Gynec. 10:664-668, December, 1957.

As labor progresses the speed of the infusion is decreased and fluids may be stopped temporarily near the end of the 1st stage of labor in the multipara to avoid precipitous delivery.

The 3d-stage uterus usually functions best without continuous intravenous Pitocin infusion, but all Pitocin fluid left is allowed to run into the mother's vein, starting immediately after delivery of the placenta, except in those patients in whom severe hypertension might be aggravated.

Intravenous Pitocin infusion so administered has been used effectively in 170 patients during the past 4 years, 85 times for induction of labor and 85 times to modify uterine inertia. No fetal or neonatal complications could be attributed directly to this method.

Comparative Study of Ergometrine and Methergine Used in Management of Third Stage of Labor is reported by F. M. C. Forster[4] (Royal Women's Hosp., Melbourne). The clinical trial included over 4,000 deliveries and extended over 32 weeks. The drugs were used on alternate weeks, and the only patients excluded were those delivered by cesarean section. Preliminary studies showed the most satisfactory routine for use of ergometrine maleate to be intravenous injection of 0.5 mg. immediately after delivery and intramuscular injection of 0.5 mg. after expulsion of the placenta. Methergine (methylergometrine tartrate) was given in 0.2 mg. doses intravenously immediately after delivery during the first 24 weeks of the study and was supplemented by 0.2 mg. intramuscularly after expression of the placenta during the last 8 weeks.

The 3d stage was completed within 10 minutes in nearly 87% of deliveries with either drug. In the first 24 weeks of the study the postpartum hemorrhage rate with ergometrine was 2.2%; with Methergine, 3.6%. When intramuscular Methergine was given after expulsion of the placenta, the hemorrhage rate was not reduced. This was in accord with the clinical observation that blood loss with Methergine usually occurred before or during delivery of the placenta. The rate of manual removal of the placenta was 5.6% with ergometrine and 4.1% with Methergine. The postpartum hemorrhage rate with manual removal was 16% when ergometrine was used and 23% when Methergine was used. Ergometrine more often caused a rise in blood pressure than did Methergine. This was more often evident in patients who already had

(4) M. J. Australia 2:155-156, Aug. 3, 1957.

hypertension. This occasional vasopressor response may be responsible for certain atypical cases of postpartum eclampsia and even for a cerebral vascular accident occurring immediately after delivery.

Results of Oral Administration of Hydergine during the First Phase of Labor were tested by Emil Jelinek[5] (Valtice, Czechoslovakia) on 162 primiparas and 24 multiparas. Hydergine was given in doses of 15-20 drops (0.75-1 mg.) orally or in 3 tablets sublingually (0.75 mg.). Definite shortening of labor was achieved in 71% and moderate shortening in 14% of the subjects. No effect was observed in the others. In many primiparas the 1st stage of labor was shortened by one-fourth and in some by one-half. In multiparas, the average shortening of the 1st stage was by one-half. The interval from cervical dilatation of 1-3 cm. to delivery in primiparas who received no medication was 11.42 hours; after use of hydergine, it was 6.4 hours. Hydergine has a weak effect in increasing uterine tone; its principal action is in relaxing the cervix within 15-22 minutes after ingestion. Cervical relaxation occurs even in patients with severe spasm after 20-30 minutes.

In certain patients with late toxemia of pregnancy oral and parenteral hydergine was combined with a high-vitamin diet. Disappearance of symptoms was particularly striking when this treatment was combined with papaverine, phenobarbital and theobromine salicylate.

Oral or sublingual administration of hydergine caused no maternal or fetal complications. Surgical termination of labor was no more frequent than when no drugs were used.

Comparison of the duration of labor in patients treated with hydergine with that in 500 patients previously treated with dihydroergotamine (2 mg. or 20 drops) favored the former. Blood loss in the 3d stage of labor with hydergine was slightly higher than in untreated patients and those given dihydroergotamine, but this difference was not statistically significant.

► [This drug is used considerably in treatment of hypertension on the Continent but has not caught on very well in America. It contains the three ergot alkaloids, dihydroergokryptine, dihydroergocornine and dihydroergocristine, in about equal parts. In experimental animals it has a demonstrable relaxing effect on the vessels through adrenergic blocking action, but the clinical literature has never been convincing to me.—Ed.]

(5) Gynaecologia 143:414-425, June, 1957.

Refined Relaxin and Length of Labor: Preliminary Report is made by Charles H. Birnberg and Maurice M. Abitbol[6] (Brooklyn Jewish Hosp.), who find that Cervilaxin, a purified preparation of the hormone, combined with oxytocin reduces the length of labor when properly used. Consistent results are achieved if the following stipulations have been met: (1) the cervix is at least 75% effaced and not less than 3 cm. dilated, (2) membranes are ruptured, spontaneously or artificially, (3) uterine contractions are strong and regular. Oxytocin, 4-5 minims/L. of 5% aqueous glucose, should be infused intravenously, starting at about 30 drops/minute (rate and quantity to vary with intensity of contractions), and continued until after delivery of baby and placenta. When these requirements are established, 40 mg. Cervilaxin in 250 ml. of 5% aqueous glucose is administered over a 15-minute period.

Under these conditions, 16 primiparas were delivered in an average of 1 hour 20 minutes, as compared with 3 hours 25 minutes for 26 given oxytocin alone. In 10 multiparas, the average time was 26 minutes as compared with 1 hour 45 minutes for 30 oxytocin controls.

Marked softening of the cervix promptly follows Cervilaxin infusion, reducing trauma to mother and infant. Larger and repeated doses relax the perineum as well, aiding in induction of labor. After the membranes are stripped and ruptured oxytocin is administered until the cervix is 3 cm. dilated and 75% effaced. The relaxin preparation administered at this point leads to delivery in less than 1½ hours.

In patients with dystocia problems, failure to deliver within an hour after Cervilaxin-oxytocin infusion may be taken as evidence of improbability of vaginal delivery, warranting cesarean intervention.

► [It seems to me that considerable independent confirmation of such findings as these should be awaited before this drug is accepted fully as an addition to the obstetric armamentarium. Kelley and Posse were unable last year (1957-58 YEAR BOOK, p. 396) to observe striking uterine relaxing effects when a sensitive tocometric technic was employed.—Ed.]

Prepartum Nausea and Vomiting: New Approach to Treatment. William G. Caldwell and Kenneth Hobbs[7] (St. Anne's Maternity Hosp., Los Angeles) report that a controlled study of 101 patients indicated that a combination of

(6) Obst. & Gynec. 10:366-370, October, 1957.
(7) California Med. 88:149-150, February, 1958.

amphetamine and rauwolfia was effective in the treatment of prepartum nausea and vomiting.

The medication used contained in a single tablet 1 mg. of the alseroxylon fraction of Rauwolfia serpentina and 5 mg. amphetamine sulfate. The initial prescription was 1 tablet 3 times daily ½ hour before meals. Dosage was later adjusted to the individual, some patients finding 2 tablets daily adequate for maintenance of effect.

Good to excellent results were obtained in 53 (83%) of 64 patients who received the combination. Five patients reported fair results and 6 were not benefited. Only 5 of a control group of 37 patients who received placebos reported good results.

In addition to relief from nausea and vomiting, concomitant emotional disturbances, notably anxiety and depression, were alleviated by this drug combination. There was almost complete lack of side effects. Also, the combination produced no adverse effect on fetus or mother.

Use of a Long-Acting Estrogenic Hormone Preparation, Estradiol Valerate (Delestrogen®), for Inhibition of Postpartum Breast Engorgement. Gordon Rosenblum and Pearl L. Ginsburg[8] (Cedars of Lebanon Hosp., Los Angeles) obtained excellent results with this drug, estradiol-17-β-N-valerate, given as a single intramuscular injection at or just before delivery. The short-acting estrogens, if used for a few days, are unsatisfactory because of mammary congestion when treatment is discontinued; if used longer, severe uterine bleeding, persistence of lochia, retarded involution of the uterus and delay in resumption of cyclic ovarian function are encountered. Androgens present the hazard of masculinization.

Delestrogen is supplied in sesame oil, 10 mg./cc. Intramuscular injection of 1-2 cc. provides potent estrogenic action for about 3 weeks. In a group of 150 women, injection was made in the buttock during the latter part of labor or immediately after delivery, with the exception of a few who attempted breast feeding for a few days. In these, injection was made immediately after nursing ceased. No other therapy such as tight breast binders or ice bags was used.

In 90%, breast engorgement and leakage were completely

(8) West. J. Surg. 65:234-238, July-Aug., 1957.

prevented. Moderate engorgement and slight leakage on the 7th postpartum day, with discomfort lasting less than 24 hours, occurred in the rest of the patients, except those with established lactation; these did did not respond to the treatment. No excessive uterine bleeding or abnormalities in time or amount of postpartum menstruation developed.

Good results depend on early administration, preferably in the delivery room; a delay of even a few hours limits the extent of inhibition of lactation which may be achieved. The single injection of long-acting estrogen, aside from its effectiveness and freedom from complications, may be recommended as convenient, inexpensive and well tolerated.

► [It may be that this is the slick trick in sunny Southern California, where suckling is no longer de rigueur; elsewhere in our benighted land, however, it is more often the mother who attempts nursing but must abandon it because of a sore nipple or a poor feeder, who poses the engorgement problem. In this type of individual these authors' drug seems to have failed.—Ed.]

Use of Ergometrine with Hyaluronidase to Prevent Postpartum Hemorrhage was studied by W. A. W. Dutton[9] (City Gen'l Hosp., Sheffield, England). An intramuscular injection of 0.5 mg. ergometrine with 1 mg. hyaluronidase (Ergorondase) was given to 500 selected normal patients in the 2d stage of labor with the birth of the anterior shoulder. Results were compared with those of 707 control patients. The incidence of primary postpartum hemorrhage in primigravidas was significantly reduced from 6.2 to 2.5%. The incidence of postpartum hemorrhage in normal multigravidas (gravidas 2-5) was not reduced but the severity of the bleeding was less, as with the primigravidas.

The incidence of manual removal of the placenta was not significantly increased, but the blood loss in the treated group was reduced. The average blood loss and duration of the 3d stage in normal patients was reduced in the treated group. Puerperal anemia in the patients with abnormal 3d stages was less in the treated than in the control group. No local or general undesirable side effects were noted.

It is felt that the routine intramuscular injection of this drug in normal hospital primigravidas is a worthwhile procedure. It may also be applied to multigravidas in understaffed hospitals.

---

(9) J. Obst. & Gynaec. Brit. Emp. 65:315-320, April, 1958.

Therapy of Late Toxemia of Pregnancy with Blood Pressure Depressants. Protoveratrine, dihydrazinophthalazine and reserpine were the drugs used by Lutwin Beck[1] to treat 78 patients with pre-eclampsia. In general, the blood pressure was successfully reduced and by improvement of circulation, symptoms were favorably influenced in many mothers. Prognosis for the fetus was also improved.

Good results (i.e., pregnancy continued to term with birth of a mature infant) were obtained when symptoms appeared near the end of gestation and functional disturbances had not progressed into organic changes, especially in women with no previous hypertension. In all but 1 of 16 patients with severe late toxemia (group I), the pregnancy was successfully completed without risk to the infant. Good results were also obtained in the patients in group IIA, in whom blood pressure had been elevated before pregnancy but had not become worse during pregnancy and was not accompanied by edema or albuminuria. With slowly increasing doses of depressant drugs, transition to a superimposed toxemia was prevented. This is of special significance, since intercurrent toxemia in such patients presents an unfavorable prognosis for the fetus.

Partial results (i.e., the condition did not improve sufficiently after several days' treatment to allow pregnancy to continue without danger to the infant) were seen in patients whose first symptoms (blood pressure over 160/100, albuminuria) appeared before the 36th week of gestation, usually in those with previous hypertension. Duration of treatment with depressants in 12 patients was 2-4 weeks. In 25% of these, pregnancy was terminated 1-2 and even 3 weeks before term by cesarean section. Through medical treatment, the pregnancy could be continued long enough to produce a live infant.

Failures are to be expected if the first severe symptoms (blood pressure increased to 180/110 or over, edema, albuminuria) appear before the 32d week of gestation, mostly in patients with pre-existing hypertension. In 2 patients of group IIB observed during the 7th month, the fetuses died in utero and therapy produced only slight improvement in the mothers. Conversely, 1 patient with severe chronic glo-

(1) Geburtsh. u. Frauenh. 17:1010-1023, November, 1957.

merulonephritis treated from the 24th week with arterial depressants was delivered of an infant weighing 2,320 Gm. in the 37th week by cesarean section.

► [In reviewing the use of antihypertensive agents in eclampsia last year, in conjunction with their own study of reserpine here in the United States, Landesman *et al.* (1957-58 YEAR BOOK, p. 413) found that none of these drugs alters the fetal outcome, though maternal protection may be afforded. In contrast, the present German observer feels that prognosis for survival of the infant is improved.—Ed.]

Antihypertension Therapy in Toxemia of Pregnancy: A 30-Month Progress Report is presented by Charles Farris, Jr., and Philip J. Krupp[2] (Charity Hosp., New Orleans). The study included 196 patients with toxemia of pregnancy (mild pre-eclampsia, severe pre-eclampsia, eclampsia and hypertension with superimposed pre-eclampsia). Treatment started on admission with protoveratrine. Basal medication consisted of 0.5-1 mg. orally every 2-4 hours until the desired responses were obtained, then as indicated for maintenance. Usually this was the only medication required in mild pre-eclampsia. Average duration was 7.5 days. For intravenous medication, 0.1-0.5 mg. in 1,000 cc. of 5% dextrose in distilled water was infused at the rate of 30-50 drops/minute. If there was no significant response, 1 ampule (0.1 mg.) was given directly into the infusion tubing, 2 minutes being taken for the injection and the dose repeated if necessary. Apresoline®, 20 mg., was given intravenously when indicated. Absolute bed rest was required. Routine laboratory tests were made. Fluids were given orally and intravenously, amounting to output plus insensible loss. A salt-free, high-protein diet was prescribed. Magnesium sulfate, 2 cc. of a 50% solution, was given intramuscularly every 2 hours for 4 times. Diuretics were given as necessary. Evacuation of the uterus was performed as indicated by the clinical course when labor did not begin during the control period.

The use of protoveratrine and protoveratrine-Apresoline combinations was found safe, effective and advantageous. Complications arising from hypertension were definitely reduced. Nursing care was greatly simplified. During the hospital stay, the patients were alert and able to handle their respiratory secretions adequately while at bed rest and to take oral feeding and medication. Oliguria was not observed after 24 hours of treatment.

(2) Am. J. Obst. & Gynec. 74:1043-1047, November, 1957.

Of the 196 patients, 177 had vaginal delivery and 19 (9.6%) cesarean section. In the entire series there were 10 (5.1%) sets of twins. One (0.51%) maternal death occurred after vaginal delivery, but the medication used seemed in no way implicated in the death. Fetal mortality consisted of 6 (3%) stillbirths; 2 were due to abruptio placentae, and no satisfactory reason other than toxemia could be found for 4. Three (1.5%) neonatal deaths occurred; 2 of these were due to prematurity and congenital heart disease.

Toxic manifestations were infrequent and usually easily reversible. Vomiting was the commonest reaction, recorded in 36 (18%) patients. In several instances, vomiting seemed to have been caused by other than the alkaloid under study. When vomiting was due to protoveratrine, it could be corrected by reducing the total dose or by adjusting the schedule of medication. Atropine reduced the incidence of vomiting, as did aluminum hydroxide given with protoveratrine. Bradycardia occurred 17 (8.5%) times and was uniformly corrected by atropine. Hypotension occurred in 4 (2%) patients because of overenthusiastic therapy, but was corrected by reducing protoveratrine dosage or by using a sympathomimetic drug.

Tolerance to protoveratrine has been noted infrequently, and it is in these patients and those who require further reduction in blood pressure that Apresoline found its greatest usefulness.

Management of Toxemia of Pregnancy with Reserpine: II. The Newborn Infant. Murdina M. Desmond, Stanley F. Rogers, John E. Lindley and John H. Moyer[3] (Baylor Univ.) studied the perinatal mortality and neonatal morbidity among infants born to 293 mothers with toxemia of pregnancy who were treated according to a plan which included use of the antihypertensive agents reserpine and hydralazine.

The total infant loss at all stages of gestation was 6.8% and the neonatal death rate 1.8%. Total fetal loss was least in mild or moderate pre-eclampsia (3%). In severe pre-eclampsia it was 7.7%, in essential hypertension complicated by toxemia 16.7% and in eclampsia 30.8%. Fetal mortality in groups other than eclampsia appeared to be lower than that

(3) Obst. & Gynec. 10:140-145, August, 1957.

reported by other authors, whereas in eclampsia it approximated the standard mortality figure.

Of 278 infants born alive, 69 showed some variation from normal behavior. Mild or transient abnormalities were observed in 40 infants, including 24 with reserpine effects. Major signs of difficulty occurred in 29, including 5 with reserpine effects. Five infants died in the neonatal period, and 2 were discharged with a diagnosis of probable cerebral palsy.

Hydralazine has not been shown to have any effects on the infant in studies previously reported. Reserpine appears to be transferred to the infant in utero. An estimated 10.4% of infants in this study showed reserpine effects. The side effects of the drug appear to be nasal congestion, lethargy, decreased briskness of the Moro reflex, bradycardia, excessive secretions and, in some instances, a tendency to lowering of body temperature. Nasal congestion and lethargy are most common. The former may be present for 5 or 6 days, the latter usually less than 24 hours. Effects of reserpine on infants could not be correlated with the presence of side effects in the mother or the dosage. The effects were less clearly seen in premature infants.

Use of reserpine in the treatment of toxemia, though associated with a significant degree of neonatal morbidity, does not appear to result in increased fetal mortality.

Protoveratrine in Toxemia of Pregnancy. Edward G. Winkler and Vincent W. Cangello[4] (Buffalo) report their experience with this highly purified preparation of Veratrum album in 31 patients with toxemia of pregnancy. The dose of protoveratrine used was individualized, depending on the patients' response. Those with mild pre-eclampsia were treated usually with oral medication, 1-2 tablets every 2-4 hours for blood pressure readings above 140/90. The smaller dose was given initially, then increased by ½ or 1 tablet every 2-4 hours until the desired response was obtained. Patients with severe pre-eclampsia or eclampsia were treated by intravenous titration, as set up by Finnerty and Fuchs in 1935 for other veratrum preparations.

In 19 patients the protoveratrine regimen was instituted after delivery (1-12 hours post partum) ; in 4 because the disease was post partum in onset, in 1 who had eclampsia be-

(4) Am. J. Obst. & Gynec. 75:433-443, February, 1958.

cause an intravenous magnesium sulfate and barbiturate regimen was begun before delivery and in the other 14 because active labor had begun before admission to the hospital and delivery was imminent. All these patients were delivered vaginally, after spontaneous onset of labor in 18 and an intravenous Pitocin® induction in the patient with eclampsia.

All but 1 patient responded adequately to protoveratrine therapy. An average blood pressure reduction of 41.3 mm. Hg systolic and 28.9 mm. Hg diastolic was obtained in the 30 patients. The desired pressure response occurred within an average of 25.3 minutes when protoveratrine was given intravenously (15 patients) and within an average of 5 hours when given orally (15). Eleven of 12 patients with edema showed a steady decline in amount once treatment was started. Albumin was noted in the urine of 29 of the 30 patients on admission; the degree declined after treatment was started, but all were reported to have from a trace to 3+ albumin when discharged.

Urinary output records were available for 26 patients. Average daily urine output was 2,600 cc.; the patient with eclampsia averaged 400 cc. urine daily before delivery and 3,100 cc. after delivery.

Average duration of therapy for all patients was 4.3 days, although 1 was given protoveratrine for 15 days. Individual doses were noted to be effective from 1 to 16 hours (average, 5.4 hours).

Toxic effects from protoveratrine were infrequent and not severe. At no time was it necessary to discontinue the drug.

Protoveratrine is a potent hypotensive agent and when carefully administered will usually control the cardinal manifestations of toxemia of pregnancy without the hazards of heavy sedation or interference with adaptive reflexes.

Evaluation of Chlorothiazide (Diuril®) in Toxemias of Pregnancy: Analysis of 144 Patients is presented by Frank A. Finnerty Jr., Joachim H. Buchholz and John Tuckerman[5] (Washington, D.C.). Excessive sodium retention is implicated in the pathogenesis of toxemia of pregnancy. Experience with 2,500 patients in a toxemia clinic showed that sodium diuresis is the most useful and effective therapy for

(5) J.A.M.A. 166:141-144, Jan. 11, 1958.

combating fluid retention in pregnancy. Its prompt institution can frequently prevent toxemia. When a small amount of edema is present, ammonium chloride is an excellent diuretic. However, with increasing edema toxemic women show a decreased sensitivity to ammonium chloride. Mercurials are contraindicated in toxemia because of their direct toxic action on renal tubular elements. Acetazolamide (Diamox®) is a potent carbonic anhydrase inhibitor. No serious toxic manifestations were noted in over 1,000 patients given 500 mg. Diamox every 2d, 3d or 4th day.

Early in the study on the 144 pregnant women with hypertension, edema, albuminuria or other manifestations of toxemia, the average effective dose of chlorothiazide was found to be 1,000 mg./day; less did not produce sufficient initial diureses and more did not enhance the diuretic response. The average weight loss with chlorothiazide was 3-4 lb. The ensuing fall in arterial pressure was frequently striking. The only side effect was occasional mild nausea.

Chlorothiazide is the ideal diuretic for prevention and treatment of the toxemias of pregnancy. When given alone at the first sign of excessive weight gain or transient elevation of the arterial pressure, it frequently reverses the toxemic process. Absence of drug resistance allows therapy to be continued throughout pregnancy. It may be instituted at the first antepartum visit of the hypertensive patient (history of hypertension before pregnancy) in whom toxemia is more likely to develop. Preliminary experience with chlorothiazide and acetazolamide given intravenously suggests that this mode of administration is superior and should be used in the patient with severe toxemia. When given in combination with veratrum or hydralazine in severe toxemia, chlorothiazide, in addition to exerting its diuretic effect, greatly enhances the potency of these antihypertensive agents.

Toxemia of Pregnancy: New Treatment for Controlling Edema. W. F. B. James and A. P. Johnson[6] (Meharry Med. College) treated 180 patients with neo-Bromth®, a combination of an 8-bromotheophyllinate compound and pyrilamine maleate. All patients presented classic signs of developing edema when first treated. All but 18 responded satisfactorily. Weight gain was arrested, blood pressure was reduced and

(6) Am. J. Obst. & Gynec. 74:1054-1058, November, 1957.

edema and albuminuria were reduced or eliminated. No side actions attributable to the preparation occurred. A few patients responded to 2 or 3 tablets twice a day, but most required more. A few were given 12 or more tablets daily, but usually 8-10 tablets daily were effective. Each tablet contained 50 mg. 2-amino-2 methyl-1-propenol 8-bromotheophyllinate and 30 mg. pyrilamine maleate.

In each of the 18 patients who failed to respond to neo-Bromth treatment weight gain continued to increase above desirable limits. Most of them had increased blood pressure and albuminuria. Treatment with ammonium chloride and magnesium sulfate was also ineffective. In these patients the more rigorous regimen of a low-salt diet, increased fluid intake and bed rest was found necessary. One patient had full-blown eclampsia but recovered after delivery of a stillborn infant.

Although neo-Bromth is not a hormone, it appears to possess a specific antidiuretic hormone antagonism. Besides its usefulness in treatment of edema of pregnancy it is effective in preventing premenstrual edema.

Treatment of Toxemias of Pregnancy with Chlorpromazine-Phenergan® is recommended by J. Ruzicska and B. Zsolnai[7] (Debrecen, Hungary) after an experience including 16 cases of pre-eclampsia, 8 of eclampsia during labor and 7 of eclampsia post partum. Chlorpromazine is not specific therapy, but it can prevent crises in the pre-eclamptic stage, arrest puerperal eclampsia and control threatening attacks during labor. With this treatment, surgical trauma can be avoided and risk of maternal and fetal mortality decreased. In this series, there was no fetal loss. The 1 maternal death could not be attributed to chlorpromazine.

Of 16 patients with pre-eclampsia late in pregnancy, 12 delivered spontaneously. Forceps delivery was required in 2 and cesarean section was performed in 2.

CASE 1.—Primigravida, 23, had marked edema of the ankles, legs and abdomen on admission. Blood pressure was 140/100, and the urine contained a flaky precipitate. Symptoms increased with development of oliguria (120 cc. in 24 hours) the following day, when blood pressure rose to 185/100. Intravenous perfusion of 100 mg. chlorpromazine, vitamin B_1 and vitamin C in 200 cc. of 5% glucose was combined with Phenergan intramuscularly. Blood pressure fell

(7) Gynéc. et obst. 56:420-427, Aug.-Oct., 1957.

rapidly to 125/90 and urinary output increased to 180 cc. Perfusions of chlorpromazine were repeated twice in the days preceding delivery when blood pressure was increasing. Until then, chlorpromazine (25 mg. twice daily) with an ampule of Phenergan controlled arterial pressure satisfactorily. Oliguria regressed after the second perfusion and urinary excretion reached 800 cc. Edema decreased moderately, and urinalysis showed albumin 2+ before delivery, with absence of nephrotic elements. Specific gravity was 1.020 and 1.028, and Eschbach's reaction was 1.5-3.3%. A healthy infant weighing 3,060 Gm. was delivered spontaneously 11 days after admission.

Among 8 patients with eclampsia during delivery, the condition was successfully controlled in 3 by chlorpromazine-Phenergan treatment, with cessation of convulsions followed by spontaneous delivery. These patients were treated after only 2 or 3 convulsions and attacks ceased promptly and completely as soon as treatment was begun. In 2, delivery had to be completed by forceps after suppression of convulsions. Further convulsions were not averted, even by repeated perfusions of chlorpromazine-glucose in 3 patients admitted after 6, 9 and 11 convulsions, in whom cesarean sections were eventually done.

CASE 2.—Primigravida, 22, admitted at onset of labor, had intact membranes, moderate edema, blood pressure of 130/110, oliguria and opalescent urine due to albumin. A few hours after admission, a typical eclamptic convulsion occurred, lasting 2½ minutes. Oliguria increased and the urine showed a flaky precipitate. Blood pressure increased to 140/120. A half hour later, another shorter eclamptic attack occurred during chlorpromazine perfusion. After another 50-mg. dose of chlorpromazine, the patient was quiet for 6 hours. Blood pressure continued to rise, however, and 2 convulsions occurred. After another perfusion of chlorpromazine (100 mg. in 150 cc. of 5% glucose) with magnesium sulfate, Phenergan and vitamins B_1 and C intramuscularly, the attacks ceased. Delivery was terminated by forceps 8 hours later. The male infant weighed 3,450 Gm. The patient's general condition improved rapidly thereafter. Chlorpromazine, 25 mg. twice daily, was continued for several days. Blood pressure was 130/80. The urine still contained albumin, but urinary output was satisfactory.

Of 7 patients with postpartum eclampsia, 2 had attacks after cesarean section. Five others were referred after 4-11 convulsions. After one or two perfusions of chlorpromazine, crises ceased. In 1 patient, 6 weeks after delivery and five previous crises, repeated infusions of chlorpromazine (300 mg.) were necessary to control the eclampsia.

Action of Chlorpromazine on Uterine Contractility and Arterial Pressure in Normal and Toxemic Pregnant Women was studied by R. Caldeyro-Barcia, J. J. Poseiro, H. Alvarez and P. Tost[8] (Montevideo, Uruguay). Chlorpromazine was administered to 22 pregnant women, of whom 8 had spontaneously started normal labor at full term, 8 had labor induced

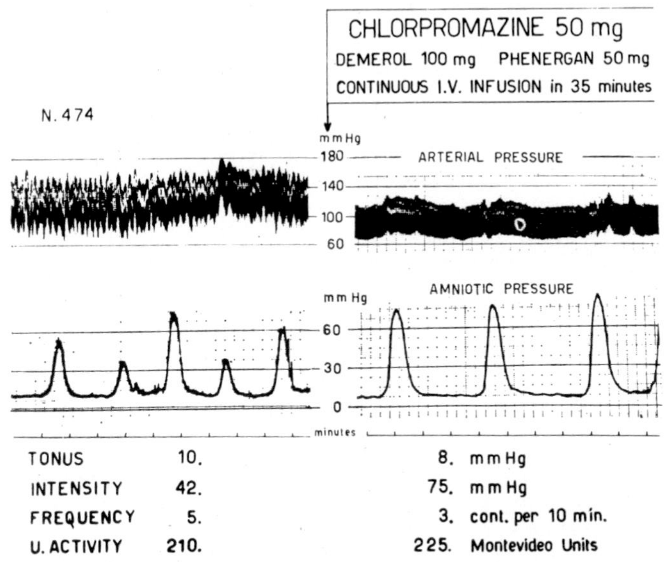

Fig. 36.—Effect of continuous intravenous infusion of chlorpromazine, Demerol and Phenergan in eclamptic patient in 26th week of pregnancy, showing reduction of arterial blood pressure to normal values but no depression in uterine contractility. (Courtesy of Caldeyro-Barcia, R., *et al.*: Am. J. Obst. & Gynec. 75:1088-1095, May, 1958.)

and 6 were toxemic. Eleven were given 50 mg. and 6 were given 25 mg. intramuscularly. Two received an intravenous injection of 50 mg. over 4 minutes and 2 a continuous infusion of 100 mg. Demerol®, 50 mg. Phenergan® and 50 mg. chlorpromazine over 35 minutes. One patient received the drug orally, 50 mg. in 2 divided doses.

Uterine contractility—spontaneous or induced by continuous intravenous infusion of oxytocin—was studied by direct recording of amniotic fluid pressure. Administration of chlorpromazine did not modify uterine activity (Fig. 36) during any of the three stages of labor.

(8) Am. J. Obst. & Gynec. 75:1088-1095, May, 1958.

Labor did not appear to be slowed by chlorpromazine. Arterial pressure, recorded by catheterization of the femoral artery, was not modified in normal pregnancy. In most instances of toxemia of pregnancy, the drug caused the arterial pressure to drop to normal values.

Toxemia of Pregnancy Treated with Progesterone during Symptomatic Stage. In view of the similarities between premenstrual syndrome and toxemia, and the fact that treatment of the former with progesterone not only relieved the symptoms but also prevented edema, hypertension and albuminuria in the premenstrum, Katharina Dalton[9] (London) decided to carry out a trial with large doses of progesterone in patients having early minor symptoms of toxemia in an attempt to arrest full development of that condition. The investigation was carried out in a maternity hospital and midwife training center with 71 beds. Patients complaining of nausea and/or vomiting, lethargy, irritability, depression, vertigo, fainting and paresthesia (generally between the 16th and the 28th weeks, but sometimes earlier) were given a test dose of 100 mg. progesterone in oil, injected deep into the buttock. If relief was obtained for 1 or 2 days, symptoms were considered those which might later lead to toxemia. Toxemia was defined as the presence, on one or more occasions, of blood pressure of 140/90 mm. Hg or over, together with edema or albuminuria in a catheter specimen after the 28th week and before onset of labor, provided the blood pressure before the 28th week had been below 140/90 mm. Hg and there had been no albuminuria.

The initial dose for continued treatment was determined by the severity of symptoms, degree of relief obtained from the test injection and the presence of excessive weight gain. Thus a patient with four different symptoms and a weekly weight gain of 1½ lb. over the previous month was given 100 mg. progesterone daily or on alternate days. If she remained symptom-free when seen a week later, the dose was reduced to 75 mg. daily or on alternate days; if the symptoms recurred, it was increased to 125, 150 or 200 mg. Another patient with few symptoms and a weight gain of 1 lb. weekly was given 25 mg. progesterone, the dose being increased if and when necessary. When the patient remained symptom

(9) Brit. M. J. 2:378-381, Aug. 17, 1957.

free for 2 or 3 weeks the dose was gradually reduced. If symptoms did not recur, treatment was ultimately discontinued; if they recurred, it was immediately resumed.

Ethisterone (anhydrohydroxyprogesterone or ethinyl testosterone) an oral progestogen, is of some value in treating selected patients, but its action is not always identical with that of progesterone. In the prophylaxis of toxemia, its use was limited to patients with mild progesterone-responsive symptoms, with no excessive weight gain, history of previous abortion or hirsutism. In all, 87 patients with progesterone-responsive symptoms were given a week's trial of 100

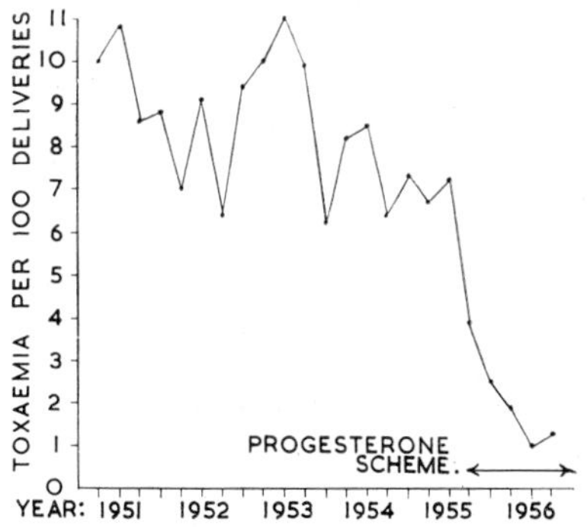

Fig. 37.—Quarterly incidence of toxemia. (Courtesy of Dalton, K.: Brit. M. J. 2:378-381, Aug. 17, 1957.)

mg. ethisterone daily. Of these, 52 (59.8%) reported symptomatic relief. As with progesterone, the dosage of ethisterone was determined on a symptomatic basis, ranging from 50 to 200 mg. daily. If the symptoms recurred late in pregnancy, indicating the need for a larger dose, progesterone was substituted.

Before the introduction of the experimental scheme in June 1955, the quarterly incidence of toxemia had varied between 6.2% and 11%—an average of 9% for 5,307 deliveries. This incidence is similar to that for local maternity hospitals. The first progesterone-treated patients were delivered in September 1955, and in the third quarter of that year the incidence fell from 7.2 to 3.9%, with further declines in subsequent quarters to 2.5, 1.9, 1% and 1.3% (Fig. 37). Before the progesterone regimen there were 12 deliveries for every toxemic patient, whereas after its introduction the rate was 47.6 deliveries.

Progesterone therapy is essentially prophylactic and effective only if started during the early symptomatic stage and before onset of signs. If signs of toxemia develop in patients not taking progesterone, even massive doses of up to 300 mg. intravenously usually prove ineffective and the toxemia pursues its uninterrupted course.

Comparison of Ocular Reactions Using Penicillin and Bacitracin Ointments in Ophthalmia Neonatorum Prophylaxis. A. M. Margileth[1] (US Naval Hosp., Corona, Calif.) reports that over 50% of 2,250 newborn infants had mild to severe chemical conjunctivitis after instillation of 1% silver nitrate for ophthalmia neonatorum prophylaxis. Of 5,394 newborn infants in whom penicillin ointment was used (1,000 units/Gm.), only 1.08% showed a mild to moderate local reaction and none showed a severe reaction. Bacteriologically proved infections occurred in 0.11% while they were still in the hospital, and in 3.1% possible infections were reported by the parents after the infant left the hospital (on the 4th day). No infant had to be detained in the hospital or readmitted because of an ocular infection or reaction. Of 2,380 newborn infants in whom bacitracin ointment (500 units/Gm.) was used for prophylaxis, 0.88% showed mild to moderate reactions, 0.37% had proved infections and 1.26% had possible infections. All bacteria cultured in the bacitracin-treated group were gram negative. The differences in reaction rate and infection rate between the two ointments are not significant. No serious reaction or infection occurred in the total of 7,774 infants studied.

The author concludes that bacitracin is a safe, effective and nonirritating bactericidal ophthalmic ointment for ophthalmia neonatorum prophylaxis. He believes, however, that the best prophylaxis would be to observe the newborn infant's eyes carefully for evidence of infection for several days after delivery without touching or using anything in the eyes at birth. If gonorrhea conjunctivitis should occur, it could be treated effectively with penicillin given intramuscularly.

Long-Acting Estrogens in Amenorrhea and Menopause were studied by Angel Isaac Gurtman, Juan Angel Andrada,

(1) J. Pediat. 51:646-651, December, 1957.

Meyer H. G. Blatt, Jeanne A. Epstein and Herbert S. Kupperman[2] (New York Univ.-Bellevue Med. Center), who judged the efficacy of two preparations by means of numerical indexes representing clinical evaluations. With values from 1 (staining) to 4 (normal flow) assigned to the extent of bleeding, the amenorrhea index was calculated by multiplying the duration of bleeding by the extent and dividing by the days to onset of bleeding after administration of the compound for a prescribed period followed by 100 mg. progesterone. The higher the index, the more potent the estrogen. A summation of numerical descriptions of the severity of symptoms was used as the index for menopause. Estrogens and placebos were administered by the double-blind method.

On this basis, 53 patients with spontaneous menopause, 28 with surgical castration and 2 with radiation castration were found to respond to 10 mg. estradiol-17-β-N-valerate every 2 weeks or to 5 mg. estradiol-17-cyclopentylpropionate every 2 weeks in a manner comparable to that observed with 329 women receiving daily oral doses of standard estrogen compounds. Of 45 controls receiving placebo injections, only 77% showed excellent response.

Similarly, intramuscular injections of the two oil-soluble compounds every 2 weeks in 19 women with secondary and 8 with primary amenorrhea led to essentially identical results with the two drugs and with conjugated equine estrogens, Tace® or oral ethinyl estradiol. The long-acting preparations may be considered effective and convenient. They offer more precise control since the physician is not dependent on the patient's reliability in taking daily oral medication.

Review of Prolonged Use of Estrogens and Androgens in Postmenopausal and Senile Osteoporosis. In 13 of 15 reported complete balance studies significant calcium retention was produced in the postmenopausal woman by estrogen therapy and in the senile man by testosterone. The available balance studies suggest that combined estrogen and androgen therapy are more effective than either alone in the senile man, but without additive effect in the postmenopausal woman.

(2) Obst. & Gynec. 10:261-265, September, 1957.

On the basis of these observations, Philip H. Henneman and Stanley Wallach[3] (Harvard Med. School) formulated the following program for treatment of postmenopausal women: 1-3 mg. diethylstilbestrol daily for 4-5 weeks, no estrogen for 7-10 days, then resumption of treatment in a cyclic fashion. Such intermittent or interrupted estrogen therapy is necessary to permit desquamation of the proliferated endometrium and to prevent metropathia hemorrhagica. Such therapy also mimics the normal cyclic pattern of estrogen secretion and avoids the pattern of continuous estrogen secretion seen in patients with granulosa cell tumors, with the associated high incidence of cervical and endometrial carcinoma.

Since diethylstilbestrol is poorly tolerated by some postmenopausal women, the best-tolerated estrogen, Premarin® (conjugated estrogenic substances), is substituted in doses of 1.25-5 mg. daily in similar cyclic fashion. Testosterone is not routinely administered to postmenopausal women, since more than 5 mg. methyltestosterone daily often produces undesirable and sometimes irreversible masculinization, with deepening of the voice, facial hirsutism, acne and excessive stimulation of libido. Testosterone is added to estrogen therapy only if the postmenopausal woman is senile, severely debilitated, anorectic or extremely osteoporotic.

Senile men with osteoporosis have been treated with 30 mg. methyltestosterone daily by Linguets®, or buccal tablet. The use of estrogens is often limited because of the development of gynecomastia and loss of libido and potentia in men treated with significant amounts. This therapy has been reserved for those men with extreme osteoporosis.

The tendency of estrogens and androgens to cause salt and water retention and mild to moderate edema in older patients can often be prevented or corrected with salt restriction and diuretics. Estrogen withdrawal menstruation is no problem if the likelihood and reasons for this phenomenon are explained to the patient.

Prolonged administration of estrogens to postmenopausal women always relieves the hot flashes characteristic of the menopause and often causes a striking return to normal of emotional stability, sleep patterns and sense of energy.

(3) A.M.A. Arch. Int. Med. 100:715-723, November, 1957.

These changes are impossible to quantitate but constitute such an important dividend of estrogen therapy of postmenopausal osteoporosis that the authors have accepted them as sufficient reason for the general use of prolonged estrogen replacement in the postmenopausal woman.

Of about 200 postmenopausal women treated with estrogen for 1-20 years, the progress of osteoporosis was arrested in nearly all, as judged by measurements of total height and by x-ray examination of the spine. The incidence of carcinoma of the breast, cervix and endometrium was low in this treated group and should allay the fear that prolonged estrogen therapy produces cancer of these tissues in women.

► [Might the new compound, norethandrolone (Nilevar®), that is the subject of the next article, be effectively substituted for testosterone in some of these cases?—Ed.]

Anabolic Effects of Norethandrolone, a 19-Nortestosterone Derivative. Androgens promote protein metabolism, but their tendency to produce sodium and water retention often has prevented effective use, and the androgenic effect is undesired by women. In 1953, a report on 19-nortestosterone indicated that it was nearly equal to testosterone in anabolic effect but had only one-tenth the androgenic effect. A derivative, norethandrolone, is available as Nilevar®, which is described as 17α-ethyl-17-hydroxynorandrostenone and is structurally intermediate between testosterone and estradiol. Pharmacologic studies have shown that Nilevar has anabolic activity equal to that of testosterone propionate but about only one-sixteenth the androgenic activity.

Alvin F. Goldfarb, E. Edward Napp, Martin L. Stone, Marvin B. Zuckerman and Julius Simon[4] (New York Med. College) studied the effect of Nilevar in 11 patients, selected from the geriatric gynecology service, who had been hospitalized primarily for chronic diseases. All were kept on a constant diet and given Nilevar, 25 mg. intramuscularly 3 times weekly for 10 weeks. All reported feeling more vigorous and experiencing an increase in appetite. Three patients with cervical cancer required less narcotics during therapy with Nilevar. Urinary nitrogen excretion decreased an average of 10-60%, and within a week nitrogen retention was evident.

(4) Obst. & Gynec. 11:454-458, April, 1958.

No change was noted which indicated androgenic activity. No major side effect was noted. In 1 patient, urticarial reaction developed at the injection site. Two patients, who had amenorrhea before therapy, had withdrawal bleeding.

The lack of androgen activity in Nilevar is an important clinical advantage, particularly in women who require anabolic therapy.

Local Hydrocortisone Therapy of Vaginal and Vulvar Pruritus. Rita S. Finkler[5] (Newark, N.J., Beth Israel Hosp.) studied the effect of locally applied hydrocortisone on genital pruritus in 40 consecutive females, aged 17-74, seen in office practice. The pruritus was associated with a heterogeneous group of disorders such as allergy, anxiety, neurodermatitis, diabetes and trichomoniasis. Most patients had a substantial history of previous, largely unsuccessful, therapy.

Vaginal tablets containing 10 mg. hydrocortisone free alcohol in a Carbowax® base were given with instructions to insert 1 tablet deep into the vagina once daily. In more severe cases, 1 tablet twice daily was prescribed for the first 2 or 3 days, after which the dosage was reduced if possible.

Regardless of the primary disorder, hydrocortisone was effective in approximately equal numbers of patients. In several, a vaginal discharge was associated with pruritus; this was equally responsive to hydrocortisone. In over 77% of the 40 patients, pruritus was practically eliminated, whereas in an additional 7% a degree of benefit was ultimately achieved.

Undesirable effects of hydrocortisone were almost absent. In no patient was there evidence of systemic absorption with its attendant complications, nor was there any sign of local irritation due to the hydrocortisone or its base.

Relief from pruritus usually occurred dramatically within the first 24 hours of treatment. It is noteworthy that while the period of therapy in half the patients was 10 days or less, pruritus did not return when hydrocortisone was discontinued, except in 3 patients who had been treated for 10 days or longer.

Hydrocortisone therapy appeared to be equally effective in all age groups studied. Neither onset of the menopause nor senile atrophic changes in the genitals were correlated with

(5) Am. J. Obst. & Gynec. 75:319-321, February, 1958.

detectable differences in response, nor was any other factor detected that could be correlated with success or failure of therapy.

Effect of Local Treatment with Trichomycin in Monilia and Trichomonas Vaginitis. In vitro studies have shown that trichomycin, whose active substance was isolated from the genus Streptomyces, is active against several fungi, including Candida albicans, and certain protozoa, particularly Trichomonas vaginalis, but has no effect on most bacteria. Clinically, excellent results have been obtained in trichomonas and monilia vaginitis.

N. Wiqvist, G. Carlström and S. Brody[6] (Karolinska Hosp., Stockholm) extended these investigations to include 45 outpatients who sought medical advice for leukorrhea and vaginitis. Thirty were pregnant. Diagnosis of monilia vaginitis was based on vaginal discharge or irritation, reddened vaginal mucosa showing yellowish white patches and positive fungus culture of vaginal secretion. Trichomonas vaginitis was diagnosed by reddened vaginal mucosa and abundant frothy vaginal discharge containing many trichomonads.

After the vaginal samples were collected, the vagina was thoroughly dried and a suppository containing trichomycin inserted. The patient then inserted two suppositories daily, morning and evening, for 7 days and reported back on the 9th day. If the patient was unimproved, therapy was continued another 7 days. If asymptomatic, she returned for follow-up in 2 weeks and subsequently for variable periods. In cases of recurrence, another course of trichomycin therapy was given.

Of 25 patients with monilia vaginitis, 18 were cured after 1 week's treatment and the other 7 were considerably improved. The incidence of recurrence was comparatively high, but further treatment resulted in maintaining 17 of the 25 patients symptom free until delivery. The others improved or were symptom free for variable periods. Of 8 patients with trichomonas vaginitis, 6 were cured and 2 improved. Of 12 patients with vaginitis from whom neither fungi nor trichomonads could be cultured, the 7 who were

(6) Acta obst. et gynec. scandinav. 37:102-111, 1958.

pregnant improved with trichomycin treatment, but the other 5 did not.

The results confirm the antifungal properties of trichomycin demonstrated in vitro and agree with the results reported by others. Trichomycin can be successfully used in both monilia and trichomonas vaginitis.

Nystatin in Office Treatment of Vaginal Moniliasis. In this antibiotic era, leukorrhea with pruritus is more likely to be caused by monilia (Candida albicans) vaginitis than by trichomonas vaginitis, in a ratio of about 3:1. A fungus etiology should be suspected in all patients of menstruating age with pruritus vulvae. Local therapy with nystatin vaginal tablets attacks the problem of vaginitis simply and directly with a high concentration of the medication at the site of infection.

Lawrence J. Caruso[7] (New York Polyclinic Med. School) prescribed this treatment for 26 patients who had laboratory-proved moniliasis. Eleven were pregnant. Average duration of symptoms was 1 month. All had leukorrhea and pruritus. The most frequent gross findings were edema and/or redness of the vaginal mucosa and vulva. White or yellowish white discharge was visible, with white, flaky, cheeselike exudates on the vaginal wall.

Treatment consisted solely of insertion of 1 nystatin vaginal tablet when the patient retired. This regimen was continued for 14 days. If the condition were uncured, a second course was given. Clinical and mycologic cure was obtained in 24 (92%) of the 26 patients; 21 were cured after the initial course and 3 after a second. The other 2 patients were improved but not cured. Reinfection from the husband and failure to use the vaginal tablets correctly were probably responsible for the failures. Nystatin was equally effective in pregnant and nonpregnant women. No untoward reactions occurred.

Trichomonas Vaginalis Urethritis in Male Patients and Its Treatment with Local Oxophenarsine Hydrochloride (Mapharsen®). Luis Angel Garza[8] (Monterrey, Mex.) reports that this drug, in solution, applied by a simple technic

(7) New York J. Med. 58:1688-1690, May 15, 1958.
(8) Antibiotic Med. & Clin. Therap. 5:36-38, January, 1958.

to the infection sites permanently cleared trichomonas infection of long or short term in all of 24 males.

TECHNIC.—The contents of an 0.06-Gm. ampule of oxophenarsine hydrochloride is dissolved in 0.5 L. of sterile water at 45 C. (113 F.). The solution is then transferred to an irrigator. It must be prepared at the time of use and not in advance because the compound is relatively unstable in solution.

After the patient urinates, the preputial cavity, when present, and the anterior urethra are washed with solution. When the posterior urethra is also infected, as it is in most instances, the entire urethrovesical field is washed. Usually it is possible to pass the solution to the bladder by asking the patient to relax while the urethral cannula is in the meatus with the pressure turned on from the irrigator. When the bladder is full, the patient is allowed to expel the solution.

If nervousness prevents the patient from relaxing the vesical sphincter, a Nélaton catheter of medium thickness is used to fill the bladder. Any visible paraurethral canals or fistulous canals are washed with the solution, using a 2-ml. hypodermic syringe fitted with a blunt needle. After the washing is finished and the bladder has been emptied, the patient is instructed to abstain from urinating for at least 3 hours. Twenty-four hours after the first treatment, the trichomonas is not noted at the microscopic examinations. Nevertheless, it is advisable to repeat the applications once daily for 3-5 days.

In patients in whom microscopic examinations show associated bacteria, the treatment is continued for a few more days, using the same technic, but substituting 500 mg. chloramphenicol for the oxophenarsine hydrochloride.

If the patient is married, his wife, if infected, should be treated at the same time.

Effect of Vaginal Administration of Aureomycin® in Monilia Vaginitis was found by G. Carlström and N. Wiqvist[9] (Karolinska Hosp., Stockholm) to be quite the opposite of what might be expected. Candida albicans is not sensitive to Aureomycin, and in numerous patients in which this antibiotic has been used a high incidence of mycotic infection has followed treatment of vaginitis from various causes. Nevertheless, 8 of 14 patients with typical and pronounced C. albicans infections, who were given 2 suppositories (0.1 Gm. Aureomycin with no fungicidal substance) daily for 2 days, were free from all subjective symptoms. The 8 patients had a normal vaginal epithelium and 6 were free from C. albicans, as shown in culture tests. Of 4 who showed marked improvement, 3 had negative cultures. The other patients showed unchanged vaginal flora. Results indicate that Aureomycin so

(9) Acta obst. et gynec. scandinav. 36:250-256, 1957.

changed bacterial flora that it was incompatible with monilial growth. There should be little risk in using Aureomycin for a short period in severe cases which do not respond to other therapy.

OPHTHALMOLOGIC DISORDERS

Management of Endophthalmitis Following Cataract Extraction is reviewed by Guillermo Pico[1] (Univ. of Puerto Rico). Sulfonamides apparently penetrate the blood-aqueous barrier satisfactorily, but their antibacterial spectrum is narrow. Penicillin, even when given systemically in massive doses, does not penetrate sufficiently into the vitreous to produce adequate concentrations to control intravitreous infections. Streptomycin is useless for the same reason. Chlortetracycline and oxytetracycline penetrate the intraocular fluids poorly, but chloramphenicol is suitable since it can penetrate in sufficient quantity to control most infections. Tetracycline has a spectrum about the same as that of chloramphenicol and its ability to penetrate intraocular fluids is only slightly less.

To date only a few cases are recorded in which endophthalmitis complicating cataract extraction has been successfully treated. With chloramphenicol or tetracycline, prognosis is somewhat improved, but only if treatment is begun early and the appropriate antibiotic is used in adequate doses. Use of a corticosteroid with the antibiotic is recommended to diminish the inflammation quickly and prevent destruction of the retina and choroid.

Five cases of endophthalmitis followed cataract extraction. Two treated before chloramphenicol and tetracycline were available were absolute failures. One patient treated with chloramphenicol, tetracycline and prednisone had vision limited to finger counting. The other 2 treated with hydrocortisone and massive doses of chloramphenicol had excellent final vision.

Chlorpromazine in Ocular Surgery was studied, in the search for a suitable sedative, by Lalit P. Agarwal, R. B. L.

(1) A.M.A. Arch. Ophth. 59:381-385, March, 1958.

Gupta and S. R. K. Malik[2] (Med. College, Agra, India), who find the Indian patient unlikely to be co-operative in intraocular surgery. In 95 cases of intracapsular cataract extraction and 10 of iridencleisis, patients were given ¾ gr. Nembutal® 1 hour before operation and 50 mg. chlorpromazine 30 minutes later. The operation was performed under 2% anethaine local surface anesthesia. Facial block and retrobulbar injection of 2% Novocain® were used in each case. Postoperatively chlorpromazine was continued for 2 days.

Apprehension and mental tension were relieved, but muscular relaxation might have been more satisfactory if curare had been used as well. Pain was not eliminated, but it was restricted to the period of stimulus and did not persist thereafter. Fall in blood pressure, while evident particularly in hypertensive patients, was not excessive. Intraocular pressure remained unchanged or was reduced in 99 patients but rose in 6. Congestion of the eyball and excessive hemorrhage during preparation of the conjunctival flaps were troublesome and may have been due to peripheral vasodilatation, which might be controlled with promethazine or a similar agent to counteract the adrenolytic activity.

Chlorpromazine reduces the incidence of vitreous prolapse and postoperative complications which may result from nonco-operation on the part of the patient. Serious reactions were not encountered.

Comparative Study of Ophthalmic Decongestants in Allergic Conjunctivitis. When a specific allergen is introduced into a sensitized conjunctival sac, a reaction is indicated by hyperemia, lacrimation and chemosis. Untreated, the hyperemia gradually disappears in 1-2 hours or longer. Removing all remaining particles of the test allergen by a cotton-tipped applicator and/or flushing the sac with sterile saline will hasten disappearance of the hyperemia. Congestion can be lessened by instilling 1-2 drops of an ophthalmic decongestant.

Many solutions have been advocated for instillation for allergic conjunctivitis, most of which have included singly or in combination: epinephrine, phenacaine, ephedrine, cortisone and hydrocortisone, usually prepared in boric acid, rose water, saline or Estivin®. Louis Tuft and Donald D. Neish

(2) Brit. J. Ophth. 41:565-569, September, 1957.

Jr.[3] (Temple Univ.) tested each of these drugs in patients in whom specific allergens had induced hyperemia, lacrimation and chemosis. Two drops of the solution being tested were instilled into the conjunctival sac and the effect noted for 10 minutes.

The most effective drug was epinephrine. Almost immediately after its instillation, there was rapid blanching and obliteration of congestion and, except in marked allergic reactions, all symptoms and signs were relieved in less than 5 minutes. No mydriasis was noted. Rose water provided the best vehicle.

Phenacaine did not reduce congestion, though most patients noted lessening of burning and itching. However, since this in itself is a potential sensitizer, it is questionable whether its use is warranted, especially if relief can be obtained by other means. Corticoid preparations induced no blanching or lessening of the congestion, nor did any patient obtain relief. Though these agents are valuable in chronic inflammatory ocular disorders of varied etiology, no benefit could be seen in use for the acute, self-limited allergic reaction. Estivin is a proprietary product popular with persons with hay fever. Its exact composition is unknown, but is believed to contain an extract of roses. It has been claimed to relieve eye and nasal symptoms associated with hay fever, but actual testing showed it to have no more benefit than a simple diluent like rose water. Instillation of 0.5% ephedrine solution uniformly provided such little relief and was so ineffective compared with other agents that it was abandoned early.

No combination of active ingredient or various diluents was any more effective than was the same quantity of epinephrine alone. The studies showed that 1:1000 epinephrine, 4 cc., to 30 cc. rose water, was the best ophthalmic decongestant. The solution should be freshly prepared because solutions stored in dark-colored, tightly-closed bottles for 6-12 months significantly deteriorated in therapeutic effectiveness.

Effect of Rauwolfia Serpentina Derivatives on Intraocular Pressure in normal and glaucomatous eyes was studied by

(3) J.A.M.A. 167:60-62, May 3, 1958.

Melvin R. Kaplan and Irvin S. Pilger[4] (Univ. of California, Los Angeles). In a double-blind test, oral rauwolfia preparations (crude root, alseroxylon fraction or crystalline reserpine) were alternated with placebos at 12-20 week intervals. Results were based on reactions of individual eyes, each serving as its own control. Conventional therapy was continued without change throughout the period of observation. In 1 patient rauwolfia had no effect on intraocular pressure until concentration of the miotic, pilocarpine nitrate was increased from 1 to 4%. One eye then showed reduced pressure.

Of 24 nonglaucomatous eyes, 22 were not influenced by the rauwolfia alkaloids, while 2 (in the same patient) showed a reduction in pressure. Of a total of 38 glaucomatous eyes, 11 showed a response, 4 a possible response and 23 no response. Only 2 of these had consistently high blood pressure during placebo administration, suggesting that arterial hypertension is not a factor in responsiveness to the drug. Most, but not all, had a wide filtration angle, but some were completely occluded, suggesting that the effectiveness of the drug does not depend on the integrity of the aqueous outflow apparatus. A considerable lag in response to initiation of treatment and to dissipation of the effect after its termination was observed in several instances.

Reserpine was administered intravenously in 20 hospitalized patients, using doses of 73-295 μg./kg. Half of the eyes in this group were initially normotensive. Some were tested more than once. In 25 trials with eyes showing an initial pressure of 30 mm. mercury or less, a fall in pressure was noted in 22. In 20 of 27 trials with the hypertensive eyes, pressure was reduced from 7 to as much as 86 mm. In 19 of these the pressure reached a normotensive level. Reduction in arterial pressure began at about the same time as reduction in intraocular pressure but reached a maximum sooner and returned to the baseline in about half the time required by the intraocular pressure.

Experiments on control of arterial pressure with norepinephrine suggested that the response of intraocular pressure to intravenous reserpine may be due to the effect on arterial pressure in the case of normotensive eyes but that another factor is also operative in eyes which are hypertensive ini-

(4) Am. J. Ophth. 43:550-574, April, 1957.

tially. Further study of the problems of dosage, mode of action of the drug and means of selecting responsive patients is indicated.

Pre- and Postoperative Acetazolamide (Diamox®) in Glaucoma Surgery. Fifty cases of iridencleisis in which acetazolamide was given pre- and postoperatively form the basis of this study reported by L. P. Agarwal and S. R. K. Malik[5] (Med. College, Agra, India). On admission, besides the routine treatment of glaucoma, each patient was given a single daily dose of 500-1,000 mg. acetazolamide, depending on initial intraocular pressure. The treatment was continued 2-3 days. One hour before operation the patient was given a 250-mg. tablet and a delayed-action capsule of 250 mg. acetazolamide. This dosage was continued for a week after operation. The patient was subjected to a postplaced valvular iridencleisis. Fifty other patients were used as controls and received no acetazolamide until the 5th postoperative day. If the chamber had not formed by then, 250 mg. acetazolamide was given daily.

Administration of acetazolamide, particularly in patients with high intraocular pressure, lowered the tension and diminished congestion, so enabling the surgeon to carry out the operative procedures with greater ease. The incidence of flat chamber was considerably reduced (from 42 to 6%). The drainage bleb formed, though less cystic than in control cases, was adequate, and drainage of aqueous humor was satisfactory.

► [In an effort to decrease the intraocular pressure by decreasing the formation of aqueous, and thus prevent until the wound was more firmly healed the "critical moment" after cataract surgery in which wound reopening and hemorrhage into the anterior chamber and in some cases into the vitreous occurs, D. Vail (Am. J. Ophth. 44:637, 1957) gave Diamox® to 100 patients for 5 days, beginning on the 3d day after cataract surgery had been performed. The effort failed.—Ed.]

Epinephrine and Acetazolamide in Therapy of Chronic Glaucomas. Bernard Becker and Albert P. Ley[6] (Washington Univ.) investigated the effects of epinephrine and acetazolamide administered both separately and simultaneously on the rate of secretion of aqueous humor and on intraocular pressure. The study included 45 eyes of 23 patients—5 eyes with chronic secondary glaucoma and 40 with chronic sim-

(5) Brit. J. Ophth. 41:613-615, October, 1957.
(6) Am. J. Ophth. 5:639-643, May, 1958.

ple (open-angle) glaucoma. All patients were receiving pilocarpine therapy, which was continued without change during the study.

First, 22 patients (41 eyes) were treated with acetazolamide. After pressures were stabilized at new levels, topical epinephrine was added to their therapy. Secondly, 20 eyes were treated with topical epinephrine and when intraocular pressures reached stable levels the 10 patients were given acetazolamide systemically. The epinephrine was made up as a 4.5% solution of the bitartrate in bisulfite as follows: epinephrine bitartrate, 90 mg.; sodium bisulfite, 10 mg.; sodium chloride, 5 mg.; chlorobutanol, 10 mg.; and distilled water, 2 ml. It was kept in a cool, dark place (refrigerator) and was given to all patients as a single drop in the conjunctival sac of the affected eye or eyes once a day at bedtime. The application was accompanied by transient burning and irritation of the eye but was tolerated by all patients. No pupillary dilatation nor systemic side effects were noted. Acetazolamide was given orally, 250 mg. every 6 hours. Tonography was performed on all patients.

The rate of secretion of aqueous humor can be suppressed partially by topical epinephrine (37% inhibition) or systemic acetazolamide (50% inhibition). These agents are useful additions to miotic therapy in lowering intraocular pressure in eyes with chronic simple or secondary glaucoma. When topical epinephrine and systemic acetazolamide are used together the decrease in rate of formation of aqueous humor is greater than with either agent alone (averaging 66%). The additive effect of these two secretory inhibitors affords further opportunities for the control of some of the chronic glaucomas medically.

► [The group of sympathomimetic amines, to which epinephrine belongs, is generally considered harmless from the standpoint of systemic toxicity when used locally in ophthalmology. However, the potentialtiy of major reactions is present: last year, W. U. McReynolds *et al.* (1957-58 Year Book, p. 427) reported a case of acute subarachnoid hemorrhage associated with the local use of phenylephrine (Neo-Synephrine®) in a case of acute iritis in which posterior synechiae had formed.—Ed.]

Glaucoma in Medical Practice: Danger of Use of Systemic Antispasmodic Drugs in Patients Predisposed to or having Glaucoma is emphasized by Mortimer Cholst, Seymour Goodstein, Conrad Berens and Alfonse Cinotti[7] (New York

(7) J.A.M.A. 166:1276-1280, Mar. 15, 1958.

Eye and Ear Infirm.). Chronic simple glaucoma is one of the most important causes of blindness among adults. Onset usually is insidious, with little ocular discomfort or pain and usually is ignored by the patient until damage becomes irreparable. In acute glaucoma, intraocular tension rises acutely, accompanied by severe pain that cannot be ignored and must be lowered immediately to prevent blindness. The accepted cause for this sudden rise in ocular tension is dilatation of the pupil, occurring in eyes with shallow anterior chambers, which crowds the iris into the anterior chamber angle and obstructs outflow of fluid from the eye.

Dilating the pupil by atropine, scopolamine (Hyoscine) hydrobromide, belladonna or belladonna-like drugs taken orally causes relatively little change in the normal eye. In persons with chronic glaucoma or predisposition to glaucoma, the same drugs may induce dangerous increase in intraocular tension and cause an acute attack of glaucoma. Blurred vision is common when antispasmodic drugs are taken and is due to paralysis of the ciliary muscles with loss of accommodation. Paralysis of the sphincter of the iris causes dilatation of the pupils. Occasionally, the patient is instructed to increase the belladonna dose until vision becomes blurred, using this as the titration end point to relieve symptoms in the gastrointestinal tract.

Dicyclomine (Bentyl®) hydrochloride, tested in 37 patients with normal tension and in 17 with chronic simple glaucoma, did not significantly increase intraocular pressure, affect pupil size nor accommodation. This drug is somewhat safer than other antispasmodics.

Before atropine, its derivatives or synthetic parasympatholytic agents are prescribed for relief from gastrointestinal disorders or parkinsonism, the physician should carefully investigate for glaucoma or a family history of glaucoma. The patient should be questioned about blurred vision, partial or complete halos seen around a bared electric light bulb, pain in the eyeball or around the eyes, difficulty with the field of vision and discomfort with close work. Tests should be made for dilated pupils, reaction to light, presence of a shallow anterior chamber, constriction of visual fields and increased intraocular pressure with a standard tonometer.

Methylprednisolone (Medrol®) in Ophthalmology. Dan M. Gordon[8] (Cornell Univ.) used oral methylprednisolone in treating ophthalmic conditions, principally uveitis, for about 11 months.

Acute iridocyclitis (anterior uveitis) was treated in 5 patients with 20 mg. daily in 4 divided doses, decreasing dosage rapidly as the disease responded. In all patients, topical corticosteroids were used every 1-3 hours with the systemic therapy. Frequently, the systemically administered steroid controls the uveitis, as observed by slit-lamp examination, and yet the eye is injected. Here, the topically used steroid immediately controls the injection of the globe and pales the eye. In all patients, the topical steroids were continued for about 2 weeks after discontinuance of the methylprednisolone.

Methylprednisolone was given to 14 patients with chronic generalized uveitis. All had previously been treated with other corticosteroids. These patients took methylprednisolone for 2-11 months, in initial doses of 24-48 mg. The drug was given 4 times daily, if possible. Lowest maintenance doses were 4-6 mg. daily.

On long-term corticosteroid therapy, the only serious problem was that of water retention. This was handled with diuretics such as ethoxzolamide (Cardrase®), with or without the addition of mercurial diuretics. Routine use of potassium chloride as prophylaxis was not helpful. All patients were instructed to drink at least 1 large glass of orange juice daily to satisfy potassium requirements. All but 1 patient was well controlled.

Ocular allergies, occurring in 7 patients, and uncontrolled by topically administered corticosteroids, were controlled with small doses of methylprednisolone. These patients rarely required more than 4-8 mg. daily, and then not every day. None required the medication for longer than 2 months.

Neomycin in Ophthalmology is discussed by Arnold Sorsby and Joseph Ungar.[9] The wide use of penicillin drops and ointment has prevented the development of ocular infections due to penicillin-sensitive organisms. Thus, many ocular infections today are due to penicillin-resistant strains

(8) Metabolism 7 (pt. 2):569-573, July, 1958.
(9) Ann. Roy. Coll. Surgeons England 22:107-116, February, 1958.

of Staphylococcus aureus or to gram-negative bacilli insensitive to penicillin.

In rabbits with intraocular infections induced by penicillin-resistant Staph. aureus, preliminary trials led to the exclusion of Magnamycin® and bacitracin because of inefficacy; erythromycin and neomycin were the only agents that showed any promise.

Soluble erythromycin salts administered in subconjunctival injection gave better results than oral administration of the drug, but the injections were not well tolerated. Subconjunctival injection of neomycin in doses of 500 mg., proved both well tolerated and effective against three strains of penicillin-resistant Staph. aureus and corneal infection due to Pseudomonas pyocyanea.

Neomycin subconjunctivally did not control an intraocular infection produced by inoculating Bacillus proteus into the anterior chamber; the infection ran a fulminating course. Control was, however, obtained when the animal was pretreated with neomycin subconjunctivally 1 hour before inoculation, or when the infection was introduced by intracorneal inoculation.

Neomycin subconjunctivally proved as effective as penicillin in treating intraocular infections produced by pneumococcus, Streptococcus hemolyticus or penicillin-sensitive Staph. aureus. In these observations, epinephrine was added to the solution of both agents.

Assessment of corneal and intraocular levels of concentration reached by subconjunctival injection of 0.5 Gm. neomycin showed that high levels are reached for 16 hours and therapeutic levels persisted for probably 24 hours. Addition of epinephrine to the solvent increased the initial levels markedly, but had no such effect on concentrations subsequently.

Clinical trials established that neomycin, 0.5 Gm. in 0.75 ml. water and 0.25 ml. epinephrine 1:1000 are fairly well tolerated and can be repeated at 24-hour intervals 3-4 times without marked discomfort or toxic effect. Likely, neomycin so used is a satisfactory standard method of treatment of the intraocular infections seen today.

Clinical and Blood Chemical Studies with Ascriptin: With Particular Reference to Headaches and Arthritic Pains. Theodore M. Feinblatt, Henry M. Feinblatt, Edgar A. Ferguson, Jr. (Brooklyn), Alison H. Price, John E. Healey, Jr., and William Allison[1] (Philadelphia) determined blood salicylate levels in a group of apparently healthy medical students after giving them a single dose, respectively, of 10 gr. Ascriptin, 10 gr. aspirin and a special aspirin buffered with aluminum glycinate and magnesium carbonate. Ascriptin tablets contain 5 gr. acetylsalicylic acid USP buffered with 2.5 gr. magnesium aluminum hydroxide.

The average blood salicylate level after a single dose of 10 gr. Ascriptin compared with that after aspirin was 160% higher after 10 minutes, 250% higher after 20 minutes, 264% higher after 30 minutes, 134% higher after 1 hour and 60% higher after 24 hours (Fig. 38). The average level after a single dose of 10 gr. Ascriptin compared with that after the aspirin buffered with a mixture of aluminum glycinate and magnesium carbonate was 8% higher after 10 minutes, 17% higher after 20 minutes, 20% higher after 30 minutes, 3% higher after 1 hour and 33% higher after 24 hours.

Therapeutic values of Ascriptin and aspirin, respectively, were compared in 2 groups of 20 patients each. One group had arthritis and the other headaches (mainly due to fatigue or overindulgence). A single dose of 10 gr. Ascriptin relieved headaches in an average of 9 minutes compared with 16 minutes for aspirin. Ascriptin relieved arthritic pain in an average of 17 minutes compared with 25 minutes for aspirin.

Eight of the 40 patients experienced gastric irritation, including burning in the stomach and belching, after taking aspirin. All took Ascriptin without discomfort. Patients with duodenal ulcer complicating arthritis, in whom aspirin

(1) New York J. Med. 58:697-700, Mar. 1, 1958.

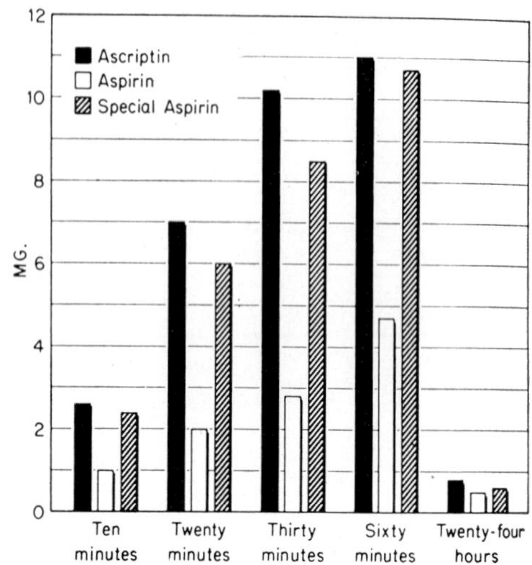

Fig. 38.—Average blood salicylate levels (mg./100 cc.) after single dose containing 10 gr. aspirin. Special aspirin used was buffered with mixture of aluminum glycinate and magnesium carbonate. (Courtesy of Feinblatt, T. M., *et al.*: New York J. Med. 58:697-700, Mar. 1, 1958.)

was known to cause gastric irritation, took Ascriptin without disturbance.

► [This evidence seems almost too pat. At any rate one will want to see independent confirmation, particularly as such studies as those reported in the next 2 articles fail to show any sort of advantage for buffered aspirin. —Ed.]

Laboratory and Clinical Studies with Buffered and Nonbuffered Acetylsalicylic Acid are reported by G. A. Cronk[2] (Syracuse Univ.). Blood salicylic acid curves were determined in a cross-over study in 20 healthy volunteers after administration of 0.6 Gm. buffered and nonbuffered acetylsalicylic acid. Blood samples were obtained at 0, 10, 20 and 60 minutes. The average blood salicylic acid levels after administration of buffered acetylsalicylic acid were 0, 0.9, 1.8, 2.3 and 2.8 mg./100 ml. The average levels after administration of nonbuffered acetylsalicylic acid were 0, 0.9, 1.9, 2.2 and 2.8 mg./100 ml.

In a double-blind study, 667 doses of nonbuffered acetylsalicylic acid (0.6 Gm.) and 757 doses of buffered acetylsalicylic acid (0.6 Gm.) were administered to patients hospital-

(2) New England J. Med. 258:219-221, Jan. 30, 1958.

ized with painful conditions. No statistical difference was demonstrated between the two agents studied in the time required for relief of pain or duration or degree of relief. In about 30% of both groups discomfort was not relieved. Most failures occurred in cases of severe pain associated with such conditions as ulcerative pharyngitis and sinusitis.

Gastrointestinal symptoms followed administration of buffered acetylsalicylic acid in 3 patients (0.4%) and of nonbuffered acetylsalicylic acid in 5 patients (0.7%). In all 8, buffered and nonbuffered acetylsalicylic acid was administered subsequently without occurrence of gastrointestinal symptoms, suggesting that the underlying disease affected production of these symptoms.

Comparison of Buffered and Unbuffered Acetylsalicylic Acid. The therapeutic value of acetylsalicylic acid in analgesia, anti-rheumatic and anti-pyretic properties and its safety are well established. A few persons manifest gastrointestinal symptoms on oral administration, which can be eased by concomitant sodium bicarbonate. Relatively small amounts of dihydroxyaluminum aminoacetate and magnesium carbonate have been combined with acetylsalicylic acid and reported to lessen gastric distress caused by acetylsalicylic acid alone.

Robert C. Batterman[3] (New York Med. College) compared analgesic effectiveness of and gastrointestinal tolerance for a rapidly disintegrating unbuffered 0.3 Gm. (5 gr.) tablet and a buffered 0.3 Gm. (5 gr.) tablet containing small amounts of dihydroxyaluminum aminoacetate and magnesium carbonate (Bufferin®). Both were supplied as identical-appearing tablets; identity of the tablets was unknown to the investigators, the staff and the patients until after the data had been tabulated. The 2 medications were tested in single-dose studies, single-day comparisons, and short- and long-term therapy in 160 hospital and outpatients. In none of 4 types of cross-over comparisons was it possible to distinguish between the 2 medications either in analgesic effectiveness or in gastrointestinal tolerance. The time required for analgesia, degree of analgesia and frequency of gastrointestinal intolerance was identical.

The present data do not support the contention that salicy-

(3) New England J. Med. 258:213-219, Jan. 30, 1958.

lates appear in the blood faster with simultaneous use of buffering antacids in the quantities used in these tablets. Similar effectiveness for both types of tablets was noted for various types of pain, acute and chronic. These antacids, in the quantities included, serve no useful purpose as constituents of the tablets studied. Inclusion with acetylsalicylic acid offers no advantage over aspirin alone.

Comparison of Anileridine, Morphine and Meperidine in Man was made by Robert D. Dripps, Ronald A. Millar and Dorothy H. Kneale[4] (Univ. of Pennsylvania). The ability of these drugs to relieve immediate postoperative pain and restlessness was recorded in 415 patients. The respiratory and circulatory effects of anileridine [Leritine] were measured in normal volunteers. The drug was also given intravenously to patients during spinal anesthesia to produce somnolence and to patients receiving nitrous oxide anesthesia to increase the potency of this anesthetic. Anileridine proved to be midway between morphine and meperidine [Demerol®] as an analgesic or in giving relief from restlessness. It did not appear to liberate histamine and caused less circulatory depression than either of the other analgesics. Respiratory depression was evident but was briefer than after morphine or meperidine.

After intramuscular injection, equipotent dosage ratios appeared to be: morphine 1, anileridine 2-2.5, meperidine 3.5-5. Average duration of relief after intramuscular administration was 50 minutes for anileridine, 58 minutes for meperidine and 72 minutes for morphine. Even small doses of the drugs produced a relatively high incidence of relief after intravenous injection. Duration of this effect tended to be briefer than after intramuscular use, i.e., 20-25 minutes. As with other narcotics, itching, nausea, vomiting and euphoria were noted after administration of anileridine. The present data did not permit quantitative comparison. Anileridine deserves continued evaluation, primarily because of diminished side actions.

Studies of Analgesic Drugs: Anileridine Dihydrochloride. Anileridine [Leritine] is a derivative of meperidine (Demerol®) in which a phenethyl group has been substituted for a methyl group in the meperidine molecule. A. S. Keats, J. Tel-

(4) Surg., Gynec. & Obst. 105:322-326, September, 1957.

ford and Y. Kurosu[5] (Baylor Univ.) estimated the analgesic potency of anileridine in postoperative patients. Dose levels of 10, 20, 40, 50 and 75 mg./70 kg. body weight were studied. Anileridine was alternated in individual patients with 50 mg. meperidine/70 kg. body weight. In one group of patients, 50 mg. anileridine was alternated with 100 mg. meperidine. A dose was considered analgesic when "most of the pain" was relieved at 45 and 90 minutes after administration.

Anileridine proved to be about 2½ times as potent as meperidine on a milligram basis, i.e., 40 mg. anileridine was the analgesic equivalent of 100 mg. meperidine. A dose of 75 mg. anileridine/70 kg. body weight produced pain relief less frequently than did 40 or 50 mg. This has been observed in studies of other potent analgesics. Although the explanation for this decrease is not known, it does suggest that an optimal dose for analgesia has been exceeded.

Anileridine depressed the respiration of normal persons to the same degree as meperidine, but respiration returned to normal more rapidly after anileridine. Meperidine produced sedation and sleep oftener than did anileridine. Incidence of nervousness, restlessness and stimulation was higher after anileridine. Differences in incidence of nausea, vomiting and sweating were not significant.

Analgesic Effectiveness of Orally Administered Ethoheptazine in Man was studied by Robert C. Batterman, Maurice Golbey, Arthur J. Grossman and Paul Leifer[6] (New York Med. College). Ethoheptazine in doses of 50 or 100 mg. 4 times a day was given to 330 patients requiring analgesia for a wide variety of medical and surgical conditions. A combination of ethoheptazine and aspirin was given to 127 other patients.

Satisfactory analgesia was achieved in 73% of ambulatory patients with the 50-mg. dose; 62% of the hospitalized patients responded but required the higher dosage. The greatest effectiveness was in relief from musculoskeletal pain, usually associated with arthritis. Satisfactory analgesia was observed in 50% of patients with early neoplastic disease, but the medication was ineffectual in any condition with severe pain where ordinarily morphine or meperidine would be re-

(5) Anesthesiology 18:690-697, Sept.-Oct., 1957.
(6) Am. J. M. Sc. 234:413-419, October, 1957.

quired. Thus, in terminal phases of neoplastic disease and in renal disease and myocardial infarction there was no effective relief from pain. Headaches were also unresponsive. A satisfactory response was obtained in neurologic patients with neuritis, tabes dorsalis and postoperative or surgical patients with mild pain.

Postpartum pain was satisfactorily controlled in 82% of patients treated with ethoheptazine alone and in every patient treated with combined ethoheptazine and aspirin. In rheumatoid arthritis, the combination of ethoheptazine and aspirin was more effective than ethoheptazine alone.

Untoward reactions occurred in 4% of patients taking ethoheptazine. They consisted of nausea, anorexia or dizziness and were mild and insignificant. There was no evidence of tolerance or physical dependence, and prolonged administration proved to be safe. Over-all response was similar to the authors' experiences with codeine, but the low incidence of untoward reactions and lack of cumulative toxicity favored ethoheptazine. There was no disturbance in bowel or urinary function and no depression of the cough reflex. Ethoheptazine satisfies to a high degree the need for a moderately potent analgesic for oral administration.

► [While visiting a ward recently in which an analgesic study was under way I saw in use a clever device for determining at suitable intervals the amount of pain the patient was experiencing: he was simply handed without remark a small board in which he shifted the peg to one of the four holes respectively labeled "none," "a little," "a lot," "it's terrible."

In a recent statistical study, unfortunately not easily presentable in the YEAR BOOK, in which both a completely blind study technic and a single-blind method and sequential analysis were used, Cass *et al.* (J.A.M.A. 166:1829, Apr. 12, 1958) found ethoheptazine to be more active than aspirin as an analgesic when each drug was used alone; in combination, the two were as effective as codeine plus aspirin.—Ed.]

Evaluation of New Analgesic Combination: Report of Use in Postoperative Gynecologic Patients and in Postpartum Period. Ethoheptazine, a racemic mixture of the d and l isomers of 1-methyl-4-carbethoxy-4-phenyl hexamethylenimine, is a moderately potent analgesic. Jacob S. Roden and Harold M. Haugen[7] (Univ. of Missouri) tried a combination of ethoheptazine citrate and acetylsalicylic acid for the relief of pain in the postpartum period and for pain following gynecologic operations. The study included 53 obstetric and 39 gynecologic patients, aged 15-72. The routine dosage was 2

(7) Missouri Med. 55:128-129, February, 1958.

tablets every 4 hours as needed for pain. Each tablet of Zactirin® contained 75 mg. ethoheptazine citrate and 325 mg. acetylsalicylic acid. For postpartum pain, 2 tablets were prescribed after delivery, to be administered only when something for the relief of pain was requested. In the gynecologic patients subjected to major procedures, the first dose was

TABLE 1.—OBSTETRIC PATIENTS

Type of Pain	No. Patients	Degree of Relief COMPLETE %	50% OR MORE %	50% OR LESS %	NONE %
"Afterbirth pains"	38	84	13	3	0
Hemorrhoids	2	66	33	0	0
Breast engorgement	2	100	0	0	0
Postspinal cephalalgia	6	0	100	0	0
Dysuria due to cystitis	1	50	50	0	0
Episiotomy	4	100	0	0	0

TABLE 2.—GYNECOLOGIC PATIENTS

Type of Pain	No. Patients	Degree of Relief COMPLETE %	50% OR MORE %	50% OR LESS %	NONE %
Vaginal surgery (hysterectomy with A-P colporrhaphy, perineorrhaphy, etc.)	13	92	0	8	0
Abdominal hysterectomy	11	50	43	0	7
Dilatation and curettage	2	100	0	0	0
Cystoscopy	1	100	0	0	0
Abortions, spontaneous	3	100	0	0	0
Radiation proctitis	4	0	100	0	0
Arthritis	1	0	100	0	0
Psychic factors	4	0	25	0	75

administered usually on the 3d postoperative day; after minor procedures, at any time the patient experienced pain.

The obstetric patients received 1-8 doses over 1-6 days and the gynecologic patients 1-12 doses over 1-7 days. The types of pain and the degree of relief in the 2 groups are presented in Tables 1 and 2. During the study, 300 doses of the combination of ethoheptazine and acetylsalicylic acid were given. The incidence of side effects was as follows: nausea after 0.3% of the doses, drowsiness after 5% and epigastric distress after 4%.

Value of Aminopyrine. As a potent antipyretic, aminopyrine is well known but has been discredited for years because of overemphasis on its use in relation to the development of agranulocytosis. It may be effective where other antipyretics fail and may even be lifesaving, according to Leonard Cardon, Oscar H. Comess, Thomas A. Noble and Mark M. Pomaranc[8] (Northwestern Univ.). Its antipyretic effects are due to direct action on the hypothalamus through the thermoregulating centers in the brain and not to any changes in heat production or dissipation. Aminopyrine relieves pain, particularly that of headache, neuralgia and myalgia, without affecting consciousness. For some patients, aminopyrine may be more analgesic than are opiates. In rheumatic fever symptoms refractory to salicylates, some physicians consider aminopyrine the drug of choice.

Fever carries with it malaise, headache, arthralgia, chills, diaphoresis, anorexia, nausea, restlessness, sleep disturbance, delirium and stupor which, if prolonged, may result in debility and exhaustion. Ideally, the cause of fever should be removed, but occasionally the cause is unknown or not susceptible to definitive therapy. The effect of aminopyrine is most striking in the virus, collagen, neoplastic and other nonbacterial diseases associated with fever.

The danger of agranulocytosis, although real, is no greater than with the use of many drugs: sulfonamides, chloramphenicol, streptomycin, thiouracil derivatives, Mesantoin and Tridione® and antihistamines. Its actual incidence is small. In 1934, an estimated total of 30 million prescriptions for aminopyrine were written in the United States alone, in addition to the large quantity purchased over the counter, yet only a total of 145 new cases of agranulocytosis were reported. The possibility of producing agranulocytosis in any patient is therefore remote. It need not occur if the drug is given under strict supervision with frequent blood studies.

Corticosteroids are now the most commonly used alternatives for symptomatic treatment of fever and associated symptoms. Morbidity and mortality related to their use are yet untallied. The danger of edema, hypertension, heart failure, diabetes, perforation and massive hemorrhage from ulcerations, exacerbation of healed and latent tuberculosis, psychosis and other serious complications is real and fre-

(8) Ann. Int. Med. 48:616-634, March, 1958.

quent. Where fever per se is an essential problem and other metabolic and alternative effects of corticosteroids are not particularly required, a preliminary trial of aminopyrine may be of value.

Aminopyrine, although acting in a nonspecific manner, was probably lifesaving in 2 cases reported. The prolonged fever probably was due to acute exacerbation of rheumatic carditis in 1. Many millions of units of penicillin and many Grams of streptomycin had no effect. Symptomatic therapy and aminopyrine controlled the fever along with its disabling and debilitating concomitant symptoms and supported the patient until the disease resolved spontaneously.

Woman, 43, had chills, fever, abdominal pain and diarrhea for a week. Daily temperatures of 101-103 F. did not respond to penicillin. Pulse was 104 and irregular. She had mitral stenosis and regurgitation. Laboratory findings and cultures were negative. Fever and other symptoms did not respond to salicylates or to massive doses of penicillin and streptomycin given for 1 month. Aminopyrine was started, 10 gr. 4 times daily, and the temperature became normal within 24 hours, with concomitant symptomatic improvement. At no time did symptoms recur. She continued taking maintenance doses of aminopyrine, 5 gr. 3 times daily, for 4 months. At follow-up 1 year later she was still well.

► [I think many of us would agree that aminopyrine is a valuable drug whose use was abandoned on evidence that nowadays does not always condemn other drugs out of hand. But just try to get it used here in Milwaukee where the original work establishing its etiologic relationship to agranulocytosis was done!—Ed.]

Intrathecal Phenol for Intractable Pain: Safety and Dangers of Method are reported by P. W. Nathan and T. G. Scott[9] (Nat'l Hosp., London). Preparations used were a 7.5% solution of phenol in myodil (ethyl iodophenylundecylate), in amounts of 0.75, 1 or 1.5 ml., and silver nitrate dissolved in as small a quantity of water as possible and added to a 5% solution of phenol in glycerin, of which 0.75 ml. was given. These solutions were injected intrathecally caudal to the 12th thoracic vertebra in all cases, except in 3, in which the injections were made immediately caudal or cranial to the 7th cervical vertebra.

In none of 30 patients given phenol in myodil did any weakness of the musculature follow the injection, even when invasion of the peripheral nerves by cancerous tissue had already caused some weakness. One patient had retention of

(9) Lancet 1:76-80, Jan. 11, 1958.

urine and extreme diminution in anal sensation. Seven eventually died of cancer and in none was there any macroscopic abnormality which could be attributed to the injection. Cerebrospinal fluid taken from 9 patients after injection of phenol in myodil showed few consistent changes and these were mild.

Of 13 patients given silver nitrate in phenol and glycerin there was a slight increase in weakness of an already affected limb in 6, an increase in already disturbed control of micturition in 2 and an increase in already disturbed control of defecation in 1. In 1 patient who had carcinoma of the breast with metastases, anemia and diabetes mellitus, injection was followed by a severe meningeal reaction; 2 days after the injection the patient died. Leptomeningitis was found at autopsy.

These studies and those of the rate of diffusion of phenol out of myodil into the cerebrospinal fluid lead the authors to conclude that at least 1 ml. of 7.5% solution of phenol in myodil can safely be injected intrathecally. The solution of silver nitrate in phenol and glycerin is less safe.

POISONING (ACUTE)

Treatment of Cadmium Poisoning with Edathamil Calcium Disodium in 3 patients is reported by Lawrence H. Cotter[1] (Columbia Univ.). The mechanism of the process is replacement of the calcium ion in the chelating agent by a cadmium ion and excretion of the chelate in a nonirritating form through the kidneys. There were no unpleasant side actions encountered in these patients, and oral administration of the drug proved effective.

Man, 35, who worked for 3 months with finely powdered cadmium acquired a hacking cough after 1 month's exposure and about 2 weeks later had digestive disturbances, with mild jaundice and marked mental irritability. On physical examination, he was pale and slightly icteric. Respiration was rapid, and the mucous membranes of nose and pharynx were congested; there was incessant coughing and many crepitant rales at both bases. Blood analysis showed the hemoglobin level to be 13.2 Gm./100 cc. There were 3,100,000 red blood cells and

(1) J.A.M.A. 166:735-736, Feb. 15, 1958.

4,000 white blood cells/cu. mm., with neutrophils 54%, monocytes 2%, lymphocytes 39%, eosinophils 4% and basophils 1%. Urinalysis revealed 2+ albumin and many red blood cells.

The patient was given 0.5 Gm. edathamil calcium disodium (calcium disodium versenate) as a pill every 2 hours while he was awake for 1 week. He returned for re-examination at the end of 3 weeks. He was then asymptomatic; his chest was clear and his color good. He said he felt better 24 hours after medication was started. Blood analysis showed a hemoglobin level of 14 Gm./100 cc. and 4,100,000 red blood cells and 6,200 white blood cells/cu. mm., with neutrophils 68%, monocytes 2%, lymphocytes 28%, eosinophils 1% and basophils 1%. Urinalysis was normal. The patient was fitted with a suitable mask and returned to work.

Chemical determinations of the amount of cadmium in the blood and urine should be made in each case 1 week after the end of treatment and medication resumed for another week, and this routine should be repeated until the patient is metal free.

► [Ca-EDTA exchanges its calcium for yttrium, americium, plutonium, copper, nickel and lead. L. Friberg (A.M.A. Arch. Indust. Health 13: 18, 1956) found that a demonstrable reduction in the cadmium content of organs could not be achieved in rabbits or rats, but it appears from the present report that it can be done in man.—Ed.]

Diagnostic and Therapeutic Use of Edathamil Calcium Disodium (EDTA, Versene) in Excessive Inorganic Lead Absorption is discussed by W. J. H. Leckie and S. L. Tompsett[2] (Univ. of Edinburgh). Seven subjects with excessive lead absorption were treated with intravenous EDTA in different ways and the resulting levels of lead excretion compared. One patient whose symptoms suggested lead poisoning but whose work did not was similarly treated before and after lowering the plasma pH. Eight control subjects received a single dose of intravenous EDTA and the resulting rise in urinary lead excretion was estimated.

The results indicated that optimum excretion of lead in the urine in a case of excessive lead absorption could be achieved by giving 2 Gm. EDTA by intravenous infusion over 6 hours daily. After such an infusion all patients with excessive lead absorption excreted lead in the urine at a rate of over 1.5 mg. in 24 hours. Lead excretion in subjects not so exposed and similarly treated varied between 0.22 mg. and 0.65 mg. in 24 hours. This information appears to be of use in diagnosing excessive lead absorption where urinary lead values are not significantly raised and other blood and bio-

(2) Quart. J. Med. 27:65-82, January, 1958.

chemical findings are not conclusive. It is, however, suggested that in cases of severe lead poisoning intravenous EDTA should be given continuously for at least 48 hours or administered in 6 hour infusions over the same period twice daily. After 48 hours it should be safe to resume intermittent daily therapy as described, in 5-day courses separated by 3 or 4 days. When lead excretion in the second 24 hours of a course is less than 1.5 mg., it indicates that the available lead stores are becoming exhausted.

It appears that urinary excretion of lead after administration of EDTA is not influenced by a single dose of parathormone and is actually depressed by hydrocortisone. Lowering plasma pH by ammonium chloride and acetazolamide, though it increased lead excretion without EDTA, appeared to depress excretion when EDTA was used. Renal elimination of EDTA was accelerated.

Two patients who had been longest exposed to the risk of excessive lead absorption had lowered creatinine clearances. In these cases excretion of EDTA was significantly delayed. In nearly 100 intravenous infusions of EDTA no toxic effects were noted.

► [The title of this article is unfortunate but the mistake is a careless one that is frequently made. Edathamil calcium disodium is Ca-EDTA but it is not Versene. Versene is the proprietary name for the tetrasodium salt of EDTA before the chelation with calcium; it is theoretically useful to decrease hypercalcemic toxicity but is not the compound that is used in treating heavy metal poisoning.

The article contains valuable information regarding use of other compounds while using Ca-EDTA—Ed.]

Clinical Studies on Action of Bemegride in Barbiturate Overdosage are hampered by lack of an accurate criterion to determine the moment of wakening. Thomas J. Thomson[3] (Univ. of Glasgow) first studied the effects of bemegride or of saline in terminating thiopentone anesthesia in 20 women, using the double-blind technic. The interval between injection and the ability of the patient to respond to questioning was accepted as the "wakening time." There was no significant difference in wakening times with these substances.

The effect of adding bemegride (ββ-methylethyl glutarimide) to an established saline intravenous drip was then studied in volunteers sleeping under the influence of sodium amylobarbitone while bipolar EEG recordings were made.

(3) Brit. M. J. 1:976-978, Apr. 26, 1958.

Bemegride roused patients, but no change in deep sleep patterns preceded wakening. In 3 patients who showed barbiturate activity on the EEG pattern, the activity was not dispelled by the bemegride.

Although this suggests that bemegride is not a specific barbiturate antagonist, it is possible that the EEG record, which indicates only cerebral cortical activity, may fail to show antagonism if both the barbiturate and bemegride act on the hypothalamus.

Accidental Digitoxin Poisoning in Children: Report of Case and Review of Literature. Digitalis intoxication is common and its incidence is on the increase, paralleling the

DATA FROM SERIAL ELECTROCARDIOGRAMS ON CHILD, AGED 2

HOURS AFTER INGESTION	P-R* INTERVAL (SEC.)	Q-T† INTERVAL (SEC.)	ATRIAL RATE	VENT. RATE	COMMENT
6	0.14	0.28	88	88	Normal sinus rhythm
9	0.23	0.24	107	107	First degree A-V block, rare dropped beat
11	0.18–0.23	0.28	107	54	Second degree A-V block
14	0.25	0.24	103	90	First degree A-V block, occasional dropped beat
18	0.24	0.24	107	107	First degree A-V block
23	0.24	0.24	103	103	First degree A-V block
28	0.19	0.24	109	90	First degree A-V block, occasional dropped beat
33	0.18	0.24	100	100	First degree A-V block
72	0.16	0.24	100	100	Normal sinus rhythm

*Upper limits of normal for child, 2, at rate of 90-110 is 0.16 second.
†Lower limits of normal for child, 2, at rate of 88 is 0.28 second; at 100, 0.27 second; at 109, 0.26 second.

increasing number of older people. Accidental digitalis poisoning is rare, especially in children, with only 2 cases previously reported. A third case is reported by Curtis C. Drevets[4] (Iowa City).

Boy, 2, began retching and vomiting and soon became seriously ill. An empty bottle of digitoxin was found from which an estimated 12-15 tablets of 0.1 mg. digitoxin had been taken by the boy. Heart rate was 96, urine showed acetone. Serial electrocardiograms during the next 3 days showed changes from normal sinus rhythm to 2d-degree block, then back to normal sinus rhythm (table). He received intravenous fluids containing potassium, recovered and was discharged.

In experimental animals, the first manifestations of digitalis poisoning are strong vagal stimulation: bradycardia, cardiac irregularities, diastolic pauses and an idioventricular rhythm. Muscular irritability may or may not follow, and ventricles may become independent of the atria. As toxicity

(4) J. Pediat. 52:577-583, May, 1958.

progresses, the ventricles fibrillate and death then follows.

In man, symptoms of digitalis poisoning usually begin with anorexia, nausea and vomiting. Occasionally there may be diarrhea, salivation, abdominal discomfort, substernal pain and, rarely, hemorrhagic gastritis. Disorders in color vision are common, and often the eyes cannot focus. Other effects in various combinations are fatigue, drowsiness, restlessness, irritability, disorientation, hallucinations, delirium, headaches, tremors, myalgias, arthralgias, convulsions, diplopia, amblyopia and scotomas. The electrocardiogram first shows flattened T waves which later become inverted. As toxicity increases, the P-R interval is prolonged and the Q-T interval diminished.

Treatment of digitalis poisoning is chiefly supportive and symptomatic. No definite conclusion is possible about potassium therapy, but it appears to have beneficial effect, at least according to electrocardiographic signs of digitalis toxicity.

PAM (Pyridine-2-Aldoxime Methiodide) Therapy for Alkylphosphate Poisoning is recommended by Tatusji Namba and Kiyoshi Hiraki[5] (Okayama, Japan). Alkylphosphate compounds have been used recently both as medicine (diisopropyl fluorophosphate) and as insecticides (parathion). Since parathion is widely used in rice fields of Japan, poisoning has become an important problem. Atropine treatment has been used but is not specific. The introduction of PAM as a reactivator of alkylphosphate-inhibited acetylcholinesterase by I. B. Wilson of Columbia University led to studies of PAM as a possible specific antidote.

Aqueous 5% solutions were tried. The LD_{50} for 2 kg. white rabbits was about 10 mg./kg. body weight, subcutaneously, producing symptoms of muscular fasciculation, salivation and noisy breathing. Intravenous injection in rabbits previously given large doses of parathion emulsion produced dramatic remission of symptoms temporarily, followed by death in about 24 hours. Repeated injections of PAM maintained the blood cholinesterase activity successfully, although later doses were less effective. Oral PAM was also effective.

Five farmers who acquired severe parathion poisoning

(5) J.A.M.A. 166:1834-1839, Apr. 12, 1958.

from spraying rice fields were treated by intravenous injections of PAM. Symptoms included nausea, vomiting, salivation, dizziness, sweating, muscular fasciculation and coma. Two received atropine therapy, 1 of whom had already recovered and a third man, not seen until the 8th day after poisoning, had minimal symptoms. At first, 0.1 Gm. PAM was given intravenously, with the dose repeated until 1 Gm. had been given in 3½ hours. All symptoms were controlled and no evidence of toxicity was observed. Two patients were given 1 Gm. intravenously in a single dose, with prompt and complete relief of symptoms. Cholinesterase activity of red cells was restored at once whereas the serum cholinesterase was restored only transiently. PAM exerts no action on cholinesterase of normal blood. No serious side effects were observed.

Accidental Ingestion of Estrogens by Children is reported in 2 families, with 2 affected siblings in each family, by Roy Hertz[6] (Nat'l Inst. of Health).

Cases 1 and 2.—Boy, 5, and his sister, 7, had distinct enlargement and nodularity of the breasts. In the girl there was distinct stimulation of the areolae, but the mammary glands were not especially prominent on direct inspection. No secretion could be expressed from either breast. There was a fine fuzz of pubic hair but no axillary hair. The labia showed distinct enlargement and the vaginal mucosa was unduly moist and vascular. Rectal examination revealed no uterine enlargement. There was a fine but unquestioned increase in the hair on the upper lip and the mother felt this was of recent origin. The skin was clear.

Besides breast enlargement, the boy had recent enlargement and increased turgidity of the penis. There was also slight development of pubic hair. Rectal examination revealed a dubious enlargement and unusual firmness of the prostate. The skin was clear.

An epidemiologic study of the family revealed that the children were taking vitamin capsules which contained the equivalent of 150 μg estrone each. During the next 6 weeks without vitamin capsules, both children had complete regression of all signs and symptoms. The girl had no menstrual bleeding on withdrawal of the medication.

Cases 3 and 4.—Brothers, 8 and 10, had shown recent and simultaneous development of obvious gynecomastia and marked sensitivity of the breasts. No effect on the penis, prostate or pubic hair was apparent. Assay of vitamins which the boys had been taking revealed that each capsule contained substantial estrogen activity. Discontinuance of the vitamins caused regression of gynecomastia.

Investigation of pharmaceutical factories producing the

(6) Pediatrics 21:203-206, February, 1958.

vitamins ingested by these patients revealed that contamination with estrogenic material was due to lack of proper cleaning of equipment used alternately for processing the vitamins in the capsules and estrogens.

RHEUMATIC DISORDERS

Empire Rheumatism Council Multicenter Controlled Trial Comparing Cortisone Acetate and Acetylsalicylic Acid in Long-Term Treatment of Rheumatoid Arthritis: Results of Three Years' Treatment.[7] One hundred patients with rheumatoid arthritis of any duration were selected after excluding those with gross irreversible changes in the joints and those under age 17 and over 60, together with any known to have mental instability, gastric disease or hypertension, those unlikely to co-operate and those who were unable to walk or had major degrees of flexion deformity. The patients were allocated to one of the two treatment groups at random. Both groups were shown to be similar initially in all relevant respects, whether the 99 patients who were started on the trial, or the 77 available at the end of the 1st year or the 53 available at the end of the 3d year only were considered.

The treatment schedule consisted of a basic regimen of general care, including use of splints and physical therapy plus cortisone acetate for one group and aspirin for the other. The drugs were given during the year at the lowest individual dosage levels that would keep each patient largely symptom free and restore maximal functional efficiency with minimal side effects.

The gradual change in mean cortisone dosage from the 75 mg./day stipulated at start of therapy became significantly less statistically at the 24th month (67.5 mg./day) and again at the 36th month (67.1 mg./day). Therapeutically, this was a comparatively small decrease. Only 1 patient on cortisone improved sufficiently to discontinue the drug entirely throughout the 3d year. No other patient was receiving less than 25 mg. or more than 100 mg./day at the end of the 3d

(7) Ann. Rheumat. Dis. 16:277-289, September, 1957.

year. There was no significant change in the aspirin dosage (52-61 gr./day) over the 3 years.

The effect of this dosage of cortisone acetate in treatment of rheumatoid arthritis was similar in most respects to that of aspirin; little advantage was shown by either drug at the end of the 1st, 2d or 3d year in any of the functional tests. Subjective well-being was slightly better maintained in the cortisone than in the aspirin group. Hemoglobin levels showed transient improvement at the end of the 1st year in the cortisone group and at the end of the 3d year in the aspirin group. Both groups showed radiologic deterioration; this was more pronounced at the end of the 2d year in the aspirin group, but the difference did not reach significant levels. In all other respects, both groups showed improvement at the 3-year assessment compared with the condition at start of the trial.

Cortisone and Salicylates in Chronic Relapsing Rheumatic Carditis. Previous clinical studies have shown this combined therapy to be more effective in the acute stages than either alone. J. Lorber, K. S. Holt, John Rendle-Short and R. S. Illingworth[8] (Univ. of Sheffield) report its effects in 6 children who had one or more previous attacks of rheumatic fever. Rheumatic activity had been continuous for several months before hormone treatment was started and each patient had gross cardiac damage. All 6 received cortisone or prednisolone in high doses with salicylates until three consecutive weekly normal erythrocyte sedimentation rates had been obtained, or longer if considered necessary.

Three children, aged 9, 9 and 11, responded well to treatment with prednisolone combined with salicylates in low dosage. The erythrocyte sedimentation rate returned to normal in all 3 on the 7th day and in 2 remained normal for 5 and 8 weeks until treatment was discontinued when a short rebound occurred followed by a subsequent uneventful course. The third had a rebound when the dose of prednisolone was reduced to 5 mg. daily. None had any significant change in heart size or signs. In 2 other children, aged 11 and 13, the course was similar to that in the first 3, except that shortly after discontinuance of treatment, both relapsed and relapses continued to recur. Each time treatment was

(8) Ann. Rheumat. Dis. 16:481-484, December, 1957.

reinstituted, remission again ensued. In the sixth child, response as measured by the sedimentation rate was doubtful and treatment was complicated by hematemesis.

The combined therapy improved the general health of these children. Long-standing cardiac lesions were not expected to regress and none did. Response to treatment, judged by the sedimentation rate, was not as uniformly satisfactory as in children treated in their first attack. The marked tendency to relapse was disappointing. Perhaps the disease was so well established that therapy could only be suppressive and not curative. It may indicate that early treatment is desirable in children with rheumatic fever. The tendency to relapse in chronic cases may indicate that combined treatment should be continued for longer periods than is necessary in children in their initial attacks treated early. Combined therapy is useful in children with smouldering rheumatic carditis, but treatment may have to be prolonged.

Aspirin as Gastric Irritant. Edward M. Schneider[9] (Univ. of Oklahoma) studied the effect of aspirin and a "buffered" aspirin preparation on gastric secretion, using the paired control-placebo-double-blind-randomization technic, with neither patients nor technician knowing the agents being used.

In all subjects a Levin tube was placed in the stomach. After 30 minutes of baseline gastric acidity determination, one of the drugs or a similar-appearing placebo was introduced into the stomach in aqueous solution. Aspiration of the stomach was resumed 90 minutes after administration of the test agents and continued at 30-minute intervals for another 210 minutes. Ten patients received 10 gr. aspirin or a similar-appearing placebo on the 1st day of study. The alternative agent was then given on a subsequent day. Nine patients received a buffered aspirin preparation containing 10 gr. aspirin and 2 gr. magnesium oxide or a similar-appearing placebo on the initial study day. The alternate agent was given on the 2d day of study.

In 6 of the 10 subjects who received aspirin, gross blood was noted in every specimen of gastric juice obtained after its administration. This occurred despite absence of change in gastric acidity subsequent to its administration. The pla-

(9) Gastroenterology 33:616-620, October, 1957.

cebo produced no bleeding or acidity alterations. Aspirin buffered with magnesium oxide caused a significant increase in gastric acidity compared with the placebo effect, but no gross blood was noted in any specimen of gastric juice obtained after its administration.

The occurrence of hemorrhage after administration of aspirin and the apparent protection provided by buffering agents strongly support the concept that aspirin is a gastric irritant. Apparently, this irritation is not related to dramatic changes in gastric acidity.

Aspirin should be used with extreme caution, if at all, in patients with known upper gastrointestinal lesions, and aspirin-induced gastric mucosal irritation should be considered in any patient with unexplained gastrointestinal hemorrhage. When aspirin is to be administered, it would be prudent to prescribe simultaneously small quantities of a buffering material, such as magnesia or sodium bicarbonate.

Polymeric-Coated Aspirin in Treatment of Aspirin-Sensitive Arthritic Patients. Paul Giovinco[1] (Hempstead, N. Y.) reports that none of 31 arthritic patients with a history of aspirin sensitivity had gastric disturbance on receiving equal or higher doses of an enteric-coated preparation. In 20 patients given higher doses of the enteric-coated aspirin than the plain aspirin tolerance of daily doses of the enteric-coated preparation averaged 53% higher than that of the plain aspirin. When dosages of plain aspirin ranged from 5 to 60 gr./day, dosages of the coated aspirin ranged from 30 to 60 gr./day.

Of 15 patients given equal doses of plain and coated aspirin, 11 said that the analgesia derived from the enteric-coated form was superior to that from plain aspirin. Two factors may account for this phenomenon: (1) The subjective impressions of these patients may have been influenced by the gastric pains, i.e., the arthritic pains may have seemed worse because of the concomitant abdominal distress. Therefore, when this distress was eliminated, the arthritic pains may have seemed less severe. (2) These patients, fearing nausea, may not have taken the prescribed doses of plain aspirin. Three patients considered the analgesia obtained from the plain and coated aspirin to be equal, and 1 inferior.

(1) New York J. Med. 58:356-358, Feb. 1, 1958.

Two patients complained of slow onset in action of the coated aspirin, especially in the morning. They were advised to take a small dose of plain aspirin on rising to gain more rapid symptomatic relief.

Phenolic Compounds in Chemotherapy of Rheumatic Fever. Treatment of rheumatic fever has been little improved since the introduction of salicylic acid 80 years ago. In an attempt to find improved compounds, Norman E. Clarke, Charles N. Clarke and Robert E. Mosher[2] (Providence Hosp., Detroit) investigated related compounds, the diphenols gentisic acid, protocatechuic acid, pyrocatechuic acid, beta resorcylic acid and gamma resorcylic acid, and the triphenols phloroglucinol carboxylic acid and 2,3,6-trihydroxybenzoic acid (table).

Data support the importance of chelation and demonstrate that potency is greatly increased by a 2d hydroxy group in the 6-position. The compound 2,3,6-trihydroxybenzoic acid had lower toxicity, acted more promptly to suppress manifestations of rheumatic fever and lower elevated blood sedimentation rates than did all other phenolic compounds. Like other double chelating phenols, it usually decreased urinary excretion of sulfur and glucuronic acid conjugates except in patients with malignant or submalignant rheumatic fever.

Superior antirheumatic qualities were associated with a 2d or 3d hydroxy group in the 3-position on the benzene ring. The ingested 2,3-dihydroxybenzoic acid improved antirheumatic activity without prompting detoxication mechanisms, and the excretion of phenolic conjugates of sulfur and glucuronides were decreased.

The toxicity of a phenol is reduced by a 2d hydroxy group, least when in the 4,6-position and most in the 3,5-position. Toxicity of phenolic compounds with a 2d hydroxy group in the 4- or 6-position is abolished by a 3d hydroxy group. The highest toxicity was found in the diphenol, protocatechuic acid, which is not a chelating compound.

The smaller amounts of gamma resorcylic, pyrocatechuic and triphenolic acids required to suppress manifestations of rheumatic fever, compared with those of salicylic acid, support the concept of antirheumatic metabolites. Compounds with reversible quinone hydroquinone systems manifested

(2) Am. J. M. Sc. 235:7-22, January, 1958.

COMPARISON OF CLINICAL RESPONSE AND METABOLISM OF MONO-, DI- AND TRIPHENOLIC COMPOUNDS IN RHEUMATIC FEVER

Structure	Compound	*Antirheumatic Potency*	*Toxicity in Therapeutic Doses*	*Urinary Excretion of Conjugates* — *Total Sulfur*	*Urinary Excretion of Conjugates* — *Glucuronides*	*Urinary Excretion 17-Ketosteroids*	*Eosinopenia 50% Plus*	*Action on Circulating Lymphocytes*	*Prevention of Heart Damage with Early Use*
HOOC, HO	Salicylic Acid	1.	High	No change	Increased	No change	Yes	Increased	No
HOOC, HO, OH	Pyrocatechuic Acid	2.	Absent	Decreased	Decreased	Decreased	Yes	Increased	No
HOOC, HO, OH	Beta Resorcylic Acid	1.	Low	No change	Increased	No change	Yes	Increased	No
HOOC, OH, HO	Gentisic Acid	1.	Absent	Increased	Increased	—	Yes	Increased	No
OH, HOOC, HO	Gamma Resorcylic Acid	5.	Low	Decreased	Decreased	Decreased	Yes	Increased	No
HOOC, OH, OH	Protocatechuic Acid	None	High	No change	Increased	No change	No	No change	No
OH, HOOC, HO, OH	Phloroglucinol Carboxylic Acid	8.	Absent	Decreased	Decreased	Decreased	No	Increased	Possible
OH, HOOC, HO, OH	2,3,6-Trihydroxy Benzoic Acid	10.	Absent	Decreased	Decreased	Decreased	No	Increased	Probable

superior antirheumatic qualities. The most important hydroxy group outside the 2- or 6-positions was the 3-position of pyrocatechuic acid, the only diphenol that decreased urinary excretion of sulfur and glucuronic acid conjugates.

The new compound, 2,3,6,-trihydroxybenzoic acid, had

maximum antirheumatic potency, was nontoxic and decreased the urinary excretion of sulfur and of glucuronic acid. When used early in the first attack of rheumatic fever, it seemed to prevent damage to the heart.

Steroid Therapy for Rheumatic Fever. Carolyn Moore McCue[3] (Med. College of Virginia) studied 94 patients with acute rheumatic fever who received varying doses of cortisone and prednisone. Of 24 given a maximum of 150 mg. cortisone daily, 47% were improved or had no heart disease at

RESULTS OF THERAPY AS JUDGED BY DISAPPEARANCE OF MURMURS OR DECREASE IN HEART SIZE ON PATIENTS TREATED IN FIRST 28 DAYS OF ILLNESS

Dosage	Patients Treated	No Heart Disease at End of Therapy	Improved (Less Murmur or Smaller Heart)	Total %, No Heart Disease or Better
200 mg. cortisone	26	12	7	73
300 mg. cortisone	12	6	3	75
60 mg. prednisone	4	2	1	75
Total	42	20	11	73.8

the end of treatment, 33% were the same or worse and 20% died. Illness had been present for 42 days or longer in 55% at the time treatment was started.

Another 45 patients received 200 mg. cortisone daily for 14 days, then the dose was reduced gradually during 61 days. There were 3 deaths; 2 patients had further progression of murmur when the drug was started after more than 28 days of illness. Sixteen patients had no heart disease at the end of treatment, and only 3 were without it at onset. The drug was considered lifesaving in 5 cases.

A maximum daily dose of 300 mg. cortisone was given 17 patients for 21 days, followed by gradual reduction of dosage over 61 days. Of 8 patients treated in the first 14 days of illness, 6 had no residual heart disease. Only 1 death occurred. The patient had had rheumatic fever for several years with a recent exacerbation.

A group of extremely ill patients received 60 mg. prednisone daily. Dosage was gradually reduced over 61 days. Of 8 patients, 6 had pericarditis or failure. There were 2 deaths and the drug was considered lifesaving in 3 cases.

Among patients receiving 200 mg. cortisone, 300 mg. cor-

(3) J. Pediat. 51:255-261, September, 1957.

tisone or 60 mg. prednisone daily, 36 had heart disease at onset of therapy and were treated within the first 28 days of illness. Of these, 13 had no residual heart disease. The percentage of patients in this group with no residual heart disease is about twice that observed among 132 patients treated before 1948 without steroids.

About half the patients on any of the large-dosage schedules treated within 28 days had no heart disease at the end of therapy and 73.8% were much improved or had no heart disease at the end of therapy (table).

Effects of Prolonged Adrenocortical Stimulation on Patients with Rheumatoid Arthritis. H. F. West[4] (Sheffield, England) reviewed the records of 110 rheumatoid arthritic patients who received adrenocortical stimulation during 4½ years. The patients fell into two categories. The 44 patients in group A had completed 3-6 weeks of therapy. In none was therapy withdrawn because of ineffectiveness or complications. Included were patients receiving adrenal restimulation after prolonged oral corticosteroid therapy and those with acute exacerbations of the disease not thought to need prolonged therapy. Group B consisted of 66 patients in whom therapy exceeded 3 months and continues to date or in whom it had to be withdrawn (42 patients).

Generally, HP Acthar® Gel was used. An intramuscular dose large enough to raise the daily urinary output of 17-ketosteroids or 17-hydroxycorticosteroids from 20 to 35 mg. was given daily. The level aimed at varied with severity of the disease and clinical response. Frequent urinary assays were made until a steady therapeutic level was achieved.

In group A, every patient showed evidence of adrenocortical stimulation after intramuscular administration of corticotropin, provided they had not previously received corticotropin and acquired the ability to destroy it. Raising the output of 17-ketosteroids or 17-hydroxycorticosteroids 50-100% above the starting level resulted in amelioration or disappearance of symptoms and regression of physical signs.

In 42 patients of group B, adrenal stimulation therapy did not eradicate the disease. Therefore, it was necessary to compare the progress of these patients with that of a similar group who did not have adrenal stimulation therapy.

(4) Ann. Rheumat. Dis. 16:322-333, September, 1957.

Adrenocortical stimulation therapy, providing a daily urinary output of 20-30 mg. 17-hydroxycorticosteroids favorably affected the course of severe rheumatoid arthritis over prolonged periods in most patients. Comparison showed that the adrenal stimulation group started treatment with no advantage which could be revealed by erythrocyte sedimentation rate, hemoglobin level, strength of grip of physical ability, yet ended with relative advantages in each characteristic. The most objective evidence of advance in the disease was in the x-ray appearance of bone erosions. In this respect, patients in this group fared better than those treated with cortisone and aspirin. If it is assumed that the latter treatments had no unfavorable affect on the course of the disease, then it must be concluded that adrenal stimulation therapy had a favorable effect, at least during the observation periods.

The major complications lay in the allergenic nature of the corticotropin used. This was the commonest cause of withdrawal and was responsible for some alarming and dangerous anaphylactic reactions. The possibility that repeated injections of foreign protein may add disease to disease cannot be excluded. These complications should disappear with the advent of purer corticotropins. The other complications fell into two classes: those such as hypertension and fluid retention that were reversible and harmless if therapy were withdrawn, and those such as psychosis and congestive heart failure that could be avoided if the degree of adrenal stimulation were well controlled. With pure corticotropin and proper control of therapy there should be no deleterious effects to set against the benefits.

Clinical Course and Corticosteroid Excretion of Patients with Rheumatoid Arthritis during Long-Term Treatment with Corticotropin. According to Oswald Savage, Leslie Chapman, J. Douglas Robertson, Peter Davis, A. J. Popert and W. S. C. Copeman[5] (West London Hosp.), treatment of severe rheumatoid arthritis with self-injected corticotropin (ACTH) over long periods is a practical procedure, and when used with biochemical estimations has certain advantages over oral cortisone and its newer analogues. (1) The level of adrenal stimulation produced by ACTH can be es-

(5) Brit. M. J. 2:1257-1262, Nov. 30, 1957.

timated by measuring the total urinary excretion of 17-hydroxycorticosteroids. This can be done for outpatients and hospital patients. (2) When corticosteroid excretion is seen to fall, the dose of ACTH can be raised before severe clinical relapse occurs. (3) When corticosteroid excretion is seen to rise, the dose of ACTH may be reduced before excessive adrenal stimulation occurs.

With help of biochemical estimations, the authors studied 41 patients. In all, suppression of activity with fall in sedimentation rate followed administration of ACTH in a dose that proved sufficient to raise urinary excretion of 17-hydroxycorticosteroids significantly. In 23 patients, excretion was doubled and in 17, it was increased by over 50%. In all patients, clinical suppression of the disease was accompanied by a significant increase in corticosteroid excretion.

After the initial response, dosage had to be adapted to fluctuation of the disease activity or development of an altered sensitivity to the hormone. A high level of adrenal stimulation was not needed to obtain continued clinical improvement. Adequate clinical and biochemical response can be maintained for years with only minor adjustments of steroid dosage. Occurrence of remission is recognized if at any time during a period of satisfactory clinical response a fall in the patient's 17-hydroxycorticosteroid excretion is noted, without concurrent relapse of the disease. One difficulty in use of ACTH is the variation in strength of the batches.

Severe side effects, such as hypertension and glycosuria, occurred only when a high level of hydroxycorticosteroid excretion had existed for some weeks. They were reversible, however. Androgenic side effects, particularly acne, occurred commonly in women before the menopause with only slight adrenal stimulation. Absence of dyspepsia was impressive. In only 1 patient did peptic ulceration develop, whereas among 83 patients treated with oral steroids during the past 5 years, gastric or duodenal ulceration developed in 13. When ACTH was withdrawn, relapse of the arthritis followed, but this was not accompanied by the distressing general symptoms that attend withdrawal of cortisone and other oral steroids.

Biochemical control during long-term treatment of severe rheumatoid arthritis with ACTH resulted in a more accurate and less dangerous dosage regimen than was formerly practicable. If a simple method were devised for testing urinary corticosteroid excretion within a fairly wide range, it would bring this additional method of control into the realm of routine clinical medicine.

Two Years' Experience of Prednisone in Rheumatoid Arthritis are reviewed by George R. Fearnley, Geoffrey V. Balmforth and Roy Blatchley[6] (Gloucestershire Royal Hosp.). Of 167 patients with rheumatoid arthritis treated with 15 mg. prednisone daily, 15 (10%) were thought to require prednisone initially; but at the end of 2 years, 47 (30%) were receiving the drug; the increase was accounted for by the failure of other drugs. Improvement of functional status occurred in about 50% of patients given prednisone; subjective improvement was reported by 90%.

The commonest complication of prednisone therapy was dyspepsia which occurred in 11 patients, in 2 of whom peptic ulcers developed. Other symptoms, such as obesity, hypertension and diabetes occurred in a much smaller percentage of patients.

Despite the risks and complications, the authors believe it justified to give prednisone to the wage earner on the point of incapacity, the housewife unable to look after a young family and the patient who is deteriorating rapidly despite all other measures. Whether steroids should be given to patients with milder disease or less arduous commitments cannot be decided until much more experience throughout the world has been gained. This may not need to be decided if research produces a better and safer remedy.

Prednisone and Prednisolone Therapy in Rheumatoid Arthritis: Clinical Evaluation with Emphasis on Gastrointestinal Manifestations in 156 Patients Observed for Periods of 4-14 Months is presented by Bertrand L. Stolzer, James H. Barr Jr., Carl H. Eisenbeis Jr., Richard L. Wechsler and Harry M. Margolis[7] (Univ. of Pittsburgh). Initial dosage ranged from 10 to 40 mg./day, given in divided doses about every 6 hours. In most patients, 10 mg. or less sufficed for maintenance. Most patients had relatively far-advanced, severe forms of rheumatoid arthritis, and most had been re-

(6) Brit. M. J. 2:1263-1266, Nov. 30, 1957.
(7) J.A.M.A. 165:13-17, Sept. 7, 1957.

ceiving hydrocortisone ineffectually before substitution of prednisone.

Measurable decrease in total severity of the disease was observed in 57% of the patients. In 41% there was measurable improvement in functional capacity, and 9 of 30 men who were not working returned to work some time during the course of treatment.

Side effects of prednisone or prednisolone were, in general, not disturbing, but the incidence of gastrointestinal symptoms increased from 11% before therapy to 21% during therapy. Definite peptic ulcer was noted in 7 of 43 patients with dyspepsia in whom gastrointestinal x-rays were made because of digestive distress. In 5 others, gastric hemorrhage or a perforated ulcer occurred. When absolutely essential for maintenance of the patient's functional capacity or self-sufficiency, administration of prednisone may possibly be continued, despite peptic ulcer, if a strict ulcer regimen is followed.

Rheumatoid Arthritis: Therapeutic Experiences with 6α-Methylprednisolone (Medrol®) in 49 women and 25 men is presented by Edward F. Rosenberg.[8] All patients were ambulatory, received physical therapy and were encouraged to take antacids. Salicylates were not limited.

Initial dosages of Medrol were determined on the basis of the rough relation of the potency of this compound to that of hydrocortisone and prednisone which was demonstrated in animal tests. Thus, for most adults, 8 mg. was used as the initial dose. This dose represents one tenth of the maximal amount of hydrocortisone and two fifths of the maximal dose of prednisone used during previous studies. The daily dose was divided, generally into 3 or 4 doses given at about equal intervals during the day. The oral route was used exclusively. After initial observation with 8 mg., various alterations were made in dosage schedules. Initial periods were sufficiently long, usually 2-4 weeks, to permit an estimate of general effectiveness of the preliminary dose. Among 34 women with rheumatoid arthritis previously treated with steroids, the daily dose during early weeks of the treatment was 10 mg.

Administration of Medrol generally resulted in prompt

(8) Metabolism 7 (pt. 2):487-496, July, 1958.

amelioration of symptoms. In some instances, this effect was noted within a few hours after the 1st dose. The benefits were greater among patients showing early manifestations of arthritis.

Among 12 patients who completed 6 months of therapy, 1 recovered so completely that no signs of articular inflammation were detectable. In 8, articular and functional status showed outstanding improvement, although residual defects were still recognizable. Among 11 patients completing 8 months of therapy, a complete remission appeared to have ensued in 1 patient; 7 showed improvement designated incomplete but of good quality; and 3 showed slight or poor response.

Comparative studies of sodium, potassium, chloride and CO_2 blood levels in 22 patients at onset of therapy and after 3-7 months' continuous treatment showed no significant alterations in any electrolyte component.

The side effects were generally mild, and their incidence compared favorably with those experienced with other steroid compounds. A rounded face and increased fat deposit were noted in 11 of 49 women. Hirsutism did not appear in severe form. Mild acne was observed in 8 women. No notable incidents involving the circulatory system were observed. The diabetogenic effect of Medrol appeared about equivalent to that of cortisone, hydrocortisone and the "metisteroids." No gross gastrointestinal hemorrhage nor perforation occurred. Psychic disturbances were minimal. No notable disturbances resulted from gradual withdrawals.

Triamcinolone in Treatment of Rheumatoid Arthritis. Edward F. Hartung[9] (New York Univ.) used a new synthetic steroid, 9α-fluoro-16α-hydroxy-Δ^1-hydrocortisone, and its diacetate ester, triamcinolone (Aristocort®), in treating 67 patients with rheumatoid arthritis. In 23, the drug was stopped before 6 months for the following causes, some patients showing two or more of them: weakness and fatigue, tachycardia, leg cramps, minor gastrointestinal complaints, recurrence of old duodenal ulcer symptoms, emotional unrest, headache, hirsutism, persistent respiratory infection, glucose tolerance decrease, excessive weight gain, no improvement and unrelated death.

(9) J.A.M.A. 167:973-976, June 21, 1958.

Twenty-three patients received the drug for over 6 and up to 11 months. They were well advanced in disease, mostly in stages 3 and 4. Therapeutic results were good; 16 had a grade 2 and 6 a grade 3 response.

The average dose of triamcinolone necessary to maintain adequate antirheumatic effect was 10 mg./day in 4 divided doses. The suppressive effects of triamcinolone and prednisone were about equal. As a rule, therapy was started with larger dose: the initial dose was commonly about 24 mg./day. Triamcinolone appeared to have these advantages over other steroids: lack of production of edema; fewer gastrointestinal symptoms, particularly the peptic ulcer syndrome; less psychic irritation; and no effect on arterial blood pressure.

Peptic Ulceration Occurring during Therapy for Rheumatoid Arthritis. According to Fred Kern, Jr., Glenn M. Clark and Jack G. Lukens[1] (Univ. of Colorado), peptic ulceration may increase 20- to 60-fold over the expected incidence during therapy with adrenocortical hormones or phenylbutazone. Among 169 patients attending clinic because of rheumatoid arthritis, 18.2% of the men and 8.7% of the women had peptic ulcer. Six of the 12 men and all 9 women acquired the ulcer after onset of arthritis. The relation between therapy and ulcer formation is demonstrated in Table 1.

TABLE 1.—ASSOCIATION BETWEEN TYPE AND DURATION OF THERAPY AND DEVELOPMENT OF PEPTIC ULCER

Duration of Therapy*	Type of Therapy†		
	Salicylates	Phenylbutazone	Adrenal steroids
mo.			
Less than 6	29	48 (3)	44 (1)
6–11	20	24	25 (2)
12–23	16	19 (3)	35 (4)
24–35	11	4	10
36–59	8	5 (1)	9
60+	7	—	1
Total	91	100	124
Number of patients developing new ulcer		(7)	(7)

*Periods of less than 1 month omitted.
†Numbers in parentheses indicate number of patients acquiring new ulcer.

(1) Gastroenterology 33:25-33, July, 1957.

TABLE 2.—EFFECT OF RHEUMATOID ARTHRITIS THERAPY ON RISK OF ACQUIRING PEPTIC ULCER*

Treatment	Sex	No. Patients	No. Man-Years Treated	No. Ulcers Expected	Actual No. Ulcers	Ratio of Actual to Expected Ulcers
Adrenal steroid...........	M	43	47	0.153	3	19:1
Adrenal steroid...........	F	77	88	0.144	4	27:1
Phenylbutazone..........	M	40	28.7	0.093	2	21:1
Phenylbutazone..........	F	67	51.5	0.084	5	59:1

*Though number of man-years in each group is small, ratio of actual to expected ulcer is similar in each instance.

The dosage of phenylbutazone which might lead to ulcer could not be determined, but ulcers were likely to occur in patients receiving over 50 mg./day cortisone or 20 mg./day prednisone. Lower doses appeared relatively safe. The incidence of ulcer during therapy with either agent greatly exceeded that in the general population (Table 2). The tendency to form ulcers appeared to increase with duration of the arthritis.

Intra-articular Administration of Hydrocortisone in High Concentration: Use in Treatment of Arthritic Knees was investigated by Bernard M. Norcross[2] (Univ. of Buffalo). Results of administration of 25-50 mg. hydrocortisone acetate into the knees of 11 patients with osteoarthritis and 49 with rheumatoid arthritis were compared with results of injection of 25-50 mg. hydrocortisone tertiary butylacetate, 150-300 mg. hydrocortisone acetate, 250 mg. hydrocortisone acetate/cc. of suspension and 25-50 prednisolone acetate.

Improvement occurred in 45 of 60 patients given 25-50 mg. hydrocortisone acetate, 51 of 60 given hydrocortisone tertiary butylacetate, 56 of 60 given 150-300 mg. hydrocortisone acetate, 38 of 40 given 250 mg./cc. hydrocortisone and 40 of 50 given prednisolone. With the larger doses of hydrocortisone, the degree of relief was greater than that obtained with 25-50 mg. Duration of improvement rose from an average of 6 to 34 days.

Coincident with the quantitative and qualitative improvement observed with the larger doses of hydrocortisone was an increase in the incidence of systemic manifestations. Of the 60 patients, 5 showed subjective improvement in other affected but untreated joints after administration of 25-50

(2) J.A.M.A. 167:839-841, June 14, 1958.

mg. hydrocortisone, whereas 40 or more showed such improvement after larger doses. A reduction in total eosinophil count and an increase in the 17-hydroxycorticosteroids in the urine was also noted. There were no flare-ups after systemic relief disappeared.

In some instances, 25-30 mg. neomycin was injected into the knees besides the hydrocortisone. No toxic or untoward effects occurred as a result. Addition of neomycin affords effective antibacterial protection against possible septic infection of the joint.

The findings in this study suggest that the larger joints such as the knee have a greater capacity than heretofore believed to hold a larger quantity of hydrocortisone in the cells. Thus greater and more intense improvement and longer lasting relief may be achieved by larger doses of the steroid.

Intra-articular Hydrocortisone Acetate in Interphalangeal and Metacarpophalangeal Joints of Fingers. Injection of hydrocortisone acetate into the larger joints of patients with rheumatoid arthritis is of established value. Little such therapy seems to have been used in smaller joints, such as the proximal interphalangeal or metacarpophalangeal joints of the fingers, yet commonly one or two of these joints are active in a patient whose arthritis is otherwise quiescent and can cause considerable discomfort and disability. V. Wright[3] (Univ. of Leeds) reports that of 37 proximal interphalangeal and 10 metacarpophalangeal joints of the fingers treated by injection of hydrocortisone acetate, a good result was obtained in 29 of the former and 9 of the latter. The results were examined in the light of clinical and x-ray features.

About 10 mg. hydrocortisone acetate was used. The average time before improvement after injection was 48 hours. Improvement lasted from 7 days to over 10 months. The result was not influenced by whether the injection was peri- or intra-articular. Neither the age of the patient, duration of arthritis nor systemic therapy appeared to affect the response to the hydrocortisone. Neither did the general activity of the disease judged clinically and by blood sedimentation rate. The joints of both hands responded equally well. Tenderness and pain in the joint before injection did not affect the

(3) Acta rheumat. scandinav. 4:40-48, 1958.

response, but all the joints with marked swelling responded well, whereas joints which did not improve had minimal swelling. The x-ray appearance gave no indication of those which would do well.

Value of Chloroquine in Rheumatoid Disease: Four-Year Study of Continuous Therapy is reported by Arthur W. Bagnall[4] (Vancouver, B. C.). Seventeen patients with Marie-Strümpell spondylitis and 108 with rheumatoid arthritis were followed clinically and hematologically. Four patients had less than 6 months' treatment, but were included because toxicity necessitated withdrawal of chloroquine. All other patients had 8 months or more of continuous therapy: 75% for more than 1 year, 50% for more than 2 years and 20% for more than 3 years. The normal dosage was 1 tablet (250 mg.) of chloroquine diphosphate given daily at bedtime. In 36%, a lower dosage was at some time necessary for a considerable period to avoid toxicity. Permanent withdrawal for this reason was eventually required in 10%.

RESULTS OF CHLOROQUINE THERAPY (A.R.A. CRITERIA)

	R.A. (108 patients)*		*M.S.S.** (17 patients)*	
Grade I (Remission)	39 patients (36%)	71%	4 patients (24%)	71%
Grade II (Major improvement)	38 patients (35%)		8 patients (47%)	
Grade III (Minor improvement)	12 patients (11%)	28%	2 patients (12%)	29%
Grade IV (Unimproved)	19 patients (17%)		3 patients (17%)	

*R.A.—Rheumatoid arthritis.
**M.S.S.—Marie-Strümpell spondylitis.

Over-all results are summarized in the table. Results were considered good in 70%; half of these patients achieved remission. Improved work performance, sedimentation rate and hemoglobin levels paralleled the objective gain in the patients with good results. Classic peripheral rheumatoid arthritis, spondylitis, arthritis of juvenile onset and rheumatoid disease with psoriasis appeared to respond equally well.

Patients who failed to show major objective improvement were rated as failures (30% of the total), though many were subjectively improved. Toxic reactions, seriously affecting the dosage of chloroquine, were responsible for less than half the failures. Among the rest of the patients, many

(4) Canad. M. A. J. 77:182-194, Aug. 1, 1957.

had prolonged, consistent, and severe rheumatoid activity.

In rheumatoid disease, failure of relapse after withdrawal of what is thought to be an effective remedy would arouse suspicion that the previous improvement was merely coincidental. Of patients with good response, 90% are still on long-term chloroquine therapy. However, in 7, treatment was apparently stopped too soon because of seeming remission. All 7 underwent relapse, but in each the relapse subsided with resumption of treatment. In another 6, relapse subsided without further chloroquine with symptomatic treatment only, such as a short course of steroid. Eight patients were unable, because of toxicity, to resume significant doses of chloroquine, and in these relapse persisted. Most relapses occurred within 3 months of withdrawal, but 9 of 21 were delayed for up to 1 year.

No definite serious toxic effects were noted, but the number of minor toxic reactions was higher than expected from previous reports, probably because this is the first large chronic chloroquine toxicity study in humans in the dosage used. Of the 125 patients treated, 70 had a total of 105 reactions which might have been due to chloroquine. However, 76% of these "reactors" were later able to take the full dosage of chloroquine consistently. Drug dermatitis was the only reaction significantly restricting dosage and treatment; this occurred in 16% of patients. It usually occurred after several months of therapy and subsided rapidly when the drug was withdrawn. Exfoliative dermatitis was not seen.

Seasickness (nausea, giddiness, frontal headache and/or blurring of vision) was common, tended to occur early in the course of treatment and usually subsided with temporary lowering of dosage. Only 2 patients had to stop the drug permanently because of this syndrome.

Agranulocytosis was not encountered, but leukopenia (with a normal differential count), rising after some weeks to normal despite continued full-dosage chloroquine therapy, occurred 6 times. A number of other reactions occurred which were probably coincidental. These included metrorrhagia in 5 patients, lymphedema of the forearm and hand in 4, serum sickness (?) in 2 and irritation of existing psoriasis in 4.

Hydrochloroquine (Plaquenyl®) is under trial as a substitute for chloroquine in the treatment of patients with persistent chloroquine toxicity. In some patients there appears to be a complete overlap of toxicity; others tolerate hydrochloroquine without evidence of reaction.

A long-term study using the double-blind technic is reported. There was no difficulty in determining from the results which drug was the placebo, but the group was too small for statistical analysis. Of 12 patients receiving the placebo, none showed a major response, whereas 12 of 19 (63%) receiving chloroquine showed considerable improvement.

The optimum dosage of chloroquine appears to be 250 mg. daily. In a few patients this dosage was increased without adding to the benefit, but with a tendency to increased toxicity. Relapse was frequent, especially in the female, when dosage was reduced below 250 mg. daily. The importance of persistence in treatment is emphasized. There is a latent period of 1-3 months before chloroquine begins to show its favorable effects, and maximum benefit may be delayed for 6-12 months or even more in the severe arthritic with long-lasting activity. Short courses of chloroquine are, therefore, of no value.

It is suggested that chloroquine comes closer to the ideal for long-term, safe control of rheumatoid disease than any other agent now available. However, little is known of its mechanism of action.

Further Observations on Use of 4-Aminoquinoline Compounds in Patients with Rheumatoid Arthritis or Related Diseases are presented by Arthur L. Scherbel, John W. Harrison and Martin Atdjian.[5] Chloroquine phosphate or hydroxychloroquine sulfate was given to 805 patients for up to 3 years. Of these, 716 patients had arthritis of the rheumatoid type, of whom 627 had typical rheumatoid arthritis, 53 arthritis of the rheumatoid type with a positive test for lupus erythematosus, 23 rheumatoid arthritis with psoriasis and 13 juvenile rheumatoid arthritis. Other disorders of the connective tissue, including arteritis, dermatomyositis, progressive scleroderma, Reiter's syndrome and systemic lupus erythematosus, were present in 89 patients. Originally an initial dose of 500 mg. chloroquine phosphate was administered daily, but later the maximum daily dose was 250 mg.

(5) Cleveland Clin. Quart. 25:95-111, April, 1958.

The initial dose of hydroxychloroquine sulfate was 600 mg. daily in divided doses. After major improvement had been maintained at least 1 year, dosage was reduced to 400 mg. daily.

Of 106 patients with rheumatoid arthritis who were given only a 4-aminoquinoline drug, there was major improvement in 62%. Variation in response was wide: less than 25% of patients obtained major improvement within the first 3 months, 37% obtained major improvement after 12 months and 38% showed an insignificant response after 18 months.

Initial improvement appeared more rapidly when a small dose of a corticosteroid was simultaneously given with a 4-aminoquinoline compound, but eventual over-all improvement after 1 year was not significantly better than in patients who received only 4-aminoquinoline compounds. In this group, major improvement occurred in 54% of the patients after the 1st month of therapy and in 61% after 6 months. Major improvement was obtained in 67% after 1 year, during which time corticosteroid dosage was reduced by one-half or administration of the drug was stopped in 47%. Corticosteroids should be considered only as temporary adjuncts in treating rheumatoid arthritis. They should be given in small doses equivalent to 3-7.5 mg. prednisone/day and should be reduced or stopped as improvement appears.

Though 55% of patients taking one of the 4-aminoquinoline compounds exhibited some reaction to the drug, 67% of these reactions cleared spontaneously while medication was continued. Withdrawal of the compound was necessary in 7% of patients because of the severity of the reaction. Neurovascular reactions, including difficulty in visual accommodation, vascular headaches, vestibular dysfunction, tinnitus, nervousness, insomnia and/or mental confusion, occurred in 49% of patients exhibiting toxic manifestations. Gastrointestinal symptoms occurred in 19% of patients taking chloroquine and in 11% of those receiving hydroxychloroquine. The most serious were anorexia with loss of weight (41 patients), diarrhea (11) and vomiting (4). Skin reactions were the most distressing and most serious of all drug reactions. They occurred with about equal frequency with chloroquine and hydroxychloroquine and accounted for 12% of all drug reactions. They included dryness of the skin, itching, urticaria, morbilliform and maculopapular eruptions, desquamating and exfoliating lesions, increased pigmentation, alopecia and graying or bleaching of the hair. Pre-existing psoriatic lesions were susceptible to exacerbation. Skin reactions were serious in about half the patients exhibiting such manifestations.

The pharmacologic action of the 4-aminoquinoline drugs is not known, though biochemical alterations occur within the central nervous system and peripheral tissues. The desirable features of therapy using these compounds are the low incidence of serious drug reactions and of chronic toxicity, ease of administration, compatibility with other therapeutic agents and low incidence of relapse after maximum improvement has been obtained. The undesirable features are the delayed onset of major improvement, persistence of minor disease fluctuations and lack of major improvement that is observed in one third or more of the patients and sometimes an apparent susceptibility to skin reactions that may be serious, though not necessarily frequent.

Present Status of Phenylbutazone Therapy in Rheumatic Disease is discussed by R. M. Mason and R. R. P. Hayter[6] (London Hosp.). The main therapeutic effect of phenylbutazone is analgesic. It is slowly absorbed but maintains a constant blood level thereafter when taken 3 times daily. This makes it more suitable for chronic painful conditions. It has a slight uricosuric effect. With blood levels below the therapeutic 10 mg./100 ml. range, it may lead to urate retention.

In rheumatoid arthritis, phenylbutazone should be given early in the disease course. The daily maximum dose is 400 mg. It should be tried before beginning deep x-ray therapy in ankylosing spondylitis. Smaller doses of the drug are more effective in this disease than in others; many patients may be controlled with 200 mg. or less a day. It is of special value in osteoarthritis of the hip where, by permitting proper use of the joint in allowing smoother walking, the development of contracture and deformity may be prevented. Nocturnal pain is also conveniently relieved due to its prolonged action.

Although the exact mechanism of its action is unknown, phenylbutazone may well supersede colchicine in acute gout.

(6) Practitioner 181:23-28, July, 1958.

The suggested daily dose is 600 mg./day until the acute attack is controlled, usually within 2-3 days, after which 400 mg./day is sufficient until the attack has completely subsided. It is especially valuable if colchicine is ineffective because therapeutic doses are prevented by gastrointestinal upset.

About 60% of the toxic reactions appeared in the first 6 weeks of administration. Among these were nearly all the cases of rash, stomatitis, buccal ulcers, edema and vertigo. Onset of gastrointestinal reactions, however, was often more delayed: in 16 patients, they developed after 6-48 months of continuous phenylbutazone therapy. The drug should be discontinued as soon as there is any apparent toxicity, no matter how long the patient has been taking it, and it is wise to abandon its use for that particular patient rather than resume its administration, even cautiously, when the symptoms have settled down.

Unfortunately, low dosage is not the whole answer to the prevention of serious reactions, and among the reported fatal cases are some in which the maximum dose never exceeded 400 mg./day.

Phenylbutazone in Small Doses in Treatment of Joint Diseases. Egon Jesting, Poul Bastrup-Madsen and Poul Bechgaard[7] (Aarhus, Denmark) report their experiences with 180 patients, some of whom were treated for 1-3 years continuously. The dosage schedule was 800 mg. the 1st day, then 200 mg. daily, which maintained a concentration in the blood of 3-4 mg./100 ml. If improvement was not noted in 1 week, the drug was withdrawn. The best effect was obtained in 9 patients with gout; all were symptomatically relieved. Seven had subsequent attacks that responded to repeated administration. In 24 of 71 patients with osteoarthritis, beneficial effect was obtained for 2-33 months. Some remained asymptomatic after the drug was stopped, presumably indicating that the disease had passed into a quiescent phase during therapy. Of 52 patients with rheumatoid arthritis, 10 benefited from treatment for 4-36 months. Of 20 with atypical arthritis, 8 showed good response for 1-13 months; after the drug was stopped, benefit persisted in 6 of these. A strikingly

(7) Acta med. scandinav. 160:305-314, 1958.

good effect was obtained in psoriatic arthritis and ankylosing spondylitis.

Reactions occurred in 27 (15%) of the patients. Only 3 continued using the drug despite side effects. Melena occurred in 2: in 1 after 12 days and in the other after 21 months of treatment. In 4, skin rash developed; in 6, dryness of the mouth and throat; in 4, epigastric oppression; in 3, nausea; in 4, diarrhea; and in 1 each, dizziness, nightmares, palpitation and neutropenia. Thus, most of the reactions were mild and insignificant. None developed agranulocytosis.

Many clinicians hesitate to use phenylbutazone because of the reactions, but these are all reversible, and even the risk of agranulocytosis is slight if promptly recognized. The advantages and disadvantages, however, must be closely considered in each patient. When no response is obtained from a maintenance dose of 200 mg., it should be increased to 400/ mg. daily before therapy is abandoned. This drug should be used only in patients with severe joint disease and in whom response is definite.

Gastrointestinal Complications of Colchicine Therapy in Gout. Colchicine is considered the drug of choice for gout and has been used since the 15th century. Poisoning produces a characteristic clinical picture, mostly involving the gastrointestinal tract, even if the drug is given parenterally. Typically, several hours elapse between administration and onset of symptoms which begin with pharyngeal burning, increased salivation, nausea, dysphagia and abdominal pain and proceed to severe vomiting, colic, diarrhea and tenesmus. At the start the stools may be normal, but then they become mucoid and bloody. With progression of this dysentery phase, the clinical picture may resemble cholera with exhaustion, collapse and increasing muscular paralysis. Autopsy in these instances reveals marked inflammation of the gastrointestinal tract.

Edward Shanbrom and Leonard Rapoport[8] (Yale Univ.) report 2 cases in which surgical exploration was performed for acute onset of abdominal symptoms while the patients were taking colchicine. In 1, symptoms began only a few hours after colchicine was taken. At operation diffuse inflammatory lesions of the bowel were found with hemor-

(8) Ann. Int. Med. 48:655-660, March, 1958.

rhages, ecchymoses and bleeding areas which seemed to fan out along the mesenteric vessels as they emerged from the intestines and in the subserosal layer of the intestinal wall, particularly the mesenteric surface. The whole picture suggested specific irritation of the bowel wall and its blood vessels, caused by absorption of some toxic agent. That such toxic manifestations have not been previously reported in patients taking colchicine may be because surgery is rarely done at the opportune time to observe such changes.

Treatment of Acute Gouty Arthritis with Demecolcine is reported by Jacob Colsky, Stanley Wallace and Morris M. Banowitch[9] (Brooklyn) in 26 patients. Demecolcine differs from colchicine chemically in having a methyl group substituted for the acetyl group in the colchicine molecule. A total dose of 8-10 mg. was given orally to 20 patients for a single attack, 5 received a total dose of 5-6 mg. and 1 received only 2 mg. The dose of 8-10 mg. was chosen empirically, and because initial responses were good, this dosage plan was retained for treatment of most patients.

Response was satisfactory in 18 patients. In 3, partial improvement occurred. Three of the 5 who failed to respond favorably were later treated with colchicine, which was also ineffective. Most patients who responded favorably to demecolcine noted improvement beginning within 4-6 hours after starting treatment and after 12-18 hours had obtained maximal subjective and objective improvement although the latter was delayed as long as 24-36 hours in some instances. Mild nausea was noted in 2 patients and mild diarrhea in 2.

Two patients received several courses of 8 mg. demecolcine interspersed during the period when they were given daily maintenance doses of 1-3 mg. In both, pancytopenia and generalized loss of hair developed. When therapy was discontinued, the peripheral blood elements returned to normal. Regrowth of hair also occurred after several weeks.

Because of its potent bone-marrow-depressing activity, demecolcine should not be used for chronic maintenance therapy in patients with gouty arthritis, nor in those with frequent recurrent attacks. It may retain a place in treatment of the patient with an occasional attack who cannot tolerate colchicine. It may also be used as a diagnostic thera-

(9) A.M.A. Arch. Int. Med. 100:765-773, November, 1957.

peutic agent for gout in patients in whom the gastrointestinal effects of colchicine are to be avoided.

In the small group of patients treated, the authors have not been able to define the necessary dose of demecolcine needed to induce improvement. Much smaller doses than were used in this study may be sufficient to induce improvement and may thereby reduce the chances of undesirable side effects.

Zoxazolamine—A Potent Uricosuric Agent: Preliminary Report is presented by Elizabeth B. Reed, Thomas V. Feichtmeir and Forrest M. Willett[1] (VA Hosp., Fort Miley, Calif.), who treated a patient with chronic traumatic arthritis and

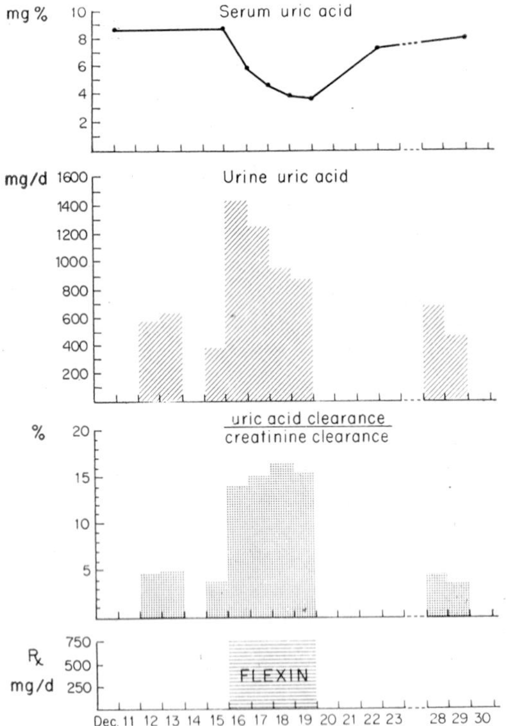

Fig. 39.—Results of zoxazolamine therapy on serum and urinary uric acid. (Courtesy of Reed, E. B., *et al.*: New England J. Med. 258:894-896, May 1, 1958.)

(1) New England J. Med. 258:894-896, May 1, 1958.

gout, using 250 mg. zoxazolamine 3 times daily. The drug showed a potent uricosuric effect (Fig. 39).

Zoxazolamine has been widely used to decrease spasm of skeletal muscle, presumably by a depressant effect on polysynaptic pathways in the central nervous system. Occasional side effects, such as drowsiness, lightheadedness, dizziness, abdominal discomfort, vomiting, headache and transient blotting of skin are transitory. Gastrointestinal symptoms, the most troublesome side effects, are usually avoided by giving this drug with food. No changes in blood pressure, respiration, blood count, urinalysis, hepatic or renal function have been noted.

Unlike the uricosuric agents, salicylates, cinchophen and ethyl biscoumacetate, zoxazolamine does not affect production of prothrombin or factor VII, at least in the doses used, over a short period. In this respect, and also in its tendency to produce few side effects, except for occasional gastrointestinal symptoms, zoxazolamine resembles probenecid.

During administration of this drug, an adequate urine volume and alkaline urine are desirable to minimize the possibility of urate precipitation in the urinary tract.

Gold in Treatment of Rheumatoid Arthritis. L. Maxwell Lockie, Bernard M. Norcross and Daniel J. Riordan[2] (Univ. of Buffalo) treated 507 patients who had rheumatoid arthritis with gold, supplemented by a minimum initial period of 3 weeks' complete bed rest, physical therapy, psychotherapy, analgesics, sedation, orthopedic aids and, when indicated, steroid therapy. Of these, 369 were given more than 300 mg. gold salts. The same regimen, except for gold salts, was offered to 566 control patients.

The gold preparation used generally was gold sodium thiomalate (Myochrysine®), given into the deltoid muscle at weekly intervals, beginning with a dose of 10 mg., then 20 mg. and then 40 mg. If no signs of sensitivity appeared, treatment was continued until 500 mg. had been given. At this point, weekly dosage was determined on the basis of the patient's clinical status. Those with moderate or severe arthritis usually required weekly injections of 40 mg. until 800 mg. had been administered, then 20 mg. for 4 weeks, 10 mg. for 4 weeks, 10 mg. at increasing intervals and, finally, 10 mg.

(2) J.A.M.A. 167:1204-1207, July 5, 1958.

once every 4 weeks for years. Those with mild symptoms were not given as much gold salts after the first 500 mg., since the dosage was cut more rapidly to be leveled eventually at 10 mg. monthly for years. While 10 mg./month is given, should exacerbation occur, the dose should be increased and the intervals between injections shortened to control symptoms.

Gold salts afford patients a 20% better chance of complete recovery or of major improvement (table). Apparently, more than 300 mg. must be given to influence the disease course favorably. Sensitivity to gold may appear at any time during

TOTAL GROUP COMPARISON OF RESPONSE TO THERAPY OF PATIENTS WITH RHEUMATOID ARTHRITIS, WITH COMPARISON OF PATIENTS RECEIVING MINIMUM OF 300 MG. GOLD SALTS AND THOSE RECEIVING LESS

	Gold-Treated					
	300 Mg. or More		Less Than 300 Mg.		Controls	
Response	No.	%	No	%	No.	%
Excellent	31	8 } 57	4	3 } 38	20	3 } 38
Major	182	49	48	35	199	35
Minor	130	35	57	41	270	48
None	26	7	29	21	77	11
Total	369		138		566	

therapy. A few patients may have manifestations after the first few injections; others may not have any until 500 mg. or more has been given. A high percentage of these manifestations are mild; any serious reaction is rare. The sensitivity reactions most commonly seen are glossitis and dermatitis; albuminuria, gastrointestinal reaction, eosinophilia, colitis, tracheitis and purpura are less frequent. Mild albuminuria may occur, but if it does not increase, the gold salts may be continued. The rare serious reactions are apt to occur when administration of the gold salts is continued despite the warning appearance of glossitis and dermatitis. They can usually be controlled by stopping the gold salts. If necessary, antihistamines and oral therapy with steroids are used for the uncomfortable manifestations. Dimercaprol (BAL) occasionally is needed for the severely affected. As many as 50% of patients who have had a mild reaction may be given further gold therapy in a smaller dose.

dl-Methionine in Urinary Incontinence. Using the double-blind technic, Gilbert Rosenberg[3] (Montreal) gave 10 mentally deteriorated and incontinent subjects, aged 74-88, gelatin capsules containing 0.2 Gm. dl-methionine 3 times daily for 1 week. Uriniferous odor markedly decreased and in most cases disappeared entirely after 3 or 4 days. Any skin irritation in the genital and perineal areas also markedly improved. Three men with cerebral arteriosclerosis showed a 50% reduction in frequency of wetting; the others showed no appreciable change in this respect. Relapse to the initial state began in all instances 2 or 3 days after medication was stopped. No noticeable effects were observed when an inert capsule was given.

► [This appears to be very welcome independent confirmation of last year's report by M. Bergman (1957-58 YEAR BOOK, p. 471) which involved a much larger number of patients.—Ed.]

Study of Long-Acting Muscle Relaxant (Tubadil®) in Anorectal Surgery. Control of pain after anorectal surgery still presents a challenge. The source of pain is thought to be spasm of the anal sphincter musculature. Locally injected anesthetics in oil and anesthetic ointments and creams have been ineffective. Prevention of muscle spasm with curare-like preparations which have a peripheral paralyzing action at the myoneural junction has been of value in treatment of painful spasm from trauma to the spine and shoulder and in other orthopedic problems as well as in anal sphincter muscle spasm. Tubadil is a crystalline tubocurarine alkaloid slowly absorbed from a repository menstruum of white wax and peanut oil.

Harold Rovner and Benjamin Haskell[4] (Jefferson Med. College) studied 66 patients undergoing hemorrhoidectomy, 33 of whom received 0.5 mg./kg. Tubadil (usual dose 1.2-1.6 cc., equivalent to 30-40 mg. tubocurarine chloride). The other 33 patients were used as controls. Narcotic requirements, anal sphincter spasm and pain during examination of the anal canal and after the first bowel movement were compared in the two groups.

(3) Canad. M. A. J. 79:123, July 15, 1958.
(4) Surg., Gynec. & Obst. 105:488-490, October, 1957.

In the first 72 hours following hemorrhoidectomy, treated patients required an average of only 1.8 injections of morphine and 1.5 doses of codeine, compared to 2.7 and 2.4, respectively, in the control group. There was less sphincter spasm in the group receiving Tubadil, but subjective pain was more difficult to evaluate accurately. There was no respiratory embarrassment in any patient receiving the drug, but 2 patients originally in the control group were so uncomfortable after hemorrhoidectomy that Tubadil was given on the 3d and 5th postoperative days, respectively, with untoward effects. Ninety minutes after administration of the drug, 1 patient had diplopia and muscular weakness of the upper extremities with loss of fine co-ordination while pain and spasms were relieved, but there was no respiratory difficulty. One hour after 1 cc. prostigmine 1:2000 was given, diplopia disappeared and normal muscle function returned to the upper extremities. The other patient had diplopia and marked muscle weakness in all extremities 35 minutes after Tubadil administration. Because of near hysteria accompanying the symptoms, evaluation of the relief of pain was difficult. These side effects were alleviated within 3 hours of administration of prostigmine. The first patient had been given the recommended dosage accurately calculated by body weight; the latter received less because of advanced age.

► [It may be just as well to remember that curare may occasionally cause peripheral circulatory depression through (*a*) widespread muscular relaxation with consequent impairment of venous return, (*b*) a direct relaxing action on the smooth muscles of the arterioles, (*c*) the capillary dilating effect of the histamine which the drug causes to be released from the tissues, (*d*) and possibly an action on the peripheral ganglions of the vasoconstrictor nerves.—Ed.]

Role of Digitalis in Mitral Valvuloplasty is a major one, as shown by the experience of Bernard Burack, John B. Schwedel and Dennison Young[5] (Montefiore Hosp., New York) with 50 consecutive patients. All the patients who had received no digitalis or an insufficient amount before surgery, including 9 with regular sinus rhythm preoperatively, acquired auricular fibrillation, often with congestive heart failure, within a few days. Those with auricular fibrillation before surgery had rapid ventricular rates and congestive failure. Of 11 patients with regular sinus rhythm and 15 with auricular fibrillation who had been taking digitalis for 3

(5) Am. Heart J. 54:863-874, December, 1957.

months to 10 years, only 5 showed increased arrhythmias. Of the 11, 9 maintained regular sinus rhythm postoperatively.

Anesthesia led to rapid ventricular rates and congestive heart failure in 4 patients who could subsequently withstand anesthesia and surgery after a period of intensified digitalis administration.

Comparison of the time of onset of auricular fibrillation among those who had no digitalis and those who had an insufficient amount indicated that myocardial irritability during surgery is not increased by digitalis. One of the 3 deaths in this series may have been influenced by overdigitalization, however. The ventricular response to exercise during the preoperative preparatory period provides a criterion for adequate digitalization. Potassium limits toxic manifestations and allows increased digitalis intake. It is recommended that all patients, regardless of the rhythm or lack of congestive failure, have prolonged and full digitalization to combat the increased left ventricular filling following valve fracture, decreased stroke volume output due to tachycardia and the positive fluid balance occurring postoperatively.

Abnormalities of Calcium Metabolism in Patients with Idiopathic Urinary Calculi: Effect of Oral Administration of Sodium Phytate. William H. Boyce, Fred K. Garvey and Carol E. Goven[6] (Bowman Gray School of Medicine) compared the daily excretion of calcium in 148 patients who had urinary calculi with that in 37 healthy persons who had no personal or familial history of calculi. Urinary calculi are composed of an organic matrix (2.5%) and an inorganic crystalline body (97.5%) which almost always is calcigerous. At least 95% of stones are idiopathic. Patients with idiopathic renal calculous disease in the active stages excrete significantly greater amounts of calcium while taking diets that contain as little as 350 mg. calcium/24 hours. In initial stages of calculus formation they have no bone or renal disease. They absorb from the intestine and excrete in the urine a greater quantity of calcium than persons in whom stones have never formed. Many factors, including high calcium, high protein and high vitamin D intake, greatly accelerate calcium absorption in these patients. The metabolic de-

(6) J.A.M.A. 166:1577-1583, Mar. 29, 1958.

rangement of this disorder is unknown, but hypercalciuria is one important aspect. Attempts to prevent recurrent stone formation by reducing calcium intake and absorption are indicated.

Sodium phytate forms an unabsorbable complex with calcium in the intestinal tract. When given orally with low-calcium diet (150 mg./24 hours) and low-vitamin D diet, it effectively reduces urinary excretion of calcium to quantities unobtainable by any tolerable diet alone. The sodium phytate powder is dissolved in distilled water and given orally in a cherry syrup vehicle, initially 125 mg. phytate/kg. body weight/24 hours in 3 divided doses, then gradually increased as tolerated until calcium excretion is reduced to 50 mg. in 24 hours or the maximum dose of 200 mg./kg./24 hours is reached.

No complications or resistance to the low-calcium and oral sodium phytate routine occurred in the patients even after more than 2 years of therapy. In selected patients carefully followed, this program is safe and beneficial in preventing urinary calculus formation. The regimen is particularly valuable in differentiating idiopathic hypercalciuria from metabolic or bone disease, in preoperative preparation of patients with renal calculi and in postoperative prevention of recurrent calculus formation.

Acetylsalicylic Acid and Salicylamide: Effect on Renal Calculosis in Patients with Spinal Cord Injury. This is a prominent complication. Of 1,187 patients with traumatic cord lesions, 100 had had renal calculi. While patients are hospitalized, a large fluid intake and weight bearing are stressed to reduce the incidence of calculosis, but few follow this schedule after discharge. Stones removed from these patients are mixtures of calcium phosphate (carboxyl apatite) and magnesium ammonium phosphate, the type reportedly slowed in their growth by use of salicylates. Therefore, A. Estin Comarr and Herbert O. Carne[7] (College of Med. Evangelists) prescribed aspirin, 10 gr. 3 times daily, to 6 and salicylamide, 10 gr. 3 times daily, to 9 men who had spinal cord injuries. All had passed stones spontaneously, had them surgically removed or had them in situ at the start of the

(7) J. Urol. 79:911-916, June, 1958.

study. The urine in each was infected and strongly alkaline. The predominant organism was Proteus vulgaris and the next most common were Pseudomonas aeruginosa, Aerobacter aoerogenes, paracolon and staphylococcus. Most were relatively insensitive to antibiotics. Duration of therapy was 3-11 months.

Of the 6 who received aspirin, only 1 showed no new stone formation or increase in size of existing stones. The other 5 showed continual growth of existing stones or formed new ones. Of the 9 who received salicylamide, 4 remained free from stones, 2 showed no further growth and 3 continued to have growth of stones. Thus in 53% of the patients the calculi continued to grow or recurred. In fact, the growth and development of new calculi during therapy were greater than previously observed for the same type of patient without therapy. Similar unfavorable results have been reported in persons with renal calculosis who had no cord damage when treated with acetylsalicylic acid. Glucuronic acid excretion was found to be naturally higher in patients who had calculi, which refutes the theory of protection against calculus growth that had previously been attributed to the ability of salicylates to increase glucuronide excretion. Salicylates are without merit in preventing new growth of urinary calculi in patients with spinal cord injury.

► [This is terribly disappointing because the study of Prien and Walker (1956-57 YEAR BOOK, p. 469) was so promising. However, Baker and Connelly (same YEAR BOOK, p. 470) had already rejected the idea of increased glucuronide content of the urine and proposed that the beneficent action of salicylate was merely a part of the antiphlogistic (anti-inflammatory) action since they look on urolithiasis as one of the collagen diseases. But now it appears that there is no action at all. Progress can sometimes be very hard to take!—Ed.]

Experiences in Use of Cordex® in Urethral Strictures: Preliminary Report. Cortisone has been very successful in treatment, but there has been lack of acceptance of this therapy because of the side effects after administration of the recommended dosages for 3-4 weeks. Prednisolone [Meticortelone®] and prednisone [Meticorten®] cause less sodium and water retention and are more potent corticosteroids. In treatment of rheumatoid arthritis, prednisolone and aspirin did not give as dramatic results as large doses of cortisone, but relief from pain and increased mobility were good and quite definite. For this reason, William H. Morse, Frank J. Malone, Jr., and Samuel L. Raines[8] (Univ. of Tennessee) believed that this combination might be of value in inhibiting recurrent scar formation after dilatation of urethral stricture.

An arbitrary dosage of 1.5 mg. prednisolone and 300 mg. aspirin (Cordex Forte) 4 times a day was chosen because this dosage had been successful in rheumatoid arthritis. Most urethral strictures were dilated and broken with use of only local anesthesia. An indwelling catheter was not necessarily used after dilatation though in some patients catheter drainage was necessary. In hope of preventing overwhelming infection while on steroid therapy, the patients were given 1 Gm. sulfisoxazole daily. Among 16 patients so treated and observed for 3-9 months, only 2 failures occurred. One was in a boy, aged 11, with a long irregular dense stricture of the membranous urethra secondary to a shearing rupture of the urethra at the apex of the prostate. The other was in a patient with a long, dense stricture after transurethral resection.

Although the follow-up was short, all had been selected because of previous history of rapid recurrence of symptoms and frequent dilatations. With this as a criterion for selection, the patients served as their own controls, and only those in whom symptoms did not recur and in whom calibration by bougie à boule revealed no decrease in the caliber of the urethra in the normal recurrent period were considered as showing good results. Of the 16 patients, 12 met these criteria and were definitely improved. In 2 others, follow-up was inadequate. This treatment may prove to be a relatively safe and inexpensive adjunct in the routine therapy of urethral strictures.

► [Why not prescribe the 2 drugs separately instead of in the fixed proportions of the proprietary preparation? While it might not be advisable in most instances to increase the prednisolone dosage when the agent is given continuously during a long period, it does seem undesirable to hold the aspirin dosage at a fixed 300 mg. (5 gr.) 4 times daily when many persons will tolerate more than this with the advantage to be gained from a higher blood salicylate titer.—Ed.]

Surgery during Long-Term Treatment with Adrenocortical Hormones carries no increased risk of complications, provided there is no gross sign of overdosage and administration is not interrupted, according to A. J. Popert and P. S.

(8) South. M. J. 50:1130-1133, September, 1957.

Davis.[9] The records were reviewed of 19 patients who had 36 surgical operations while under treatment with adrenocortical hormones. Of these, 15 had chronic rheumatoid arthritis and 1 each had ankylosing spondylitis, disseminated lupus erythematosus, polyarteritis nodosa and breast cancer. Wound healing was uneventful after 33 of the operations. Bone repair was normal apart from nonunion of the fractured neck of a femur. After gastrectomy for gastrointestinal hemorrhage, 2 patients died and 1 recovered. Three elective operations for peptic ulceration, 3 emergency operations for perforation and 5 operations in the presence of sepsis were uneventful. Postoperative complications were insignificant.

Steroid therapy was continued over the period of operation and postoperatively in all but 1 patient; additional cortisone was given routinely to patients receiving this drug or an analogue. Most of the operations in which no additional cortisone was given were minor. The precise schedule of this dosage varied somewhat. Usually, for operations not involving the gastrointestinal tract, 75-100 mg. cortisone acetate was given intramuscularly 24 hours and 1 hour preoperatively, or a single injection of 150 mg. an hour preoperatively, oral administration being continued until the time of operation and resumed as soon as possible afterward. For partial gastrectomy 100-150 mg. cortisone was given intramuscularly 24 hours and 1 hour preoperatively and a further 100 mg. 12 hours postoperatively; intramuscular administration was continued for the next 3 days, with daily dosage of 100, 100 and 75 mg., and oral administration was resumed on the 4th postoperative day.

No additional dose was given to patients receiving corticotropin because the variation in strength between the batches of corticotropin at present available and the individual variation in responsiveness make the nominal dosage meaningless. All these patients, however, showed clinical evidence of suppression of their disease, and those in whom urinary excretion of 17-hydroxycorticosteroids was estimated showed evidence of adrenal stimulation; corticotropin was continued over the operation, but no additional dose was given.

► [According to R. M. Salassa *et al.* (Proc. Staff Meet. Mayo Clin. 28:

(9) Lancet 1:21-24, Jan. 4, 1958.

662, 1953), one may safely presume that a patient who has received significant quantities of cortisone or one of the analogues within 3 to 6 months of coming to surgery should be given prophylactic treatment with the drugs.—Ed.]

Use of Trypsin (Intramuscular) in Treatment of Edema Due to Intestinal Anastomosis. A. Lee Lichtman[1] (New York Polyclinic Med. School) gave 59 patients trypsin intramuscularly after operations involving anastomosis in the stomach, small intestine or colon. Immediately after surgery, 5 mg. crystalline trypsin in 1 cc. sesame oil was given by deep intramuscular injection and repeated every 8 hours for 9 doses. Indwelling duodenal suction was used until flatus was passed by rectum, and fluids and electrolyte balance were maintained. A control group of 59 postoperative patients who had had similar surgical procedures was treated similarly except that trypsin was not administered.

Of the 59 patients treated with trypsin, 55 responded favorably. They passed gas in 48-72 hours. Four patients took 80-96 hours. These patients were more comfortable and had less distention than those in the control group. The latter passed gas in 70-120 hours.

Three patients with malfunction of a gastroenterostomy stoma secured release of retention within 24 hours when given trypsin intramuscularly. Duration of gastric retention was 3-9 days before treatment was started.

Trypsin was used in 10 patients with acute intestinal obstruction due to diverticulitis or carcinoma of the descending colon. When a tumor mass obstructs the colon, it is a sudden increase in the inflammatory edema that finally causes the obstruction. Decompression occurred in these patients within 54 hours. It was the consensus of those who observed these patients that release of obstruction occurred earlier than in similar patients under previous therapy.

Buccally Administered Streptokinase: Clinical and Experimental Observations. Proteases given parenterally have a definite anti-inflammatory effect of proved value in edema, cellulitis and particularly hemorrhagic extravasations in the tissues. The postulated mechanism is an increase in tissue permeability, which suggested to Irving Innerfield, Harold Shub and Linn J. Boyd[2] (New York Med. College) that a buc-

(1) Am. J. Surg. 94:781-783, November, 1957.
(2) New England J. Med. 258:1069-1074, May 29, 1958.

cal route for streptokinase might be as effective as parenteral administration. Tablets of 20,000 units of streptokinase were given buccally 4 times daily to 14 patients with diabetes, 51 with recent trauma or acute inflammation, including hematoma, cellulitis, abscess, upper respiratory infection and thrombophlebitis, and 23 who had chronic thrombotic or inflammatory conditions or both such as indolent leg ulcer, retinal vein thrombosis, chronic bronchitis and bronchiectasis. Tablets were retained sublingually or in the buccal pouch.

Significantly greater serum antithrombin activity was present in 7 patients treated with streptokinase as compared with untreated, healthy control subjects, and studies of antithrombin activity indicated an augmented effect in those receiving streptokinase. The most conspicuous and consistent clinical response was the rapid control of inflammatory edema and tenderness, especially in patients who had had recent trauma with pain and local collections of edema fluid, blood and tissue fluid. In patients with acute or chronic respiratory tract infection, previously thick, tenacious, stringy secretions thinned considerably, and coughing became loose and productive.

Side effects were minimal. No local irritative signs developed in the mouth in any of the 88 patients. The only systemic side effect was occasional mild gastrointestinal disturbance characterized by brief, moderate fulness or rumbling. Patient acceptance of buccal administration was excellent.

The mechanism of the anti-inflammatory or thrombolytic effects of proteases is unknown, but the end result is dramatic. Buccal streptokinase therapy provides an effective, simple, convenient means for reversing inflammation.

Case 1.—Woman, 84, had acute iliofemoral thrombophlebitis. Absolute bed rest and tetracycline orally for 4 days had no appreciable effect. Buccal streptokinase was then started, 1 tablet of 20,000 units every 4 hours. Within 6 hours she could move the involved extremity more freely and had less discomfort along the involved venous segment. Edema and redness were significantly decreased 24 hours later. Streptokinase was continued for 10 days. She was ambulatory on the 4th treatment day.

Case 2.—Woman, 79, had diabetes and massive ulceration at the stump of a midthigh amputation, with ragged edges and purulent, thick, green material at the base, from which was cultured Pseudomonas aeruginosa. Antibiotics, prolonged bed rest, topical streptokinase, crystalline trypsin and 2 weeks of intramuscular streptokinase were ineffective. After 4 weeks' observation, buccal streptokinase, 1 tablet every 4 hours, was started. At the end of 1 week, the ulcer seemed cleaner and less inflamed and by the 3d week was considerably improved. Treatment was stopped after 13 weeks, when the base of the ulcer was perfectly clean and had granulated considerably and only a scanty serous discharge was occasionally noted. A prosthetic device was then applied and the patient became ambulatory.

Clinical Experience with Streptokinase Administered Buccally: Treatment of Infection and Edema is discussed by Joseph M. Miller, George C. Godfrey, Milton Ginsberg and Constantine J. Papastrat[3] (VA Hosp., Fort Howard, Md.). The ability of streptokinase, given intramuscularly in conjunction with one of the antibacterial drugs, to influence the inflammatory reaction has been demonstrated. It is assumed that plasmin, an active lytic agent, is the fundamental force in the reaction. Plasmin apparently lyses fibrin in the inflammatory barrier about an area of infection. The viscosity of the edema fluid is reduced, fibrin clots in the local vascular and lymphatic circulations are dissolved and edema fluid is resorbed. Improvement in the local vascular and lymphatic systems results.

The authors used 10,000 units of streptokinase buccal tablets derived from streptokinase-streptodornase. One tablet was placed in the buccal pouch twice a day for 3 days or longer if necessary; it dissolved in about 2 minutes. The patients were cautioned not to swallow for about 5 minutes. All were given one of the antibacterial drugs concurrently with the streptokinase. Sixty-two maladies were treated in 57 patients, and attempts to prevent or allay edema were made 19 times in 18 patients.

Case 1.—Man, 66, was hospitalized with thrombophlebitis of varicosities of the right leg of about 2 weeks' duration. Tetracycline, 0.25 Gm., was given orally every 6 hours for 8 days and streptokinase every 12 hours during the first 4 days. Pain, tenderness and edema were gone by the 2d, and erythema by the 3d day of treatment. High ligation and stripping of the right greater saphenous vein were done about 3 weeks later. After surgery, tetracycline was given every 6 hours for 1 week. The wound healed rapidly.

Case 6.—Man, 59, was hospitalized with thrombophlebitis and cellulitis of about 10 days' duration. Tetracycline, 0.25 Gm., was given orally every 6 hours and streptokinase every 12 hours for 5 days. On the 2d day erythema and induration disappeared; the edema was gone from the thigh and was only slight in the lower leg the following day.

(3) J.A.M.A. 166:478-481, Feb. 1, 1958.

Aggravation of the infection did not occur in any patient. Healing of granulating wounds was hastened by reduction of the surrounding induration. Rise in temperature attributable to the streptokinase was not noted, nor were pain and tenderness in the mouth, sore throat, chills, cyanosis, hemorrhage, hematomas, petechiae or allergic responses.

The streptokinase reduction of inflammation and edema may permit dissemination of bacteria. It is mandatory, therefore, that patients suspected of having infection be treated concurrently with an antibacterial drug. Streptokinase should not be given to patients with defects in the clotting mechanism.

► [E. Davidson *et al.* (Harlem Hosp. Bull. 11:5, 1958) gave the commercially available streptokinase-streptodornase preparation (Varidase®) in 20,000-unit tablets buccally to 35 patients with traumatic edema or chronic inflammation. In all instances except 1 (a case of scleroderma) there was reversal of edema and inflammation and rapid resorption of hematomas. There was no local irritation or toxic side action.—Ed.]

Erythromycin and Erythromycin-Neomycin for Intestinal Antisepsis were evaluated by Isidore Cohn, Jr., and Alfred B. Longacre[4] (Louisiana State Univ.) as part of a program investigating various antibacterial agents for preoperative preparation of the colon. Preoperative conditions were simulated by combining antibiotic administration with mechanical cleansing, using a low-residue diet, a laxative and daily enemas.

Erythromycin was administered in doses of 500 mg. every 6 hours for 72 hours. The drug proved unsatisfactory for preoperative preparation of the colon because of inadequate control of streptococci, staphylococci, coliform organisms and bacteroides. Erythromycin-neomycin was administered according to the following schedule: 250 mg. erythromycin and 1 Gm. neomycin were given every hour for 4 hours, then every 6 hours for 72 hours. Rapid disappearance of streptococci, coliform organisms and bacteroides, plus control of staphylococci in patients in whom they were found, made this one of the most satisfactory combinations so far studied for preoperative intestinal antisepsis. This combination is not recommended for routine use, because such use might lead to establishment of a bacterial flora in the hospital patient population that might not be responsive if micrococcic enteritis should develop. As preoperative preparation in a

(4) Am. J. Surg. 94:402-408, September, 1957.

patient who has been on prolonged antibiotic therapy, this combination might prove useful in reducing the number of strains that have become resistant to the antibiotic previously used.

Comparison of Complications Following Intestinal Surgery After Oral and Parenteral Preoperative Antibiotic Preparation. Donald F. Phillips, William H. Dearing and John M. Waugh[5] (Mayo Clinic and Found.) divided patients into 3 groups according to the antibiotic they received before intestinal surgery. One group received an average of 4 doses of 750 mg. chlortetracycline by mouth daily for 3 or 4 days before operation. A second group received oxytetracycline by mouth in average doses of 500-750 mg. 4 times a day for 3 or 4 days before operation. Patients in both groups received penicillin and dihydrostreptomycin on the day of operation and daily thereafter for a variable period, depending on the postoperative course. The third group was given parenterally 0.5 Gm. streptomycin, 0.5 Gm. dihydrostreptomycin and 400,000 units of penicillin on the evening before operation and received daily 1 Gm. streptomycin, 1 Gm. dihydrostreptomycin and 800,000 units of penicillin for varying periods after operation.

The incidence of postoperative complications differed little between the groups receiving a 3 or 4 day preparation of the intestine with orally administered tetracycline (total of 261 patients) and the group receiving parenteral penicillin, streptomycin and dihydrostreptomycin (total of 243 patients) the evening before operation. The data indicate that, with modern methods of managing patients with various types of surgical intestinal lesions, it is not absolutely necessary to alter the flora of the intestines with antibiotics.

► [In discussing a presentation of I. Cohn, Jr., on certain experimental aspects of antibiotics and colon surgery (Am. J. Gastroenterology 28:298, 1957) O. H. Wangensteen expressed himself as not persuaded that antibiotics have been an important factor in the reduction of mortality in acute intestinal obstruction and he felt that in colic resection nothing is as good as overcoming the obstruction without spillage of intestinal content. "If spillage occurs during an anastomosis, all the drugs in New York City are not as good as though the anastomosis had been made without spillage." —Ed.]

Treatment of Benign Prostatic Hypertrophy with Estrogen Administered Intravenously: Report of 17 Cases is pre-

(5) Surg., Gynec. & Obst. 106:145-152, February, 1958.

sented by Milton Ende and Philip Jacobson[6] (Petersburg, Va.). All patients had complete urinary retention and were poor surgical risks because of recent myocardial infarction, congestive heart failure and general debilitation. Estrogen was given intravenously, 20 mg. daily for 3 days to 1 week. Conjugated estrogens were also given orally, 1.25 mg. 3 times a day for 1 week and 1.25 mg. once a day thereafter. Most patients were able to void on the 3d or 4th day of therapy, and 16 of the 17 patients have retained this ability without further difficulty for a year or more since treatment. Occasionally enlargement of the breasts has occurred after prolonged therapy, but this complication subsides if the estrogen is stopped for 10-14 days. Therapy can then be resumed.

Use of intravenous estrogen offers an initial therapeutic method which may bring temporary if not permanent relief in patients with benign prostatic hypertrophy and urinary retention. Estrogen therapy has advantages which can be used even if operation is contemplated. The opportunity to delay operation provides a period for rehabilitation and strengthening of the cardiovascular system. Estrogen reduces postoperative bleeding. It also induces an elevation in mood and a feeling of fitness and vigor.

Intravenous administration of estrogen produces effects which are much more reliable, rapid and constant than those observed following administration by any other route. The authors have no explanation for the action of estrogen in prostatic hypertrophy, unless it corrects the supposed hormone imbalance which originally created the enlargement of the prostate. The authors' first case is described here.

Man, 72, presented with complete obstruction of the urethra. Rectal examination disclosed a symmetrically enlarged prostate. Operation was advised but the patient refused. He was catheterized every 8-12 hours during the next 3 days but was unable to resume voiding. He was then hospitalized and a retention catheter was inserted for 3 days. When the catheter was removed, he was still unable to void and again refused operation. Catheterization was resumed when necessary, and 20 mg. intravenous estrogen was given daily for 4 days, augmented by 1.25 mg. conjugated estrogens 3 times a day orally. After 48 hours the patient began voiding. During the next 16 months there was no recurrence of obstruction and the patient had no nocturia. The prostate diminished to almost normal size. A maintenance dose of 1.25 mg. estrogen daily was continued.

(6) J. Am. Geriatrics Soc. 5:676-680, July, 1957.

Muscle Relaxants in Management of Orthopedic Back Injury are discussed by M. C. Cobey[7] (Georgetown Univ.). Meprobamate appears unique; its interneuronal blocking action relaxes skeletal muscles without impairment of their function. It also acts in the subcortical area to assuage anxiety and calm the patient chronically irritable from pain. Meprobamate, 400 mg. 4 times daily as adjunct to conventional therapy, was given to 129 patients with a median age of 45 (28-60) years having typical symptoms of injury to the muscular or ligamentous structures of the cervical, dorsal or lumbosacral spine but without bone damage. Therapy usually began within 2 days of diagnosis and in accident cases 2-7 days after the injury. It lasted 1-31 days, according to the severity of the disorder, and continued for about 2 weeks after discharge from hospital in the severe cases.

The results were excellent. Abused muscular and ligamentous structures were relaxed, patient anxiety was reduced, response to physical therapy was enhanced and the rehabilitation program was accelerated. Most patients returned to their occupations in less time than under conventional therapy. Transient drowsiness occurred occasionally and was considered an advantage. Urticaria developed in 2 patients but subsided on withdrawal of the drug. No other side effects or evidences of intolerance appeared.

Management of Postphlebitic Syndrome: Dynamic Pathologic Physiology and Medical Therapy. Eugene J. Chesrow, Sigmund S. Winton and R. Taher Qureshi[8] (Oak Forest, Ill.) studied 30 ambulatory patients (25 men and 5 women aged 54-87) with stasis ulcer. The diagnosis of iliofemoral thrombosis in 25 patients was obtained from the clinical records; in 5, the onset of deep thrombophlebitis was vague.

The measures used were (1) removal of necrotic tissue, (2) reduction of infection to a minimum, (3) reduction of fibroplasia of the ulcer base, (4) reduction of local intercellular edema, and (5) reduction of cellular necrosis by decreasing local tissue hypersensitivity to bacterial toxins. The patients were treated while ambulatory.

All patients were given an oral antibiotic (Tetracyn-SF®,

(7) Am. Surgeon 24:350-353, April, 1958.
(8) Geriatrics 12:444-451, July, 1957.

1 capsule 4 times daily) until the pus disappeared. Ulcers showing gross necrotic material were treated with crystalline Tryptar® dispensed from a salt shaker. Applications were made every half hour for 2-8 hours, depending on the amount of debris at the ulcer base. After this preliminary treatment, an ointment containing Terramycin® and hydrocortisone (Terra-Cortril®) was applied once daily to the ulcer and surrounding tissue showing dermatitis, the area then being covered with vaseline gauze strips followed by dry sterile dressings and an elastic Ace bandage. Efficient bandaging was very important; it extended from the base of the toes, included the heel, to just below the knee. The patient was encouraged to walk to assist venous circulation.

The rate and extent of healing of the ulcer depended on its duration, size and degree of fibrosis. Fourteen ulcers which had existed less than 6 months and were shallow and had minimal fibrosis healed completely within 8 weeks; 2 which had existed 6-12 months healed within 14 weeks; 5 which had existed 1-5 years healed within 30 weeks. The remaining 9 ulcers had a duration of more than 5 years and healed only moderately; the edges became thickened, rolled and hyperemic, while the central portion remained deep and densely fibrotic.

Reactions to Intravenous Organic Iodine Compounds and Their Immediate Treatment are discussed by John F. Weigen and Sydney F. Thomas[9] (Med. Clinic, Palo Alto, Calif.). For cardiovascular collapse, the following measures are suggested at the first indication of a fall in blood pressure:

Step 1. Remove all encumbrances, such as an abdominal compression band, etc. Give oxygen, with the patient in a 10-20 degree head-down position. Make sure the airway is clear. Call for assistance by a prearranged signal. Record blood pressure.

Step 2. Give Aramine®, 2-3 mg. intravenously (0.2-0.3 cc.). This dose may be repeated after 1 minute if the pressure does not rise. It may be repeated and 2-10 mg. may be given intramuscularly (0.2-1 cc.) if the pressure falls after rising.

Step 3. If the blood pressure is not sustained, give Aramine, 50 mg. in an intravenous infusion of 500 cc. physiologic saline, at a rate necessary to sustain systolic pressure at 90-120 mm. Hg. If the blood pressure does not rise in 1-5 minutes after administration of Aramine, give Solu-Cortef®, 100 mg. intravenously (2 cc. Mix-o-vial®).

(9) Radiology 71:21-27, July, 1958.

If cardiac arrest ensues, one must decide whether or not to perform a thoracotomy and massage the heart.

At the first indication of central nervous system stimulation, such as marked restlessness, twitching or convulsions, action should be taken:

Step 1. Remove encumbrances. Give oxygen. Call for assistance. Record blood pressure.

Step 2. Treat hypotension as described for cardiovascular collapse.

Step. 3. If convulsions continue, give Nembutal®, 25 mg. intravenously (0.5 cc.), at 2-minute intervals until they are controlled.

With the beginning of an asthmatic attack, the following is suggested:

Step 1. Give epinephrine, 0.3-1 cc. of a 1:1000 aqueous solution subcutaneously.

Step 2. If complete relief is not obtained, give aminophylline, 250-500 mg. intravenously (10-20 cc.).

Step 3. Give Benadryl®, 20 mg. intramuscularly (2 cc.) if mild symptoms persist. Give Solu-Cortef, 100 mg. intravenously, if severe symptoms continue, or if status asthmaticus develops.

In laryngeal edema, the following course of action is suggested:

Step 1. Give oxygen by positive pressure. Give epinephrine, 0.05-0.1 cc. of a 1:1000 aqueous solution intravenously. Give Benadryl, 10 mg. intravenously.

Step 2. If these measures fail, perform a tracheotomy, but only if Step 1 is unsuccessful after an adequate trial.

If what appears to be pulmonary edema should be the dominant process of a reaction, the following measures are suggested:

Step 1. Remove encumbrances. Give oxygen and call for assistance.

Step 2. Give epinephrine, 0.05-0.1 cc. of a 1:1000 aqueous solution intravenously. Give Demerol®, 50 mg. intravenously (1 cc.). Give Solu-Cortef, 100 mg. intravenously.

Step 3. Treat associated cardiovascular or central nervous system reactions.

The following emergency equipment is suggested: oxygen tank and mask, and pharyngeal airways; Aramine, 1-cc. ampule (10 mg.) and 10-cc. ampule (100 mg.); epinephrine chloride, 1:1000 aqueous solution, 1-cc. ampule; aminophylline, 10-cc. ampule (25 mg./cc.); Benadryl, 10-cc. ampule (10 mg./cc.); Solu-Cortef, 100 mg. (2 cc. Mix-o-vial®); Nembutal sodium, 5-cc. ampule (25 mg./cc.); aromatic ammonia, crushable vial; amyl nitrite, crushable vial; Demerol, 2-cc. ampule (50 mg./cc.); tuberculin, 2, 5 and 20-cc. tuber-

"CARDIOVASCULAR COLLAPSE"	ARAMINE R	I.V.	0.2-0.3 cc.	(2-3 mgms)
		I.M.	0.2-1.0 cc.	(2-10 mgms)
		I.V.	5 cc. in 500 cc. SALINE	(50 mgms)
CONVULSIONS	NEMBUTAL R	I.V.	0.5 cc. q. 2 MINUTES	(25 mgms)
BRONCHIAL ASTHMA	ADRENALIN R	S.C.	0.3 cc. 1/1000 AQUEOUS	
	AMINOPHYLLINE	I.V.	10 cc.	(250 mgms)
	BENADRYL R	I.M.	2 cc.	(20 mgms)
STATUS ASTHMATICUS	SOLU-CORTEF R (IN ADDITION TO ABOVE)	I.V.	2 cc.	(100 mgms)
LARYNGEAL EDEMA	ADRENALIN R	I.V.	0.05-0.1 cc. 1/1000 AQUEOUS	
	BENADRYL R	I.V.	1 cc.	(10 mgms)
PULMONARY EDEMA	ADRENALIN R	I.V.	0.1 cc. 1/1000 AQUEOUS	
	DEMEROL R	I.V.	1.0 cc.	(50 mgms)
	SOLU-CORTEF R	I.V.	2 cc.	(100 mgms)

Fig. 40.—Drugs and dosages for treatment of acute reactions to intravenous organic iodine compounds. Chart should be prominently displayed on cover of emergency kit to avoid errors which might occur under stress which prevails during reaction. (Courtesy of Weigen, J. F., and Thomas, S. F.: Radiology 71:21-27, July, 1958.)

culin syringes; 1-in. needles of various sizes; 4-in. needle, no. 20; rubber tubing adapter; 30 cc. physiologic saline; 500 cc. physiologic saline and venoclysis set; sphygmomanometer and stethoscope; padded tongue depressor; instruction card (Fig. 40); suture kit, including scalpel; and tourniquet.

Pain Control Following Hemorrhoidectomy was studied by Howard D. Trimpi and Guy L. Kratzer[1] (Allentown, Pa.) in 150 patients in three randomized groups of 50 to determine the efficacy of dihydromorphinone (Dilaudid®) hydrochloride, meperidine (Demerol®) hydrochloride, and levorphanol (Levo-Dromoran®) tartrate, respectively. Dosages were based on body weight. Doses under 2 mg. dihydromorphinone hydrochloride, 75 mg. meperidine hydrochloride or 2 mg. levorphanol proved ineffective in the immediate postoperative periods. Doses over 4 mg. dihydromorphinone hydrochloride, 150 mg. meperidine hydrochloride and 4 mg. levorphanol tartrate were unnecessary.

Levorphanol provided faster, more complete and longer

(1) A.M.A. Arch. Surg. 76:123-127, January, 1958.

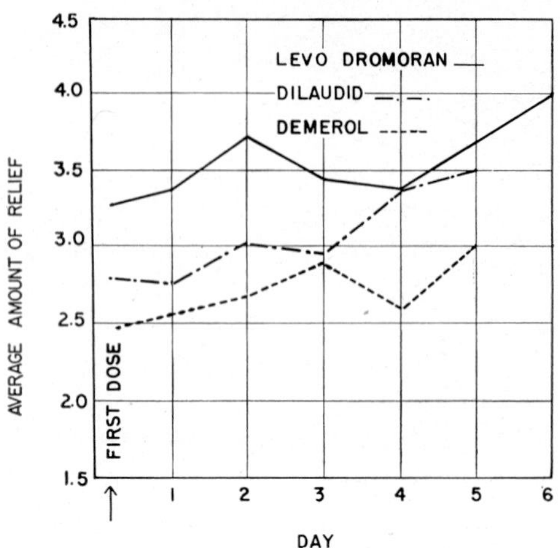

Fig. 41.—Amount of relief obtained from analgesic drugs different days after operation. (Courtesy of Trimpi, H. D., and Kratzer, G. L.: A.M.A. Arch. Surg. 76:123-127, January, 1958.)

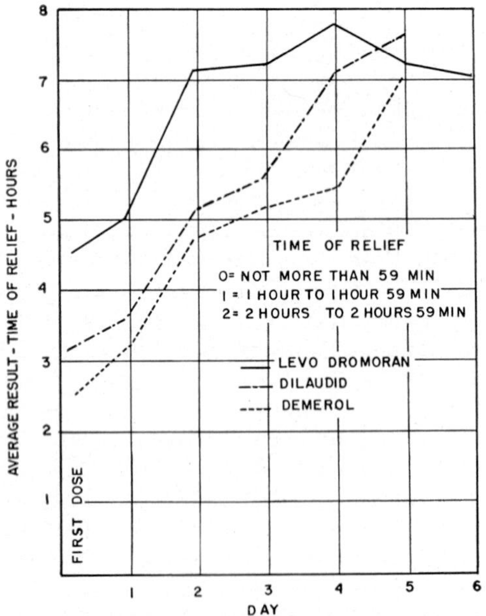

Fig. 42.—Duration of relief from analgesic drugs according to day after operation. (Courtesy of Trimpi, H. D., and Kratzer, G. L.: A.M.A. Arch. Surg. 76:123-127, January, 1958.)

pain relief per dose than did dihydromorphinone or meperidine (Figs. 41 and 42). In the 150 patients studied, the only untoward reactions seen that could be attributed partially or totally to the pain suppressants were nausea and constipation. In no instance did blood pressure fall; in none was there respiratory depression, drug addiction, pruritus or other complication. Undoubtedly, the operative procedure itself contributed to both nausea and constipation in many patients; however, there were differences in the groups. Nausea was slightly less in the meperidine group than in the others, whereas constipation was markedly less in the levorphanol group.

Palliative Treatment of Benign Prostatic Hypertrophy: Value of Glycine-Alanine-Glutamic Acid Combination, suggested by a chance observation, is discussed by Henry M. Feinblatt and Julian C. Gant.[2] While a group of allergic patients were being given an amino acid mixture, 1 patient volunteered that all his urinary symptoms had disappeared. Glycine-alanine-glutamic acid, 2 capsules 3 times daily after meals for 2 weeks and then 1 capsule 3 times daily, was given to 40 patients with benign prostatic hypertrophy. This regimen was continued for 3 months. As controls, the same patients were given a placebo for a comparable 2 months.

Glycine-alanine-glutamic acid reduced the size of the enlarged prostate in 93% of patients, including 33% in whom the gland was restored to normal size. With the placebo only 5% showed partial reduction of prostatic enlargement, in no instance to normal size. Treatment relieved nocturia in 95% (complete relief in 72%), urgency in 81%, frequency in 73%, discomfort in 71% and delayed micturition in 70%. With the placebo, nocturia was relieved in 15% (complete relief in 5%), urgency in 11%, frequency in 15%, discomfort in 9% and delayed micturition in 4%. No untoward effects were observed. The modus operandi appears to be an antiedemic (diuretic) action, which reduces edematous swelling of the prostate and surrounding perineal tissues. A special metabolic activity may be a factor.

(2) J. Maine M. A. 49:99-101, March, 1958.

Treatment of Juvenile Thyrotoxicosis with Potassium Perchlorate. In general, subtotal thyroidectomy is the treatment of choice for adults with hyperthyroidism, and medical treatment is reserved for those deemed unsuitable for surgery. In childhood, however, endocrine balance is easily deranged. To remove part of the thyroid at this age is somewhat speculative and hazardous, and the ultimate outcome cannot be accurately assessed. Treatment by external radia-

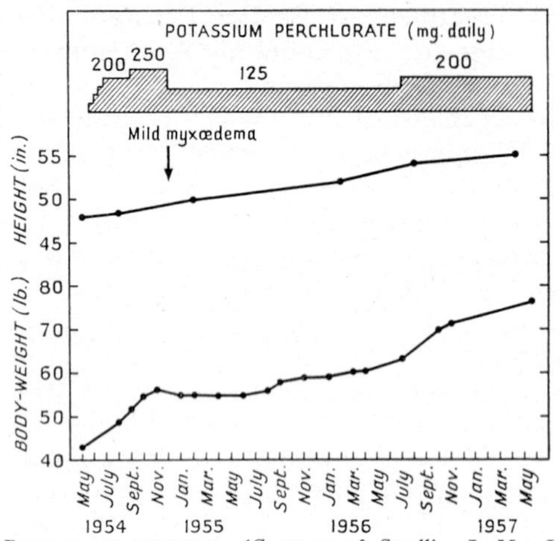

Fig. 43.—Response to treatment. (Courtesy of Smellie, J. M.: Lancet 2:1035-1036, Nov. 23, 1957.)

tion or radioactive iodine is unsuitable, because of possible sequelae. Thiouracil and its derivatives are effective, but may produce dangerous toxic reactions. Potassium perchlorate has been shown to displace iodine from its position in the thyroid gland, and thus far treatment of 132 adults for hyperthyroidism with this drug has been reported. J. M. Smellie[3] (Univ. of Birmingham) reports effective treatment of 6 children.

Girl, 8, had typical clinical hyperthyroidism for 5 months, confirmed by highly active uptake of I^{131} by the thyroid. Her mother, maternal uncle, great-aunt and grandfather had all had partial thyroidectomy for thyrotoxicosis. Figure 43 shows the patient's response to treat-

(3) Lancet 2:1035-1036, Nov. 23, 1957.

ment with potassium perchlorate. When she had had 250 mg. daily for 3 months, her mother reported she had become dull, uninterested, drowsy and had complained of feeling cold. When the dose was reduced well-being and good health returned. After treatment for 3 years, she is well and appears stabilized on 200 mg. daily. Exophthalmos and enlarged gland are evident. The dose of potassium perchlorate is being cautiously reduced.

Potassium perchlorate has a place in treating juvenile thyrotoxicosis. Apart from hypothyroidism, easily recognized, no untoward side effects have occurred in treatment for as long as 3 years. It takes about 6 weeks of perchlorate therapy to induce euthyroid function, similar to the time required of propylthiouracil. Treatment apparently is needed for 2-3 years, perhaps through puberty. If it can delay partial thyroidectomy it will render any operation safer and sounder. Iodide-containing medication is contraindicated in any patient taking perchlorate, because sudden raising of the blood iodide level is liable to induce relapse.

WORM INFESTATIONS

Treatment of Enterobiasis with One Oral Dose of Promethazine Hydrochloride or another phenothiazine derivative, pyrathiazine, did not produce as many spontaneous cures as might be expected among 127 infected children treated by Thomas S. Bumbalo, Lois J. Plummer and John R. Warner[4] (Univ. of Buffalo). Those receiving promethazine [Phenergan®] were among 184 children in an orphanage, 107 of whom showed pinworm eggs on cellophane tape smears taken before bathing on 2 consecutive mornings. The other 20 diagnosed as infected were among 24 hospitalized children. Both infected and noninfected subjects were given 125 mg. of the drug at bedtime. After 10 days, cellophane tape smears were again examined; negative smears on 7 consecutive days was the criterion of cure. Among the 107 children on promethazine, only 5 were cured; of the 20 on pyrathiazine, 3 were cured. The dosage could not be increased safely, since at this level a few showed side effects, including enuresis, disorientation, nausea and vomiting.

(4) J.A.M.A. 164:1651-1653, Aug. 10, 1957.

Although the relative lack of toxicity of these drugs was confirmed, the high cure rate reported by others could not be confirmed, and the authors see no reason to use them since more efficient oxyuricides are available.

► [In the article in which he originally described the use of this drug in treating enterobiasis, J. L. Avery (J.A.M.A. 161:681, 1956) mentioned that 5% of the children aged 4-10 experienced nightmares on the night of medication, which he suggested might evidence the release of toxic by-products of the drug's anthelmintic action. In the 2 children and 1 adult treated by T. James (South African M. J.: July 5, 1958) these nightmares were quite violent and followed by very deep sleep.—Ed.]

Treatment of Enterobiasis in Children: Comparative Study of Piperazine (Antepar®) and Pyrvinium Chloride (Vanquin) was made by Thomas S. Bumbalo, Lois J. Plummer, and J. Roger Warner[5] (Univ. of Buffalo). Among 34 infected children treated with a single daily dose of 3 Gm. piperazine for 3 days, the cure rate was 90.6%; and among 34 others treated similarly for 2 days, the cure rate was 86.2%. Of 35 children treated with 1.5 mg./kg. pyrvinium chloride in 2 equal doses daily for 6 days, the cure rate was 100%; whereas, of 36 treated with 2.1 mg./kg., the cure rate was 97.1%.

No patient treated with piperazine or pyrvinium chloride received any previous preparation, posttreatment enemas or cathartics. Except for the usual hygienic measures, no special cleanliness or hygiene was practiced during treatment. Both piperazine and pyrvinium chloride were well accepted and tolerated and no untoward or toxic reactions were noted.

The authors believe that if piperazine therapy had been continued for 6 days, the results would compare favorably with those obtained with pyrvinium chloride. Piperazine is still the drug of choice for the short single-dose regimen.

Piperazine and Male Fern in Expulsion of Tapeworms was studied by L. G. Goodwin and O. D. Standen[6] (London) in the Shirati area of Tanganyika. Patients averaged 2 tapeworms. One group was given piperazine citrate (equivalent to 3 Gm. hexahydrate) and instructed to return the next morning without breakfast. They were then given 5.3 ml. extract of male fern shaken with milk, followed 2 hours later by 2 oz. magnesium sulfate dissolved in water. If no stool resulted within 2 hours, a further dose of 2 oz. magnesium sul-

(5) Am. J. Trop. Med. 7:212-214, March, 1958.
(6) Brit. M. J. 1:133-134, Jan. 18, 1958.

fate was given. A second group was treated with extract of male fern and purge only.

More persons with tapeworm heads in the stools were found in the first group than in the control group treated with male fern alone, but the difference was not statistically significant. Piperazine, used alone, caused some large segments of worm to be expelled, but did not cause the scolex to detach itself from the mucosa.

Dithiazanine, Effective Broad-Spectrum Anthelmintic: Results of Therapy of Trichuriasis, Strongyloidiasis, Enterobiasis, Ascariasis and Hookworm Infection are reported by J. Clyde Swartzwelder, William W. Frye, John P. Muhleisen, Joseph H. Miller, Ralph Lampert, Antonio Peña Chavarria, Stanley H. Abadie, Samuel O. Anthony and Robert W. Sappenfield.[7] Dithiazanine was given by mouth to patients with various helminthiases.

Trichuriasis in 164 patients was treated with doses of 200 mg. 3 times daily. This dosage, continued 5 days, cured 97% of them. Ascariasis was treated in 42 persons with up to 600 mg. daily in divided doses. The egg count of these patients was reduced 97% and 27 showed complete elimination of the infection. Strongyloidiasis was eliminated in 16 of the 18 patients treated for 5-21 days with 200 mg. dithiazanine 3 times daily. Enterobiasis was treated in 35 boys; 100 mg. dithiazanine 3 times daily for 5 days cured all cases.

Hookworm infection was found in 39 of the patients being treated for these other helminthiases. Treatment incidentally caused reductions of the hookworm egg counts. A similar reduction was observed in a separate group of 8 patients with hookworm, but better results were obtained by giving subcurative doses of tetrachloroethylene with the dithiazanine.

The side effects of the drug were minimal, and its usefulness for the mass therapy of trichuriasis was demonstrated.

► [In a subsequent publication, the same group of investigators (Swartzwelder, J. C., *et al.*: Am. J. Trop. Med. 7:329, 1958) reported that the only adverse reaction to this drug in their experience was vomiting, which occurred in 9 of 37 children, usually being limited to one episode during a course of treatment. In no instance was the reaction severe enough to stop therapy.—Ed.]

Acute Urticarial Reaction to Piperazine Citrate. The increasing use of piperazine compounds for treatment of

(7) J.A.M.A. 165:2063-2067, Dec. 21, 1957.

threadworm infestation will probably lead to more reports of sensitivity reactions at variance with claims that the drug has no significant toxic manifestations in the recommended dose of 50-75 mg./kg. A case of acute urticaria is reported by Brian H. R. Hill[8] (Napier).

Boy, 5, with no family history of allergy and no previous illnesses had oxyuris infestation. He was given Antepar® Elixir for 7 days, with no ill effects on 1,000 mg./day piperazine citrate. Three months later another infestation of oxyuris was noted and a second course of Antepar Elixir, 1,000 mg./day in 2 doses of 500 mg. night and morning, was started. On the 2d day of treatment large, irritable, urticarial, erythematous swellings appeared on the face, eyelids and penis and smaller urticarial wheals on the trunk and legs. The drug was stopped and within the next 48 hours the swelling, irritation and gross edema increased. These gradually subsided in the succeeding 2 days.

This is considered to have been an allergic reaction to Antepar Elixir, occurring on second exposure to the drug.

► [Piperazine appears to be of established value in ascariasis (roundworm) and enterobiasis (pinworm) infestations, but its usefulness in other helminthiases is less well substantiated. L. G. Goodwin and O. D. Standen (Brit. M. J. 1:135, Jan. 18, 1958) recently reported it noncurative in hookworm cases that were subsequently treated effectively with tetrachlorethylene.—Ed.]

Effective Use of Piperazine for Treatment of Human Helminthiases is reported by Clyde Swartzwelder, Joseph H. Miller and Robert W. Sappenfield[9] (Louisiana State Univ.). Diagnosis of enterobiasis was established in 82 patients by demonstration of pinworm eggs on Scotch tape and swabs. Piperazine citrate was administered in total daily dosage of 30-35 mg./lb. body weight. When given as a single daily dose, after breakfast, for 6 days, results were as satisfactory as when given for 14 days in divided doses. This represents the shortest effective treatment schedule for enterobiasis with piperazine citrate yet reported. The reduction in duration and cost of medication without loss of effect are significant factors in the treatment of this common, often familial, infection.

An effective schedule for treating patients with ascariasis is initially 70 mg. (hexahydrate equivalent) piperazine citrate/lb., (maximum 3 Gm.; 30 cc. syrup of Antepar®), repeated a week later. No fasting or purgation is required. Worms are passed alive, nonmotile and intact after treat-

(8) New Zealand M. J. 46:572, October, 1957.
(9) Gastroenterology 33:87-96, July, 1957.

ment. Piperazine citrate, adipate and phosphate are equally effective in eliminating ascarides.

Piperazine citrate syrup may be useful in treating partial intestinal obstruction due to Ascaris lumbricoides. Parenteral fluids, abdominal decompression to relieve distention and vomiting, intubation of piperazine citrate through the drainage tube and physiologic saline enemas are all valuable adjuncts. Such conservative management may obviate the necessity for surgery in patients who have this complication of ascariasis.

No significant untoward reactions were observed in over 150 patients treated with piperazine citrate in the dosage described, although abdominal cramps, nausea and diarrhea occasionally occurred.

Trichinosis Involving Central Nervous System: Treatment with Corticotropin (ACTH) and Cortisone. The manifestations of trichinosis vary with the number of parasites and with the susceptibility of the host. The disease is often asymptomatic. The most heavily infected areas are the diaphragm, intercostal muscles, tongue, eyes, larynx and neck. The most serious complications involve the myocardium and central nervous system. Two types of central nervous system involvement appear clinically. (1) Such features as nonspecific headache, neck pain, stiffness, apathy, confusion and diminished to absent deep tendon reflexes occur in 10-17% of cases. Prognosis is good and complete recovery is to be expected. (2) Specific focal cerebral damage is probably more common than is usually realized. It is often confused with meningitis, poliomyelitis, polyneuritis, collagen diseases, encephalitis, and psychoses, among other entities.

No specific therapy is available, though combined cortisone and corticotropin have been used recently. Lawrence E. Meltzer and Albert A. Bockman[1] (Gen'l Hosp., Philadelphia) report a case of clearly defined focal cerebral damage due to trichinosis in which the neurologic signs and symptoms were rapidly reversed by combined steroid therapy.

Man, 43, had headache, weakness, malaise and fever for 10 days and when hospitalized was confused, lethargic, semistuporous and unable to use his left hand. He was incontinent and had expressive aphasia. He had many splinter hemorrhages under all the finger-nails,

(1) J.A.M.A. 164:1566-1569, Aug. 3, 1957.

and he was unable to abduct or adduct the fingers or oppose the thumb of the left hand. The flexor muscles of the left upper and lower extremities were weak. Plantar response was extensor bilaterally, and abdominal reflexes were absent. Admission diagnosis was poliomyelitis. A differential white blood cell count showed 50% eosinophils. A detailed history then revealed ingestion of raw pork 3 weeks before admission and 1 week before onset of symptoms. Muscle biopsy showed several foci of invasion with polymorphonuclear leukocytes and proliferation of cells resembling the reaction elicited by trichinae. No parasites were observed.

Diagnosis was thus established within 12 hours of admission. The patient was given 300 mg. cortisone and 80 units of corticotropin daily for 3 days, which was reduced to 200 mg. and 60 units, respectively, for the next 3 days, and then maintained on prednisone in decreasing doses for 10 days. Within 24 hours of the start of therapy temperature was normal, and the patient no longer appeared acutely ill. He cleared mentally within 48 hours and became more alert and then expressive. He remained incontinent for 7 days. Muscle strength improved 5 days after treatment was started and was normal by 13 days. Eosinophils decreased from 50 to 6% while steroid therapy was given, rose again to 47% within a week after medication was stopped, gradually decreased during the next 2 months, and have remained at about 23%. Recovery was complete.

Much of the clinical picture of trichinosis suggests an antigen-antibody reaction or toxic and allergic elements. Rapid recovery and reversal of focal neurologic damage by steroid therapy may be related to these aspects.

► [N. M. Greenstein and D. Steinberg (A.M.A. J. Dis. Child. 95:261, 1958) reported the successful use of corticotropin in 3 cases of trichinosis in children under 12 years of age. High dosage for a short period was employed; a child aged 10 received 80 units intramuscularly 3 times daily for 3 days, then 40 units 3 times daily for another 3 days.—Ed.]

INDEX TO AUTHORS

T

U

V

W

SUBJECT INDEX

B

C

E

N

O

P

Q

R

T

U